ACUTE PHASE PROTEINS AS EARLY NON-SPECIFIC BIOMARKERS OF HUMAN AND VETERINARY DISEASES

Edited by **Francisco Veas**

Acute Phase Proteins as Early Non-Specific Biomarkers of Human and Veterinary Diseases
Edited by Francisco Veas

Published by InTech
Janeza Trdine 9, 51000 Rijeka, Croatia

Publishing Process Manager Davor Vidic

Technical Editor Teodora Smiljanic

Cover Designer InTech Design Team

Additional hard copies can be obtained from orders@intechopen.com

Acute Phase Proteins as Early Non-Specific Biomarkers of Human and Veterinary Diseases, Edited by Francisco Veas
p. cm.
ISBN 978-953-307-873-1

For EU product safety concerns:
IN TECH d.o.o., Prolaz Marije Krucifikse Kozulić 3, 51000 Rijeka, Croatia,
info@intechopen.com or visit our website at intechopen.com.

Meet the editor

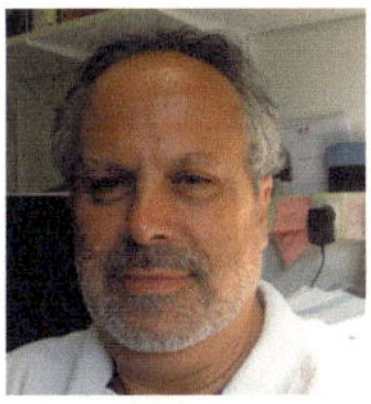

Dr. Francisco Veas, Ph.D. is a Viral Immuno-Physiopathologist and is currently a Research Professor at the Health Department of the French Institute for Development (IRD). He is also in charge of Comparative Molecular Immuno-Physiopathology Lab and Deputy Director of the research unit UMR-MD3-Université Montpellier 1 in Montpellier, France. Professor Veas received his PhD in Comparative Pathology in 1986 at the University Montpellier II. Between January 1987 and June 1988 he held a post-doctoral position on molecular biology of the protozoan Leishmania sp and Trypanosoma cruzi at the Research Centre on Macromolecular Biology of the centre National de la Recherche Scientifique (CNRS), Montpellier. In 1988, he was a laureate of the Fondation pour la Recherche Médicale and from July 1988 up to 1990 he served as Assistant Professor in the Parasites' population genetics lab at the IRD in Montpellier. From 1991-1995 he was in charge of viral experimental research of the AIDS program at IRD. From 1996 to 2000, he was director of the Retroviral Immunology Lab at the IRD CNRS Unit 5087 in Montpellier. In 2000, he cofounded the ApoH-Technologies biotech spin-off of IRD. From 2001 to 2009 he was in charge of studies on viral physiopathology of HIV and Dengue virus at the IRD research Unit "Viral Emerging Diseases Unit". In 2009, Professor Veas has been appointed CSO of ApoH-Technologies and in 2010 has been appointed head of Comparative Molecular Immuno-Physiopathology Lab at the Unit MD3 which he co-directs. From 1998, different French institutions, including Foundation pour la Recherche Médicale, SIDACTION, ANRS, CNRS, IRD, Region Languedoc Roussillon, have been supporting and funding his research. Recently, he was promoter, member of the executive board and reporter of the USDEP European Project (Ultrasensitive detection of emerging pathogens, 2006-2010). Professor Veas has also created several technological platforms including sequencing, high biosafety labs (BSL2 and BSL3), proteomics, etc. His scientific activities and publication and patents have been mainly dedicated to conserved aspects of host and pathogens including innate immunity, viral physiopathology, vaccines and diagnostics.

Contents

Preface

A dynamic physiological equilibrium known under the name of homeostasis is determined by endogenous factors and by interactions of organisms with their exogenous environment. To preserve this equilibrium state, which reflects a healthy state of the individual, the organism is constantly sensing and adjusting levels of factors involved in these mechanisms participating to the equilibrium. Most of these homeostatic factors are well preserved because of their highly relevant functional importance for life.

Depending on species, some of them could vary in their expression, and will be adapted to the encountered situations. These conserved innate strategies will not only have effects on individuals, but also on populations and moreover in their relations with the environmental stimuli (temperature, humidity, chemical, infections, diet).

A broad and conserved response to internal or external stimuli will very quickly be induced, in a matter of minutes, to generate a cascade of inflammatory processes in order to reestablish the homeostatic state in the organism as soon as possible. Stimuli inducing homeostatic changes can be of different nature: trauma, toxin, infection, genetic dysfunction, childbirth, etc.

The process of acute inflammation is initiated by cells already present in all tissues, including macrophages, dendritic cells, Kupffer cells. These cells harbor surfaces pattern recognition receptors (PRRs), which recognize at the beginning of the infectious process, exogenous molecules broadly shared by pathogens (pathogen-associated molecular patterns, PAMPs), but not by the host. Important addition to PAMPs, but to a lesser extent, are non-pathogenic microorganisms which also harbor the highly conserved molecules recognized as non-self that will induce a very low level of local inflammation. This response is amplified by endogenously released mediators and by co-factors or concomitant stressful events (burn, trauma, apoptosis, etc.) as well as molecular mechanisms involved in the vicious circle of destruction-reconstruction of vessels and tissues, acting through injury-associated signals known as Damage-Associated Molecular Patterns (DAMPs or Alarmins) and acute phase proteins. Moreover, some of the APP are also antimicrobials exhibiting a wide range of defensive functions, that alongside their repair functions help to reduce pathologic damage, and consequently help to restore the homeostasis.

The maintaining of homeostasis requires rapid and short acute inflammatory responsiveness. Inflammatory mediators, including APP, exhibit short half-lives, which ensures that the inflammatory phenomenon ceases as soon as the stimulus disappears. In contrast, the presence of APP at increased levels can be considered as sensitive sensor of homeostasis disruption. Persisting levels of APP are observed in chronic diseases.

The inflammation process is strongly associated with vascular changes as vasodilation and its resulting increased blood flow causes the redness (*rubor*) and increased heat (*calor*) as well as an augmented permeability resulting in a plasma protein leakage into the tissue causing edema, observed as swelling (*tumor*) and pain (*dolor*). Activated cells will then migrate the injury site. Depending on the intensity of inflammation and the organ in question, it is possible to observe the fifth component of inflammation as described by Aulus Cornelius Celsus in his treatise *On Medicine* (1st century BC) - loss of function (*functio laesa*) that results from cross talk between inflammation process and the central nervous system.

The two volumes of Acute Phase Proteins book consist of chapters that give a large panel of fundamental and applied knowledge on one of the major elements of the inflammatory process during the acute phase response, i.e., the acute phase proteins expression and functions that regulate homeostasis. We have organized this book in two volumes - the first volume, mainly containing chapters on structure, biology and functions of APP, the second volume discussing different uses of APP as diagnostic tools in human and veterinary medicine.

By using an open access publishing model, we wanted to facilitate a large access to readers from different places all over the world, notably developing countries, with the aim of contributing to a better world of knowledge. We also wanted to dedicate this book to our colleagues from both academia and industry in order to create values of knowledge in the field of control of inflammatory processes occurring in diverse diseases to improve the management efficacy of a more personalized medicine.

At present, CRP and SAA are the most responsive APP during inflammatory processes in humans. In most cases they are associated with the erythrocyte sedimentation rate (ESR) marker, which strongly depends on high fibrinogen concentration allowing the sticking between erythrocytes. In mice, some changes are also reported for SAA. Despite the fact that the field of inflammation and its associated factors, including APP, cytokines antimicrobial peptides, etc., have been observed and studied from very ancient times, a detailed and updated knowledge is urgently needed as well as pivotal in future research for an integrative personalized medicine that takes into account several parameters including nutritional and systemic factors. Particularly, with the help of large-scale identification methods, such as proteomics, transcriptomics, metabolomics and interactomics, it should be important to get more precise data on kinetic and on the individual role of each APP within the network of the acute phase responsive elements. Thus, it should be important, in this research, to consider organs involved in this complex network - the central nervous system that reflects its involvement by fever, somnolence, anorexia, over-secretion of some hormones, liver being the main provider of APP, epithelial cells that produce cationic antimicrobials, bone being the site of erythropoiesis suppression and thrombosis induction, and the adrenal gland that produces cortisol to regulate inflammatory inducers, adipose tissue that induces changes in lipids metabolism.

As a final note, I would like to thank InTech's editorial staff, particularly Mr. Vidic who managed, with patience, difficult tasks in helping the organization of chapter reviewing and finalization process.

Francisco Veas, PhD
Comparative Molecular Immuno-Physiopathology Lab
UMR-MD3 Faculty of Pharmacy, University Montpellier 1, Montpellier
France

1

Acute Phase Proteins as Cancer Biomarkers

W. Shannon Orr[1], Linda H. Malkas[2],
Robert J. Hickey[2] and John A. Sandoval[1]
[1]*St. Jude Children's Research Hospital, Memphis TN*
[2]*City of Hope Cancer Center, Duarte, CA*
United States of America

1. Introduction

Interactions between tumor cells and the host microenvironment have been shown to play a significant role in the initiation, progression, and invasiveness of human cancer. The complex changes in the tumor microenvironment have been shown to modulate the activation of the different arms of the host immune system including the acute phase response. Acute phase changes are mediated by several serum proteins [acute phase proteins (APP)] whose concentrations may increase (positive APP) or decrease (negative APP) as a result of varied clinical conditions, including cancer. To date, a body of evidence suggests APP may have a profound impact on cancer growth and appear to court a protective immune response by co-opting the body's innate immune system. In this review, we discuss the impact of the host tumor response in relation to acute phase proteins and examine literature characterizing APP as helpful cancer biomarkers. Insights gained into the mechanism of action of acute-phase reactants towards malignancy and how they are induced could be exploited for the future development of more specific and targeted cancer biomarker strategies.

2. Microenvironment and cancer

In recent decades, the tumor microenvironment has received much attention as compelling evidence has demonstrated that a battery of various components interact to play a critical role in establishing fertile ground for tumor growth and progression. The neoplastic microenvironment roughly includes immune cells (lymphocytes, natural killer cells, and antigen presenting cells), stromal cells (including myofibroblasts), and vasculature (see Fig.1). Tumor microenvironment has been shown to contribute to tumor growth. Stromal cells stimulate cancer cell growth and invasion through the chemokine–chemokine receptor axis.(Orimo et al 2005;Polyak & Hahn 2006) Tumor vasculature allows nutrients and oxygen uptake by tumors and tumor-infiltrating immune cells anergize the immune effectors. In the present work, we will review the relevant interactions between tumor microenvironment and solid tumors that aid in creating the conditions for supporting tumor cell survival and metastasis. In particular, one important response is the host reaction to a cancer that promotes an inflammatory microenvironment. It is clear that this inflammatory environment associated with solid tumors can exert pro-and and anti-tumor functions and this response can play a central role in modulating cancer development.

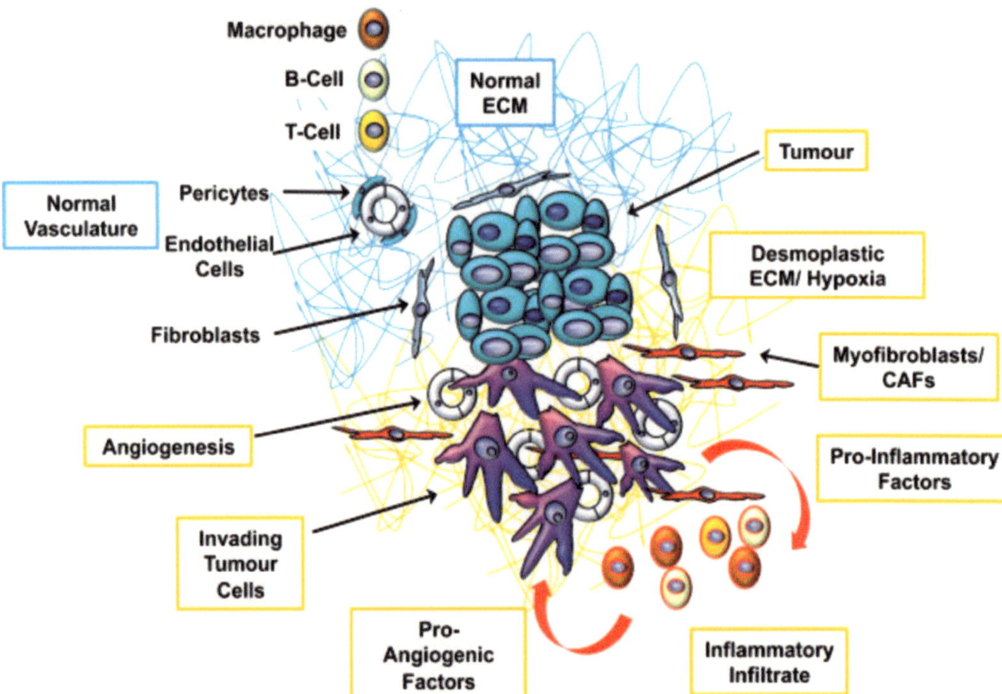

Fig. 1. Representation of the microenvironment alterations in response to tumor growth. Adapted from (Allen & Louise 2011)

2.1 Cancer microenvironment and acute phase proteins

As the tumor microenvironment plays a fundamental role in both the organization of and the escape from anticancer immune responses, the dynamic interplay of the proinflammatory mediators has long supported the notion that inflammation and cancer are interelated. Links between cancer and inflammation were first made in the nineteenth century, on the basis of observations that tumors often arose at sites of chronic inflammation and that inflammatory cells were present in biopsied samples from tumours.(Balkwill & Mantovani 2001) The idea that these processes are connected was out of favour for more than a century, but there has been a recent resurgence in interest. Several lines of evidence(Balkwill et al 2005;Balkwill & Mantovani 2001;Coussens & Werb 2002;Karin 2006) – based on a range of findings, from epidemiological studies of patients to molecular studies of genetically modified mice have led to a general acceptance that inflammation and cancer are linked. General hallmarks of cancer-related inflammation include the presence of inflammatory cells and inflammatory mediators (for example, chemokines, cytokines and prostaglandins) in tumour tissues, tissue remodelling and angiogenesis similar to that seen in chronic inflammatory responses, and tissue repair. These signs of 'smoldering' inflammation (Balkwill, Charles, & Mantovani 2005;Roxburgh & McMillan 2010) are also present in tumors for which a firm causal relationship to inflammation has not been established. Indeed, inflammatory cells and mediators are present in the microenvironment of most, if not all, tumors, irrespective of the trigger for development. The cytokines interleukin-6 (IL-6), tumor necrosis factor alpha (TNFα) and interleukin-1 beta (IL-1β) are critical mediators of the systemic inflammatory response. As a result, these cytokines are main stimulators for the synthesis of an acute-phase response. A variety of other modulators may affect APP responses, which include glucocorticoids, insulin and growth factors such as epidermal growth factor, hepatocyte growth factor and transforming growth factor β. To this effect, the presence of a systemic inflammatory response detected through the measurement of acute-phase reactants is considered a poor prognostic factor for various cancers.

3. Acute phase proteins in cancer

A number of well characterized APP have been linked to distinct cancer types and stages of malignancy (See Table 1). C-reactive protein (CRP), serum amyloid A (SAA), α-1 glycoprotein (AGP), haptoglobin (HAP), α-1 antichymotrypsin (ACT), and complement proteins represent major positive host response reactants that play different functional roles and have relevance to different types of cancer in humans. The following sections describe compiled data showing support for APPs in distinct human cancers in addition to prognostic significance.

APRP	Type of cancer	Response	Method
AAT	Liver cancer	↑	Radial immunodiffusion
	Cervical cancer	↑	Immunochemical assay
			Trypsin inhibitory capacity; immunodiffusion
	Colorectal cancer	↑	Immunological methods and nephelometry
	Gastric cancer	↑	Immunological method and nephelometry
	Lung cancer	↑	Immunological methods
	Multiple myeloma	↑	Nephelometry
	Ovarian cancer	↑	Radial immunodiffusion
	Pancreatic cancer	↑	Radial immunodiffusion
	Prostate cancer	↑	Radial immunodiffusion
ACT	Colorectal cancer	↑	Rocket immunoelectrophoresis
	Gastric cancer	↑	Rocket immunoelectrophoresis
	Lung cancer	↑	Immunological methods
	Pancreatic cancer	↑	Radial immunodiffusion
AHS	Liver cancer	↓	Radial immunodiffusion
CLU	Urinary bladder cancer	↑	ELISA
CPL	Cervical cancer	↑	Radial immunodiffusion
			Nephelometry
	Chronic lymphocytic leukemia	↑	Nephelometry
	Endometrial cancer	↑	Radial immunodiffusion
	Gastrointestinal cancer	↑	Immunological methods and nephelometry
	Kidney and urinary tract cancer	↑	Radial immunodiffusion
	Lung adenocarcinoma	↑	Biochemical assays
	Melanoma	↑	Nephelometry
	Solid malignant tumors	↑	Nephelometry
HAP	Cervical cancer	↑	Nephelometry
	Ovarian cancer	↑	Immunochemical assay
			ELISA
KNG	Gastrointestinal cancer	↓	Immunochemical assay

↑ = increase in expression; ↓ = decrease in expression

Table 1. Acute phase protein expression levels in various cancer types [AAT, *a*1-antitrypsin; ABG, *a*1-B glycoprotein; ACT, *a*1-antichymotrypsin; AHS, *a*2-HS glycoprotein; ATR, Antithrombin III; CFB ,Complement factor B; CLU, Clusterin; CPL, Ceruloplasmin; CRP, C-reactive protein; HAP, Haptoglobin; KNG, Kininogen; LRG, Leucine-rich glycoprotein; ZAG, Zinc *a*2-glycoprotein] Adapted from (Pang et al 2010).

3.1 Gastrointestinal (esophagus, stomach, pancreatic, and colorectal)

3.1.1 Esophagus

Worldwide, esophageal carcinoma affects approximately 480,000 people per year.(Jemal et al 2011) The prognosis of esophageal cancer remains poor. Most patients are still diagnosed with advance stage disease. Advances in neoadjuvant therapy and surgical technique have improved the 5 year survival up to 40-50% in patients with localized disease. Patients with advanced disease have a 5 year survival of 15%. Accurate staging therefore is essential in patients with esophageal cancer. Many investigators have correlated CRP with esophageal cancer. Acute phase protein levels are thought to reflect the host response to the biological behavior of a tumor. The mean CRP level in patients with esophageal cancer has been found to be elevated compared to patients with benign pathology.(Guillem & Triboulet 2005) CRP has been shown to be elevated in both adenocarcinoma (AC) and squamous cell carcinoma (SCCA) of the esophagus.(Gockel et al 2006;Nozoe et al 2001;Wang et al 2009) Nozoe et al showed there was no statistical difference in the CRP levels between AC and SCCA.(Nozoe, Saeki, & Sugimachi 2001) Elevated CRP in both AC and SCCA correlates with tumor depth, lymph node invasion and metastasis.(Gockel, Dirksen, Messow, & Junginger 2006;Ikeda et al 2003;Nozoe, Saeki, & Sugimachi 2001;Shimada et al 2003;Wang, Hsieh, Chiu, Li, Huang, Fang, & Huang 2009) Patients with upper third esophageal cancer have a higher CRP level than patients with middle and lower third cancers.(Wang, Hsieh, Chiu, Li, Huang, Fang, & Huang 2009) An elevated pretreatment CRP is also associated with decrease survival compared to patients with normal CRP levels(Gockel, Dirksen, Messow, & Junginger 2006;Ikeda, Natsugoe, Ueno, Baba, & Aikou 2003;Nozoe, Saeki, & Sugimachi 2001;Shimada, Nabeya, Okazumi, Matsubara, Shiratori, Aoki, Sugaya, Miyazawa, Hayashi, Miyazaki, & Ochiai 2003;Wang, Hsieh, Chiu, Li, Huang, Fang, & Huang 2009;Zingg et al 2010). Zingg et al showed that an elevated serum CRP level independent prognostic indicator for survival in patients with esophageal cancer. In patients that underwent neoadjuvant therapy followed by esophagectomy, patients with normal CRP levels had a significant survival advantage compared to patient with an elevated CRP (median survival 65.4 moths and 5-year survival 52.1% compared to median survival 18.7 months vs 5-year survival 23.3%, $p=0.027$).(Zingg, Forberger, Rajcic, Langton, & Jamieson 2010) Data for other acute phase proteins in esophageal cancer is limited. An et al showed in a small study that SAA and HAP were elevated in patients with esophageal cancer.(An et al 2004)

3.1.2 Stomach

Worldwide, an estimated total of 989,600 new stomach cancer cases and 738,000 deaths are estimated to have occurred in 2008. Over 70% of new cases and deaths occur in developing countries. (Jemal, Bray, Center, Ferlay, Ward, & Forman 2011) The prognosis for gastric cancer is poor because of advanced disease at diagnosis. (Collard et al 2003) To improve the poor survival outcome and help identify earlier diagnosis, there is a need for new and more sensitive biomarkers.

CRP has been shown to be elevated in patients with gastric cancer compared to healthy controls. (Ilhan et al 2004;Kim et al 2009;Lukaszewicz-Zajac et al 2010;Tsavaris et al 2005) Elevated CRP (>3mg/L) is associated with infiltrative type, larger tumors, serosal invasion, lymph node metastasis, distant metastasis. (Chang et al 2010;Kim, Oh, Kwon, Lee, Kwon, Kim, Kim, Kim, Jang, Kim, Kim, Han, & Kim 2009;Lukaszewicz-Zajac, Mroczko, Gryko, Kedra, & Szmitkowski 2010) Chang et al showed that 5-year survival rate of patients with an

elevated CRP was significantly worse than those without (<3.0mg/L).(Chang, Sun, Pai, Wang, Hsieh, Kuo, & Wang 2010)
SAA has been shown to be elevated in gastric cancer. Elevated SAA was associated with tumor size, depth of tumor, lymph node metastasis, and tumor location.(Chan et al 2007;Chang, Sun, Pai, Wang, Hsieh, Kuo, & Wang 2010) Chang et al showed that SAA increased 2.10mg/L for each 1mm increase in tumor size and SAA concentration was higher in patients with tumors located in the upper portion of the stomach compared to the lower stomach. SAA was also elevated in patients with recurrent cancer compared to those who did not recur.
AAT has been reported to be elevated in patients with gastric cancer compared to healthy controls. There has not been any correlation with an elevated AAT and disease status or patient outcome. Several reports have corroborated elevated levels of AAT in gastric juice in patients with gastric cancer compared with healthy controls. (Hsu et al 2007;Lee et al 2004)

3.1.3 Pancreas

Pancreatic cancer is the fourth most common cause of cancer-related death in the United States. The five-year survival is about 4%, which is the lowest among all cancers. The high mortality rate is due to patients presenting with advanced stage of the disease due to the early aggressiveness of this cancer, the inability to diagnose it early and the currently lack of effective therapies. Surgical resection is the only potentially curative treatment for pancreatic cancer. Only 10-20% of patients diagnosed with pancreatic cancer are able to undergo surgical resection due to advanced presentation at diagnosis. Advances are needed to help accurately detect pancreatic cancer early in its disease process.
Circulating levels of CRP have been found to be significantly elevated in patients with pancreatic cancer compared to healthy controls.(Mroczko et al 2010;Orchekowski et al 2005) There was a significant increase in CRP levels with more advanced stages of pancreatic cancer. Patients with an elevated pre-operative CRP level were found at surgery to have an increase in tumor size, vascular invasion, and poor differentiated tumors.(Jamieson et al 2005) Serum levels of CRP have been found to be independent predictor of survival in both patients with resectable pancreatic adenocarcinoma and metastatic disease.(Falconer et al 1995;Jamieson, Glen, McMillan, McKay, Foulis, Carter, & Imrie 2005;Pine et al 2009;Tingstedt et al 2007) Falconer et al in a respective review of 102 patients with unresectable pancreatic cancer found the presence of an acute-phase response to be the most significant independent predictor of survival duration.(Falconer, Fearon, Ross, Elton, Wigmore, Garden, & Carter 1995) The median survival of those was an acute-phase response was 66 days compared to 222 days for those with no acute phase response.
Other APP, SAA, AAT, APE, and HAP have been reported as being elevated in patients with pancreatic cancer but the correlation with tumor pathology and survival data is lacking.(Deng et al 2007;Firpo et al 2009;Koomen et al 2005;Orchekowski, Hamelinck, Li, Gliwa, vanBrocklin, Marrero, Vande Woude, Feng, Brand, & Haab 2005;Trichopoulos et al 1990;Yu et al 2005) Firpo et al demonstrated that HPT and SAA were both elevated in patients with pancreatic cancer compared to healthy controls and patients with other benign pancreatic diseases. The addition of HAP and SAA improved detection of pancreatic cancer when they were added to a screening panel.(Firpo, Gay, Granger, Scaife, DiSario, Boucher, & Mulvihill 2009) Trichopoulos et al demonstrated that patients with an elevated AAT at the time of diagnosis had a significantly shorter survival.

3.1.4 Colorectal

Yearly, there are approximately 1.2 million new colorectal cancer cases and 608,700 deaths are estimated to occur. (Jemal, Bray, Center, Ferlay, Ward, & Forman 2011) Colorectal cancer is curable if detected early. New methods are needed to help detect colorectal cancer and patients that are at high risk for developing metastatic disease and reoccurrence.

The association of serum CRP levels with risk of colorectal cancer has been examined in several prospective studies. The results of these studies have been inconsistent. (Aleksandrova et al 2010;Erlinger et al 2004;Gunter et al 2006;Ito et al 2005;Zhang et al 2005) In several prospective studies, patients with an elevated baseline CRP were at a higher risk for developing colon cancer compared to rectal cancer.(Aleksandrova, Jenab, Boeing, Jansen, Bueno-de-Mesquita, Rinaldi, Riboli, Overvad, Dahm, Olsen, Tjonneland, Boutron-Ruault, Clavel-Chapelon, Morois, Palli, Krogh, Tumino, Vineis, Panico, Kaaks, Rohrmann, Trichopoulou, Lagiou, Trichopoulos, van Duijnhoven, Leufkens, Peeters, Rodriguez, Bonet, Sanchez, Dorronsoro, Navarro, Barricarte, Palmqvist, Hallmans, Khaw, Wareham, Allen, Spencer, Romaguera, Norat, & Pischon 2010;Erlinger, Platz, Rifai, & Helzlsouer 2004;Gunter, Stolzenberg-Solomon, Cross, Leitzmann, Weinstein, Wood, Virtamo, Taylor, Albanes, & Sinha 2006) In these studies, persons in the highest quartile of CRP concentration had greater than a 3-fold increase risk of developing colon cancer compared with those in the lowest quartile. Erlinger et al found persons who subsequently developed colon cancer, the median CRP was 2.69 vs 1.97mg/L for matched controls (P<.001).(Erlinger, Platz, Rifai, & Helzlsouer 2004) CRP has been shown to be elevated in patients with colorectal cancer compared to controls.(Aleksandrova, Jenab, Boeing, Jansen, Bueno-de-Mesquita, Rinaldi, Riboli, Overvad, Dahm, Olsen, Tjonneland, Boutron-Ruault, Clavel-Chapelon, Morois, Palli, Krogh, Tumino, Vineis, Panico, Kaaks, Rohrmann, Trichopoulou, Lagiou, Trichopoulos, van Duijnhoven, Leufkens, Peeters, Rodriguez, Bonet, Sanchez, Dorronsoro, Navarro, Barricarte, Palmqvist, Hallmans, Khaw, Wareham, Allen, Spencer, Romaguera, Norat, & Pischon 2010;Kaminska et al 2000;Kemik et al 2010) Elevated CRP concentrations are associated with tumor length, poorly differinated histology, tumor depth, lymph node metastasis, liver metastases, and Duke's stage.(Nozoe et al 1998;Nozoe et al 2008) There has been controversy as to an elevated CRP is an independent prognostic indicator.(Chung & Chang 2003;McMillan et al 2003;Nielsen et al 2000;Nozoe, Mori, Takahashi, & Ezaki 2008;Simpson et al 1995) Nozoe et al showed the 5-year survival rates in patients with elevated CRP levels was 28.8% compared to 94.3% in patients with normal CRP levels.(Nozoe, Mori, Takahashi, & Ezaki 2008)

SAA has been found to be elevated in patient with colorectal cancer compared to healthy controls.(Glojnaric et al 2001) Glojnaric et al showed that mean pre-operative SAA concentration was 38mg/l in patients with Dukes stage B and C colorectal carcinoma. SAA concentrations have been shown to increase with advanced stage in colorectal cancer.(Biran et al 1986) Several studies have shown that patients with colorectal cancer have higher levels of circulating HAP and AAT.(Park et al 2010;Ward et al 1977) Patients that developed recurrence within 2 years or developed hepatic metastases had elevated HPT and AAT.(Ward, Cooper, Turner, Anderson, & Neville 1977)

3.2 Lung

In 2008, lung cancer was the most commonly diagnosed cancer and the leading cause of cancer death in males. In females, it is the fourth most diagnosed cancer and the second leading cause of cancer death. (Jemal, Bray, Center, Ferlay, Ward, & Forman 2011) The expected 5-year survival for all patients diagnosed with lung cancer is 15%. Surgical resection of non-small cell lung cancer (NSCLC) offers the potential for cure, but there is often difficulty in selecting suitable patients for surgical resection. Newer approaches are needed to aid in earlier diagnosis.

The Rotterdam Study (Siemes et al 2006) found that high levels (>3mg/L) of CRP were associated with an increased incidence of lung cancer. There was an age-, sex-, and smoking-adjusted hazard ratio for incident lung cancer of 2.8 when CRP levels were elevated. After the 5-year latent period, the hazard ratio was reduced to a 2.1 fold risk increase. Elevated pre-operative CRP levels have been found to be an independent and significant prognostic indicator in patients with NSCLC. Elevated pre-operative CPR level is associated with increase maximum pathologic tumor size, lymphovascular invasion, and inability to achieve complete resection in patients with NSCLC.(Hara et al 2007;Jones et al 2006;Lee et al 2009) Disease specific survival and overall survival were significantly decreased in patients with elevated pre-operative CRP compared to non-elevated CRP patients, which is independent of TNM stage. (Hara, Matsuzaki, Shimuzu, Tomita, Ayabe, Enomoto, & Onitsuka 2007;O'Dowd et al 2010)

SAA was found to be higher in patients in patients with NSCLC compared to healthy controls.(Benson et al 1986;Dowling et al 2007;Gao et al 2005;Howard et al 2003;Liu et al 2007) Howard BA et al found SAA to elevated at 286ng/mL in serum of lung cancer patients compared to 34.1ng/mL in serum of control patients. Elevated levels of SAA correlated with increase in the clinical stages I-IV and were higher in patients with squamous cell carcinoma.(Liu, Wang, Zhang, Dai, Liu, Liu, Wu, Yang, Fu, Xiao, & He 2007) SAA has been shown to be a prognostic biomarker. Patients with a survival ≥ 5years had a significantly lower SAA than patients with a survival < 5 years.(Cho et al 2010)

Circulating levels of HAP has been shown to be elevated as high as three-fold in patients with SCLC compared to healthy controls.(Bharti et al 2004;Dowling, O'Driscoll, Meleady, Henry, Roy, Ballot, Moriarty, Crown, & Clynes 2007) Bharti et al showed a tendency of increased survival when HAP was <1.9. AAT and apolipoprotein A-1 (ApoA-1) have been also shown to be elevated in lung cancer compared to healthy controls. (Dowling, O'Driscoll, Meleady, Henry, Roy, Ballot, Moriarty, Crown, & Clynes 2007;Gao, Kuick, Orchekowski, Misek, Qiu, Greenberg, Rom, Brenner, Omenn, Haab, & Hanash 2005)

3.3 Melanoma

Malignant melanoma is a cutaneous neoplasm known for its highly aggressiveness, early dissemination, and poor prognosis once metastasized. It is estimated that 68, 130 cases of invasive malignant melanoma and at least 48,000 cases of melanoma in-situ will be diagnosed in the US this year. (Rigel 2010) Numerous biomarkers help determine exist to help determine the prognosis of patients with distant metastases; S100B and lactate dehydrogenase (LDH)are the most widely distributed clinical markers, yet these fail to predict disease progression, relapse or metastasis in early-stage melanoma.(Findeisen et al 2009)

CRP levels have been found to be elevated in all stages of melanoma. High levels of circulating CRP has been associated with a reduced overall survival in early disease stages (stage I to III) and late stage (stage IV).(Findeisen, Zapatka, Peccerella, Matzk, Neumaier, Schadendorf, & Ugurel 2009) Circulating levels of CRP correlate with clinical response to interleukin-2 (IL-2) based immunotherapy. (Tartour et al 1994) Tartour et al found patients with CRP levels >10 has a poor clinical response to IL-2 therapy and poor survival compared to patients with lower CRP levels. In a prospective study by Deichman et al, CRP

was significantly elevated in stage IV melanoma patients compared to stage I to stage III, whereas LDH was not. (Deichmann et al 2004) They concluded that LDH provided no additional information to CRP.
Circulating levels of SAA was found to be prognositic in melanoma patients.(Findeisen, Zapatka, Peccerella, Matzk, Neumaier, Schadendorf, & Ugurel 2009) SAA levels less than 10mg/mL showed favorable survival complared to patients with high serum levels. SAA levels were prognostic when patients were analyzed separately in stage I-III and stage IV. ACT has been shown to be elevated in metastatic melanoma. Patients with stage III melanoma with low ACT levels, survived 43.4 months compared to 18.5 months in patients with high levels of ACT, p = 0.048).(Wang et al 2010) Similar results were seen with stage IV disease.

3.4 Renal cell

Renal cell carcinoma (RCC) is difficult to diagnose due to lack of clinical symptoms. Approximately 40% of patients with RCC have a metastasis at the time of diagnosis and approximately 25-30% of patients will develop metastatic tumors within 5 years after nephrectomy.(Cohen & McGovern 2005) Metastatic RCC has a poor prognosis with a median overall survival of about 1 year.(Bleumer et al 2003) The need for reliable markers for diagnosis and follow-up of RCC remains.
CRP has been shown to be elevated in patients with localized and metastatic RCC. (Casamassima et al 2005;Cho et al 2011;Ito et al 2006;Jagdev et al 2010;Komai et al 2007;Saito et al 2009) Patients with localized RCC and elevated CRP levels have been found to have larger tumors, higher percentages of lymph node metastasis, higher histological grade and higher percentages of microvascular invasion.(Cho, Kim, Lee, Ahn, Kim, & Kim 2011;Ito, Asano, Yoshii, Satoh, Sumitomo, & Hayakawa 2006;Komai, Saito, Sakai, & Morimoto 2007) Elevated circulating levels of CRP have been shown to be independent factor of disease specific survival (DSS) and recurrence free survival (RFS).(Cho, Kim, Lee, Ahn, Kim, & Kim 2011;Ito, Asano, Yoshii, Satoh, Sumitomo, & Hayakawa 2006;Jagdev, Gregory, Vasudev, Harnden, Sim, Thompson, Cartledge, Selby, & Banks 2010;Komai, Saito, Sakai, & Morimoto 2007) Komai Y et al showed the 5- and 10-year DSS rates with patients with elevated CRP were 75% and 30% compared to both 93% in patients with normal CRP ($p<0.001$) Circulating levels of CRP have been shown to be elevated in patients with metastatic RCC and predictive of overall survival.(Casamassima, Picciariello, Quaranta, Berardino, Ranieri, Paradiso, Lorusso, & Guida 2005;Saito, Tatokoro, Fujii, Iimura, Koga, Kawakami, & Kihara 2009) Saito et al showed overall survival was significantly different in patients with elevated CRP levels who did not normalize while on treatment. Patients with metastatic non-elevated CRP levels had a 2-year survival of 69% compared to 4% in patients with elevated CRP that did not normalize.
Circulating levels of SAA has been shown to be elevated in patients with RCC.(Engwegen et al 2007;Kimura et al 2001;Ramankulov et al 2008;Tolson et al 2004;Wood et al 2010) Elevated levels of SAA correlated with increased tumor stage, tumor grade, and metastasis.(Kimura, Tomita, Imai, Saito, Katagiri, Ohara-Mikami, Matsudo, & Takahashi 2001;Ramankulov, Lein, Johannsen, Schrader, Miller, Loening, & Jung 2008) In relation to histological features, median SAA concentration in clear cell, papillary and chromophobe subtypes were not statistically different.(Ramankulov, Lein, Johannsen, Schrader, Miller, Loening, & Jung 2008)

SAA concentrations have been shown to be an independent prognostic factor for outcome in patients with RCC. Patient with high circulating levels of SAA had shorter survival times compared to patients with non-elevated SAA.(Kimura, Tomita, Imai, Saito, Katagiri, Ohara-Mikami, Matsudo, & Takahashi 2001;Ramankulov, Lein, Johannsen, Schrader, Miller, Loening, & Jung 2008;Wood, Rogers, Cairns, Paul, Thompson, Vasudev, Selby, & Banks 2010)

3.5 Ovarian

Worldwide, there is approximately 225,000 new cases of ovarian cancer diagnosed yearly.(Jemal, Bray, Center, Ferlay, Ward, & Forman 2011) The 5-year survival for patients with early-stage ovarian cancer is approximately 95%, but it is 25% for advanced-stage disease. In 80% of patients with ovarian cancer, the disease is already advanced at the time of initial diagnosis. This highlights the need for early diagnosis to decrease the morbidity and mortality of ovarian cancer.

Ovarian cancer risk is positively associated with increasing serum levels of CRP concentration.(McSorley et al 2007) In a multicenter, nested, case-control study, McSorley et al found a significant increased risk of developing ovarian cancer with increasing serum CRP levels. There was a two -fold risk of developing ovarian cancer was observed among women with CRP levels within a range of 3 to 10mg/L, as compared to women with CRP levels less than 1mg/L. CRP has been shown to be significantly elevated in patients with ovarian cancer.(Bertenshaw et al 2008;Edgell et al 2010;Hefler et al 2008;Hefler-Frischmuth et al 2009;Kodama et al 1999;Maccio et al 1998) Circulating levels of CRP have been shown to correlate with International Federation of Gynecologists and Obstetricians stage (FIGO), post-operative residual tumor.(Hefler, Concin, Hofstetter, Marth, Mustea, Sehouli, Zeillinger, Leipold, Lass, Grimm, Tempfer, & Reinthaller 2008;Hefler-Frischmuth, Hefler, Heinze, Paseka, Grimm, & Tempfer 2009) Hefler et al demonstrated patients with platinum-resistant epithelial ovarian cancer (EOC) had a significantly higher CRP serum levels compared with patients with platinum-sensitive EOC. Elevated serum CRP is a significant prognostic factor in patients with EOC. Hefler et al found women with an elevated CRP (>1mg/L) had a 5-year overall survival of 58.5% versus 82% in women with normal CRP (<1mg/L).

Several other AAP have been reported to be elevated in ovarian cancer, but the correlation with tumor stage and prognosis is lacking. SAA has been shown to be elevated in patients with ovarian cancer.(Edgell, Martin-Roussety, Barker, Autelitano, Allen, Grant, & Rice 2010;Helleman et al 2008; Moshkovskii et al 2007a;Moshkovskii et al 2007b) Edgell et al found the mean SAA in patients with ovarian cancer to be 113ng/mL compared to 5ng/mL in healthy controls. HAP has been demonstrated to be elevated in patients with ovarian cancer.(Bertenshaw, Yip, Seshaiah, Zhao, Chen, Wiggins, Mapes, & Mansfield 2008;Ye et al 2003) Bertenshaw et al found AAT to be elevated in patients with ovarian cancer compared to controls.(Bertenshaw, Yip, Seshaiah, Zhao, Chen, Wiggins, Mapes, & Mansfield 2008)

Circulating levels of ApoA-1 has been shown to be decreased compared to healthy controls.(Bertenshaw, Yip, Seshaiah, Zhao, Chen, Wiggins, Mapes, & Mansfield 2008;Nosov et al 2009;Su et al 2007;Zhang et al 2004) Nosov V et al demonstrated that patients with late stage ovarian cancer had an ApoA-1 level of 88.10mg/dL compared to 154.36mg/dL for healthy controls.

3.6 Breast

Worldwide breast cancer is the most frequently diagnosed cancer among women and the leading cause of cancer death in females. In 2008, breast cancer accounted for 1.38 million (23%) o the total new cancer cases and 458,000 (14%) of the total cancer deaths in females.(Jemal, Bray, Center, Ferlay, Ward, & Forman 2011) Chronic inflammation has been shown to contribute to breast cancer development and progression. Chronic inflammation promotes mammary tumor development through mechanisms involving chronic activation of humoral immunity and infiltration of Th2 cells and polarized innate inflammatory cells.(DeNardo & Coussens 2007) Inflammatory status is suggested to be a prognostic factor for breast cancer.

The association between circulating concentrations of CRP levels have been widely analyzed. There is conflicting reports between baseline levels of CRP and developing breast cancer. Rotterdam Study reported a 28% increase in breast cancer risk was associated with 1-unit increase of CRP levels above baseline.(Siemes, Visser, Coebergh, Splinter, Witteman, Uitterlinden, Hofman, Pols, & Stricker 2006) There was no statistically significantly associated breast cancer risk in studies conducted by Il'yasova et al and Trichopoulos et al.(Il'yasova et al 2005;Trichopoulos et al 2006) Results from studies assessing the association of NSAIDs and statins, which are also known to lower CRP levels, and breast cancer risk have also been mixed. The circulating levels of CRP have been found to be higher in patients with breast carcinoma compared to healthy controls. (O'Hanlon et al 2002) Significant increases in circulating levels of CRP correlate with increase tumor size, lymph node involvement and distant metastasis. As the stage of the disease increased, CRP levels increased proportionally. (O'Hanlon, Lynch, Cormican, & Given 2002;Ravishankaran & R K 2011) Results from several studies have shown an association between CRP and survival in patients with metastatic disease.(Al Murri et al 2007;Albuquerque et al 1995;Pierce et al 2009) Pierce et al also found that elevated CRP levels were associated with reduced disease-free survival.(Pierce, Ballard-Barbash, Bernstein, Baumgartner, Neuhouser, Wener, Baumgartner, Gilliland, Sorensen, McTiernan, & Ulrich 2009)

3.7 Neuroblastoma

Neuroblastoma (NB) is the most common extracranial solid tumor of childhood. Despite treatment which may involve multimodality approaches, children with high-risk disease still have an overall survival rate of less than 40% despite multi-modality therapy.(Maris et al 2007) This highlights the need for earlier detection of advanced stage NB.

While limited in number, studies have corroborated circulating levels of several acute phase proteins to be elevated in children with NB. Serum concentrations of apolipoprotein A-IV (ApoA-IV), HAP, AAT and SAA have been shown to be elevated in children with NB compared to healthy controls.(Combaret et al 2005;Gerson et al 1977;Lipinska et al 1992;Sandoval et al 2007) Work from our laboratory demonstrated that ApoA-IV, HAP, and SAA were increased in patients with advanced stage neuroblastoma compared to healthy controls (Sandoval et al 2007). Others have shown CRP, HP and AAT were higher in patients with poor prognosis patient compared to good prognosis patients (Lipinska et al1992). Finally, work by Gerson et al demonstrated the APP response returned to normal in all patients that responded to treatment by surgery, radiation and chemotherapy, but rose again with recurrence of disease. These studies support the notion of an inflammatory response to the tumor maybe detected and potentially used as complementary cancer markers.

4. Profiling acute phase proteins

Advances in proteomics technologies have provided an important tool that can systematically identify and quantify steady-state or perturbation-induced changes in a complex biological system in a high throughput fashion. There has been a great interest in applying this technology to cancer biomarker discovery. Yet the clinical translation of proteomic technology and bioinformatics tools to human samples, such as in the area of cancer biomarkers, represents one of the major opportunities and challenges facing this field. An ongoing challenge in proteomics continues to be the analysis of the serum proteome due to the vast number and complexity of proteins estimated to be present in this biofluid. The enormous diversity in protein species and post-translational modifications of proteins, and the vast differences in protein abundance, create major challenges, as well as a great opportunity, in employing quantitative plasma proteomics for biomarker discovery. Nonetheless, an active area of interest includes enrichment strategies for optimal biomarker candidates from serum and plasma.

As proteomics aims for the full identification and quantification of all expressed proteins, profiling strategies usually are applied on sub-sets of the proteome. The expression of serum proteins can be analyzed concurrently by using the gel-based proteomic technology. This is appropriate for studying the acute-phase response, which involves the simultaneous altered expression of serum proteins in association to inflammation, infection, injury or cancer. Many proteomic studies on serum or plasma have been performed using samples that were depleted of albumin and/or immunoglobulins in order to analyze serum proteins of lower abundance. However, a number of serum proteins including those that have been used clinically or experimentally have been demonstrated to adhere strongly to albumin and immunoglobulins. These serum proteins were also removed in experiments involving depletion of the high abundance proteins, and thus, may affect interpretation of the results. Moreover, recent studies using rat plasma have revealed that depletion of high abundance proteins only reduced the dynamic range of plasma proteome by two to three orders of magnitude. Removal of albumin, IgG, IgM, transferrin, fibrinogen, HAP and AAT from rat plasma leads to the unmasking of only a few proteins and was still far from being able to detect the low abundance proteins (Linke et al 2007). Given these barriers, applied approaches to simplify and increase the depth of serum proteomic analysis include fractionation strategies, targeted protein subpopulation enrichment (phosphoproteins, glycoproteins, etc.), and differential quantifying protein methods such as isobaric tags for relative and absolute quantification (iTRAQ). In addition, other novel work in biomarker discovery involves proximal fluid proteomics. (Teng et al 2010) Proximal fluid, the fluid derived from the extracellular milieu of tissues, contains a large repertoire of shed and secreted proteins that are likely to be present at higher concentrations relative to plasma/serum. It has been hypothesized that many, if not all, proximal fluid proteins exchange with peripheral circulation, which has provided significant motivation for utilizing proximal fluids as a primary sample source for protein biomarker discovery. Finally, opportunities in the exploration of the nano-scale open new strategies for serum protein analysis. For example, Pujia and colleagues recently described a tool based on biodegradable nanoporous nanoparticles (NPNPs) that allows the harvesting of low-molecular-weight fractions of crude human serum/plasma. (Pujia et al 2010) NPNPs with a diameter of 200 nm and pore size of a few nm were obtained by ultrasonication of nanoporous silicon. When incubated with a solution, the NPNPs harvest only the molecules small enough to be absorbed into the nanopores. These in turn can be recovered by centrifugation and dissolved in water, making the harvested molecules available for further analyses. The development and utilization of novel methods in serum APP biomarker discovery may include novel strategies including nanostructured materials and other high throughput methods like protein arrays, multiplexed protein assays, and chip-based proteomic platforms.

5. Acute phase proteins as biomarkers

Blood-based protein biomarkers have been used in clinical laboratories for decades to aid in the diagnosis and prognosis of many diseases, including a variety of cancers. As shown in this chapter, circulating levels of APPs have been confirmed to coincide in patients with many solid malignancies. However, these acute phase reactants are not specific for cancer, and these serum APP concentrations need to be interpreted in the context of a full clinical examination and the presence of other signs and symptoms of malignancy. Nevertheless, an ongoing emerging theme clearly supports the role of a bidirectional tumor-host response and the ensuing concept of inflammation as a biomarker for cancer.

While the analysis of the serum proteome has challenges, we envision contemporary serum proteomics studies using high-throughput proteomic methodologies and bioinformatics will enable the identification of a subset of acute phase protein markers for the unequivocal discrimination of malignancy. While many of these APP are found within the inflammatory cascade, an important distinctive feature may include protein glycosylation. Glycosylation-related changes represent one of the major post translational modifications and can have significant effects on protein function. Moreover, changes in the carbohydrate structure are increasingly being recognized as an important modification associated with cancer. (Hakomori 1996;Hakomori 2002) These differences can be further explored using techniques such as microarray platform to characterize glycan structure and to study glycosylation-related biological interactions using probes as a means to interrogate the spotted or captured glycosylated molecules on the arrays. The high-throughput and reproducible nature of the microarray platforms allow simultaneous assessment of a number of defined proteins on a single platform. For instance, Zeng et al using an integrated system based on multiple lectin affinity chromatography (M-LAC) that partions serum proteins based on glycan characteristics, found proteins such as ABG, complement C3, ATT, and transferrin accurately identified patients with breast cancer. As the field of inflammatory biomarkers continues to evolve, we feel the host immune response can be further exploited to better integrate these APPs into the design of personalized biomarkers for the noninvasive diagnosis of cancer. (Zeng et al 2010)

6. Conclusions

Inflammation appears to play a dominant role in the pathogenesis of various cancer types. This review has focused on the current understanding of the dynamic role of the host-tumor interaction with regards to inflammation and the developing field of acute phase reactants as circulating cancer biomarkers. The field of acute phase proteins as cancer biomarkers has tremendous potential. The identification of specific proteomic expression patterns in acute phase proteins related to cancer as well as a more thorough understanding of this proinflammatory response in tumor pathogenesis offers promise not only for novel molecular diagnostic markers but also for new therapy strategies in the treatment of solid malignancies.

7. Acknowledgements

The authors of this chapter wish to acknowledge Mrs. Gailya Taylor for her assistance in the preparation of this work.

8. References

Al Murri,A.M., Wilson,C., Lannigan,A., Doughty,J.C., Angerson,W.J., McArdle,C.S., & McMillan,D.C. (2007) Evaluation of the relationship between the systemic inflammatory response and cancer-specific survival in patients with primary operable breast cancer. *Br.J.Cancer* 96, 891-895.

Albuquerque,K.V., Price,M.R., Badley,R.A., Jonrup,I., Pearson,D., Blamey,R.W., & Robertson,J.F. (1995) Pre-treatment serum levels of tumour markers in metastatic breast cancer: a prospective assessment of their role in predicting response to therapy and survival. *Eur.J.Surg.Oncol.* 21, 504-509.

Aleksandrova,K., Jenab,M., Boeing,H., Jansen,E., Bueno-de-Mesquita,H.B., Rinaldi,S., Riboli,E., Overvad,K., Dahm,C.C., Olsen,A., Tjonneland,A., Boutron-Ruault,M.C., Clavel-Chapelon,F., Morois,S., Palli,D., Krogh,V., Tumino,R., Vineis,P., Panico,S., Kaaks,R., Rohrmann,S., Trichopoulou,A., Lagiou,P., Trichopoulos,D., van Duijnhoven,F.J., Leufkens,A.M., Peeters,P.H., Rodriguez,L., Bonet,C., Sanchez,M.J., Dorronsoro,M., Navarro,C., Barricarte,A., Palmqvist,R., Hallmans,G., Khaw,K.T., Wareham,N., Allen,N.E., Spencer,E., Romaguera,D., Norat,T., & Pischon,T. (2010) Circulating C-reactive protein concentrations and risks of colon and rectal cancer: a nested case-control study within the European Prospective Investigation into Cancer and Nutrition. *Am.J.Epidemiol.* 172, 407-418.

Allen,M. & Louise,J.J. (2011) Jekyll and Hyde: the role of the microenvironment on the progression of cancer. *J Pathol* 223, 162-176.

An,J.Y., Fan,Z.M., Zhuang,Z.H., Qin,Y.R., Gao,S.S., Li,J.L., & Wang,L.D. (2004) Proteomic analysis of blood level of proteins before and after operation in patients with esophageal squamous cell carcinoma at high-incidence area in Henan Province. *World J.Gastroenterol.* 10, 3365-3368.

Balkwill,F., Charles,K.A., & Mantovani,A. (2005) Smoldering and polarized inflammation in the initiation and promotion of malignant disease. *Cancer Cell* 7, 211-217.

Balkwill,F. & Mantovani,A. (2001) Inflammation and cancer: back to Virchow? *Lancet* 357, 539-545.

Benson,M.D., Eyanson,S., & Fineberg,N.S. (1986) Serum amyloid A in carcinoma of the lung. *Cancer* 57, 1783-1787.

Bertenshaw,G.P., Yip,P., Seshaiah,P., Zhao,J., Chen,T.H., Wiggins,W.S., Mapes,J.P., & Mansfield,B.C. (2008) Multianalyte profiling of serum antigens and autoimmune and infectious disease molecules to identify biomarkers dysregulated in epithelial ovarian cancer. *Cancer Epidemiol.Biomarkers Prev.* 17, 2872-2881.

Bharti,A., Ma,P.C., Maulik,G., Singh,R., Khan,E., Skarin,A.T., & Salgia,R. (2004) Haptoglobin alpha-subunit and hepatocyte growth factor can potentially serve as serum tumor biomarkers in small cell lung cancer. *Anticancer Res.* 24, 1031-1038.

Biran,H., Friedman,N., Neumann,L., Pras,M., & Shainkin-Kestenbaum,R. (1986) Serum amyloid A (SAA) variations in patients with cancer: correlation with disease activity, stage, primary site, and prognosis. *J.Clin.Pathol.* 39, 794-797.

Bleumer,I., Oosterwijk,E., De,M.P., & Mulders,P.F. (2003) Immunotherapy for renal cell carcinoma. *Eur.Urol.* 44, 65-75.

Casamassima,A., Picciariello,M., Quaranta,M., Berardino,R., Ranieri,C., Paradiso,A., Lorusso,V., & Guida,M. (2005) C-reactive protein: a biomarker of survival in patients with metastatic renal cell carcinoma treated with subcutaneous interleukin-2 based immunotherapy. *J.Urol.* 173, 52-55.

Chan,D.C., Chen,C.J., Chu,H.C., Chang,W.K., Yu,J.C., Chen,Y.J., Wen,L.L., Huang,S.C., Ku,C.H., Liu,Y.C., & Chen,J.H. (2007) Evaluation of serum amyloid A as a biomarker for gastric cancer. *Ann.Surg.Oncol.* 14, 84-93.

Chang,C.C., Sun,C.F., Pai,H.J., Wang,W.K., Hsieh,C.C., Kuo,L.M., & Wang,C.S. (2010) Preoperative serum C-reactive protein and gastric cancer; clinical-pathological correlation and prognostic significance. *Chang Gung.Med.J.* 33, 301-312.

Cho,D.S., Kim,S.J., Lee,S.H., Ahn,H.S., Kim,Y.S., & Kim,S.I. (2011) Prognostic significance of preoperative C-reactive protein elevation and thrombocytosis in patients with non-metastatic renal cell carcinoma. *Korean J.Urol.* 52, 104-109.

Cho,W.C., Yip,T.T., Cheng,W.W., & Au,J.S. (2010) Serum amyloid A is elevated in the serum of lung cancer patients with poor prognosis. *Br.J.Cancer* 102, 1731-1735.

Chung,Y.C. & Chang,Y.F. (2003) Significance of inflammatory cytokines in the progression of colorectal cancer. *Hepatogastroenterology* 50, 1910-1913.

Cohen,H.T. & McGovern,F.J. (2005) Renal-cell carcinoma. *N.Engl.J.Med.* 353, 2477-2490.

Collard,J.M., Malaise,J., Mabrut,J.Y., & Kestens,P.J. (2003) Skeletonizing en-bloc gastrectomy for adenocarcinoma in Caucasian patients. *Gastric.Cancer* 6, 210-216.

Combaret,V., Bergeron,C., Brejon,S., Iacono,I., Perol,D., Negrier,S., & Puisieux,A. (2005) Protein chip array profiling analysis of sera from neuroblastoma patients. *Cancer Lett.* 228, 91-96.

Coussens,L.M. & Werb,Z. (2002) Inflammation and cancer. *Nature* 420, 860-867.

Deichmann,M., Kahle,B., Moser,K., Wacker,J., & Wust,K. (2004) Diagnosing melanoma patients entering American Joint Committee on Cancer stage IV, C-reactive protein in serum is superior to lactate dehydrogenase. *Br.J.Cancer* 91, 699-702.

DeNardo,D.G. & Coussens,L.M. (2007) Inflammation and breast cancer. Balancing immune response: crosstalk between adaptive and innate immune cells during breast cancer progression. *Breast Cancer Res.* 9, 212.

Deng,R., Lu,Z., Chen,Y., Zhou,L., & Lu,X. (2007) Plasma proteomic analysis of pancreatic cancer by 2-dimensional gel electrophoresis. *Pancreas* 34, 310-317.

Dowling,P., O'Driscoll,L., Meleady,P., Henry,M., Roy,S., Ballot,J., Moriarty,M., Crown,J., & Clynes,M. (2007) 2-D difference gel electrophoresis of the lung squamous cell carcinoma versus normal sera demonstrates consistent alterations in the levels of ten specific proteins. *Electrophoresis* 28, 4302-4310.

Edgell,T., Martin-Roussety,G., Barker,G., Autelitano,D.J., Allen,D., Grant,P., & Rice,G.E. (2010) Phase II biomarker trial of a multimarker diagnostic for ovarian cancer. *J.Cancer Res.Clin.Oncol.* 136, 1079-1088.

Engwegen,J.Y., Mehra,N., Haanen,J.B., Bonfrer,J.M., Schellens,J.H., Voest,E.E., & Beijnen,J.H. (2007) Validation of SELDI-TOF MS serum protein profiles for renal cell carcinoma in new populations. *Lab Invest* 87, 161-172.

Erlinger,T.P., Platz,E.A., Rifai,N., & Helzlsouer,K.J. (2004) C-reactive protein and the risk of incident colorectal cancer. *JAMA* 291, 585-590.

Falconer,J.S., Fearon,K.C., Ross,J.A., Elton,R., Wigmore,S.J., Garden,O.J., & Carter,D.C. (1995) Acute-phase protein response and survival duration of patients with pancreatic cancer. *Cancer* 75, 2077-2082.

Findeisen,P., Zapatka,M., Peccerella,T., Matzk,H., Neumaier,M., Schadendorf,D., & Ugurel,S. (2009) Serum amyloid A as a prognostic marker in melanoma identified by proteomic profiling. *J.Clin.Oncol.* 27, 2199-2208.

Firpo,M.A., Gay,D.Z., Granger,S.R., Scaife,C.L., DiSario,J.A., Boucher,K.M., & Mulvihill,S.J. (2009) Improved diagnosis of pancreatic adenocarcinoma using haptoglobin and serum amyloid A in a panel screen. *World J.Surg.* 33, 716-722.

Gao,W.M., Kuick,R., Orchekowski,R.P., Misek,D.E., Qiu,J., Greenberg,A.K., Rom,W.N., Brenner,D.E., Omenn,G.S., Haab,B.B., & Hanash,S.M. (2005) Distinctive serum protein profiles involving abundant proteins in lung cancer patients based upon antibody microarray analysis. *BMC.Cancer* 5, 110.

Gerson,J., Evans,A.E., & Rosen,F.S. (1977) The prognostic value of acute phase reactants in patients with neuroblastoma. *Cancer* 40, 1655-1658.

Glojnaric,I., Casl,M.T., Simic,D., & Lukac,J. (2001) Serum amyloid A protein (SAA) in colorectal carcinoma. *Clin.Chem.Lab Med.* 39, 129-133.

Gockel,I., Dirksen,K., Messow,C.M., & Junginger,T. (2006) Significance of preoperative C-reactive protein as a parameter of the perioperative course and long-term prognosis in squamous cell carcinoma and adenocarcinoma of the oesophagus. *World J.Gastroenterol.* 12, 3746-3750.

Guillem,P. & Triboulet,J.P. (2005) Elevated serum levels of C-reactive protein are indicative of a poor prognosis in patients with esophageal cancer. *Dis.Esophagus.* 18, 146-150.

Gunter,M.J., Stolzenberg-Solomon,R., Cross,A.J., Leitzmann,M.F., Weinstein,S., Wood,R.J., Virtamo,J., Taylor,P.R., Albanes,D., & Sinha,R. (2006) A prospective study of serum C-reactive protein and colorectal cancer risk in men. *Cancer Res.* 66, 2483-2487.

Hakomori,S. (1996) Tumor malignancy defined by aberrant glycosylation and sphingo(glyco)lipid metabolism. *Cancer Res.* 56, 5309-5318.

Hakomori,S. (2002) Glycosylation defining cancer malignancy: new wine in an old bottle. *Proc.Natl Acad.Sci.U.S.A* 99, 10231-10233.

Hara,M., Matsuzaki,Y., Shimuzu,T., Tomita,M., Ayabe,T., Enomoto,Y., & Onitsuka,T. (2007) Preoperative serum C-reactive protein level in non-small cell lung cancer. *Anticancer Res.* 27, 3001-3004.

Hefler,L.A., Concin,N., Hofstetter,G., Marth,C., Mustea,A., Sehouli,J., Zeillinger,R., Leipold,H., Lass,H., Grimm,C., Tempfer,C.B., & Reinthaller,A. (2008) Serum C-reactive protein as independent prognostic variable in patients with ovarian cancer. *Clin.Cancer Res.* 14, 710-714.

Hefler-Frischmuth,K., Hefler,L.A., Heinze,G., Paseka,V., Grimm,C., & Tempfer,C.B. (2009) Serum C-reactive protein in the differential diagnosis of ovarian masses. *Eur.J.Obstet.Gynecol.Reprod.Biol.* 147, 65-68.

Helleman,J., van,d., V, Jansen,M.P., Luider,T.M., van der Burg,M.E., Stoter,G., & Berns,E.M. (2008) Serum proteomic patterns for ovarian cancer monitoring. *Int.J.Gynecol.Cancer* 18, 985-995.

Howard,B.A., Wang,M.Z., Campa,M.J., Corro,C., Fitzgerald,M.C., & Patz,E.F., Jr. (2003) Identification and validation of a potential lung cancer serum biomarker detected by matrix-assisted laser desorption/ionization-time of flight spectra analysis. *Proteomics.* 3, 1720-1724.

Hsu,P.I., Chen,C.H., Hsieh,C.S., Chang,W.C., Lai,K.H., Lo,G.H., Hsu,P.N., Tsay,F.W., Chen,Y.S., Hsiao,M., Chen,H.C., & Lu,P.J. (2007) Alpha1-antitrypsin precursor in gastric juice is a novel biomarker for gastric cancer and ulcer. *Clin.Cancer Res.* 13, 876-883.

Ikeda,M., Natsugoe,S., Ueno,S., Baba,M., & Aikou,T. (2003) Significant host- and tumor-related factors for predicting prognosis in patients with esophageal carcinoma. *Ann.Surg.* 238, 197-202.

Il'yasova,D., Colbert,L.H., Harris,T.B., Newman,A.B., Bauer,D.C., Satterfield,S., & Kritchevsky,S.B. (2005) Circulating levels of inflammatory markers and cancer risk in the health aging and body composition cohort. *Cancer Epidemiol.Biomarkers Prev.* 14, 2413-2418.

Ilhan,N., Ilhan,N., Ilhan,Y., Akbulut,H., & Kucuksu,M. (2004) C-reactive protein, procalcitonin, interleukin-6, vascular endothelial growth factor and oxidative metabolites in diagnosis of infection and staging in patients with gastric cancer. *World J.Gastroenterol.* 10, 1115-1120.

Ito,K., Asano,T., Yoshii,H., Satoh,A., Sumitomo,M., & Hayakawa,M. (2006) Impact of thrombocytosis and C-reactive protein elevation on the prognosis for patients with renal cell carcinoma. *Int.J.Urol.* 13, 1365-1370.

Ito,Y., Suzuki,K., Tamakoshi,K., Wakai,K., Kojima,M., Ozasa,K., Watanabe,Y., Kawado,M., Hashimoto,S., Suzuki,S., Tokudome,S., Toyoshima,H., Hayakawa,N., Kato,K., Watanabe,M., Ohta,Y., Maruta,M., & Tamakoshi,A. (2005) Colorectal cancer and serum C-reactive protein levels: a case-control study nested in the JACC Study. *J.Epidemiol.* 15 Suppl 2, S185-S189.

Jagdev,S.P., Gregory,W., Vasudev,N.S., Harnden,P., Sim,S., Thompson,D., Cartledge,J., Selby,P.J., & Banks,R.E. (2010) Improving the accuracy of pre-operative survival prediction in renal cell carcinoma with C-reactive protein. *Br.J.Cancer* 103, 1649-1656.

Jamieson,N.B., Glen,P., McMillan,D.C., McKay,C.J., Foulis,A.K., Carter,R., & Imrie,C.W. (2005) Systemic inflammatory response predicts outcome in patients undergoing resection for ductal adenocarcinoma head of pancreas. *Br.J.Cancer* 92, 21-23.

Jemal,A., Bray,F., Center,M.M., Ferlay,J., Ward,E., & Forman,D. (2011) Global cancer statistics. *CA Cancer J.Clin.*

Jones,J.M., McGonigle,N.C., McAnespie,M., Cran,G.W., & Graham,A.N. (2006) Plasma fibrinogen and serum C-reactive protein are associated with non-small cell lung cancer. *Lung Cancer* 53, 97-101.

Kaminska,J., Kowalska,M.M., Nowacki,M.P., Chwalinski,M.G., Rysinska,A., & Fuksiewicz,M. (2000) CRP, TNF-alpha, IL-1ra, IL-6, IL-8 and IL-10 in blood serum of colorectal cancer patients. *Pathol.Oncol.Res.* 6, 38-41.

Karin,M. (2006) Nuclear factor-kappaB in cancer development and progression. *Nature* 441, 431-436.

Kemik,O., Sumer,A., Kemik,A.S., Hasirci,I., Purisa,S., Dulger,A.C., Demiriz,B., & Tuzun,S. (2010) The relationship among acute-phase response proteins, cytokines and hormones in cachectic patients with colon cancer. *World J.Surg.Oncol.* 8, 85.

Kim,D.K., Oh,S.Y., Kwon,H.C., Lee,S., Kwon,K.A., Kim,B.G., Kim,S.G., Kim,S.H., Jang,J.S., Kim,M.C., Kim,K.H., Han,J.Y., & Kim,H.J. (2009) Clinical significances of preoperative serum interleukin-6 and C-reactive protein level in operable gastric cancer. *BMC.Cancer* 9, 155.

Kimura,M., Tomita,Y., Imai,T., Saito,T., Katagiri,A., Ohara-Mikami,Y., Matsudo,T., & Takahashi,K. (2001) Significance of serum amyloid A on the prognosis in patients with renal cell carcinoma. *Cancer* 92, 2072-2075.

Kodama,J., Miyagi,Y., Seki,N., Tokumo,K., Yoshinouchi,M., Kobashi,Y., Okuda,H., & Kudo,T. (1999) Serum C-reactive protein as a prognostic factor in patients with epithelial ovarian cancer. *Eur.J.Obstet.Gynecol.Reprod.Biol.* 82, 107-110.

Komai,Y., Saito,K., Sakai,K., & Morimoto,S. (2007) Increased preoperative serum C-reactive protein level predicts a poor prognosis in patients with localized renal cell carcinoma. *BJU.Int.* 99, 77-80.

Koomen,J.M., Shih,L.N., Coombes,K.R., Li,D., Xiao,L.C., Fidler,I.J., Abbruzzese,J.L., & Kobayashi,R. (2005) Plasma protein profiling for diagnosis of pancreatic cancer reveals the presence of host response proteins. *Clin.Cancer Res.* 11, 1110-1118.

Lee,J.G., Cho,B.C., Bae,M.K., Lee,C.Y., Park,I.K., Kim,D.J., Ahn,S.V., & Chung,K.Y. (2009) Preoperative C-reactive protein levels are associated with tumor size and lymphovascular invasion in resected non-small cell lung cancer. *Lung Cancer* 63, 106-110.

Lee,K., Kye,M., Jang,J.S., Lee,O.J., Kim,T., & Lim,D. (2004) Proteomic analysis revealed a strong association of a high level of alpha1-antitrypsin in gastric juice with gastric cancer. *Proteomics.* 4, 3343-3352.

Linke,T., Doraiswamy,S., & Harrison,E.H. (2007) Rat plasma proteomics: effects of abundant protein depletion on proteomic analysis. *J Chromatogr.B Analyt.Technol.Biomed.Life Sci.* 849, 273-281.

Lipinska,L., Laskowska-Klita,T., & Izbicki,T. (1992) Serum acute phase proteins in neuroblastoma children at diagnosis and during the clinical treatment. A preliminary report. *Folia Histochem.Cytobiol.* 30, 205-206.

Liu,D.H., Wang,X.M., Zhang,L.J., Dai,S.W., Liu,L.Y., Liu,J.F., Wu,S.S., Yang,S.Y., Fu,S., Xiao,X.Y., & He,D.C. (2007) Serum amyloid A protein: a potential biomarker correlated with clinical stage of lung cancer. *Biomed.Environ.Sci.* 20, 33-40.

Lukaszewicz-Zajac,M., Mroczko,B., Gryko,M., Kedra,B., & Szmitkowski,M. (2010) Comparison between clinical significance of serum proinflammatory proteins (IL-6 and CRP) and classic tumor markers (CEA and CA 19-9) in gastric cancer. *Clin.Exp.Med.*

Maccio,A., Lai,P., Santona,M.C., Pagliara,L., Melis,G.B., & Mantovani,G. (1998) High serum levels of soluble IL-2 receptor, cytokines, and C reactive protein correlate with impairment of T cell response in patients with advanced epithelial ovarian cancer. *Gynecol.Oncol.* 69, 248-252.

Maris,J.M., Hogarty,M.D., Bagatell,R., & Cohn,S.L. (2007) Neuroblastoma. *Lancet* 369, 2106-2120.

McMillan,D.C., Canna,K., & McArdle,C.S. (2003) Systemic inflammatory response predicts survival following curative resection of colorectal cancer. *Br.J.Surg.* 90, 215-219.

McSorley,M.A., Alberg,A.J., Allen,D.S., Allen,N.E., Brinton,L.A., Dorgan,J.F., Pollak,M., Tao,Y., & Helzlsouer,K.J. (2007) C-reactive protein concentrations and subsequent ovarian cancer risk. *Obstet.Gynecol.* 109, 933-941.

Moshkovskii,S.A., Vlasova,M.A., Pyatnitskiy,M.A., Tikhonova,O.V., Safarova,M.R., Makarov,O.V., & Archakov,A.I. (2007a) Acute phase serum amyloid A in ovarian cancer as an important component of proteome diagnostic profiling. *Proteomics.Clin.Appl.* 1, 107-117.

Moshkovskii,S.A., Vlasova,M.A., Pyatnitskiy,M.A., Tikhonova,O.V., Safarova,M.R., Makarov,O.V., & Archakov,A.I. (2007b) Acute phase serum amyloid A in ovarian cancer as an important component of proteome diagnostic profiling. *Proteomics.Clin.Appl.* 1, 107-117.

Mroczko,B., Groblewska,M., Gryko,M., Kedra,B., & Szmitkowski,M. (2010) Diagnostic usefulness of serum interleukin 6 (IL-6) and C-reactive protein (CRP) in the differentiation between pancreatic cancer and chronic pancreatitis. *J.Clin.Lab Anal.* 24, 256-261.

Nielsen,H.J., Christensen,I.J., Sorensen,S., Moesgaard,F., & Brunner,N. (2000) Preoperative plasma plasminogen activator inhibitor type-1 and serum C-reactive protein levels in patients with colorectal cancer. The RANX05 Colorectal Cancer Study Group. *Ann.Surg.Oncol.* 7, 617-623.

Nosov,V., Su,F., Amneus,M., Birrer,M., Robins,T., Kotlerman,J., Reddy,S., & Farias-Eisner,R. (2009) Validation of serum biomarkers for detection of early-stage ovarian cancer. *Am.J.Obstet.Gynecol.* 200, 639-5.

Nozoe,T., Matsumata,T., Kitamura,M., & Sugimachi,K. (1998) Significance of preoperative elevation of serum C-reactive protein as an indicator for prognosis in colorectal cancer. *Am.J.Surg.* 176, 335-338.

Nozoe,T., Mori,E., Takahashi,I., & Ezaki,T. (2008) Preoperative elevation of serum C-reactive protein as an independent prognostic indicator of colorectal carcinoma. *Surg.Today* 38, 597-602.

Nozoe,T., Saeki,H., & Sugimachi,K. (2001) Significance of preoperative elevation of serum C-reactive protein as an indicator of prognosis in esophageal carcinoma. *Am.J.Surg.* 182, 197-201.

O'Dowd,C., McRae,L.A., McMillan,D.C., Kirk,A., & Milroy,R. (2010) Elevated preoperative C-reactive protein predicts poor cancer specific survival in patients undergoing resection for non-small cell lung cancer. *J.Thorac.Oncol.* 5, 988-992.

O'Hanlon,D.M., Lynch,J., Cormican,M., & Given,H.F. (2002) The acute phase response in breast carcinoma. *Anticancer Res.* 22, 1289-1293.

Orchekowski,R., Hamelinck,D., Li,L., Gliwa,E., vanBrocklin,M., Marrero,J.A., Vande Woude,G.F., Feng,Z., Brand,R., & Haab,B.B. (2005) Antibody microarray profiling reveals individual and combined serum proteins associated with pancreatic cancer. *Cancer Res.* 65, 11193-11202.

Orimo,A., Gupta,P.B., Sgroi,D.C., Arenzana-Seisdedos,F., Delaunay,T., Naeem,R., Carey,V.J., Richardson,A.L., & Weinberg,R.A. (2005) Stromal fibroblasts present in invasive human breast carcinomas promote tumor growth and angiogenesis through elevated SDF-1/CXCL12 secretion. *Cell* 121, 335-348.

Pang,W.W., Abdul-Rahman,P.S., Wan-Ibrahim,W.I., & Hashim,O.H. (2010) Can the acute-phase reactant proteins be used as cancer biomarkers? *Int.J Biol.Markers* 25, 1-11.

Park,S.Y., Yoon,S.J., Jeong,Y.T., Kim,J.M., Kim,J.Y., Bernert,B., Ullman,T., Itzkowitz,S.H., Kim,J.H., & Hakomori,S.I. (2010) N-glycosylation status of beta-haptoglobin in sera of patients with colon cancer, chronic inflammatory diseases and normal subjects. *Int.J.Cancer* 126, 142-155.

Pierce,B.L., Ballard-Barbash,R., Bernstein,L., Baumgartner,R.N., Neuhouser,M.L., Wener,M.H., Baumgartner,K.B., Gilliland,F.D., Sorensen,B.E., McTiernan,A., & Ulrich,C.M. (2009) Elevated biomarkers of inflammation are associated with reduced survival among breast cancer patients. *J.Clin.Oncol.* 27, 3437-3444.

Pine,J.K., Fusai,K.G., Young,R., Sharma,D., Davidson,B.R., Menon,K.V., & Rahman,S.H. (2009) Serum C-reactive protein concentration and the prognosis of ductal adenocarcinoma of the head of pancreas. *Eur.J.Surg.Oncol.* 35, 605-610.

Polyak,K. & Hahn,W.C. (2006) Roots and stems: stem cells in cancer. *Nat Med* 12, 296-300.

Pujia,A., De,A.F., Scumaci,D., Gaspari,M., Liberale,C., Candeloro,P., Cuda,G., & Di,F.E. (2010) Highly efficient human serum filtration with water-soluble nanoporous nanoparticles. *Int.J Nanomedicine.* 5, 1005-1015.

Ramankulov,A., Lein,M., Johannsen,M., Schrader,M., Miller,K., Loening,S.A., & Jung,K. (2008) Serum amyloid A as indicator of distant metastases but not as early tumor marker in patients with renal cell carcinoma. *Cancer Lett.* 269, 85-92.

Ravishankaran,P. & R K (2011) Clinical significance of preoperative serum interleukin-6 and C-reactive protein level in breast cancer patients. *World J.Surg.Oncol.* 9, 18.

Rigel,D.S. (2010) Epidemiology of melanoma. *Semin.Cutan.Med.Surg.* 29, 204-209.

Roxburgh,C.S. & McMillan,D.C. (2010) Role of systemic inflammatory response in predicting survival in patients with primary operable cancer. *Future.Oncol* 6, 149-163.

Saito,K., Tatokoro,M., Fujii,Y., Iimura,Y., Koga,F., Kawakami,S., & Kihara,K. (2009) Impact of C-reactive protein kinetics on survival of patients with metastatic renal cell carcinoma. *Eur.Urol.* 55, 1145-1153.

Sandoval,J.A., Turner,K.E., Hoelz,D.J., Rescorla,F.J., Hickey,R.J., & Malkas,L.H. (2007) Serum protein profiling to identify high-risk neuroblastoma: preclinical relevance of blood-based biomarkers. *J.Surg.Res.* 142, 268-274.

Shimada,H., Nabeya,Y., Okazumi,S., Matsubara,H., Shiratori,T., Aoki,T., Sugaya,M., Miyazawa,Y., Hayashi,H., Miyazaki,S., & Ochiai,T. (2003) Elevation of preoperative serum C-reactive protein level is related to poor prognosis in esophageal squamous cell carcinoma. *J.Surg.Oncol.* 83, 248-252.

Siemes,C., Visser,L.E., Coebergh,J.W., Splinter,T.A., Witteman,J.C., Uitterlinden,A.G., Hofman,A., Pols,H.A., & Stricker,B.H. (2006) C-reactive protein levels, variation in the C-reactive protein gene, and cancer risk: the Rotterdam Study. *J.Clin.Oncol.* 24, 5216-5222.

Simpson,W.G., Heys,S.D., Whiting,P.H., Eremin,O., & Broom,J. (1995) Acute phase proteins and recombinant IL-2 therapy: prediction of response and survival in patients with colorectal cancer. *Clin.Exp.Immunol.* 99, 143-147.

Su,F., Lang,J., Kumar,A., Ng,C., Hsieh,B., Suchard,M.A., Reddy,S.T., & Farias-Eisner,R. (2007) Validation of candidate serum ovarian cancer biomarkers for early detection. *Biomark.Insights.* 2, 369-375.

Tartour,E., Dorval,T., Mosseri,V., Deneux,L., Mathiot,C., Brailly,H., Montero,F., Joyeux,I., Pouillart,P., & Fridman,W.H. (1994) Serum interleukin 6 and C-reactive protein levels correlate with resistance to IL-2 therapy and poor survival in melanoma patients. *Br.J.Cancer* 69, 911-913.

Teng,P.N., Bateman,N.W., Hood,B.L., & Conrads,T.P. (2010) Advances in proximal fluid proteomics for disease biomarker discovery. *J Proteome.Res.* 9, 6091-6100.

Tingstedt,B., Johansson,P., Andersson,B., & Andersson,R. (2007) Predictive factors in pancreatic ductal adenocarcinoma: role of the inflammatory response. *Scand.J.Gastroenterol.* 42, 754-759.

Tolson,J., Bogumil,R., Brunst,E., Beck,H., Elsner,R., Humeny,A., Kratzin,H., Deeg,M., Kuczyk,M., Mueller,G.A., Mueller,C.A., & Flad,T. (2004) Serum protein profiling by SELDI mass spectrometry: detection of multiple variants of serum amyloid alpha in renal cancer patients. *Lab Invest* 84, 845-856.

Trichopoulos,D., Psaltopoulou,T., Orfanos,P., Trichopoulou,A., & Boffetta,P. (2006) Plasma C-reactive protein and risk of cancer: a prospective study from Greece. *Cancer Epidemiol.Biomarkers Prev.* 15, 381-384.

Trichopoulos,D., Tzonou,A., Kalapothaki,V., Sparos,L., Kremastinou,T., & Skoutari,M. (1990) Alpha 1-antitrypsin and survival in pancreatic cancer. *Int.J.Cancer* 45, 685-686.

Tsavaris,N., Kosmas,C., Kopterides,P., Tsikalakis,D., Skopelitis,H., Sakelaridi,F., Papadoniou,N., Tzivras,M., Balatsos,V., Koufos,C., & Archimandritis,A. (2005) Retinol-binding protein, acute phase reactants and Helicobacter pylori infection in patients with gastric adenocarcinoma. *World J.Gastroenterol.* 11, 7174-7178.

Wang,C.Y., Hsieh,M.J., Chiu,Y.C., Li,S.H., Huang,H.W., Fang,F.M., & Huang,Y.J. (2009) Higher serum C-reactive protein concentration and hypoalbuminemia are poor prognostic indicators in patients with esophageal cancer undergoing radiotherapy. *Radiother.Oncol.* 92, 270-275.

Wang,Y., Jiang,H., Dai,D., Su,M., Martinka,M., Brasher,P., Zhang,Y., McLean,D., Zhang,J., Ip,W., Li,G., Zhang,X., & Zhou,Y. (2010) Alpha 1 antichymotrypsin is aberrantly expressed during melanoma progression and predicts poor survival for patients with metastatic melanoma. *Pigment Cell Melanoma Res.* 23, 575-578.

Ward,A.M., Cooper,E.H., Turner,R., Anderson,J.A., & Neville,A.M. (1977) Acute-phase reactant protein profiles: an aid to monitoring large bowel cancer by CEA and serum enzymes. *Br.J.Cancer* 35, 170-178.

Wood,S.L., Rogers,M., Cairns,D.A., Paul,A., Thompson,D., Vasudev,N.S., Selby,P.J., & Banks,R.E. (2010) Association of serum amyloid A protein and peptide fragments with prognosis in renal cancer. *Br.J.Cancer* 103, 101-111.

Ye,B., Cramer,D.W., Skates,S.J., Gygi,S.P., Pratomo,V., Fu,L., Horick,N.K., Licklider,L.J., Schorge,J.O., Berkowitz,R.S., & Mok,S.C. (2003) Haptoglobin-alpha subunit as potential serum biomarker in ovarian cancer: identification and characterization using proteomic profiling and mass spectrometry. *Clin.Cancer Res.* 9, 2904-2911.

Yu,K.H., Rustgi,A.K., & Blair,I.A. (2005) Characterization of proteins in human pancreatic cancer serum using differential gel electrophoresis and tandem mass spectrometry. *J.Proteome.Res.* 4, 1742-1751.

Zeng,Z., Hincapie,M., Haab,B.B., Hanash,S., Pitteri,S.J., Kluck,S., Hogan,J.M., Kennedy,J., & Hancock,W.S. (2010) The development of an integrated platform to identify breast cancer glycoproteome changes in human serum. *J Chromatogr.A* 1217, 3307-3315.

Zhang,S.M., Buring,J.E., Lee,I.M., Cook,N.R., & Ridker,P.M. (2005) C-reactive protein levels are not associated with increased risk for colorectal cancer in women. *Ann.Intern.Med.* 142, 425-432.

Zhang,Z., Bast,R.C., Jr., Yu,Y., Li,J., Sokoll,L.J., Rai,A.J., Rosenzweig,J.M., Cameron,B., Wang,Y.Y., Meng,X.Y., Berchuck,A., van Haaften-Day,C., Hacker,N.F., de Bruijn,H.W., van der Zee,A.G., Jacobs,I.J., Fung,E.T., & Chan,D.W. (2004) Three biomarkers identified from serum proteomic analysis for the detection of early stage ovarian cancer. *Cancer Res.* 64, 5882-5890.

Zingg,U., Forberger,J., Rajcic,B., Langton,C., & Jamieson,G.G. (2010) Association of C-reactive protein levels and long-term survival after neoadjuvant therapy and esophagectomy for esophageal cancer. *J.Gastrointest.Surg.* 14, 462-469.

2

Apolipoprotein H, an Acute Phase Protein, a Performing Tool for Ultra-Sensitive Detection and Isolation of Microorganisms from Different Origins

Ilias Stefas[1], Gregor Dubois[2], Sylvia Tigrett[1], Estelle Lucarz[1] and Francisco Veas[2]
[1]*ApoH-Technologies*
Faculty of Pharmacy, University Montpellier 1, Av Charles Flahault, Montpellier
[2]*Comparative Molecular Immuno-Physiopathology Lab. UMR-MD3*
Faculty of Pharmacy, University Montpellier 1, Av Charles Flahault, Montpellier
France

1. Introduction

Apolipoprotein H (ApoH), also known as beta2-glycoprotein I (ß2-GPI), is a plasma glycoprotein of 50 kDa. ApoH is present in human plasma at a concentration of between 150 and 300 mg/ml (Bouma et al., 1999). In blood, ApoH circulate in free conformations or bound to lipoproteins: chylomicrons, very low-density lipoprotein (VLDL), low density lipoprotein (LDL) and high-density lipoprotein (HDL). In addition, ApoH has a high affinity for triglyceride-rich lipoproteins. The amount of ApoH associated with plasma lipoproteins in healthy individuals varies according to the authors from 4 to 13% (Gambino et al., 1999a) up to about 40% (Polz & Kostner, 1979). ApoH is able to activate lipoprotein lipases (Lee et al., 1983). ApoH was isolated from the fraction of plasma lipoproteins, and described for the first time in 1961 by H. Schultze E (Schultze, 1961). In a lesser extent, ApoH is also associated to ß2-globulin fraction.

ApoH is expressed in human liver, in intestinal cells and tissues (Averna et al., 1997). In rats, other sites of synthesis in low concentrations were identified as the kidney, small intestine, brain, cardiomyocytes of the heart, and at even lower in the spleen, stomach and prostate (Ragusa et al., 2006).

ApoH is an acute phase protein and because when activated, ApoH bind, with a relative high affinity, to pathogens or their proteins, ApoH is also considered as an element of the host innate immune response, particularly during the acute phase. It is difficult to classified as positive or negative acute phase protein. This property is used as a mean to drastically improve diagnostic of pathogens from different origins, including human, animal or environmental and nature, including enveloped or non-enveloped viruses, parasites, and Gram+ or Gram - bacteria. Indeed, activated ApoH coupled to solid supports is used to concentrate and "clean" pathogens (from inhibitor of detection methods) to detect pathogens with molecular or immunological methods and thus avoiding false negative diagnostics.

2. ApoH expression

2.1 Structure and localization of the ApoH gene

The gene encoding ApoH was localized by fluorescent *in situ* hybridization, on chromosome 17, locus q23-24, and extends over 18 kilobases (kb). It consists of eight exons (~ 1.2 kb) separated by large introns (~ 16.2 kb) encoding a protein of 345 amino acids (aa). This protein is subsequently cleaved at a signal peptide of 19 aa located at the N-terminal position (N-ter) to generate the matured protein (Mehdi et al., 1991; Steinkasserer et al., 1991).

Eight exons will form the matured protein constituted of five domains. Exon 1 encodes the 5'-untranslated region (5'-UTR) and the signal peptide. Exons 3 and 4 encode the domain II and exons 2, 5, 6 and 7 respectively encode domains I, III, IV and V of the protein. Exon 8 encodes the C-terminal (C-ter), the stop codon and 3'-UTR region (Fig. 1) (Okkels et al., 1999).

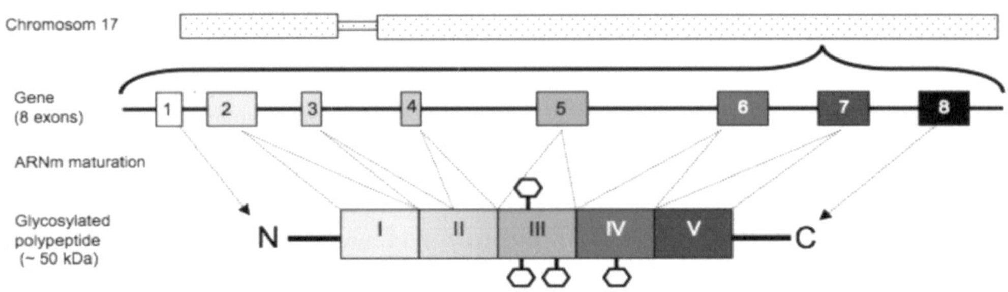

Fig. 1. ApoH gene organization (Sodin-Semrl & Rozman, 2007)

2.2 Promoter of the ApoH gene

Using the HepG2 liver cell line, deletion analyses in the 5' region of ApoH gene evidenced that its promoter is located between positions -197 and 7 (Wang & Chiang, 2004). The ApoH gene expression is governed by several transcription factors including a liver-specific atypical TATA box (TATTA) located between positions -97 and -92 and the transcription factor HNF-1 (Hepatic nuclear factor-1) located upstream of the TATTA box. The soluble transactivation factor HNF-1α interacts with HNF-1 leading to transactivation of the ApoH promoter. The gene expression increasing of endogenous ApoH is correlated with an overproduction HNF-1α.

Several transcription factors are able to bind multiple ApoH regulating sites. In liver cells, these sites are located near the promoter (up-670pb), as shown in Fig. 2. These transcription factors are:

- STAT Signal Transducer and Activator of Transcription.
- Leucine zipper domains: CREB (cAMP Response Element Binding) and C /EBPβ (CCAAT-Enhancer-Binding Proteins).
- AP-1 (Activating Protein 1) also known as TPA-responsive element (TRE)
- HNF-3β (Hepatocyte Nuclear Factor 3β) involved in embryo development

- HNF1 (Hepatocyte Nuclear Factor 1), a transcription factor that regulates the expression of several hepatic proteins, including serum albumin or α1-antitrypsin.
- The protein NFAT (nuclear factor of activated T-cells) activated in the cytoplasm by calcium-dependent phosphatase. The signal may interact with transcription factors AP-1 and NF-AT.

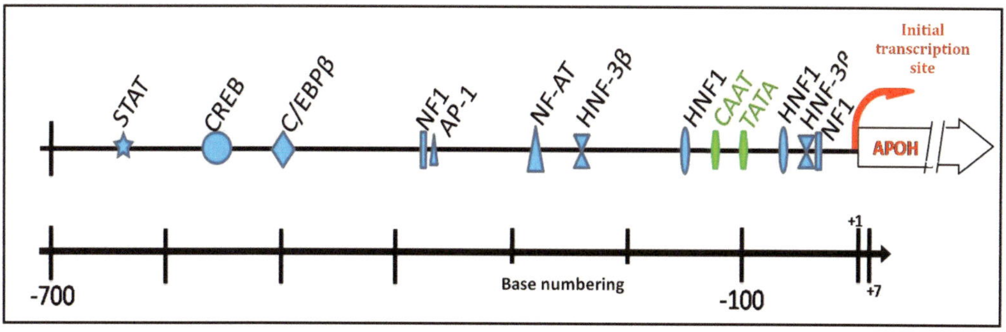

Fig. 2. Promoter region of the ApoH gene and transcription factors (Wang & Chiang, 2004). The transcription sites in the promoter (TATA and CAAT boxes) are located near the initiation of ApoH transcription site (+1). Regulatory sites (blue), CAAT &TATA boxes (green), initiation site of transcription (red).

2.3 Protein structure of ApoH

Primary structure and domain concepts

The peptide sequence of ApoH was identified in 1984. Its primary structure consists in a single polypeptide chain of 326 amino acids. With the exception of collagen and other related molecules, ApoH appears as one of the richest eukaryotic structures containing prolins, exhibiting 31 prolin residues per molecule. ApoH is also rich in lysin (30 residues), glycin (23 residues) and cystein (22 residues) (Lozier et al., 1984) amino-acids.
The peptide sequence can be divided into four continuous domains of about 60 amino acids each, called SCR (short consensus repeat) and a fifth domain in the C-ter region (Lozier et al., 1984; Steinkasserer et al., 1991). SCR domains are also known under the term of Sushi domain, or CCP (Complement Control Protein) that are motifs often found in proteins of the complement system, but also in some proteins, such as interleukin-2 receptor. These SCR confer to the ApoH sequence exhibit a homology with several proteins such as VCP (vaccinia virus protein), CD46 (binding protein of measles virus) and HI, a Drosophila protein that belongs to the family of immunoglobulins and complement proteins. As shown in Fig. 3, each SCR contains four cysteins associated by pairs, Cys-1 to Cys-3 and Cys-2 to Cys-4 linked by disulfide (S-S) bridges (Okkels et al., 1999) that confers a high structural stability to ApoH.
In contrast, the domain V of ApoH exhibits a very different structure. A sequence of six amino-acids (KNKEKK) is inserted within a highly positive charged region, an extension of 19 residues at the C-ter and the presence of an additional S-S bridge (Steinkasserer et al., 1991). A highly conserved tryptophan within the domain V will contribute to hydrophobic interactions with the ApoH partners.

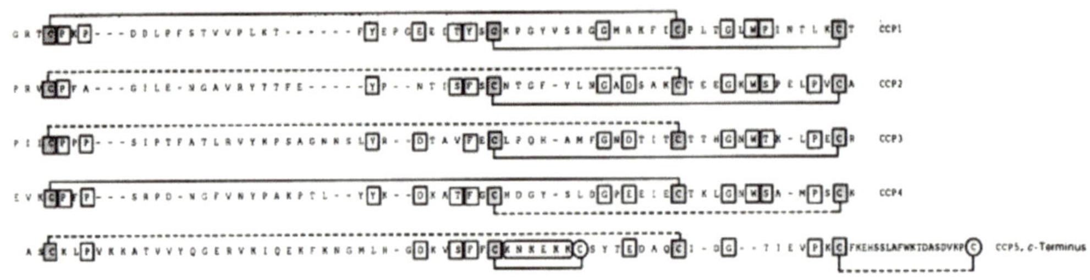

Fig. 3. Alignment and organization of the disulfide bonds of ApoH (Steinkasserer et al., 1991).

Secondary structure of ApoH

ApoH contains four N-glycosylation sites and one site of O-glycosylation linked to domain III and IV of the protein (Fig.4A). The glycosylated chains of ApoH are composed of galactose, mannose, N-acetylglucosamin, fructose, N-acetylneuraminic acid and sialic acid (Kamboh et al., 1988). They are linked to the peptide sequence *via* a nitrogen or oxygen atom (Gambino et al., 1999b).

Secondary structures of each domain are composed of several anti-parallel beta-sheets, shorts, and coiled around a hydrophobic core (Fig. 4B). Two S-S bridges, respectively located in N-ter and C-ter stabilize the structure. A long central ß-sheet is framed along of the longitudinal axis by short beta-sheets parallels anti-parallels located near the C-ter and N-ter. The fifth domain, folds into a central β -sheet composed of four anti-parallel β-sheets and two short α-helices and this domain is stabilized by three S-S bridges (Fig. 4C) (Bouma et al., 1999).

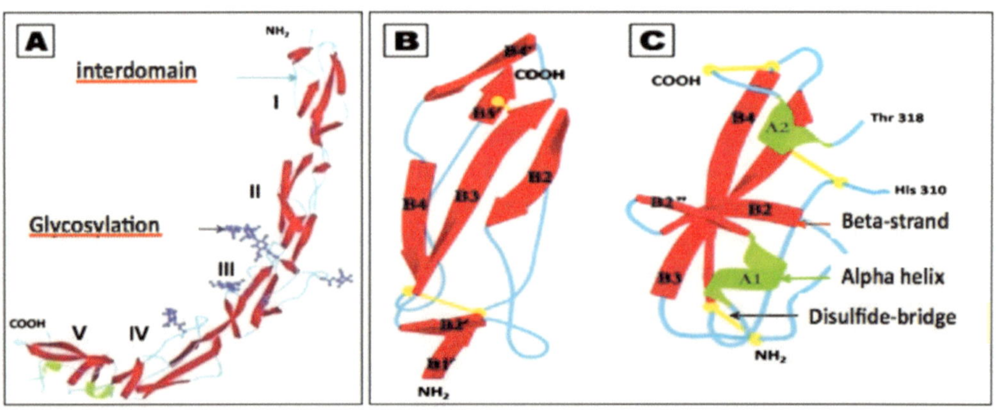

Fig. 4. The different structures of glycosylated chains of ApoH (Gambino et al., 1997)

Composition and organization of sugar chains

There are three possible structures for the glycosilated chains (Fig. 5) (Gambino et al., 1997): Complex, hybrid and Mannose-rich. These structures have a common motif consisting in two N-acetylglucosamins and three mannoses, differing in the antennas composition, and their number varies from two to five.

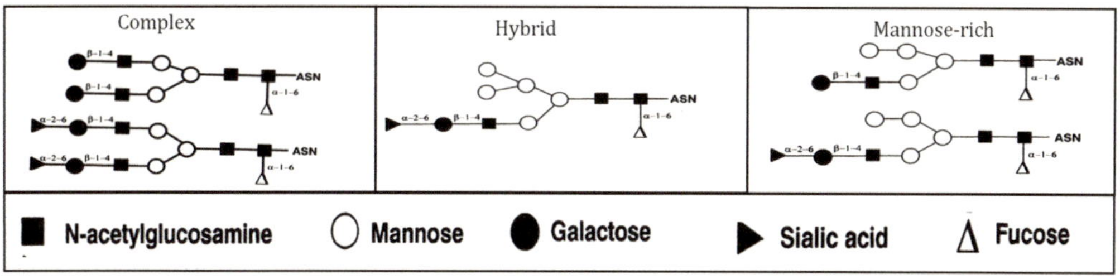

Fig. 5. Structural representation ApoH and domains (Bouma et al., 1999). (A) Secondary structure ApoH; (B) Secondary structure of domain III of ApoH; (C) Secondary structure of domain V of ApoH.

The ApoH inter-domain regions

Different ApoH domains are linked each other by sequences respectively composed of three amino-acids, between domains IV and V, and four amino-acids for other domains. Between domains II-III and III-IV residues form chains of β-sheets connecting the N-ter-B5 B4' sheet at the C-ter-sheet B1' B2'. The inter-domain represents 10-15% of the molecular surface. The inter-domain orientation varies in its inclination angle, ranging from 128 to 160° and a rotation angle ranging from 41 to 137°. Within the conserved domains, all are obtuse angles ranging from 120 to 162°, while the rotation angles vary widely between 22 and 180 ° (Bouma et al., 1999).

Tertiary structure

The analysis of crystallized structure of ApoH revealed a spatial organization to form a "J" or fishhook-like shape (Bouma et al., 1999; Schwarzenbacher et al., 1999). The four SCRs are arranged along a single axis with a slight spiral to the right to join the domain V. This very compact form suggests a certain rigidity of the protein. The X-ray analysis shows that in solution, the protein is folded, bulkier and exhibiting an "S-shape" (Fig. 6) (Hammel et al., 2002).

These differences may be explained by the absence of sugar chains in the crystallized protein and by changing the orientation of different domains due to the use of ions to form the crystal.

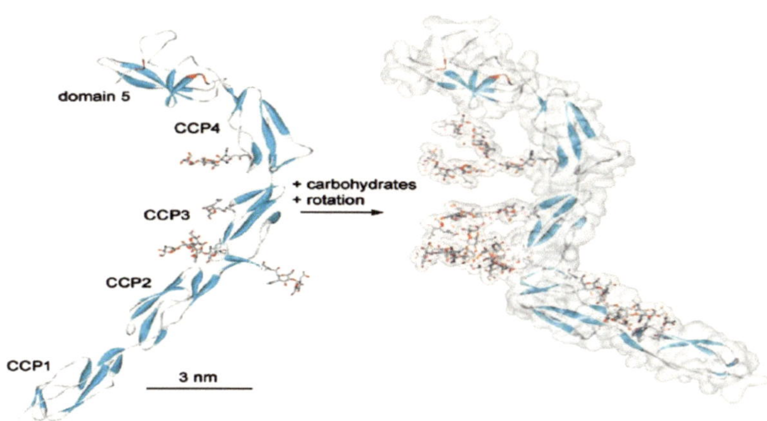

Fig. 6. The ApoH structure (Hammel et al., 2002). Crystal form (left) compared with the schematic atomic structure model in solution (right).

However, recent studies on electronic microscopy has evidenced the presence of inactive ring forms of ApoH as well as the fishhook-like active ApoH able to catch LPS present in sepsis cases (Agar et al., 2011).

3. ApoH and physiology

The role of ApoH *in vivo* remains only partially elucidated. Studies conducted *in vitro* have demonstrated that ApoH has the particularity to bind, not only to negatively charged molecules and structures, including anionic phospholipids (PL), but also binds platelets, apoptotic cells (d'Angeac et al., 2005), mitochondria, DNA as well as bile acids (Schousboe, 1983). Apart from the PL, ApoH also has the ability to bind cellular proteins such as the kidney calmodulin (Rojkjaer et al., 1997), megalin, an endocytic receptor of the renal epithelium (Moestrup et al., 1998), Annexin II (Ma et al., 2000) as well as other binding proteins or receptors including phosphatidylserine PS , LPS (Agar et al., 2011) and TLR2 (Alard et al., 2010).

Expression studies in HepG2 cells demonstrate that ApoH mRNA is regulated in a cell cycle-dependent manner, with very low expression in low cycling conditions and increasing levels in proliferating cells. p21 WAF-dependent growth arrest, induced by butyrate treatment, down-regulate ApoH mRNA levels. Immunolocalization in normal rat liver shows a non-homogeneous pattern, being mainly present in the centrolobular area; post-hepatectomy regenerating rat liver is uniformly immuno-stained and mitotic elements show the highest protein expression. Albumin gene expression, studies as control liver specific product, was not affected by sodium butyrate induced growth arrest. As previously reported for endothelial cells, ApoH behaves as survival factor for HepG2 cells: when increasing amounts of the protein (10–50 µg) have been added to serum deficient cultured liver cells a progressive reduced cell loss was observed (Averna et al., 2004).

In some autoimmune diseases, such as anti-phospholipid syndrome (APS), anti-ApoH antibodies and the complex ApoH-PL has been reported. These antibodies impact the inhibition of coagulation. They are associated with clinical manifestations of thrombotic venous or arterial type and recurrent fetal loss (Asherson & Cervera, 1993; Kandiah et al., 1998). Thus, APS may be associated with various clinical manifestations: thrombocytopenia, coronary or valve damage, neurological disorders, and autoimmune hemolytic anemia. The presence of these antibodies may also occur in infectious diseases (viral, bacterial or parasitic) and neoplasia (solid tumors, lympho-proliferative disorders)(Arnoux & Boutière, 2006; Harel et al., 2005).

ApoH is also involved in the whole process of hemostasis regulation. ApoH inhibits both the factor Xa genesis, in the presence of platelets and the activation of factor XI (Shi et al., 2005; Shi et al., 2004), as well as fibrinolysis, by preventing the generation of plasmin (Yasuda et al., 2004). ApoH also inhibits activated protein C that is an inhibitor of hemostasis (Keeling et al., 1993). ApoH therefore, exhibits both procoagulant and anticoagulant activities (McNeil et al., 1990).

The presence of antibodies to form an immune complex ApoH consisting in ApoH-oxidized LDL:anti-ApoH antibodies, complex that is phagocytized by macrophages. Thus, there would be presentation of ApoH epitopes, by major the histocompatibility complex type II (MHC II), at the macrophages surface, leading $CD4^+$ T cells activation. Moreover, it follows an excessive of macrophage lipids burden, and these macrophages are transformed into foam cells, the early stage of plaque formation.

Thus, ApoH is highly present in atherosclerotic plaques (George et al., 1999). ApoH allow binding and internalization of LDL in macrophages because of its ability to bind to LDL and oxidized LDL (Kochl et al., 1997). Moreover, ApoH is involved in apoptosis by binding to phosphatidylserine (PS), present at the surface of cells undergoing apoptosis (d'Angeac et al., 2005). Altogether, these data contribute to characterize ApoH as a scavenger-like protein. Finally, ApoH is also necessary to placental homeostasis and is involved in activation of endothelial cells and apoptotic mechanisms (Miyakis et al., 2004). However, despite available data showing pleitotropic functions of ApoH, many precise physiological roles of ApoH remain to be elucidated.

The high correlation between ApoH and CRP expression during systemic inflammation indicates that ApoH is a part of the group of acute phase proteins (Sellar et al., 1993). However, the expression of the acute phase protein, ApoH, sometimes is upregulated and sometimes is down regulated, reflecting its pleiotropic functions Then, it become difficult to classify this APP as positive or negative. Indeed, divers data are sometime contradictory such as the observation of ApoH reduction in CSF during cerebral malaria (Agar et al., 2011) and the increase of ApoH in several other infectious diseases (Gast et al., 2006; Myles et al., 2003; van Hemert et al., 2006).

Due to different results presented here, ApoH can be considered as one of the major elements of the first line of the innate immune response regulating homeostasis.

4. Interactions between ApoH and phospholipids

ApoH has a strong ability to bind anionic phospholipids (PL), such as cardiolipin or phosphatidylserine, rather than the neutral PL, such as phosphatidylcholin (Wang et al., 1998; Willems et al., 1996; Wurm, 1984). This interaction is ionic strength-dependent.

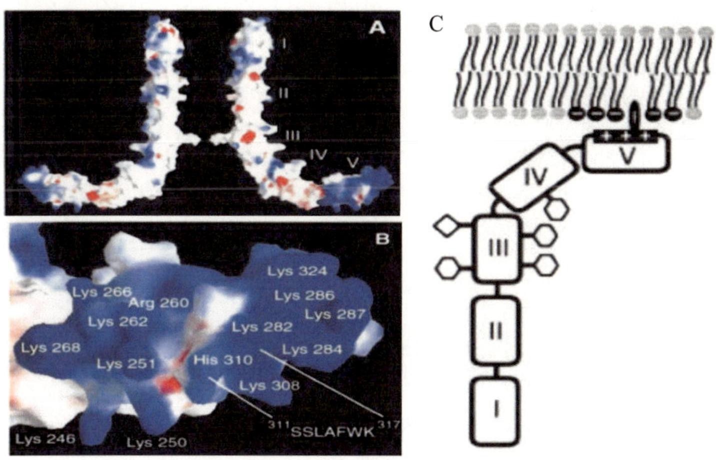

Fig. 7. Binding between ApoH and membranes (Bouma et al., 1999). (A) Representation of the electrostatic potential ApoH surface, with a view rotated 180 °. ApoH domains are numbered from I to V. negative charges (red); positive charges (blue); (B) Prominent representation of half of the domain V. The positive charges are mainly due to the presence of lysine; negative charges (red), positive charges (blue); (C) scheme of the binding between ApoH (including the Tryptophan from domain V) and phospholipids bilayer.

Mechanisms of interaction between the anionic PL and ApoH could involve two types of bonds: (i) ionic and (ii) hydrophobic, this latter involving the V domain of ApoH (Hammel et al., 2001; Wang et al., 1998). Initially, the sequence C-C-KNKEKK 281-288, highly positively charged (Steinkasserer et al., 1991), and most likely exposed on the surface of the protein would be responsible for the initiation of ionic bonds with anionic heads responsible for PL. A second step, would involves the insertion of a mobile hydrophobic loop of the protein in the PL layer (Fig. 8). The authors report a sort of anchor protein to the interface head polar/non-polar tail of PL *via* the hydrophobic (tryptophan) residue of the mobile loop region located in the position 311-SSLAFWK-317 (Hong et al., 2001; Mehdi et al., 2000).

5. ApoH-viruses binding

Enveloped and non-enveloped viruses

Human and animal viruses such as influenza have a lipid bilayer coat covering their capsid, which is a protein box protecting the nucleic acid (short or large RNA or DNA). These envelopes are derived from portions of the host cell membranes including phospholipids together with specific viral glycoproteins that frequently mature during virus development. These glycoproteins play a pivotal role in the cell entry of these viruses. The cell entry of the non-enveloped viruses is less well known. However, for some viruses, such as for rotaviruses A, trypsin plays a role in preparing the capsid to find a good "conformation" of some peptides to fuse with the cell membrane to enter cells.

6. The use of ApoH for drastic improvement of viral detection

An interesting feature of ApoH, is its ability to bind both enveloped and non-enveloped viruses. Thus, it was shown that the protein bind hepatitis B virus (HBV), and more particularly the surface antigen HBsAg (Mehdi et al., 1994). HBsAg exists in three molecular forms: S for small, small protein, M for middle, moderate protein and L for Large protein (Fig. 9). The viral anionic PL are also involved in the interaction between ApoH and HBsAg (Neurath & Strick, 1994; Stefas et al., 2001). These results are reinforced by the fact that the recombinant HBsAg protein and anionic PL share the domain V of ApoH as binding domain (Mehdi et al., 2008). When viral PL becomes oxidized, the binding affinity ApoH-HBsAg increases. It has been shown that ApoH has an affinity for infectious Dane particles

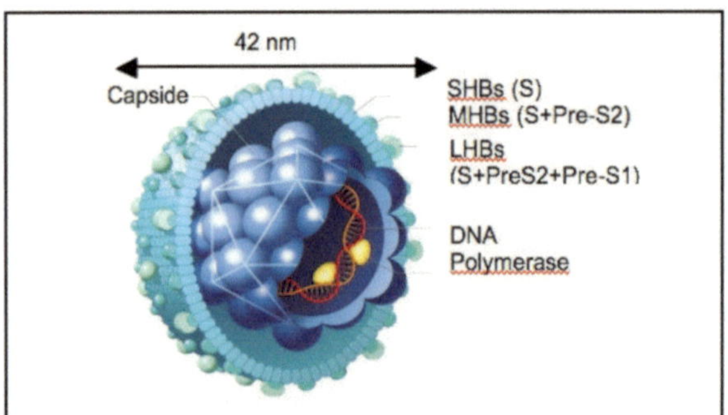

Fig. 8. Structure of hepatitis B virus (http://dicos.ens-lyon.fr/vie/viro/image/V05_2H1_Hepatites_8HBV.jpg)

that are characterized by the presence of a myristyl group on the pre-S1 domain of protein L. The presence of the myristyl group enhances its binding with ApoH (Stefas et al., 2001).
Among experiments carried out by us, four HBV/HBsAg and HBV-DNA-positive patients' sera were preincubated for 1 hr at 37°C in the presence or absence of 100 µg/mL of polymyxin B or 2 mmol/L of iron or a mixture of both. The ability of HBV+ from patient sera (diluted at 1/100) to bind to ApoH-coated ELISA wells was assessed in the following conditions: sera HBV+ alone, in the presence of either polymyxin B (PB) or in the presence of Fe3+. ApoH-coated wells preincubated with PB or Fe3+ and washed were used as controls (Fig.9).

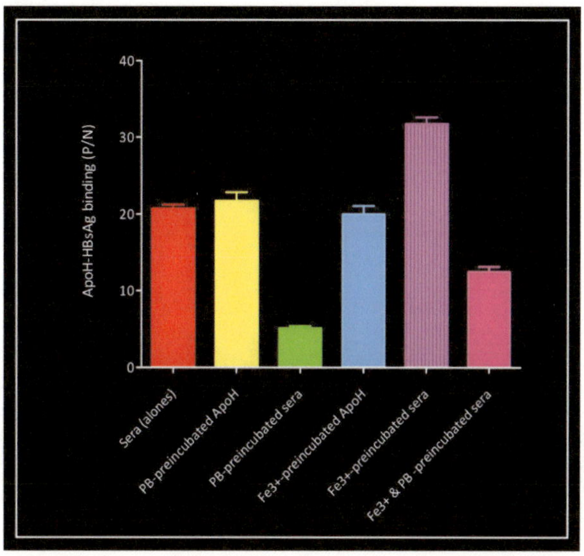

Fig. 9. Effects of polymyxin B and/or metal ions on the ApoH-HBsAg binding.

The preincubation of HBV+ sera with PB significantly reduced HBV/HBsAg binding to ApoH and this interaction was dose-dependent (data not shown). In contrast, the preincubation of HBV sera with Fe3+ increased HBV/HbsAg binding. No effect was observed when ApoH-coated wells were preincubated with polymyxin and washed, before the addition of serum. These data strongly suggest that viral phospholipids are involved in the ApoH-HBV/HBsAg interaction.
It has been also shown that ApoH interact with antigens of human immunodeficiency virus (HIV) types I and II, particularly the Gag proteins of HIV 1 and 2 of p18 and p26 of HIV-1 HIV-2 or of gp160 of HIV-1 (Stefas et al., 1997), suggesting that the interaction of ApoH with HIV proteins may result in part from the ApoH affinity for PL. According to Stefas et al. (1997), experimental conditions, such as acidic pH and/or the presence of detergent, could lead to conformational changes of ApoH or viral proteins thereby inducing the binding between ApoH and HIV-1.
More recently, within the European USDEP project (www.usdep.eu), it has been shown that ApoH capture viruses including Hantavirus in both serum and urine from infected patients (Godoy et al., 2009), and very interestingly avoiding false negative generated by conventional and standard PCR methods (Fig. 10) and from stools rotavirus-infected patients permitting a very highly immune detection as sensitive as quantitative PCR

(Adlhoch et al., 2011). Within the same project, many other viruses have been shown strongly bind to ApoH, including poxvirus virus, hepatitis C virus, pseudorabies virus, vesicular stomatitis virus, and Altogether these data clearly demonstrate that ApoH binds enveloped or non-enveloped DNA or RNA virus with high affinity permitting their ultrasensitive detection.

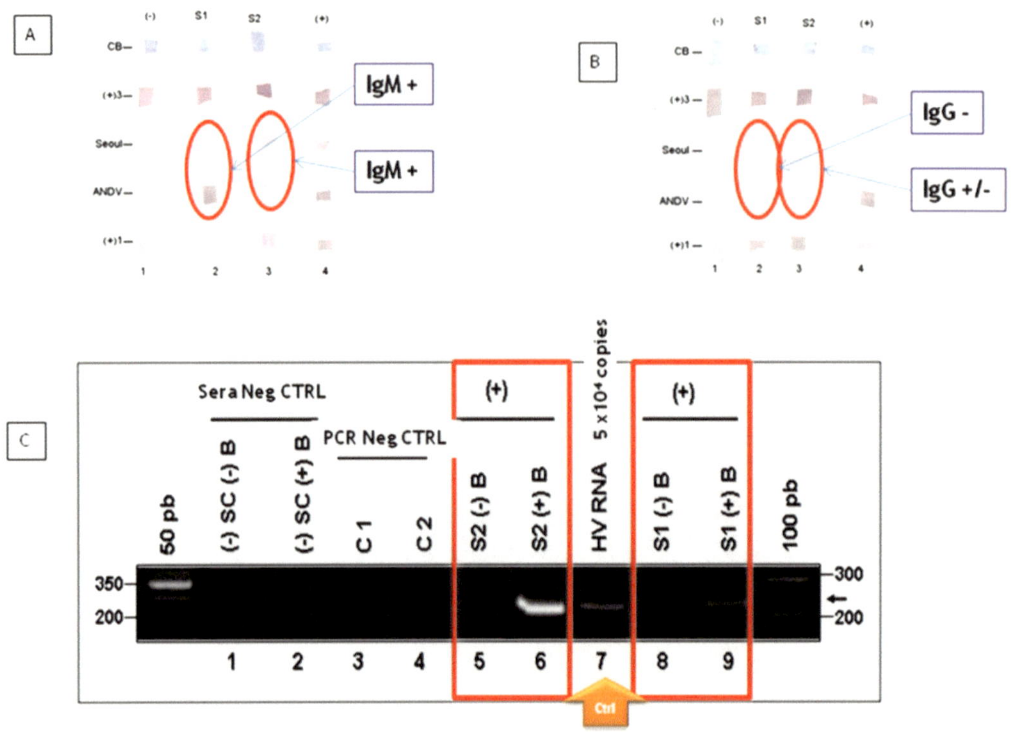

Fig. 10. ANDV binds serum-purified human ApoH (Godoy et al., 2009). Serum from patients S1 and S2 were tested for the presence of anti-hantavirus IgM (A) and IgG (B) antibodies by SIA using affinity-purified recombinant ANDV and Seoul virus N antigen. As internal controls, two levels (+1 and +3) of human IgG were applied to the blot. Serum from a negative donor (-) and of from a known HCPS-positive patient (+) were used as controls. Coomassie blue (CB) was used to determine the orientation of the strip. (C) Serum samples from patients S1 and S2 were divided in two. RNA was directly extracted from 300 μL of sample one without the addition of ApoH beads [(-) B; lanes 5 and 8]. In parallel, the second sample of each patient was submitted to an additional step of ANDV capture by ApoH-coated magnetic beads prior to RNA extraction [(+) B; lanes 6 and 9]. Extracted RNA was used as the template in a RT-PCR/heminested PCR assay. As an additional control, total RNA extracted from sera of healthy negative donors with [(-) SC (+) B; lane 2] or without [(-) SC (-) B; lane 1] a step of virus capture and concentration by ApoH-coated magnetic beads was used as the negative control. Water controls for the RT-PCR (C1; lane 3) and heminested PCR (C2; lane 4) were included. In vitro-transcribed RNA corresponding to the ANDV S segment was used as a positive control for RT-PCR (HV RNA; lane 7). The arrow indicates the expected amplicon.

7. ApoH and bacteria relationship

Circulating anti-ApoH antibodies in APS and infections

In addition to circulating anti-ApoH antibodies in serum of patients exhibiting APS, an increased amount of anti-ApoH antibodies is also associated with several bacterial infections including: (i) urinary tract bacterial infections (Stojanovic et al., 2004); (ii) presence of *Helicobacter pylori* associated to ulcers (Pellicano et al., 1999); (iii) bacteria-associated rheumatic fever (Blank et al., 2004) and some other infections summarized in Table 1.

Infection agents or pathology	Frequency (%)
Typhus	20
Mycobacterium leprae	33 - 67
Mycobacterium tuberculosis	27 - 53
Bacterial endocarditis	5 - 44
Helicobacter pylori	ND
Mycoplasma pneumoniae	20 - 53
Staphylococcus aureus	43
Streptococcus epidermidis	80
Staphylococcus pyogenes	0 - 80
Salmonella typhi	60
Escherichia coli	67
Coxiella burnetti	42 - 84
Leptospirosis	50
Borrelia burgdorferi	14 - 41
Sacharomyces cerevisiae	ND
Plasmodium falciparum	30

Table 1. Prevalence of anti-ApoH in infection associated diseases (Blank et al., 2004). *ND= undetermined

Moreover, it was shown that epitopes recognized by the anti-ApoH antibodies, exhibited similarities with peptides associated to several infectious diseases (Blank et al., 2002; Gharavi et al., 2002). The ApoH-like epitope expressed by microorganisms, might use by these latter to escape the immune response *via* molecular mimicry mechanisms. Thus, pathogen ApoH-like epitope expression could induce autoimmune response. The involvement of molecular mimicry in the induction of APS was demonstrated in a mouse experimental model. Balb/c mice immunized with pathogens having sequence homology with the peptide TLRVYK, a peptide recognized by anti-ApoH. The mouse anti-TLRVYK Ab were purified and injected into new BALB/c, which have subsequently developed an experimental APS (Blank & Shoenfeld, 2004). Synthetic peptides corresponding to the ApoH-phospholipid binding site and having a high sequence homology with cytomegalovirus, adenovirus and *Bacillus subtilis* were used to induce an APS (Gharavi et al., 2002; Gharavi et al., 1999).

Changes of ApoH amounts have been reported in some bacterial infections. In a rare clinical case showing that a *purpura fulminans* phenomenon following an infection with *Haemophilus influenzae* in an adult was associated to a drastic elevation of the ApoH plasma concentration (Gast et al., 2006). A gene expression study performed on *Helicobacter hepaticus*-infected mice showed an increased expression of the gene of ApoH three months after infection, once a chronic inflammation was established (Myles et al., 2003). The infection of chickens with *Salmonella* leads to high ApoH gene over-expression approximately 40-fold excess as compared with uninfected controls (van Hemert et al., 2006). In contrast, it has been reported that *Legionella pneumophila* produces enzymes able to cleave ApoH (Muller, 1980).

Altogether these reports suggest that increased gene expression of ApoH or even its "degradation" by enzymes induced by microorganisms may be in favor of active recognition of microorganisms by ApoH.

Some ApoH-derived peptides have shown antibacterial effects against both Gram-positive (*Staphylococcus pyogenes and S. aureus*) and Gram-negative bacteria (*Escherichia coli*), while the intact entire ApoH protein did not exhibit any antibacterial effects. At the infection site, polymorphonuclear neutrophils (PMN) active secrete proteolytic enzymes. These enzymes generate antibacterial peptides derived from ApoH that can be found in high concentrations at the infected sites. These peptides bind to released bacterial cell wall and induce bacterial lysis (Fig. 11A). Thus, ApoH contributes as a precursor to the human innate immunity.

However, it has been hypothesized that some bacteria, including *S. pyogenes*, may have developed defense mechanisms against the ApoH-derived peptides (Nilsson et al., 2008).

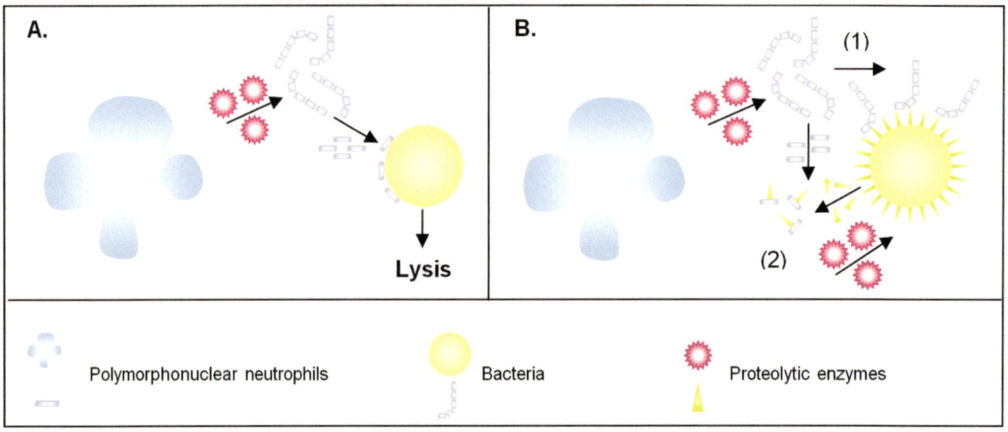

Fig. 11. Mechanisms used by *Streptococcus pyogenes* AP1 to neutralize the effect of anti-bacterial peptides derived from ApoH (Nilsson et al., 2008). (A) At the site of infection, activated neutrophils secrete proteolytic enzymes generating lytic antibacterial ApoH-derived peptides. (B) Mechanisms proposed to be used by AP1 bacteria to prevent the antibacterial activity of ApoH: (i) The binding of ApoH to *S. pyogenes* surface proteins M1 and H prevents the cleavage of the ApoH; (ii) soluble proteins M1 and H interact with ApoH-derived peptides to neutralize their anti-bacterial effects.

The first mechanism is the link between the bacterium and the ApoH. Once ApoH is bound to bacteria, proteinases from PMN cannot cleave ApoH and therefore the production of antibacterial ApoH-derived peptides is reduced (Fig. 11B1). The second mechanism circumventing host immune defenses is the binding of soluble proteins M1 and H with peptides derived from ApoH inducing the inactivation of these latter. The proteins M1 and H became soluble due to proteases from the PMN that cleaved proteins M and H of the bacterium surface (Fig. 11B2).

Thus ApoH, a precursor of antibacterial peptides, would be a mechanism of host protection against infectious agents. It is possible to speculate that certain bacteria are capable to neutralize ApoH *via* their binding mechanisms and thereby escaping the host immune responses.

General structure of bacteria

Bacteria belong to one independent branch of the tree main phyla of life (Woese, 1987). Bacteria have characteristics that are not found in other living prokaryotes (Archeae) or eukaryotes. These are bacterial surface structures, which have the most unique features, not shared with other living beings. Among these structures, the bacterial wall, the exopolysaccharides, protein structures as external S layer, pili, flagella. Most of these surface structures are involved in bacteria-host interactions through their adhesion molecules at their surfaces with host's cells. In addition, these interactions play a pivotal role in bacterial pathogenicity.

Despite their simple morphology and unicellular organization, bacteria present both large organic and structural diversities. This structural diversity is primarily expressed in surface structures. Structure and function properties of the bacteria envelope structures of are a direct consequence of their adaptive strategies.

Bacterial cell wall

Bacteria cells are particularly robust because of their cell wall, which allow them to withstand particularly high variations in osmotic pressure. The wall structure is a base for the determination of major bacterial groups mainly including: Gram-positive bacteria, Gram-positive and mycobacteria.

The common component of bacterial cell wall or murein is a peptodoglycane. Murein is a polymer of two sugar-derivatives (N-acetylglucosamin and N-acetylmuraminic) and several amino-acids and/or lipids that largely differ in a specie-depending manner.

Gram-positive's cell wall

The wall of Gram-positive bacteria is a homogeneous structure with thickness variation from 10 to 80 nm. It consists mostly of a thick layer of multimolecular murein associated with lesser amounts of other dispersed polymers, especially the teichoic and teichuronic acids).

There are a wide variety of these compounds being highly antigenic. The nature of their carbohydrate skeleton, and position of many substitutions are submitted to considerable variations.

Numerous other components are also present in some species, such as proteins or polysaccharides, and they can play an important role in the antigenic properties or pathogenicity. For example, protein A, found in over 98% of strains of *Staphylococcus aureus*, is a receptor for the Fc fragment of immunoglobulin G that when present on bacteria surface will inhibits opsonization. In addition, bacterial mutants lacking protein A present a lower virulence in mouse experimental infections.

Gram-negative's cell wall

The wall of Gram-negative bacteria is more complex. We distinguish an inner membrane and outer membrane, which defines a periplasmic space containing a thin layer of peptidoglycan. The wall is much thinner than those of Gram-positive bacteria, of about 10 nm. Murein of gram-negative bacteria does not contain teichoic acid.

Periplasmic space contains the Braun lipoproteins, which connects the outer membrane to peptidoglycan involved in the cohesion of the wall.

The outer membrane has a distinct chemical composition. Its structure is a phospholipid bilayer with the inner layer has a composition similar to that of the cytoplasmic membrane. Its outer layer, by cons, has a particular constituent embodiment in the PL: lipopolysaccharide (LPS) is a complex molecule consisting of three components: (i) The lipid A, which anchors the LPS in the outer leaflet of the outer membrane. This lipid A is also called endotoxin because of these properties highly toxic for the host. Endotoxin is responsible for septic shock in systemic infections with Gram-negative bacteria; (ii) short series of sugar in the center including: desoxyoctonoic keto-acid and heptose; (iii) long carbohydrate chain whose length is 40 sugars that constitutes the O antigen, covering the surface of the bacterium highly antigenic.

The outer membrane also contains a large number of proteins such as porins involved in the permeability of small hydrophilic molecules (<600 Da) and proteins involved in bacterial virulence (http://www.bacterio.cict.fr/bacdico/bacteriogene/structure.html).

7.1 Bacteria and ApoH binding

In vitro direct interaction has been shown between *S. aureus* and ApoH *via* the Sbi protein (Zhang et al., 1999). Furthermore, a study from a DNA library of *S. aureus* phages and on human blood proteins that adhere to implanted materials, such as catheters, showed the presence of ApoH on these biomaterials. This study attest to the connection on the *ex vivo* biomaterial ApoH *S. aureus* (Bjerketorp et al., 2004). More recently (Agar et al., 2011), it has been shown that upon interaction of LPS with domain V of ApoH, a conformational change occurs in ApoH binds LPS from the ring or close form to a "J or fishhook-like form". Thus, the 'active' fishhook-like conformation of ApoH in complex with LPS is then able to bind to the LPR receptor after which the ApoH-LPS complex is cleared (4). The scavenging of LPS by ApoH leads to a decreased binding of LPS to the TLR-4 receptor resulting in a decreased expression of the inflammatory markers TNF**α**, IL-6 and IL-8.

ApoH also interacts with *Streptococcus pyogenes*. At least two streptococcal proteins are involved in this interaction, M1 protein and H factor, which are surface proteins. M1 protein is a virulence factor, allowing the bacteria to resist phagocytosis. The M1 protein would interact with plasma proteins (fibrinogen, C4b binding protein, H factor) to avoid bacterial lysis (Nilsson et al., 2008).

7.2 The use of ApoH to drastic improvement of bacterial detection

As different bacteria are able to interact with ApoH, we used these fundamental property to propose that ApoH can be a useful tool to capture, from different complex biological media, different kinds of bacteria (Gram- or Gram+) and proceed to their detection and/or diagnostic (Fig. 12) by using different methods including ATP detection by luminometry, cultivation in an appropriated media or PCR.

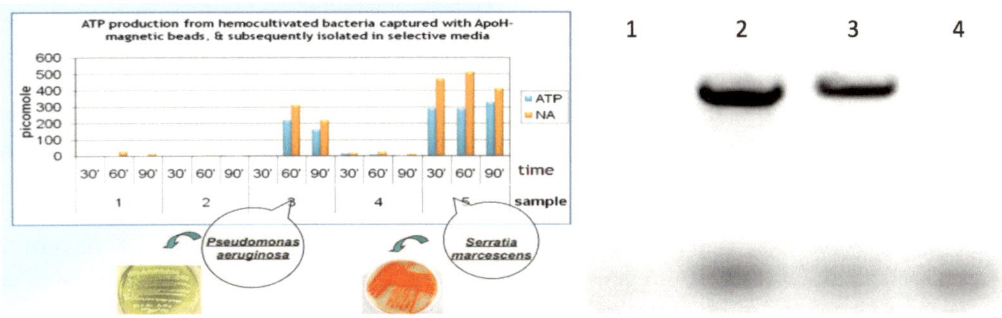

Fig. 12. Bacterial detection. (left) ATP detection and specific cultivation of *Pseudomonas aeruginosa* and *Seratia marcescens* from clinical hemocultivation; (right) 16S RNA PCR. Bacterial Luria broth (LB) Medium (1), ApoH-captured *Escherichia coli* from LB medium (2), positive PCR control, *E. coli* DNA (3), H2O (4)

8. Conclusion

Taking into account literature data and our own data, it is possible to mention that, probably one of the main roles for the acute phase protein ApoH is to be an important actor of host innate immune response through its capacity to bind with high affinity to a large panel of pathogens and or antigens from different origins. This ApoH property can be applied to face a tremendous public health problem that is the existence of (re)-emerging pathogens and their difficulties to be detected.

Indeed, according to the Center for Disease Control and Prevention in Atlanta (CDC), 70% of emerging infectious diseases in humans, are zoonotic pathogens. Most of theses human diseases are caused by the introduction of existing pathogens into human populations from other species or dissemination from endemic areas into larger populations. This process depends upon a complex interaction of factors such as ecological, environmental and/or climatic changes, the basic biology of pathogens, host and cell tropism, the route of transmission, the natural host reservoir and the vector, social behavior, international travel and commerce, political instability, breakdown in public health measures, etc.

Nucleic acid amplification is widely used for the detection and identification of pathogens. Sequencing and comparison to known microorganisms may allow identification of unidentified pathogens. Extraction and careful purification of DNA and/or RNA is an essential step for sensitivity and reliability of these diagnostic techniques, but often incompatible within high throughput screening in routine diagnostics eg. in blood transfusion centres where large series of samples have to be tested. Several major diagnostic companies have been involved in the development of universal viral nucleic acid purification systems from plasma and serum, compatible with IVD (In Vitro Diagnostics) assays. However, despite a gain in sensitivity brought by these methods, the EQA studies revealed that molecular diagnostics still showed a poor overall test proficiency compared to serological diagnostics. One of the main problems for pathogen detection in clinical but also in environmental samples is that they generate false negative results. This problem is mainly due to 3 reasons:

i. Presence of inhibitors such as heme, anticoagulants like EDTA and heparin, high concentrations of leukocyte DNA, immunoglobulins and other unknown inhibitors of nucleic acid amplification in the plasma or serum (Al-Soud et al., 2000; Al-Soud &

Radstrom, 2001; Wilson, 1997). Such an inhibition was described at a frequency of 0.34 to 2.1% of tests for patients infected with human immunodeficiency virus type 1 or hepatitis C virus, respectively (Drosten et al., 2001; Nolte et al., 2001). In the case of patients with severe viral hemorrhagic fever false-negative results are also likely to occur, especially in the acute phase of the disease where a rapid confirmation is required for the introduction of countermeasures(Drosten et al., 2002). In this scenario it is extremely important to develop methods for pathogen concentration allowing their separation from these reaction inhibitors. Such a technology is critical for the development of novel methodologies of sample préparation which would result in the reliable detection of pathogens present within complex biological samples such as blood.

ii. Absence of a universal extraction method that efficiently lyses the pathogens and allow the separation of nucleic acids (RNA or DNA) from other components of the microorganisms or cellular materials that might interfere with downstream processes. Different nucleic acid extraction techniques have shown to result in variable diagnostic outcome for viruses detected by the polymerase chain reaction (PCR). The choice of appropriate RNA and DNA extraction methods, thus, is a critical step for the successful and valid use of RT-PCR and PCR based exams on clinical samples (Fredricks et al., 2005; Labayru et al., 2005; Scansen et al., 2005),

iii. Lack of a rapid and reliable pathogen concentration methodology. Often pathogens present in clinical samples and particularly in environmental samples are diluted in large sample volumes poorly amenable for molecular methods (Brassard et al., 2005; Dreier et al., 2004; Fung et al., 2000); in this case, working with a small fraction of the sample may lead to false-negative results due to the specific sensitivity of the used detection method. Yet, simple and inexpensive methods for the concentration of pathogens, present within the samples, that could be easily introduced into the normal working scheme used by most clinical microbiology laboratories involved in the routine screening of large numbers of human samples are currently not at hand.

One of the main concerns for pathogen detection in clinical, but also in environmental samples, is that they generate false negative results that are mainly due to: (i) presence of inhibitors, (ii) absence of suitable molecular detection methods (e.g. PCR) and (iii) lack of a rapid and reliable pathogen concentration methodology.

The above-mentioned disadvantages have been compensated by the use of a matrix-bound ApoH to concentrate pathogens from biologically complex fluids (blood, feces, tissues, etc). After capture, washing of the ligand-pathogen(s) complex would allow removal of the inhibitors of the subsequent diagnostic steps. Thus, in this novel diagnostic schema the concentrated pathogen(s) would be highly accessible to any subsequent method of extraction, thus increasing the expected efficiency and sensitivity of nucleic acid detection.

Thus, ApoH-coated solid matrix is used as a generic capture method for a wide range of pathogens in order to concentrate them from large sample volumes of complex biological mixtures, otherwise poorly amenable for molecular methods and thus to improve their detection threshold (Fig. 13).

Tools and protocols have been established to use this simple, fast and broad target method adapted to different types of specimen, saliva, plasma, serum, urine and feces as well as various environmental samples. Thus, the pre-analytical sample processing by ApoH allows an efficient and ultrasensitive detection of very divers pathogens from their originated media using simple or sophisticated methods related to immunological (ELISA) or molecular (real-time RT-PCR) detection techniques, therefore drastically diminishing false negative diagnostics generated by classical standardized method.

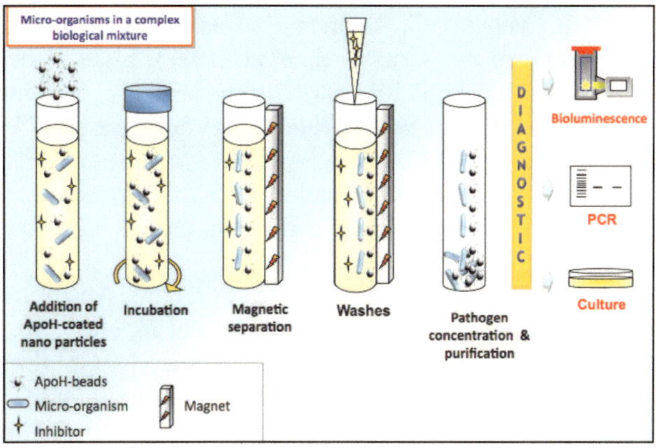

Fig. 13. A schematic representation of different steps to capture and concentrate microorganisms from complex biological fluids using ApoH-coated nano-magnetic beads to drastically improve their ultra-sensitive detection.

9. Acknowledgement

We are grateful to FP6 program of the European Commission for supporting the Ultrasensitive Detection of emerging Pathogens (USDEP, www.usdep.eu or www.apotech.com) project (2006-2010) grant # LSHB-CT-2006-037560.

10. References

Adlhoch, C., Kaiser, M., Hoehne, M., Marques, A. M., Stefas, I., Veas, F. & Ellerbrok, H. (2011). Highly sensitive detection of the group A Rotavirus using Apolipoprotein H-coated ELISA plates compared to quantitative real-time PCR. *Virology Journal* Vol.8, pp.-.

Agar, C., de Groot, P. G., Morgelin, M., Monk, S. D., van Os, G. M., Levels, J. H., de Laat, B., Urbanus, R. T., Herwald, H., van der Poll, T. & Meijers, J. C. (2011). {beta}2-glycoprotein I: a novel component of innate immunity. *Blood.*

Al-Soud, W. A., Jonsson, L. J. & Radstrom, P. (2000). Identification and characterization of immunoglobulin G in blood as a major inhibitor of diagnostic PCR. *Journal of Clinical Microbiology* Vol.38, No.1, pp.345-350.

Al-Soud, W. A. & Radstrom, P. (2001). Purification and characterization of PCR-inhibitory components in blood cells. *Journal of Clinical Microbiology* Vol.39, No.2, pp.485-493.

Alard, J. E., Gaillard, F., Daridon, C., Shoenfeld, Y., Jamin, C. & Youinou, P. (2010). TLR2 is one of the endothelial receptors for beta 2-glycoprotein I. *The Journal of Immunology* Vol.185, No.3, pp.1550-1557.

Arnoux, D. & Boutière, B. (2006). *Pathologie acquise de la coagulation*, Vol 1, (Vélizy-Villacoublay: Arnette).

Asherson, R. A. & Cervera, R. (1993). Antiphospholipid syndrome. *The Journal of Investigative Dermatololgy* Vol.100, No.1, pp.21S-27S.

Averna, M., Paravizzini, G., Marino, G., Emmanuele, G., Cefalu, A. B., Magro, G., Bartoloni, G., Ragusa, M., Noto, D., Barbagallo, C. M., *et al.* (2004). Beta-2-glycoprotein I is growth regulated and plays a role as survival factor for hepatocytes. *The international journal of biochemistry & cell biology* Vol.36, No.7, pp.1297-1305.

Averna, M., Paravizzini, G., Marino, G., Lanteri, E., Cavera, G., Barbagallo, C. M., Petralia, S., Cavallaro, S., Magro, G., Grasso, S., *et al.* (1997). Liver is not the unique site of synthesis of beta 2-glycoprotein I (apolipoprotein H): evidence for an intestinal localization. *International Journal of Clinical Laboratory Research* Vol.27, No.3, pp.207-212.

Bjerketorp, J., Rosander, A., Nilsson, M., Jacobsson, K. & Frykberg, L. (2004). Sorting a *Staphylococcus aureus* phage display library against ex vivo biomaterial. *Journal of Medical Microbiology* Vol.53, No.10, pp.945-951.

Blank, M., Asherson, R. A., Cervera, R. & Shoenfeld, Y. (2004). Antiphospholipid syndrome infectious origin. *Journal of Clinical Immunology* Vol.24, No.1, pp.12-23.

Blank, M., Krause, I., Fridkin, M., Keller, N., Kopolovic, J., Goldberg, I., Tobar, A. & Shoenfeld, Y. (2002). Bacterial induction of autoantibodies to beta2-glycoprotein-I accounts for the infectious etiology of antiphospholipid syndrome. *The Journal of Clinical Investigation* Vol.109, No.6, pp.797-804.

Blank, M. & Shoenfeld, Y. (2004). Beta-2-glycoprotein-I, infections, antiphospholipid syndrome and therapeutic considerations. *Clinical Immunology* Vol.112, No.2, pp.190-199.

Bouma, B., de Groot, P. G., van den Elsen, J. M., Ravelli, R. B., Schouten, A., Simmelink, M. J., Derksen, R. H., Kroon, J. & Gros, P. (1999). Adhesion mechanism of human beta(2)-glycoprotein I to phospholipids based on its crystal structure. *The Embo Journal* Vol.18, No.19, pp.5166-5174.

Brassard, J., Seyer, K., Houde, A., Simard, C. & Trottier, Y. L. (2005). Concentration and detection of hepatitis A virus and rotavirus in spring water samples by reverse transcription-PCR. *Journal of virological methods* Vol.123, No.2, pp.163-169.

d'Angeac, A. D., Stefas, I., Duperray, C., Rucheton, M., Graafland, H., Montero, J. L. & Chicheportiche, R. (2005). Oxidation and biotinylation of beta 2 glycoprotein I glycan chains induce an increase in its affinity for anionic phospholipids similar to that obtained by the addition of anti-beta 2 glycoprotein I or anti-cardiolipin antibodies. *Journal of Immunological Methods* Vol.300, No.1-2, pp.160-178.

Dreier, J., Kroger, M., Diekmann, J., Gotting, C. & Kleesiek, K. (2004). Low-level viraemia of hepatitis B virus in an anti-HBc- and anti-HBs-positive blood donor. *Transfusion medicine* Vol.14, No.2, pp.97-103.

Drosten, C., Panning, M., Guenther, S. & Schmitz, H. (2002). False-negative results of PCR assay with plasma of patients with severe viral hemorrhagic fever. *Journal of Clinical Microbiology* Vol.40, No.11, pp.4394-4395.

Drosten, C., Seifried, E. & Roth, W. K. (2001). TaqMan 5'-nuclease human immunodeficiency virus type 1 PCR assay with phage-packaged competitive internal control for high-throughput blood donor screening. *Journal of Clinical Microbiology* Vol.39, No.12, pp.4302-4308.

Fredricks, D. N., Smith, C. & Meier, A. (2005). Comparison of six DNA extraction methods for recovery of fungal DNA as assessed by quantitative PCR. *Journal of Clinical Microbiology* Vol.43, No.10, pp.5122-5128.

Fung, C. P., Lee, Y. M., Kuo, B. I., Yang, S. P., Chan, Y. J., Liu, C. Y., Ho, L. T. & Liu, W. T. (2000). Using buffy coat for reverse transcriptase-polymerase chain reaction in the diagnosis of dengue virus infection: preliminary study. *Journal of microbiology, immunology, and infection = Wei mian yu gan ran za zhi* Vol.33, No.4, pp.217-222.

Gambino, R., Ruiu, G., Pagano, G. & Cassader, M. (1997). Characterization and representative structures of N-oligosaccharides bound to apolipoprotein H. *Journal of Lipid Mediators and Cell Signalling* Vol.17, No.3, pp.191-205.

Gambino, R., Ruiu, G., Pagano, G. & Cassader, M. (1999a). The binding of apolipoprotein H (beta2-Glycoprotein I) to lipoproteins. *Prostaglandins and other Lipid Mediators* Vol.57, No.5-6, pp.351-359.

Gambino, R., Ruiu, G., Pagano, G. & Cassader, M. (1999b). Study of the glycosylation of apolipoprotein H. *Chemistry and Physic of Lipids* Vol.103, No.1-2, pp.161-174.

Gast, T., Kowal-Vern, A., An, G. & Hanumadass, M. L. (2006). Purpura fulminans in an adult patient with *Haemophilus influenzae* sepsis: case report and review of the literature. *Journal of Burn Care & Research* Vol.27, No.1, pp.102-107.

George, J., Harats, D., Gilburd, B., Afek, A., Levy, Y., Schneiderman, J., Barshack, I., Kopolovic, J. & Shoenfeld, Y. (1999). Immunolocalization of beta2-glycoprotein I (apolipoprotein H) to human atherosclerotic plaques: potential implications for lesion progression. *Circulation* Vol.99, No.17, pp.2227-2230.

Gharavi, A. E., Pierangeli, S. S., Espinola, R. G., Liu, X., Colden-Stanfield, M. & Harris, E. N. (2002). Antiphospholipid antibodies induced in mice by immunization with a cytomegalovirus-derived peptide cause thrombosis and activation of endothelial cells *in vivo*. *Arthritis and Rheumatism* Vol.46, No.2, pp.545-552.

Gharavi, E. E., Chaimovich, H., Cucurull, E., Celli, C. M., Tang, H., Wilson, W. A. & Gharavi, A. E. (1999). Induction of antiphospholipid antibodies by immunization with synthetic viral and bacterial peptides. *Lupus* Vol.8, No.6, pp.449-455.

Godoy, P., Marsac, D., Stefas, E., Ferrer, P., Tischler, N. D., Pino, K., Ramdohr, P., Vial, P., Valenzuela, P. D., Ferres, M., *et al.* (2009). Andes virus antigens are shed in urine of patients with acute hantavirus cardiopulmonary syndrome. *Journal of Virology* Vol.83, No.10, pp.5046-5055.

Hammel, M., Kriechbaum, M., Gries, A., Kostner, G. M., Laggner, P. & Prassl, R. (2002). Solution structure of human and bovine beta(2)-glycoprotein I revealed by small-angle X-ray scattering. *Journal of Molecular Biology* Vol.321, No.1, pp.85-97.

Hammel, M., Schwarzenbacher, R., Gries, A., Kostner, G. M., Laggner, P. & Prassl, R. (2001). Mechanism of the interaction of beta(2)-glycoprotein I with negatively charged phospholipid membranes. *Biochemistry* Vol.40, No.47, pp.14173-14181.

Harel, M., Aron-Maor, A., Sherer, Y., Blank, M. & Shoenfeld, Y. (2005). The infectious etiology of the antiphospholipid syndrome: links between infection and autoimmunity. *Immunobiology* Vol.210, No.10, pp.743-747.

Hong, D. P., Hagihara, Y., Kato, H. & Goto, Y. (2001). Flexible loop of beta 2-glycoprotein I domain V specifically interacts with hydrophobic ligands. *Biochemistry* Vol.40, No.27, pp.8092-8100.

http://dicos.ens-lyon.fr/vie/viro/image/V05_2H1_Hepatites_8HBV.jpg. In.

http://www.bacterio.cict.fr/bacdico/bacteriogene/structure.html. In.

Kamboh, M. I., Ferrell, R. E. & Sepehrnia, B. (1988). Genetic studies of human apolipoproteins. IV. Structural heterogeneity of apolipoprotein H (beta 2-glycoprotein I). *American Journal of Human Genetics* Vol.42, No.3, pp.452-457.

Kandiah, D. A., Sali, A., Sheng, Y., Victoria, E. J., Marquis, D. M., Coutts, S. M. & Krilis, S. A. (1998). Current insights into the "antiphospholipid" syndrome: clinical, immunological, and molecular aspects. *Advances in Immunology* Vol.70, pp.507-563.

Keeling, D. M., Wilson, A. J., Mackie, I. J., Isenberg, D. A. & Machin, S. J. (1993). Role of beta 2-glycoprotein I and anti-phospholipid antibodies in activation of protein C in vitro. *Journal of Clinical Pathology* Vol.46, No.10, pp.908-911.

Kochl, S., Fresser, F., Lobentanz, E., Baier, G. & Utermann, G. (1997). Novel interaction of apolipoprotein(a) with beta-2 glycoprotein I mediated by the kringle IV domain. *Blood* Vol.90, No.4, pp.1482-1489.

Labayru, C., Eiros, J. M., Hernandez, B., de Lejarazu, R. O. & Torres, A. R. (2005). RNA extraction prior to HIV-1 resistance detection using Line Probe Assay (LiPA): comparison of three methods. *Journal of clinical virology : the official publication of the Pan American Society for Clinical Virology* Vol.32, No.4, pp.265-271.

Lee, N. S., Brewer, H. B., Jr. & Osborne, J. C., Jr. (1983). beta 2-Glycoprotein I. Molecular properties of an unusual apolipoprotein, apolipoprotein H. *The Journal of biological chemistry* Vol.258, No.8, pp.4765-4770.

Lozier, J., Takahashi, N. & Putnam, F. W. (1984). Complete amino acid sequence of human plasma beta 2-glycoprotein I. *Proceedings of the National Academy of Sciences of the United States of America* Vol.81, No.12, pp.3640-3644.

Ma, K., Simantov, R., Zhang, J. C., Silverstein, R., Hajjar, K. A. & McCrae, K. R. (2000). High affinity binding of beta 2-glycoprotein I to human endothelial cells is mediated by annexin II. *The Journal of biological chemistry* Vol.275, No.20, pp.15541-15548.

McNeil, H. P., Simpson, R. J., Chesterman, C. N. & Krilis, S. A. (1990). Anti-phospholipid antibodies are directed against a complex antigen that includes a lipid-binding inhibitor of coagulation: beta 2-glycoprotein I (apolipoprotein H). *Proceedings of the National Academy of Sciences of the United States of America* Vol.87, No.11, pp.4120-4124.

Mehdi, H., Kaplan, M. J., Anlar, F. Y., Yang, X., Bayer, R., Sutherland, K. & Peeples, M. E. (1994). Hepatitis B virus surface antigen binds to apolipoprotein H. *Journal of Virology* Vol.68, No.4, pp.2415-2424.

Mehdi, H., Naqvi, A. & Kamboh, M. I. (2000). A hydrophobic sequence at position 313-316 (Leu-Ala-Phe-Trp) in the fifth domain of apolipoprotein H (beta2-glycoprotein I) is crucial for cardiolipin binding. *European Journal of Biochemistry* Vol.267, No.6, pp.1770-1776.

Mehdi, H., Naqvi, A. & Kamboh, M. I. (2008). Recombinant hepatitis B surface antigen and anionic phospholipids share a binding region in the fifth domain of beta2-glycoprotein I (apolipoprotein H). *Biochimica et Biophysica Acta* Vol.1782, No.3, pp.163-168.

Mehdi, H., Nunn, M., Steel, D. M., Whitehead, A. S., Perez, M., Walker, L. & Peeples, M. E. (1991). Nucleotide sequence and expression of the human gene encoding apolipoprotein H (beta 2-glycoprotein I). *Gene* Vol.108, No.2, pp.293-298.

Miyakis, S., Giannakopoulos, B. & Krilis, S. A. (2004). Beta 2 glycoprotein I--function in health and disease. *Thrombosis Research* Vol.114, No.5-6, pp.335-346.

Moestrup, S. K., Schousboe, I., Jacobsen, C., Leheste, J. R., Christensen, E. I. & Willnow, T. E. (1998). beta2-glycoprotein-I (apolipoprotein H) and beta2-glycoprotein-I-phospholipid complex harbor a recognition site for the endocytic receptor megalin. *The Journal of Clinical Investgation* Vol.102, No.5, pp.902-909.

Muller, H. E. (1980). Proteolytic action of *Legionella pneumophila* on human serum proteins. *Infection and immunity* Vol.27, No.1, pp.51-53.

Myles, M. H., Livingston, R. S., Livingston, B. A., Criley, J. M. & Franklin, C. L. (2003). Analysis of gene expression in ceca of *Helicobacter hepaticus*-infected A/JCr mice before and after development of typhlitis. *Infection and immunity* Vol.71, No.7, pp.3885-3893.

Neurath, A. R. & Strick, N. (1994). The putative cell receptors for hepatitis B virus (HBV), annexin V, and apolipoprotein H, bind to lipid components of HBV. *Virology* Vol.204, No.1, pp.475-477.

Nilsson, M., Wasylik, S., Morgelin, M., Olin, A. I., Meijers, J. C., Derksen, R. H., de Groot, P. G. & Herwald, H. (2008). The antibacterial activity of peptides derived from human beta-2 glycoprotein I is inhibited by protein H and M1 protein from Streptococcus pyogenes. *Molecular Microbiology* Vol.67, No.3, pp.482-492.

Nolte, F. S., Fried, M. W., Shiffman, M. L., Ferreira-Gonzalez, A., Garrett, C. T., Schiff, E. R., Polyak, S. J. & Gretch, D. R. (2001). Prospective multicenter clinical evaluation of AMPLICOR and COBAS AMPLICOR hepatitis C virus tests. *Journal of Clinical Microbiology* Vol.39, No.11, pp.4005-4012.

Okkels, H., Rasmussen, T. E., Sanghera, D. K., Kamboh, M. I. & Kristensen, T. (1999). Structure of the human beta2-glycoprotein I (apolipoprotein H) gene. *European Journal of Biochemistry* Vol.259, No.1-2, pp.435-440.

Pellicano, R., Broutet, N., Ponzetto, A. & Megraud, F. (1999). Helicobacter pylori: from the stomach to the heart. *European Journal of Gastroenterology and Hepatology* Vol.11, No.11, pp.1335-1337.

Polz, E. & Kostner, G. M. (1979). The binding of beta 2-glycoprotein-I to human serum lipoproteins: distribution among density fractions. *FEBS Letters* Vol.102, No.1, pp.183-186.

Ragusa, M. A., Costa, S., Cefalu, A. B., Noto, D., Fayer, F., Travali, S., Averna, M. R. & Gianguzza, F. (2006). RT-PCR and in situ hybridization analysis of apolipoprotein H expression in rat normal tissues. *International Journal of Molecular Medicine* Vol.18, No.3, pp.449-455.

Rojkjaer, R., Klaerke, D. A. & Schousboe, I. (1997). Characterization of the interaction between beta2-glycoprotein I and calmodulin, and identification of a binding sequence in beta2-glycoprotein I. *Biochimica et Biophysica Acta* Vol.1339, No.2, pp.217-225.

Scansen, B. A., Kruger, J. M., Wise, A. G., Venta, P. J., Bartlett, P. C. & Maes, R. K. (2005). In vitro comparison of RNA preparation methods for detection of feline calicivirus in urine of cats by use of a reverse transcriptase-polymerase chain reaction assay. *American journal of veterinary research* Vol.66, No.5, pp.915-920.

Schousboe, I. (1983). Characterization of the interaction between beta 2-glycoprotein I and mitochondria, platelets, liposomes and bile acids. *International Journal of Biochemistry* Vol.15, No.12, pp.1393-1401.

Schultze, H. E. (1961). [Glycoproteins of human plasma.]. *Bulletin der Schweizerischen Akademie der Medizinischen Wissenschaften* Vol.17, pp.77-91.

Schwarzenbacher, R., Zeth, K., Diederichs, K., Gries, A., Kostner, G. M., Laggner, P. & Prassl, R. (1999). Crystal structure of human beta2-glycoprotein I: implications for phospholipid binding and the antiphospholipid syndrome. *The Embo Journal* Vol.18, No.22, pp.6228-6239.

Sellar, G. C., Keane, J., Mehdi, H., Peeples, M. E., Browne, N. & Whitehead, A. S. (1993). Characterization and acute phase modulation of canine apolipoprotein H (beta 2-glycoprotein I). *Biochemical and biophysical research communications* Vol.191, No.3, pp.1288-1293.

Shi, T., Giannakopoulos, B., Iverson, G. M., Cockerill, K. A., Linnik, M. D. & Krilis, S. A. (2005). Domain V of beta2-glycoprotein I binds factor XI/XIa and is cleaved at Lys317-Thr318. *Journal of Biological Chemistry* Vol.280, No.2, pp.907-912.

Shi, T., Iverson, G. M., Qi, J. C., Cockerill, K. A., Linnik, M. D., Konecny, P. & Krilis, S. A. (2004). Beta 2-Glycoprotein I binds factor XI and inhibits its activation by thrombin and factor XIIa: loss of inhibition by clipped beta 2-glycoprotein I. *Proceedings of the National Academy of Sciences of the United States of America* Vol.101, No.11, pp.3939-3944.

Sodin-Semrl, S. & Rozman, B. (2007). Beta2-glycoprotein I and its clinical significance: from gene sequence to protein levels. *Autoimmunity Reviews* Vol.6, No.8, pp.547-552.

Stefas, E., Rucheton, M., Graafland, H., Moynier, M., Sompeyrac, C., Bahraoui, E. M. & Veas, F. (1997). Human plasmatic apolipoprotein H binds human immunodeficiency virus type 1 and type 2 proteins. *AIDS Research and Human Retroviruses* Vol.13, No.1, pp.97-104.

Stefas, I., Rucheton, M., D'Angeac, A. D., Morel-Baccard, C., Seigneurin, J. M., Zarski, J. P., Martin, M., Cerutti, M., Bossy, J. P., Misse, D., *et al.* (2001). Hepatitis B virus Dane particles bind to human plasma apolipoprotein H. *Hepatology* Vol.33, No.1, pp.207-217.

Steinkasserer, A., Estaller, C., Weiss, E. H., Sim, R. B. & Day, A. J. (1991). Complete nucleotide and deduced amino acid sequence of human beta 2-glycoprotein I. *Biochemistry Journal* Vol.277 (Pt 2), pp.387-391.

Stojanovic, M., Inic-Kanada, A., Popovic, Z., Zivkovic, I. & Dimitrijevic, L. (2004). Changes in pools of autoantibodies and anti-bacterial antibodies in patients suffering from recurrent infections of the urinary tract and undergoing bacterial immunization treatment. *Immunology Letters* Vol.94, No.1-2, pp.123-133.

van Hemert, S., Hoekman, A. J., Smits, M. A. & Rebel, J. M. (2006). Gene expression responses to a Salmonella infection in the chicken intestine differ between lines. *Veterinary Immunology and Immunopathology* Vol.114, No.3-4, pp.247-258.

Wang, H. H. & Chiang, A. N. (2004). Cloning and characterization of the human beta2-glycoprotein I (beta2-GPI) gene promoter: roles of the atypical TATA box and hepatic nuclear factor-1alpha in regulating beta2-GPI promoter activity. *Biochemical Journal* Vol.380, No.Pt 2, pp.455-463.

Wang, S. X., Cai, G. P. & Sui, S. F. (1998). The insertion of human apolipoprotein H into phospholipid membranes: a monolayer study. *Biochemical Journal* Vol.335 (Pt 2), pp.225-232.

Willems, G. M., Janssen, M. P., Pelsers, M. M., Comfurius, P., Galli, M., Zwaal, R. F. & Bevers, E. M. (1996). Role of divalency in the high-affinity binding of anticardiolipin antibody-beta 2-glycoprotein I complexes to lipid membranes. *Biochemistry* Vol.35, No.43, pp.13833-13842.

Wilson, I. G. (1997). Inhibition and facilitation of nucleic acid amplification. *Applied and Environmental Microbiology* Vol.63, No.10, pp.3741-3751.

Woese, C. R. (1987). Bacterial evolution. *Microbiological Reviews* Vol.51, No.2, pp.221-271.

Wurm, H. (1984). beta 2-Glycoprotein-I (apolipoprotein H) interactions with phospholipid vesicles. *The International Journal of Biochemistry* Vol.16, No.5, pp.511-515.

Yasuda, S., Atsumi, T., Ieko, M. & Koike, T. (2004). Beta2-glycoprotein I, anti-beta2-glycoprotein I, and fibrinolysis. *Thrombosis Research* Vol.114, No.5-6, pp.461-465.

Zhang, L., Jacobsson, K., Strom, K., Lindberg, M. & Frykberg, L. (1999). *Staphylococcus aureus* expresses a cell surface protein that binds both IgG and beta2-glycoprotein I. *Microbiology* Vol.145 (Pt 1), pp.177-183.

3

Diagnostic Value of Acute Phase Proteins in Periodontal, Psychosomatic and Cardiometabolic Diseases: Response to Treatment

Mena Soory[1] and Una El-Shinnawi[2]
[1]*Periodontology, King's College London Dental Institute, King's College Dental Hospital, Denmark Hill, London SE5 9RW*
[2]*Periodontology and Oral Medicine, Faculty of Dentistry, Mansoura University,*
[1]*UK*
[2]*Egypt*

1. Introduction

The host response to bacterial plaque biofilm on tooth surfaces initiates periodontal disease and its progression affecting the supporting structures of teeth. Stressor responses of the host to plaque biofilm result in markers of inflammation that are common to diabetes mellitus and coronary heart disease (Pussinen et al 2007). These inflammatory markers are relevant to periodontitis, anxiety states, associated systemic diseases and their sequelae in a bi-directional manner. The extent and clinical significance of these associations have received increasing coverage in the literature. This is largely dependent on the scale of the inflammatory loading based on the severity of periodontal inflammation at the time of examination and the number of sites involved (Norse et al 2008). Response to periodontal treatment with decreased levels of serum markers is indicative of the importance of this source of systemic inflammatory loading. The impact of inflammatory loading from the periodontium as a significant source of systemic inflammation has been an area of debate.

The extent and severity of periodontal inflammation in the presenting population determine its significance in this context. It has wider implications in the context of co-morbidities in periodontal patients. In addition to the commoner co-morbidities, coronary heart disease (CHD), diabetes mellitus and arthritis, other autoimmune conditions and anxiety states also show similar links. This chapter aims to provide such evidence, conflicting at times due to multifactorial presentations of clinical conditions and individual susceptibility. In relevant cases, given a sufficient impetus from inflammatory loading it highlights the importance of controlling periodontal disease in a systemically-ill population. Searches were done over the past 10-15 years, using keywords relevant to the title; subsequently limited to those representing key information focusing on inflammatory markers, their significance and relevance to periodontal, psychosomatic and cardiometabolic diseases with implications on treatment.

This included a systematic review and meta-analysis of C-reactive protein (CRP) in relation to periodontitis, a general overview of the acute phase reaction in infections and inflammatory diseases as the main core, using objective selection criteria and a comprehensive database (Pub Med, Science direct, Wiley-Blackwell, Springer and Ovid-Medline). Several putative risk factors/indicators involved in periodontal disease progression with emphasis on those associated with altered immune mechanisms such as markers of stress/ anxiety states, markers of periodontal disease and relevance of cardiometabolic disorders and autoimmune diseases have been discussed in the context of treatment responses, throughout the text. The search was limited to the last 10 - 15 years including reviews and original research in the subject areas of relevant acute phase reactions and their role in the progression of periodontitis, treatment responses and association with cardiometabolic disorders; and documentation was selected to represent the theme and provide insight in key areas of relevance.

Key words and phrases used for searches include: 1. Psychological stress; acute phase proteins, 2. Periodontitis; cardiometabolic diseases; atherosclerosis; periodontal treatment, 3. Risk factors; atherosclerosis; inflammation; periodontitis; treatment response, 4. Biomarkers; periodontitis; cardiovascular disease, 5. Periodontal disease; psychology; stress, 6. Inflammatory cytokines; periodontitis; atherosclerosis, 7. Aggressive periodontitis; C-reactive protein; IL-6, 8. Psychosomatic factors; stress; anxiety and periodontal disease.

The main objectives and key questions asked are:

1. The effects of psychological stress on acute phase protein profiles in periodontitis patients.
2. Are CRP levels significantly elevated in periodontitis patients and what is the effect of periodontal therapy?
3. What are the potential mechanisms implicated in the association between periodontitis and cardiometabolic disorders; and the effect of periodontal treatment on markers of coronary arterial, peripheral arterial and metabolic diseases?

The above theme has been addressed in the context of diagnostic and therapeutic relevance.

2. Anxiety states and periodontal disease

Stress-induced neurohormones play a critical role in the outcome of infections. Neuro-immune-endocrine interactions in response to stress could affect periodontal disease progression. Catecholamines (epinephrine and norepinephrine) stimulate the formation and activity of prostaglandins and proteolytic enzymes, which can indirectly produce tissue destruction. The relationship between stress and periodontal disease could be mediated by alteration in gingival crevicular interleukins, depressed polymorphonuclear leukocyte chemotaxis and phagocytosis and reduced proliferation of lymphocytes upon stimulation by a mitogen. Anxiety states could dysregulate neuro-endocrine regulatory mechanisms involved in immune regulation and thereby alter immune responses influencing the development and progression of infections and inflammatory diseases including periodontitis; with potential impact on bone density and osteoporotic changes via immune and endocrine mechanisms. Determination of levels of anxiety states in relation to disease markers would clarify cause and effect relationships in psychosomatic diseases.

Variation in severity of periodontal disease cannot be explained by a limited number of risk factors (Teng et al 2003). Associations between stress-inducing factors and periodontal disease have been examined in several studies (Wimmer et al 2002, Pistorius et al 2002).

Periodontal disease is more widespread and severe in subjects with higher levels of stress. Effects of various psychological and psychosocial factors such as emotional and other sources of stress have been the focus of documentation in the context of oral diseases. There are correlations between psychological factors and advanced periodontal disease (Wimmer et al 2002) with unfavourable effects on the progression of periodontal diseases (Pistorius et al 2002). A great deal of evidence suggests that stress-induced neurohormones play a critical role in the outcome of infections (Aviles et al 2004; Sonnenfeld et al 2002; Belay and Sonnenfeld 2002; Lyte 2004). Individual susceptibility factors could affect disease outcome and account for the variations seen.

Glucocorticoids released in the cortex of the suprarenals induce reduced secretion of pro-inflammatory cytokines such as interleukins (IL), tumour necrosis factor (TNF) and also prostaglandins. On the other hand, catecholamines (epinephrine and norepinephrine) have the opposite effect, stimulating the formation and activity of prostaglandins and proteolytic enzymes, which can indirectly produce tissue destruction. Several studies have explored the associations among stress, salivary cortisol, and periodontal disease (Rosania et al 2009; Johannsen et al 2006; Hilgert et al 2006). The relationship between stress and periodontal diseases could be mediated by alteration in gingival crevicular IL levels (Deinzer et al 1999; Mengel et al 2002; Giannopolou et al 2003; Kamma et al 2004), depressed polymorphonuclear leukocyte (PMN) chemotaxis, phagocytosis, and reduced proliferation of lymphocytes upon stimulation by a mitogen. Other possible mechanisms could involve changes in gingival circulation, alteration in salivary flow, its components and possible endocrine changes (Sheiham & Nicolau 2005). Raised serum and tissue levels of noradrenaline in patients subjected to stress could affect the composition or phenotype of subgingival periodontal pathogens.

Recent studies suggest that stress and depression may affect the onset and progression of periodontal disease through behavioral and physiologic mechanisms (Peruzzo et al 2007; Rosania et al 2009). Depression may dysregulate cerebral homeostatic mechanisms involved in immune regulation, and thereby influence the initiation and progression of infections and inflammatory diseases, including periodontitis (Pavlov & Tracey 2004; Behl et al 2008). Antidepressant treatment contributes to immune regulation in patients with major depressive disorders (Maes 2001). Venlafaxine and fluoxetine were found to exert negative immunoregulatory effects by inducing a change in lymphocyte subsets and by suppressing the interferon-γ and interleukin-10 production ratio in whole-blood cells (Kubera et al 2001; Basterzi et al 2009).

There is extensive documentation of individuals under psychological stress being more susceptible to loss of periodontal attachment and alveolar bone. Social stressors could contribute to glucocorticoid resistance and increased production of IL-1β, IL-6 and TNF-α (Powell et al. 2005), as a result of stressor-induced dysregulation of CD11b+ monocyte activity in response to microbial products (Bailey et al 2009). There is increased toll-like receptor-driven nuclear factor-kappa B (NF–κB) activity (Padgett and Glaser 2003). This could exacerbate periodontal and systemic inflammation, insulin resistance and hypertension, predictive of vascular impairment. Human stress-response studies of peripheral blood leukocytes show under-representation of genes activated by glucocorticoids which serve to suppress the immune response and an over-representation of genes regulated by NF-κB, usually suppressed by glucocorticoids. Some of these mechanisms could explain the strong psychosomatic implications of stress on periodontal disease (Hilgert et al 2006; Genco et al 1999; Ishisaka et al 2008; Ishisaka et al 2007). Other possible mechanisms include modification of patients' health behavior. Individuals with high levels of stress tend to adopt habits that are harmful to periodontal health, such as negligent oral hygiene, increased smoking or changes in dietary habits (Deinzer et al 1999) and the outcome my be modified by genetic predisposition.

Studies have reported an association between depression and low bone mineral density. Depression may induce bone loss and osteoporotic fractures, primarily via specific immune and endocrine mechanisms, while use of specific antidepressants such as the selective serotonin re-uptake inhibitors (SSRIs) are potential contributory factors (Cizza et al 2009). These factors could play a secondary role in the progression of periodontitis in patients thus afflicted.

2.1 Concept of markers for periodontal and systemic diseases, relevant to anxiety states

Based on the psychosomatic interactions discussed, markers which allow identification of susceptible individuals prior to the onset of periodontitis, have evolved. There is increasing recognition of risk factors that might be modified in order to prevent or alter the course of periodontal disease (Van Dyke 2005). An analysis of systemic and microbial factors in epidemiological studies points to several risk factors associated with periodontitis. These factors include local, systemic, demographic, and behavioural host conditions which markedly affect the resistance to infecting pathogens (Albander 2002; Genco 1999). They may be considered to be associations which amplify or abate responses but not necessarily causative. Non-environmental intrinsic factors such as genetic make-up, are not modifiable (Van Dyke 2005), but may be influenced by environmental and behavioural factors.

Associations have been established between chronic periodontitis, caused by unresolved inflammation (Pihlstrom et al 2005), and an increased risk of coronary artery disease where inflammation appears to be the main factor (Gibson lll & Genco 2007; Gibson lll et al. 2008; Paoletti et al. 2004). Interestingly, both disease entities have been associated with the stress response.

Individuals under psychological stress are more likely to develop clinical attachment loss and associated alveolar bone loss (Hugoson et al 2002; Mawhorter & Lauer 2001; Pistorius et al 2002; Wimmer et al 2002). One possible link in this regard may be increases in production of IL-6 in response to increased psychological stress (Kiecolt-Glaser et al 2003). IL-6 induces the expression of CRP, an acute-phase reactant responsible for the increase in expression of cellular adhesion molecules and vascular inflammation. Based on the biological properties of these pro-inflammatory cytokines, high plasma levels of TNF-α and IL-6 have been associated with an increased risk for developing cardiovascular events, morbidity and mortality (Abeywardena et al 2009; Ryan et al 2009). Periodontal diseases seem to act as a source of pathogenic species, virulence factors and inflammatory mediators that are conveyed systemically, creating and sustaining a chronic systemic inflammatory burden (Haraszthy et al 2000; De Nardin 2001; Beck & Offenbacher 2005). The magnitude of this inflammatory burden would depend on the degree of inflammation present at the time of examination. It has also been suggested that peripheral blood monocytes from periodontitis subjects may present a distinct profile of inflammatory mediator release in response to bacterial challenge when compared with healthy subjects (Sorensen et al 2009; Yamaguchi et al 2009).

Periodontal symptoms can be exacerbated during periods of stress, and stress could potentially increase the risk of developing coronary heart disease (Dimsdale 2008), along the mechanisms detailed above, depending on individual susceptibility factors. As a result, a thorough understanding of the diverse ways in which inflammation can be regulated is imperative in order to execute effective management to control inflammatory diseases.

In response to a stressor, host responses which provide a buffering effect are triggered. Chronic activation of stress responses results in chronic release of glucocorticoids and catecholamines due to activation of the hypothalamic-pituitary-adrenal- and sympathetic-adrenal-medullary axes. Glucocorticoids expressed in host immune cells bind cortisol and interfere with NF-kB-regulated functions of host cells which produce cytokines. The role of stress in contributing to immune dysregulation and the mechanisms involved have been reviewed (Padgett & Glaser 2003). Genes encoding for a variety of cytokines are induced by adrenergic receptors binding epinephrine and norepinephrine via a cAMP response element binding protein, a cellular transcription factor. Glucocorticoids and catecholamines mediate changes in gene expression which could cause immune dysregulation. There is good documented evidence from animal and human studies of the significant impact of stress-associated immune dysregulation on health.

2.2 Effects of stress on inflammation: Role of cytokines as a source of inflammatory loading

Psychological stress increases the expression of markers of peripheral inflammation. There is increasing evidence of an association between periodontal pathogens and systemic inflammation. The impact of social disruption (SDR) as a social stressor was investigated in mice in response to LPS derived from the periodontal pathogen *Porphyromonas gingivalis* (*Pg*) (Bailey et al 2009). Following consistent exposure to SDR over 6 days, mice were tested for anxiety-related behaviour and sacrificed. Harvested spleen cells were stimulated with *Pg*-derived LPS in the presence or absence of increasing doses of corticosterone. SDR-induced anxious behaviour was associated with the production of significant amounts of IL-1β and TNF-α, when compared with non-stressed control mice. Cultures enriched for CD11b+ cells indicate that splenic myeloid cell activity is affected by social stress. The inflammatory response to oral pathogens could play an important role in stress-associated systemic inflammation.

The social stressor SDR induces an increased inflammatory response and glucocorticoid resistance in CD11b+ monocytes. Splenic dendritic cells (DC) from SDR mice displayed increased levels of MHC1, CD80 and CD44 indicating an activated phenotype, compared with controls. Increased amounts of TNF-α, IL-6 and IL-10 are produced by DCs from SDR mice, compared with controls (Powell et al 2009). Previous work has shown glucocorticoid resistance in DCs from SDR mice. This is suggestive of DC activation by social stress in the absence of an immune challenge, with increased cytokine secretion in response to toll-like receptor activity and glucocorticoid resistance.

SDR, a murine model of social stress alters the phenotype and actions of splenic immune cells. In response to SDR, splenic CD11b+ monocytes are increased in number and are less sensitive to the negative effects of glucocorticoids on cell viability. Greater amounts of the inflammatory cytokines TNF-α and IL-6 were secreted by spleen cells from SDR mice in response to LPS, compared with controls. Secretion of TNF-α was increased by SDR in an enriched fraction of CD11+ monocytes stimulated by LPS (Avitsur et al 2005). The kinetics of TNF-α release in these cells are also altered with minor changes in attenuation of LPS-induced TNF-α secretion in response to corticosterone and norepinephrine. Responses to social stress are determined by complex immunomodulatory mechanisms which could have a varied impact on individuals, based on genetic and other environmental factors.

Both IL-1β and TNF-α are known to be important in the development of oral inflammatory diseases such as gingivitis and periodontitis; elevated levels of these cytokines have been isolated in periodontal patients at the site of active tissue breakdown (Gamonal et al 2003; Orozco et al 2006). These cytokines have diverse effects on gingival tissue, such as degradation of connective tissue matrix via an increase in matrix metalloproteinases, and activation of osteoblastic/osteoclastic responses via disruption of the balance between physiological repair and remodelling (Graves & Cochran 2003). Elevated cytokine levels, however, are not limited to the infected gingiva, and people with chronic periodontitis have been found to have increased levels of cytokines in the circulation, including IL-1β and TNF-α (Golub et al 2006). These circulatory cytokines are not likely to be the result of "spillover" from the infected gingiva, but rather, derived from peripheral cytokine producing cells, such as CD11b+ macrophages present in reticuloendothelial organs (i.e., the spleen, liver, and lungs), which are capable of producing high levels of inflammatory cytokines upon encountering *Pg* or its lipopolysaccharide (LPS).

Oral bacteria and bacterial derived products can enter the bloodstream via standard oral hygiene procedures and periodontal treatment (Kinane et al 2005) as well as through pathogen-induced ulceration and vascular permeability in the gingivae (Gibson lll et al 2008). As they circulate systemically, microbial products are recognized by cells of the reticulendothelial macrophages and other innate immune cells. These cells are able to respond to *Pg* and *Pg*-associated products, by producing a variety of inflammatory mediators, including the inflammatory cytokines IL-6, IL-1, TNF-α and CRP (Pussinen et al 2007a). These inflammatory mediators are considered to be the link between oral inflammatory diseases and associated systemic conditions.

Inflammatory loading from periodontal disease could contribute to the progression of cardiometabolic and autoimmune diseases which are driven by inflammatory mechanisms leading to oxidative stress-induced tissue and organ damage (Pussinen et al 2007b). The bidirectional relationship between periodontal disease and diabetes mellitus is well documented. Serum markers of periodontitis are derived from periodontal pathogens and host defence mechanisms. Elevated levels of serum LPS derived from periodontal pathogens, antibodies to LPS and LPS binding protein are detected in periodontitis compared with periodontally healthy subjects. Surrogate markers of immune-mediated responses to plaque antigens such as antibodies, MMPs, cytokines and markers of inflammation are detected. Antibodies to periodontal pathogens are indicative of systemic exposure to this antigenic stimulus. Serum screening methods for detection of markers for periodontitis would be useful in correlating with inflammatory markers from systemic diseases. The scale of inflammatory loading from periodontal disease would largely determine its impact on systemic diseases. This could account for variations in clinical presentation and response to treatment.

3. Acute phase proteins (APPs)

The APPs are synthesized and released from the liver and have a tendency to increase in response to various stimuli, including tissue injury and surgical stress. Activation of the sympathetic nervous system, hypothalamic-pituitary axis and the renin-angiotensin system, results in the release of various stress hormones.

An acute phase response is similar to that associated with inflammation, which is characterized by macrophage activation, the production of cytokines, other inflammatory mediators, APP, and mast cell activation, all of which promote inflammation (Black and Garbutt 2002). IL-1, released from macrophages activated at the site of injury appears to be the most important factor in this response. IL-1 initiates a variety of systemic reactions, including the production of APP by hepatocytes. C-reactive protein (CRP), alpha-1-acide glycoprotein (AAG), ceruloplasmin (CER), haptoglobulin (HPT), and alfa-1-antitrypsin (AT) have been shown to be APPs. Serum levels of the acute phase protein AAG, are elevated in response to a variety of acute and chronic inflammatory stimuli. Its function is unclear, but is used as an indicator of the acute phase response (Mc Pherson 2001). Recent documentation demonstrates the importance of CRP and cytokines such as IL-6 and TNF-α amongst others, in untreated chronic periodontal disease and their association with systemic diseases as effective markers of inflammation, showing reduction with disease control.

3.1 Implications of CRP and cytokines on periodontal and systemic diseases

A thorough understanding of diverse means of regulation of inflammation is imperative for effective control and treatment of inflammatory diseases. A spectrum of inflammatory mediators, including CRP, the inflammatory cytokines IL-6, IL-1β and TNF-α are thought to provide a link between periodontal and systemic diseases (Craig et al 2003). Periodontal disease is more prevalent and severe in subjects with greater levels of stress, associated with psychological and psychosocial factors (Hugoson et al 2002), affecting its progression and response to treatment.

CRP is one of the major acute-phase proteins synthesized in response to pro-inflammatory cytokines. The concentration of CRP increases with inflammation. Recently, CRPs have been found to activate complement in damaged vessel walls and to promote the formation of foam cells during the initiation of atheroma formation. IL-6 is an important activator of CRP production and is a key pro-inflammatory and immune-modulatory cytokine, secreted mainly by monocytes, macrophages and T lymphocytes recruited to sites of infection or inflammation. The pro-inflammatory and pro-coagulant properties of IL-6 are likely to play a significant role in the pathogenesis of coronary syndromes. The elevation of CRP and IL-6 suggests a plausible biological mechanism underlying the association between periodontitis and cardiovascular diseases (Ridker 2003).

Several parameters of systemic inflammation have been linked with CHD and diabetes. For example, serum levels of CRP are increased in diabetic patients and CRP has been shown to be a strong predictor of cardiovascular events, with reduced levels following periodontal treatment (Hussain-Bokhari et al 2009); elevated levels of IL-6 in peripheral blood have been associated with unstable angina and metabolic dysregulation. Periodontitis is associated with elevated systemic levels of CRP and IL-6. As periodontal infections may increase the risk of atherosclerosis and poor glycemic control in diabetic patients, it is postulated that CRP andIL-6 are some of the mediators involved in the association between periodontitis and cardiometabolic disorders (Freeman et al 2002).

Inflammation plays a pivotal role in destructive periodontitis and atherosclerotic complications, which could be exacerbated by stress (Dimsdale 2008). CRP, monitored as a major risk factor for complications of atherosclerosis, also demonstrates raised levels in periodontitis. Mean CRP is shown to be elevated significantly in subjects with extensive periodontal pocketing in comparison with those with shallower probing pocket depths. Body mass index (BMI) modifies the association of extensive periodontal disease with CRP. A BMI of 20 is predictive of a 2-fold difference in mean CRP levels between deep and shallow periodontal pocket groups (Slade et al 2003). This would be a relatively simple and effective tool for advising patients on improving periodontal and systemic health at baseline and in response to treatment.

It has been demonstrated that several parameters of systemic inflammation are associated with cardiovascular diseases and diabetes. For example, CRP has been shown to be a strong predictor of cardiovascular events, and the levels of CRP are increased in the serum of diabetic patients (Ridker 2003; Freeman et al 2002). In addition, elevated levels of IL-6 in peripheral blood have been associated with unstable angina and metabolic dysregulation (Biasucci et al 1996; Vozarova et al 2001).

Furthermore, periodontitis has been related to the elevation of systemic levels of CRP and IL-6 (Loos et al 2000; Yamazaki et al 2005; Noack et al 2001). As periodontal infections may increase the risk of atherosclerosis and poor glycemic control in diabetic patients (Beck et al 2005; Taylor et al 1996), it is postulated that CRP and interleukin-6 could be possible mediators involved in the association between periodontitis and systemic diseases.

CRP is one of the major acute-phase proteins, synthesized primarily in the liver in response to pro-inflammatory cytokines. The concentration of CRP increases with inflammation (Gabay and Kushner 1999). These acute phase proteins are known to activate complement in damaged vessel walls and to promote the formation of foam cells during the initiation of atheroma formation (Torzewski et al 2000; Du Clos 2000). IL-6 is an important activator of CRP production (Steel and Whitehead 1994) and is a key pro-inflammatory and immune-modulatory cytokine, secreted mainly by monocytes, macrophages and T lymphocytes recruited to sites of infection or inflammation. IL-6 has pro-inflammatory properties and procoagulant effects, and these properties are likely to play a role in the pathogenesis of coronary syndromes (Maseri et al 1996).

The elevation of CRP and IL-6 suggests a plausible biological mechanism underlying the association between periodontitis and cardiovascular diseases. Several inflammatory signals and markers including high sensitivity CRP (hsCRP), cytokines such as IL-1, IL-6 and TNF-α which are reported to be associated with periodontitis are also involved in atherothrombogenesis (Ridker et al 2000; Ridker & Silvertown 2008). An elevation of CRP is regarded as a biomarker of systemic inflammation and as a risk marker for CVD (Ridker 2003); hsCRP has been shown to be the strongest biomarker for predicting cardiovascular events. A recent meta-analysis of 10 cross-sectional studies showed that CRP in periodontitis patients is elevated in comparison with controls without periodontitis (Paraskevas et al 2008). In addition, the presence of *Pg* in periodontitis patients is associated with increased CRP levels, suggesting that elimination of this periodontal pathogen could reduce serum CRP levels (Pitiphat et al 2008).

Other biomarkers significantly associated with the risk of cardiovascular events are serum amyloid A, sICAM-1, IL-6, homocysteine, total cholesterol and low density lipoprotein (LDL) cholesterol (Ridker et al 2000). Among them, serum levels of IL-6 in the upper quartile of the considered normal range are independently predictive of an increased risk of premature death or future myocardial infarction, even after accounting for CRP levels in large prospective studies of healthy populations (Nakamura et al 2008). IL-6 is also a marker for identifying patients with unstable coronary artery disease independent of other risk indicators. It is relevant that both periodontal and coronary heart disease populations share similar risk factors in this context.

4. Associations of periodontal disease with coronary heart disease

A possible association of periodontal disease with coronary heart disease (CHD) has received attention in the literature, demonstrating a raised antibody titre to periodontopathic bacteria in CHD patients compared with healthy controls. When serum antibody levels in response to 12 periodontal pathogens were investigated amongst patients with CHD and moderate to severe periodontitis, the antibody response was most prevalent for *Pg* a major causative pathogen implicated in CHD as well as periodontitis (Yamazaki et al 2007). When the antibody response to two different strains *Pg* FDC381 and Su63 was analysed, periodontal patients were positive for both strains while CHD patients showed an elevated response to *Pg* Su63 but not for the *Pg* FDC381 strain. These findings demonstrate that periodontal pathogens with high virulence may affect atherogenesis; knowledge of the virulence factors of *Pg* Su63 could open new therapeutic modalites for *Pg*-associated atherosclerotic changes. DNA of *Pg* has been detected in atherosclerotic plaque suggestive of bacteraemias and endotoxaemias during the progression of periodontitis (Pussinen et al 2007a; Forner et al 2006; Nakano et al 2008). Direct effects of periodontopathic bacteria on host cells could contribute to the link between periodontitis and coronary heart disease (Schenkein et al 2000). A cause and effect relationship based on these concepts would be determined by the size of the inflammatory loading, genetic and environmental factors.

Destructive periodontal disease is associated with increased risk of atherosclerotic complications. Inflammation plays a pivotal role in periodontitis and atherosclerosis. CRP an acute phase protein monitored as a major risk factor for complications of atherosclerosis, also demonstrates raised levels in periodontitis. The effect of periodontal disease progression (>2mm attachment loss, 2 months post-baseline) on the acute-phase response has been investigated (Craig et al 2003). ELIZA (enzyme-linked immunosorbent assay) was used for measuring serum antibody and a high sensitivity (hs) CRP assay was used to measure CRP. Results indicated that periodontal disease status, severity and progression; also male gender and smoking were associated with serum IgG antibody to *Pg* rather than 5 other species. LDL cholesterol increased in disease, while HDL increased in health. Regression analysis indicated a correlation between IgG antibody to *Pg* and age, probing depth and hsCRP. Multiple sites of disease progression and raised antibody titre to *Pg* increased the odds ratio for elevated levels of hsCRP. It was concluded that destructive periodontal disease and its progression are characterized by an acute phase-response associated with relevant serum markers. These events are similar to those seen in cardiometabolic disorders, underscoring the impact of periodontal disease progression on systemic diseases in view of the contribution of extensive periodontal disease and BMI to raised CRP levels in susceptible subjects. Also highlighting the importance of cardiometabolic disorders in periodontal patients in evaluating the source of acute phase proteins and a bi-directional impact of treatment, beneficial in controlling both periodontal and systemic diseases.

Documented literature indicates the importance of periodontal disease as an inflammatory exposure relevant to the progression and outcome of systemic diseases in addition to being a disease entity with its own outcome. Clinical, microbiological and inflammatory components indicate risk for systemic diseases, associated with an inflammatory burden and its sequelae. These may not necessarily be the same parameters used to define periodontal disease. Temporal relationships between exposure and disease outcome are also relevant. Clinical parameters of periodontal disease have been correlated with serum levels of 2 systemic risk markers of cardiovascular disease, soluble intercellular adhesion molecule (sICAM) as a measure of vascular stress and serum CRP as a measure of an acute phase response (Beck & Offenbacher 2002). This was part of a cross-sectional study of the relationship between periodontal disease and cardiovascular disease in the Dental Atherosclerosis Risk in Communities (ARIC) study. It is relevant that while attachment loss, probing depth (PD) and bleeding on probing (BOP) were individually associated with sICAM and CRP, only BOP was significant for sICAM when all 3 were included in the model; PD was significant for CRP. Both clinical parameters PD and BOP are more robust in estimating the extent of systemic inflammation than categorization of early, moderate and severe periodontal disease based on bone support or attachment loss which may not correlate with the extent of inflammation at the time of examination. A tooth centered approach to periodontitis may not fit the mould of systemic inflammation where relevant parameters such as PD and BOP would fit the underlying mechanisms and temporal sequelae affecting systemic outcome of periodontal inflammation. Study design and parameters measured could account for some discrepancies in the reported literature, on systemic markers for periodontal and cardiometabolic disorders and response to treatment in this context.

In view of the association between systemic levels of the inflammatory markers CRP, fibrinogen and WBC with a risk of CHD, also demonstrated for periodontal disease, the effect of periodontal treatment on these systemic parameters has been investigated in subjects with or without CHD. The periodontal paramenters, bleeding on probing (BOP) and probing depths (PD) were measured in subjects with or without coronary heart disease (Hussain-Bokhari et al 2009). All subjects received non-surgical periodontal therapy including plaque control measures and thorough root surface debridement. There were significant reductions in BOP, PD and systemic inflammatory markers in both groups after periodontal therapy. This could contribute to decreased risk for CHD in treated periodontal patients. This profile is valuable in the planning of large-scale intervention trials to reduce risk for CHD with periodontal intervention.

Non-surgical periodontal treatment for periodontal pocket reduction induces systemic changes in several biochemical markers that reflect the risk for atherosclerosis. In a study where successful periodontal treatment with pocket reduction was reported in adult periodontal patients with severe periodontitis, serum glucose, lipids and markers of systemic inflammation were not significantly altered after 3 months. At one year, HDL-C concentrations were significantly increased and LDL-C concentrations decreased with concurrent reduction in IL-18 and interferon δ levels (Buhlin et al 2009). Both mechanical periodontal debridement and treatment with a nonsteroidal anti-inflammatory drug appeared to affect serum glycoprotein markers of infection and inflammation. Steroids and disease-modifying anti-rheumatic drugs are also effective in reducing levels of CRP by 30–70% which have implications for periodontal disease progression in patients presenting with co-morbidities. The results of some studies indicate that nonsteroidal anti-inflammatory drugs had minimal effects on CRP, although others have reported that flurbiprofen decreased CRP levels in a subset of patients. A change of 150% (CRP) or 70% (haptoglobin) in the levels of these acute-phase reactants indicate significance in the context of individual subject variation.

5. Periodontitis and dyslipidaemia

5.1 Psychosomatic aspects of obesity

There is growing evidence in the recent literature that obesity and periodontitis may be triggered or exacerbated by adverse social factors and certain psychological pathologies, traits and behaviors. Dental practitioners should therefore give consideration to the fact that overweight patients who present with impaired periodontal status may also be experiencing anxiety, depression, and impaired satisfaction with life.

Although periodontal disease is affected by behaviour determined by social and psychological factors, periodontists have not seriously considered psychosocial pathways in its etiology, diagnosis, and treatment. However, a sound understanding of the psychosocial pathways of behavior strongly linked to periodontal disease, and mechanisms whereby psychological factors affect the response of periodontal tissues to pathogens, is essential for diagnosis and improving the effectiveness of interventions (Sheiham & Nicolau 2005); which could also affect impact on co-morbidities.

5.2 Mechanisms affecting dyslipidaemia, diabetes and periodontitis

The inflammatory loading from periodontal disease could compromise cardiometabolic and autoimmune diseases which are driven by inflammatory mechanisms leading to oxidative stress-induced tissue and organ damage. The bi-directional relationship between periodontal disease and diabetes mellitus is well documented. Serum markers of periodontitis are derived from periodontal pathogens and host defence mechanisms. Elevated levels of serum lipopolysaccharide (LPS) derived from periodontal pathogens, antibodies to LPS and LPS binding protein are detected in periodontitis compared with periodontally healthy subjects; and surrogate markers of immune mediated responses to plaque antigens such as antibodies, matrix metalloproteinases, cytokines and markers of inflammation. Antibodies to periodontal pathogens are indicative of systemic exposure to this antigenic stimulus. Serum screening methods for detection of markers for periodontitis would be useful in correlating with inflammatory markers from systemic diseases.

Several parameters of systemic inflammation have been linked with CHD and diabetes. For example, serum levels of CRP are increased in diabetic patients and CRP has been shown to be a strong predictor of cardiovascular events; elevated levels of IL-6 in peripheral blood have been associated with unstable angina and metabolic dysregulation. Periodontitis is associated with elevated systemic levels of CRP and IL-6. As periodontal infections may increase the risk of atherosclerosis and poor glycaemic control in diabetic patients, it is postulated that CRP and IL-6 are some of the mediators involved in the association between periodontitis and cardiometabolic disorders.

Plasma fatty acids, an important cardiovascular biomarker, showed an altered profile, particularly when concentrations were measured in periodontitis patients, who presented with higher amounts of total fatty acids, saturated fatty acids, MUFA, and n-6 PUFA than controls. Dietary fat may affect immune responses and determine susceptibility of lipoprotein to oxidation, which affects the activation of adhesion molecules and other inflammatory agents (Von Schacky & Harris 2007).

Recently, a new association between lipid peroxidation, oxidative stress and periodontitis has been suggested and it is also related to the clinical periodontal status (Bullon et al. 2008). Evidence suggests an association between inflammatory markers, such as interleukins, oxidative stress-related parameters, and CHD events. It has been hypothesized that CHD may be triggered by systemic mechanisms, in addition to local inflammatory factors, and chronic periodontal infection is one of the possibilities to be considered. Here, this hypothesis is fully supported by reported results on oxidative stress status, fatty acid profile, inflammatory interleukines and adhesion molecules. Indeed, the high correlations found between plasma triacylglycerols, LDLc, saturated fatty acids, polyunsaturated fatty acids, total amount of fatty acids and coenzyme Q10; with some periodontal data such as probing depths, gingival margin location and clinical attachment levels, leads to the conclusion that there is a close association between periodontitis, plasma fatty acids profile and an increase in metabolic risk factors for CHD.

Periodontal treatment influences blood lipid levels in a manner which is consistent with a decreased risk for CHD. HDL-C concentrations increased and LDL-C concentrations decreased significantly (Pussinen et al 2004). Previous intervention studies suggest that periodontal treatment decreases the levels of inflammatory markers such as CRP, fibrinogen and IL-6 (Pussinen et al 2004; Montebugnoli et al 2005). However, these studies were fairly small and the follow-up periods were only between 3 and 6 months. It would be important to carry out large scale, long-term studies on this theme considering the potential impact of controlling periodontal disease progression on coronary heart disease.

The predictive and prognostic value of CRP and fibrinogen as risk factors for cardiovascular disease is well-documented and could be used to stratify patients for this purpose. Moreover recent data is also suggestive of a primary role for insulin resistance in the pathogenesis of metabolic syndrome and prediction of cardiovascular events. Glycaemic indices could function as significant markers of the incidence of new cardiac events in subjects who may not be diagnosed diabetics. Although the traditional markers, reduced HDL-c, elevated LDL-c, triglycerides and visceral adiposity are associated with insulin resistance, it may independently influence the progression of coronary atherosclerotic plaques in asymptomatic patients, via endothelial dysfunction. Insulin resistance seems to have a significant prognostic role and informative for preventive care in acute coronary syndrome (Caccamo et al 2010). These mechanisms could impact on periodontal disease progression and therapeutic targets.

A common pathological pathway associated with systemic inflammation and insulin resistance link cardiometabolic disorders (Pischon et al 2007; Saito & Shimazaki 2007). The non-glycosylated polypeptide leptin synthesized primarily by adipocytes has several regulatory functions, with increased production during inflammatory responses. Its dual characteristics as a hormone and a cytokine provide a link between neuroendocrine and immune systems. It plays an important role in the pathogenesis of autoimmune inflammatory conditions such as diabetes (Lago et al 2008; Soory 2010a) and rheumatoid arthritis (Otero et al 2006; Soory 2010b). Metabolic syndrome is diagnosed in individuals with a risk of cardiovascular disease, comprising a cluster of abdominal obesity, hypertension, impaired glucose tolerance, hyper-insulinaemia and dyslipidaemia (Eckel et al 2005).

A significant relationship between oxidative stress and metabolic syndrome has been demonstrated in humans when compared with normo-lipidaemic subjects. Systemic oxidative stress and insulin resistance have been shown to correlate with attenuated antioxidant capacity. The effects of a hyper-inflammatory state seen in severe uncontrolled periodontitis and its impact on organs distant from the focus of inflammation are well documented in the context of oxidative stress-inducing mechanisms and the role of antioxidants (Soory 2009). Several cytokines are involved in the mediation of insulin resistance, TNF-α in particular (Tilg and Moschen 2008). In the context of substances derived from oxidative damage, plasma lipid peroxidation plays an important role in the diabetic periodontal patient (Sonoki et al 2006) with decreased lipid peroxidation following periodontal therapy. The pathogenesis and progression of periodontal disease is escalated by advanced glycaemic end products AGE (Takeda et al 2006), receptor for AGE (RAGE) which is highly expressed in periodontal tissues and AGE/RAGE interactions in uncontrolled diabetics. Using a diabetogenic cell culture model of well characterized osteoblasts, it has been demonstrated that the oxidative effects of AGE and nicotine were overcome by the antioxidant glutathione (Rahman & Soory 2006). Preliminary studies in pro-oxidant cultures of oral periosteal fibroblasts and well characterized osteoblasts demonstrated that co-enzyme Q10, phytoestrogens and the antioxidant Pycnogenol derived from pine bark, attenuated oxidative stress induced by nicotine in this model (Figuero-Ruiz et al 2006); indicating a possible role for these antioxidants in the adjunctive therapy of inflammatory diseases characterized by a pro-oxidant profile.

An uncontrolled immune response could have a synergistic effect in periodontal patients with co-existing DM (Nassar et al 2007). Effective treatment of periodontitis could improve diabetic parameters such as glycated haemoglobin (Grossi and Genco 1998). Hyperglycaemia induces oxidative stress via protein kinase-dependent activation of enzymes that catalyse the generation of reactive oxygen species from PMNs in diabetic patients with a direct bearing on periodontitis in uncontrolled diabetics (Karima et al 2005). Fundamental mechanisms associated with an over-exuberant host response are synergized in diabetic and pre-diabetic obese subjects prone to severe periodontal disease (Nishimura et al 2007).

5.3 Role of leptin in periodontal and cardiometabolic diseases

An association between periodontal disease severity and serum and gingival crevicular fluid leptin levels is well documented (Karthekayan et al 2007a,b; Bozkurt et al 2006). There is less information on the effects of periodontal treatment on serum leptin levels. Adipose tissue cells secrete over 50 bioactive substances including TNF-α and IL-6 collectively known as adipokines (Ritchie 2007; Saxlin et al 2008). Obese individuals have raised levels of circulating TNF-α and IL-6 compared with those of normal weight, with some reduction in cytokine levels on weight reduction (Ziccardi et al 2002).

There is documented evidence of a significant association between periodontitis and dyslipidaemia and that metabolic syndrome increases the risk for periodontitis; suggesting that subjects exhibiting components of metabolic syndrome should be encouraged to undergo regular periodontal examination. There are several mechanisms whereby adipose tissue mass and secretion of adipokines including leptin affect the host response. Leptin levels correlate with increasing periodontal pocket probing depths. Visceral adipose tissue in particular is an important organ that secretes several bioactive substances known as adipocytokines, including TNF-α, which contributes to periodontal disease progression. Anxiety states could correlate with visceral fat and its association with periodontal disease.

A few reports have proposed several mechanisms by which obesity can directly affect periodontal tissue. Obesity affects host immunity (Marti et al 2001), and the relationship between adipose tissue and the immune system is believed to be related to the secretion of numerous adipokines, including leptin, amounts of which correlate with fat mass (Caspar-Bauguil et al 2006). It has been demonstrated that human leptin is present within healthy and marginally inflamed gingiva, and that it could be released coincident with vascular expansion. Gingivae, in addition to adipose tissue may be a source of circulating leptin (Johnson & Serio 2001). Recent studies have indicated that adipose tissue, especially visceral adipose tissue, is an important organ that secretes several bioactive substances known as adipocytokines, including tumor necrosis factor-α, which may enhance periodontal destruction (Saito & Shimazaki 2007).

The relationship between body mass index and events leading to risk of CHD is made complex by several factors; some of which include potential confounding factors such as smoking, medication and weight loss due to prevalent disease. The impact of body mass index on CHD is attenuated when mediators of this risk such as diabetes, hypertension and hyperlipidaemia are accounted for. It is relevant that markers of inflammation may differentiate between fatal and non-fatal events, being more strongly associated with fatal events (Logue et al 2011). The cardiovascular disease markers of inflammation, CRP and IL-6 are more significantly linked with fatal than non-fatal events (Sattar et al 2009), CRP being a weaker link than IL-6. If inflammation poses a greater risk of cardiovascular mortality, it would apply to adiposity as a source and mediator of inflammatory markers (Logue et al 2011) with important implications for treatment targets which would also apply to periodontal disease control. In addition to severity there could be subtle differences in the mechanisms involved. Treatment outcome with weight loss interventions would be a relevant area for investigation. The biological effect of obesity as a nidus of inflammation is an important one, likely to affect its role as a cardiovascular risk factor. In the context of adipose tissue functioning as an endocrine organ and releasing pro-inflammatory cytokines (Hotamisligil & Erbay 2008), obesity may be regarded as a low-grade inflammatory state (Welsh et al 2010; Cartier et al 2008).

The effects of periodontal treatment on serum levels of leptin and other cytokines adiponectin, TNF-α, IL-6 and CRP have been investigated in patients with chronic periodontitis before and after non-surgical periodontal treatment (Shimada et al 2010). The possible role of periodontal disease in producing serum leptin was investigated by determining serum leptin levels in patients with chronic periodontitis and correlated with other inflammatory markers for comparison with serum leptin levels following periodontal treatment. Serum leptin was associated with mean probing depth, clinical attachment level, alveolar bone loss and body mass index, with significant correlations between serum leptin, IL-6 and CRP levels. There were significant differences in serum leptin, IL-6 and CRP levels between healthy and chronic periodontitis patients. Non-surgical periodontal treatment was effective in reducing serum leptin, IL-6 and CRP with significant decreases in their serum levels. The efficacy of priodontal treatment in reducing these parameters is suggestive of common mediators in the progression of periodontal disease and metabolic syndrome, providing an effective therapeutic target.

Other workers have also reported that serum levels of hsCRP and IL-6 are significantly higher in periodontitis patients with decreased levels following treatment (Yamazaki et al 2005; Nakajima et al. 2010). However there was no significant association between TNF-α levels and periodontitis. An association between serum TNF-α, IL-l-6, body weight and periodontitis has been reported (Saxlin et al 2008). They suggest that IL-6 rather than TNF-α, correlated with periodontal probing depth, BMI and periodontal disease progression. The lack of significant change in serum TNF-α levels in periodontitis patients after non-surgical periodontal treatment has been reported (Ikezawa-Suzuki et al 2008), although high levels are detected in GCF or gingival tissue of periodontitis patients. It would appear that IL-6 shows clearer associations between periodontitis and systemic disease. In addition to IL-6,

IL-1 and LPS, also act as pro-inflammatory stimuli in regulating mRNA expression and circulating levels of leptin.

Leptin is also responsible for directly stimulating the production of cytokines such as IL-6 which in turn could influence the synthesis of CRP. Human CRP could inhibit receptor binding of leptin, blocking cell signalling activities; physiological concentrations of leptin stimulate CRP expression in human hepatocytes in a dose-dependent manner. This is a potential mechanism for leptin resistance whereby CRP in the circulation binds to leptin and alters its physiological functions (Chen et al 2006). It is uncertain whether changes in these cytokines reflect a common underlying cause such as obesity. A raised level of leptin during periodontal inflammation amongst other infectious / inflammatory conditions is suggestive of its role in immunolgically mediated host responses.

Leptin is also involved in modulating bone homeostasis. It stimulates bone formation directly via differentiation and proliferation of osteoblasts. It also enhances the lifespan of osteoblasts by preventing apoptosis (Gordeladze et al 2002). Leptin is implicated in bone modulatory activities in addition to local inflammation in the periodontium. Raised serum leptin levels are a risk factor for cardiovascular disease (Parhami et al 2001; Yamagishi et al 2001). Increased levels of serum leptin seen during the progression of periodontal disease, are suggestive of the influence of progressive periodontitis on cardiovascular disease. Larger studies are required to establish the connection between periodontitis and metabolic syndrome mediated by leptin.

6. Immune markers common to periodontal and cardiometabolic diseases

The effect of periodontal therapy on gene expression of peripheral blood monocytes has been investigated (Papapanou et al 2007). The time scale was 1 week before treatment, at initiation of treatment and post-treatment at 6 and 10 weeks. The periodontal status was established at baseline and subgingival plaque samples were obtained. Periodontal treatment was completed within 6 weeks. Expression profiles of monocyte RNA were determined within the stipulated time frame. Treatment resulted in improved periodontal status and reduced numbers of pathogens. About a third of patients showed significant changes in gene expression of relevance to cell signalling, apoptosis and innate immunity, consistent with a systemic anti-inflammatory effect. These responses could have a positive impact on periodontal patients presenting with cardiometabolic diseases.

There is an association between premature atherosclerosis and rheumatoid arthritis. The concept that elevated levels of inflammatory markers such as IL-6, IL-1α, TNF-α, E-selectin, ICAM-1, MMP-9 and VCAM-1 identified in atherosclerosis, are associated with the severity of coronary atherosclerosis in patients with RA, was investigated (Rho et al 2009). Levels of inflammatory mediators, clinical variables and coronary artery calcification were measured in patients with RA and in control subjects. Most of the above markers were significantly elevated in patients with RA when compared with controls; and a significant association between concentrations of IL-6 and TNF-α with greater amounts of coronary calcium. These effects were distinctly different from those of controls. It was concluded that TNF-α and IL-6 are significantly associated with the severity of sub-clinical atherosclerosis in patients with RA.

The emergence of periodontal medicine has increased interest in defining the behaviour of peripheral blood cells in periodontitis subjects in comparison with a healthy group. *E. coli* LPS-stimulated peripheral blood monocytes (PBMC) from subjects with periodontitis present a different pattern of cytokine release when compared to PBMC from healthy subjects, with significantly greater levels of TNF-α and IL-6 released by PBMC isolated from periodontitis subjects (Goncalves et al 2010). This phenomenon could have implications locally, in periodontitis as well as in systemic diseases, in response to circulating levels of LPS from periodontal pathogens.

Periodontopathic bacteria have been detected in 52% of atherosclerotic specimens. Cytomegalovirus (CMV) and / or *Chlamidophila pneumoniae* were detected in 4% of specimens (Chen et al 2008). After adjusting for age, gender, diabetes and smoking, periodontitis increased the risk of peripheral arterial disease by 5-fold. There were preliminary indications that periodontitis was associated with increased serum IL-6 and TNF-α concentrations which further reinforces a systemic link.

7. Conclusions

Psychosomatic pathways in the progression of periodontal and systemic diseases may not have received serious consideration. However, a sound understanding of psychosocial determinants have important implications on the host response to antigens and disease mechanisms instrumental in their progression. These concepts have far-reaching consequences in improving the efficacy of diagnoses and treatment interventions for periodontal and systemic diseases.

The schematic diagram below demonstrates that anxiety states could contribute to diseases with psychosomatic implications such as coronary heart disease (CHD), diabetes mellitus (DM) and periodontal disease. Progression of periodontal disease and its response to treatment could influence the progression of cardiometabolic disorders in a bi-directional manner. These pathways and their ramifications provide tremendous potential for future work, which is likely to clarify increasing interest in the relevance of these connections.

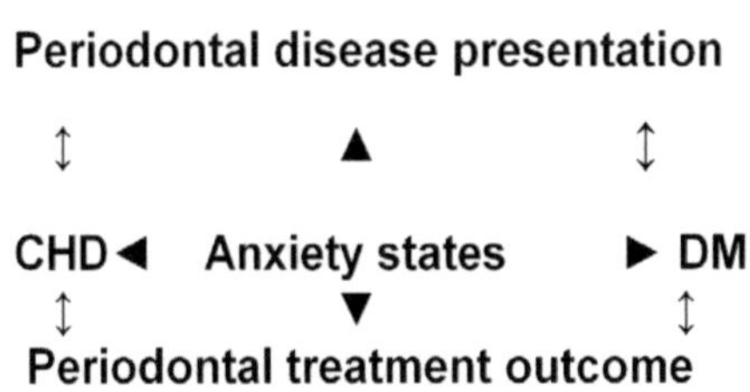

Comprehensive documentation of biological and physiological mechanisms by which psychosocial stress contributes to periodontal destruction provides biological rationale for this relationship. Psychosocial implications of cardiometabolic diseases addressed, converge on an inflammatory nidus as the driving force of disease progression, providing treatment options which attenuate the focus of inflammation. A relevant profile of inflammatory markers discussed provides common ground for targeting prognosis and therapeutic outcome in periodontal and cardiometabolic diseases with psychosomatic determinants, in a bi-directional manner.

Effects of treatment of periodontal disease show promising pointers towards reducing potential systemic inflammatory loading by reducing the levels of inflammatory mediators implicated in its pathogenesis. Considering the systemic impact of periodontal inflammation, effective periodontal treatment could enhance treatment outcome of cardiometabolic co-morbidities in periodontal patients. A composite profile of inflammatory agents is likely to be more useful than individual agents in determining periodontal treatment outcome and its systemic implications. The unique role of periodontitis as a potential core nucleus of inflammation with systemic implications as discussed and extraordinary potential for treatment outcome have global implications. This has received universal documentation in the literature, underscoring the importance of early detection and intervention. Genetic and environmental predisposition could account for some of the diversity observed, in disease presentation and treatment responses.

8. References

Abeywardena MY, Leifert WR, Warnes KE, Varghese JN & Head RJ. (2009). Cardiovascular biology of interleukin-6. *Current Pharmaceutical Design*, vol.15, No. 15,1809–21.

Albandar JM. (2002). Global risk factors and risk indicators for periodontal diseases. *Periodontology 2000*, Vol. 29, No.1,177-206.

Aviles H, Johnson MT & Monroy FP. (2004). Effects of cold stress on spleen cell proliferation and cytokine production during chronic *Toxoplasma gondii* infection. *Neuroimmunomodulation,* Vol.11, No. 2, 93–102.

Avitsur R, Kavelaars A, Heijnen C & Sheridan JF. (2005). Social stress and the regulation of tumor necrosis factor-alpha secretion. *Brain Behaviour and Immunity,* Vol.19, No. 4, 311-7.

Bailey MT, Kinsey SG, Padgett DA, Sheridan JF & Leblebicioglu B. (2009). Social stress enhances IL-1beta and TNF-alpha production by *Porphyromonas gingivalis* lipopolysaccharide-stimulated CD11b+ cells. *Physiology and Behaviour,* Vol. 98, No. 3, 351-8.

Basterzi AD, Yazici K, Buturak V, Cimen B, Yazici A, Eskandari G, Tot Acar S & Tasdelen B. (2009). Effects of venlafaxine and fluoxetine on lymphocyte subsets in patients with major depressive disorder: A flow cytometric analysis. *Progress in Neuro-psychopharmacology and Biological Psychiatry,* doi: 10.1016/ j.jpnpbp.2009.09.025.

Beck JD, Eke P, Heiss G, Madianos P, Couper D, Lin D, Moss K, Elter J & Offenbacher S. (2005). Periodontal disease and coronary heart disease: a reappraisal of the exposure. *Circulation,* Vol. 112, No. 1, 19–24.

Beck JD & Offenbacher S. (2002). Relationships among clinical measures of periodontal disease and their associations with systemic markers. *Annals of Periodontology,* Vol. 7, No. 1, 79-89.

Beck JD & Offenbacher S. (2005). Systemic effects of periodontitis: epidemiology of periodontal disease and cardiovascular disease. *Journal of Periodontology,* Vol. 76, No. 11 Suppl., 2089–100.

Behl Y, Siqueira M, Ortiz J, Li J, Desta T, Faibish D & Graves DT. (2008). Activation of the acquired immune response reduces coupled bone formation in response to a periodontal pathogen. *Journal of Immunology,* Vol. 181, No.12, 8711-8718.

Belay T & Sonnenfeld G. (2002). Differential effects of catecholamines on *in vitro* growth of pathogenic bacteria. *Life Sciences,* Vol. 71, No. 4, 447–56.

Biasucci LM, Vitelli A, Liuzzo G, Altamura S, Caligiuri G, Monaco C, Rebuzzi AG, Ciliberto G & Maseri A. (1996). Elevated levels of interleukin-6 in unstable angina. *Circulation*, Vol. 94, No. 2, 874–877.

Black PH & Garbutt LD. (2002). Stress, inflamation and cardiovascular disease. *Journal of Psychosomatic Research*, Vol. 52, No. 1, 1- 23.

Bozkurt FY, Ay ZY, Sutcu R, Delibasx N & Demirel R. (2006). Gingival crevicular fluid leptin levels in periodontitis patients with long-term and heavy smoking. *Journal of Periodontology*, Vol. 77, No. 4, 634-640.

Buhlin K, Hultin M, Norderyd O, Persson L, Pockley AG, Pirkko J. Pussinen PJ, Rabe P, Björn Klinge B & Gustafsson A. (2009). Periodontal treatment influences risk markers for atherosclerosis in patients with severe periodontitis, *Atherosclerosis*, Vol. 206, No. 2, 518–522.

Bullon P, Morillo JM, Ramirez-Tortosa MC, Quiles JL, Newman H & Battino M. (2008). Metabolic syndrome and periodontitis: is oxidative stress a common link? *Journal of Dental Research*, Vol. 87, No. 1, 79-83.

Caccamo G, Bonura F, Bonura F, Vitale G, Novo G, Evola S, Evola G, Grisanti MR & Novo S. (2010). Insulin resistance and acute coronary syndrome. *Athero*sclerosis, Vol. 211, No. 2, 672-5.

Cartier A, Lemieux I, Almeras N, Tremblay A, Bergeron J & Després JP. (2008). Visceral obesity and plasma glucose-insulin homeostasis: contributions of interleukin-6 and tumor necrosis factor-alpha in men. *Journal of Clinical Endocrinology and Metabolism*, Vol. 93, No. 5, 1931-8.

Caspar-Bauguil S, Cousin B, André M, Nibbelink M, Galinier A, Periquet B, Casteilla L & Pénicaud L. (2006). Weight-dependent changes of immune system in adipose tissue: importance of leptin. *Experimental Cell Research*, Vol. 312, No. 12, 2195-2202.

Chen K, Li FH, Li J, Cai H, Strom S, Bisello A, Kelley DE, Friedman-Einat M, Skibinski GA, McCrory MA, Szalai AJ & Zhao AZ. (2006). Induction of leptin resistance through direct interaction of C-reactive protein with leptin. *Nature Medicine*, Vol. 12, No. 4, 425-432.

Chen Y-W, Umeda M, Nagasawa T, Takeuchi Y, Huang Y, Inoue Y, Iwai T, Izumi Y & Ishikawa I. (2008). Periodontitis may increase the risk of peripheral arterial disease. *European Journal of Vascular and Endovascular Surgery*, Vol. 35, No. 2, 153-158.

Cizza G, Primma S & Csako G. Depression as a risk factor for osteoporosis. (2009). *Trends in Endocrinology and Metabolism*, Vol. 20, No. 8, 367-373.

Haffajee AD. (2003). Relationship of destructive periodontal disease to the acute-phase response. *Journal of Periodontology*, Vol. 74, No. 7, 1007-16.

Deinzer R, Forster P, Fuck L, Herforth A, Stiller-Winkler R & Idel H. (1999). Increase of crevicular interleukin 1beta under academic stress at experimental gingivitis sites and at sites of perfect oral hygiene. *Journal of Clinical Periodontology*, Vol. 26, No. 1, 1–8.

De Nardin E. (2001). The role of inflammatory and immunological mediators in periodontitis and cardiovascular disease. *Annals of Periodontology*, Vol. 6, No. 1, 30–40.

Dimsdale JE. (2008). Psychological stress and cardiovascular disease. *Journal of the American College of Cardiology*, Vol. 51, No. 13, 1237–46.

Du Clos TW. (2000). Function of C-reactive protein. *Annals of Medicine* , Vol. 32, No. 4, 274–278.

Eckel RH, Grundy SM & Zimmet PZ. (2005). The metabolic syndrome. *Lancet*, Vol. 365, No. 9468, 1415-1428.

Figuero-Ruiz E, Soory M, Cerero R & Bascones A. (2006). Oxidant / antioxidant interactions of nicotine, Coenzyme Q10, Pycnogenol and phytoestrogens in oral periosteal fibroblasts and MG63 osteoblasts, *Steroids*, Vol. 71, No. 13-14, 1062-1072.

Forner L, Larsen T, Kilian M & Holmstrup P. (2006). Incidence of bacteremia after chewing, tooth brushing and scaling in individuals with periodontal inflammation. *Journal of Clinical Periodontology*, Vol. 33, No. 6, 401-7.

Freeman DJ, Norrie J, Caslake MJ, Gaw A, Ford I, Lowe GD, O'Reilly DS, Packard CJ & Sattar N. (2002). C-reactive protein is an independent predictor of risk for the development of diabetes in the West of Scotland Coronary Prevention Study. *Diabetes*, Vol. 51, No. 5, 1596- 1600.

Gabay C & Kushner I. (1999). Acute-phase proteins and other systemic response to inflammation. *New England Journal of Medicine*, Vol. 340, No. 6, 448-454.

Gamonal J, Sanz M, O'Connor A, Acevedo A, Suarez I, Sanz A, Martinez B & Silva A. (2003). Delayed neutrophil apoptosis in chronic periodontitis patients. *Journal of Clinical Periodontology*, Vol. 30, No. 7, 616–23.

Genco RJ, Ho AW, Grossi SG, Dunford RG & Tedesco LA. (1999). Relationship of stress, distress and inadequate coping behaviors to periodontal disease. *Journal of Periodontology*, Vol. 70, No. 7, 711–23.

Giannopoulou C, Kamma JJ & Mombelli A. (2003). Effect of inflammation, smoking and stress on gingival crevicular fluid cytokine level. *Journal of Clinical Periodontology*, Vol. 30, No. 2, 145–53.

Gibson III FC & Genco CA. (2007). *Porphyromonas gingivalis* mediated periodontal disease and atherosclerosis: disparate diseases with commonalities in pathogenesis through TLRs. *Current Pharmaceutical Design*, Vol. 13, No. 36, 3665–75.

Gibson III FC, Ukai T & Genco CA. (2008). Engagement of specific innate immune signaling pathways during *Porphyromonas gingivalis* induced chronic inflammation and atherosclerosis. *Frontiers in Bioscience*, Vol. 13, No. 1, 2041–59.

Golub LM, Payne JB, Reinhardt RA & Nieman G. (2006). Can systemic diseases co-induce (not just exacerbate) periodontitis? A hypothetical "two-hit" model. *Journal of Dental Research*, Vol. 85, No. 2, 102–5.

Gonçalves TO, Costa D, Brodskyn CI, Duarte PM, Neto JBC & Nogueira-Filho G. (2010). Release of cytokines by stimulated peripheral blood mononuclear cells in chronic periodontitis. *Archives of Oral Biology*, Vol. 55, No. 12, 975 - 980.

Gordeladze JO, Drevon CA, Syversen U & Reseland JE. (2002). Leptin stimulates human osteoblastic cell proliferation, de novo collagen synthesis, and mineralization: Impact on differentiation markers, apoptosis, and osteoclastic signaling. *Journal of Cellular Biochemistry*, Vol. 85, No. 4, 825-836.

Graves DT & Cochran D. (2003). The contribution of interleukin-1 and tumor necrosis factor to periodontal tissue destruction. *Journal of Periodontology*, Vol. 74, No. 3, 391-401.

Grossi SG & Genco RJ. (1998). Periodontal disease and diabetes mellitus: a two-way relationship. *Annals of Periodontology*, Vol. 3, No. 1, 51–61.

Haraszthy VI, Zambon JJ, Trevisan M, Zeid M & Genco RJ. (2000). Identification of periodontal pathogens in atheromatous plaques. *Journal of Periodontology*, Vol. 71, No. 10, 1554-60.

Hilgert JB, Hugo FN, Bandeira DR & Bozzetti MC. (2006). Stress, cortisol, and periodontitis in a population aged 50 years and over. *Journal of Dental Research*, Vol. 85, No. 4, 324-8.

Hotamisligil GS & Erbay E. (2008). Nutrient sensing and inflammation in metabolic diseases.*Nature Reviews Immunology*, Vol. 8, No. 12, 923-34.

Hugoson A, Ljungquist B & Breivik T. (2002). The relationship of some negative events and psychological factors to periodontal disease in an adult Swedish population 50 to 80 years, of age. *Journal of Clinical Periodontology* , Vol. 29, No. 3, 247–253.

Hussain Bokhari SA, Khan AA, Tatakis DN, Azhar M, Hanif M & Izhar M. (2009). Non-surgical periodontal therapy lowers serum inflammatory markers: a pilot study. *Journal of Periodontology*, Vol. 80, No. 10, 1574-80.

Ikezawa-Suzuki I, Shimada Y, Tai H, Komatsu Y, Tanaka A & Yoshie H. (2008). Effects of treatment on soluble tumour necrosis factor receptor type 1 and 2 in chronic periodontitis. *Journal of Clinical Periodontology*, Vol. 35, No. 11, 961-968.

Ishisaka A, Ansai T, Soh I, Inenaga K, Awano S, Yoshida A, Hamasaki T, Sonoki K, Takata Y, Nishikara T & Takehara T. (2008). Association of cortisol and dehydroepiandrosterone sulphate levels in serum with periodontal status in older Japanese adults. *Journal of Clinical Periodontology*, Vol. 35, No. 10, 853–61.

Ishisaka A, Ansai T, Soh I, Inenaga K, Yoshida A, Shigeyama C, Awano S, Hamasaki T, Sonoki K, Takata Y & Takehara T. (2007). Association of salivary levels of cortisol and dehydroepiandrosterone with periodontitis in older Japanese adults. *Journal of Periodontology*, Vol. 78, No. 9, 1767–73.

Johannsen A, Rylander G, Söder B & Asberg M. (2006). Dental plaque, gingival inflammation, and elevated levels of interleukin-6 and cortisol in gingival crevicular fluid from women with stress-related depression and exhaustion. *Journal of Periodontology*, Vol. 77, No. 8, 1403–9.

Johnson RB & Serio FG. (2001). Leptin within healthy and diseased human gingiva. *Journal of Periodontology*, Vol. 72, No. 9, 1254-1257.

Kamma JJ, Giannopoulou C, Vasdekis VG & Mombelli A. (2004). Cytokine profile in gingival crevicular fluid of aggressive periodontitis: influence of smoking and stress. *Journal of Clinical Periodontology*, Vol. 31, No. 10, 894–902.

Karima M, Kantarci A, Ohira T, Hasturk H, Jones VL, Nam BH, Malabanan A, Trackman PC, Badwey JA & Van Dyke TE. (2005). Enhanced superoxide release and elevated protein Kinase C activity in neutrophil from diabetic patients: association with periodontitis. *Journal of Leukocyte Biology*, Vol. 78, No. 4, 862-70.

Karthikeyan BV & Pradeep AR. (2007a). Gingival crevicular fluid and serum leptin: Their relationship to periodontal health and disease. *Journal of Clinical Periodontology,* Vol. 34, No. 6, 467-472.

Karthikeyan BV & Pradeep AR. (2007b). Leptin levels in gingival crevicular fluid in periodontal health and disease. *Journal of Periodontal Research,* Vol. 42, No. 4, 300-304.

Kiecolt-Glaser JK, Preacher KJ, MacCallum RC, Arkinson C, Malarkey WB & Glaser R. (2003). Chronic stress and age-related increases in the proinflammatory cytokine IL-6. *Proceedings of the National Academy of Science* USA, Vol. 100, No. 15, 9090–9095.

Kinane DF, Riggio MP, Walker KF, MacKenzie D & Shearer B. (2005). Bacteraemia following periodontal procedures. *Journal of Clinical Periodontology,* Vol. 32, No. 7, 708–13.

Kubera M, Lin AH, Kenis G, Bosmans E, van Bockstaele D, Maes M. (2001). Anti-inflammatory effects of antidepressants through suppression of the interferon-gamma/interleukin-10 production ratio. *Journal of Clinical Psychopharmacology,* Vol. 21, No. 2, 199-206.

Lago R, Gomez R, Lago F, Gomez-Reino J & Gualillo O. (2008). Leptin beyond body weight regulation–Current concepts concerning its role in immune function and inflammation. *Cellular Immunology,* Vol. 252, No. 1-2, 139-145.

Logue J, Murray HM, Welsh P, Shepherd J, Packard C, Macfarlane P, Cobbe S, Ford I, Sattar N. (2011). Obesity is associated with fatal coronary heart disease independently of traditional risk factors and deprivation. *Heart,* in press [Epub ahead of print].

Loos BG, Craandijik J, Hoek FJ, Wertheim-van Dillen ME & Van Der Velden U. (2000). Elevation of systemic markers related to cardiovascular diseases in the peripheral blood of periodontitis patients. *Journal of Periodontology,* Vol. 71, No. 10, 1528–1534.

Lyte M. (2004). Microbial endocrinology and infectious disease in the 21st century. *Trends in Microbiology,* Vol. 12, No. 1, 14–20.

Maes M. (2001). The immunoregulatory effects of antidepressants. *Human Psychopharmacology,* Vol. 16, No. 1, 95-103.

Martí A, Marcos A & Martínez JA. (2001). Obesity and immune function relationships. *Obesity Reviews,* Vol. 2, No. 2, 131- 140.

Maseri A, Biasucci LM & Liuzzo G. (1996). Inflammation in ischaemic heart disease. *British Medical Journal,* Vol. 312, No. 7038, 1049–1050.

Mawhorter SD & Lauer MA (2001). Is atherosclerosis an infectious disease? *Cleveland Clinic Journal of Medicine* Vol. 68, No. 5, 449–458.

Mc Pherson RA. Specific proteins. In: Henry JB, editor. Clinical diagnosis and management by laboratory methods, 20th ed. Saunders, Philadelphia (PA), 2001. pp. 249–63.

Mengel R, Bacher M & Flores-De-Jacoby L. (2002). Interactions between stress, interleukin-1beta, interleukin-6 and cortisol in periodontally diseased patients. *Journal of Clinical Periodontology,* Vol. 29, No. 11, 1012–22.

Montebugnoli L, Servidio D, Miaton RA, Prati C, Tricoci P, Melloni C & Melandri G. (2005). Periodontal health improves systemic inflammatory and haemostatic status in subjects with coronary heart disease. *Journal of Clinical Periodontology,* Vol. 32, No. 2, 188-92.

Nakajima T, Honda T, Domon H, Okui T, Kajita K, Ito H, Takahashi N, Maekawa T, Tabeta K & Yamazaki K. (2010). Periodontitis-associated up-regulation of systemic inflammatory mediator level may increase the risk of coronary heart disease. *Journal of Periodontal Research*, Vol. 45, No. 1, 116-122.

Nakamura N, Yoshida M, Umeda M, Huang Y, Kitajima S, Inoue Y, Ishikawa I & Iwai T. (2008). Extended exposure of lipopolysaccharide fraction from *Porphyromonas gingivalis* facilitates mononuclear cell adhesion to vascular endothelium via Toll-like receptor-2 dependent mechanism. *Atherosclerosis*, Vol. 196, No. 1, 59-67.

Nakano K, Inaba H, Nomura R, Nemoto H, Takeuchi H, Yoshioka H, Toda K, Taniguchi K, Amano A & Ooshima T. (2008). Distribution of *Porphyromonas gingivalis* fimA genotypes in cardiovascular specimens from Japanese patients. *Oral Microbiology and Immunology*, Vol. 23, No. 2, 170-2.

Nassar H, Kantarci A & Van Dyke TE. (2007). Diabetic periodontitis: a model for activated innate immunity and impaired resolution of inflammation. *Periodontology 2000*, Vol. 43, No. 1, 233–244.

Nishimura S, Iwamoto Y & Soga Y. (2007). The periodontal host response with diabetes. *Periodontology 2000*, Vol. 43, 1, 245-53.

Noack B, Genco RJ, Trevisan M, Grossi S, Zambon JJ & De Nardin E. (2001). Periodontal infections contribute to elevated systemic C-reactive protein level. *Journal of Periodontology*, Vol. 72, No. 9, 1221–1227.

Norse W, Abbas F, van der Ploeg I, Spijkervet FKL, Dijkstra PU & Vissink A. (2008). Periodontal inflamed surface area: quantifying inflammatory burden. *Journal of Clinical Periodontology*, Vol. 35, No. 8, 668-673.

Orozco A, Gemmell E, Bickel M & Seymour GJ. (2006). Interleukin-1beta, interleukin-12 and interleukin-18 levels in gingival fluid and serum of patients with gingivitis and periodontitis. *Oral Microbiology and Immunology*, Vol. 21, No. 4, 256–60.

Otero M, Lago R, Gomez R, Lago F, Dieguez C, Gómez-Reino JJ & Gualillo O. (2006). Changes in plasma levels of fat-derived hormones adiponectin, leptin, resistin and visfatin in patients with rheumatoid arthritis. *Annals of the Rheumatic Diseases*, Vol. 65, No. 9, 1198-1201.

Padgett DA, Glaser R. (2003). How stress influences the immune response. *Trends in Immunology*, Vol. 24, No. 8, 444-448.

Paoletti R, Gotto Jr AM & Hajjar DP. (2004). Inflammation in atherosclerosis and implications for therapy. *Circulation*, Vol. 109, No. 23 (suppl.1), III20–6.

Papapanou PN, Sedaghatfar MH, Demmer RT, Wolf DL, Yang J, Roth GA, Celenti R, Belusko PB, Lalla E & Pavlidis P. (2007). Periodontal therapy alters gene expression of peripheral blood monocytes. *Journal of Clinical Periodontology*, Vol. 34, No. 9, 736–747.

Paraskevas S, Huizinga J & Loos B. (2008). A systematic review and metaanalyses on C-reactive protein in relation to periodontitis. *Journal of Clinical Periodontology*, Vol. 35, No. 2, 277-90.

Parhami F, Tintut Y, Ballard A, Fogelman AM & Demer LL. (2001). Leptin enhances the calcification of vascular cells: Artery wall as a target of leptin. *Circulation Research*, Vol. 88, No. 9, 954- 960.

Pavlov VA & Tracey KJ. (2004). Neural regulators of innate immune responses and inflammation. Cellular and Molecular Life Sciences, Vol. 61, No. 18, 2322-2331.

Peruzzo DC, Benatti BB, Ambrosano GMB, Nogueira-Filho GR, Sallum EA, Casati MZ & Nociti H Jr. (2007). A Systematic review of stress and psychological factors as possible risk factors for periodontal disease. *Journal of Periodontology,* Vol. 78, No. 8, 1491-1504.

Pihlstrom BL, Michalowicz BS & Johnson NW. (2005). Periodontal diseases. *Lancet,* Vol. 366, No. 9499, 1809–20.

Pischon N, Heng N, Bernimoulin JP, Kleber BM, Willich SN & Pischon T. (2007). Obesity, inflammation, and periodontal disease. *Journal of Dental Research,* Vol. 86, No. 5, 400-409.

Pistorius A, Krahwinkel T, Willerhausen B & Bockstegen C. (2002). Relationship between stress factors and periodontal disease. *European Journal of Medical Research,* Vol. 7, No. 9, 393–398.

Pitiphat W, Savetsilp W & Wara-aswapati N. (2008). C-reactive protein associated with periodontitis in a Thai population. *Journal of Clinical Periodontology,* Vol. 35, No. 2, 120-5.

Powell ND, Bailey MT, Mays JW, Stiner-Jones LM, Hanke ML, Padgett DA & Sheridan JF. (2009). Repeated social defeat activates dendritic cells and enhances Toll-like receptor dependent cytokine secretion. *Brain, Behaviour and Immunity,* Vol. 23, No. 2, 225-31.

Pussinen PJ, Jauhiainen M, Vilkuna-Rautiainen T, Sundvall J, Vesanen M, Mattila K, Palosuo T, Alfthan G & Asikainen S. (2004). Periodontitis decreases the antiatherogenic potency of high density lipoprotein. *Journal of Lipid Research,* Vol., 45, No. 1,139–47.

Sorsa T. (2007a). Serum microbial- and host-derived markers of periodontal diseases: a review. *Current Medicinal Chemistry,* Vol. 14, No. 22, 2402-12.

Pussinen P, Tuomisto K, Jousilahti P, Havulinna A, Sundvall J & Salomaa V. (2007b). Endotoxemia, immune response to periodontal pathogens, and systemic inflammation associate with incident cardiovascular disease events. *Arteriosclerosis, thrombosis and Vascular Biology,* Vol. 27, No. 6, 1433-9.

Rahman ZA & Soory M. (2006). Antioxidant effects of glutathione and IGF in a hyperglycaemic cell culture model of fibroblasts: some actions of advanced glycaemic end products (AGE) and nicotine, *Endocrine, Metabolic & Immune Disorders - Drug Targets,* Vol. 6, No. 3, 279-86.

Rho YH, Chung CP, Oeser A, Solus J, Asanuma Y, Sokka T, Pincus T, Raggi P, Gebretsadik T, Shintani A & Stein CM. (2009). Inflammatory mediators and premature coronary atherosclerosis in rheumatoid arthritis. Arthritis and Rheumatism, Vol. 61, No. 11, 1580–1585.

Ridker PM. (2003). Clinical application of C-reactive protein for cardiovascular disease detection and prevention. *Circulation,* Vol. 107, No. 3, 363-369.

Ridker P, Hennekens C, Buring J & Rifai N. (2000). C-reactive protein and other markers of inflammation in the prediction of cardiovascular disease in women. *New England Journal of Medicine,* Vol. 342, No. 12, 836-43.

Ridker P & Silvertown J. (2008). Inflammation, C-reactive protein, and atherothrombosis. *Journal of Periodontology*, Vol. 79, No. 8 Supplement, 1544-51.

Ritchie CS. (2007). Obesity and periodontal disease. *Periodontology 2000*, Vol. 44, No. 1, 154-163.

Rosania AE, Low KG, McCormick CM & Rosania DA. (2009). Stress, depression, cortisol, and periodontal disease. *Journal of Periodontology*, Vol. 80, No. 2, 260-266.

Ryan S, Taylor CT & McNicholas WT. (2009). Systemic inflammation: a key factor in the pathogenesis of cardiovascular complications in obstructive sleep apnoea syndrome? *Thorax*, Vol. 64, No. 7, 631-6.

Saito T & Shimazaki Y. (2007). Metabolic disorders related to obesity and periodontal disease. *Periodontology 2000*, Vol. 43, No. 1, 254-266.

Sattar N, Murray HM, Welsh P, Blauw GJ, Buckley BM, Cobbe S, de Craen AJ, Lowe GD, Jukema JW, Macfarlane PW, Murphy MB, Stott DJ, Westendorp RG, Shepherd J, Ford I & Packard CJ (2009). Prospective Study of Pravastatin in the Elderly at Risk (PROSPER) Study Group. Are markers of inflammation more strongly associated with risk for fatal than for nonfatal vascular events? PLoS Medicine, Vol. 6, No. 6, e1000099.

Saxlin T, Suominen-Taipale L, Kattainen A, Marniemi J, Knuuttila M & Ylostalo P. (2008). Association between serum lipid levels and periodontal infection. *Journal of Clinical Periodontology*, Vol. 35, No. 12, 1040-1047.

Sheiham A & Nicolau B. (2005). Evaluation of social and psychological factors in periodontal disease. *Periodontology 2000*. Vol. 39, No. 1, 118-31.

Schenkein H, Barbour S, Berry C, Kipps B & Tew J. (2000). Invasion of human vascular endothelial cells by *Actinobacillus actinomycetemcomitans* via the receptor for platelet-activating factor. *Infection and Immunity*, Vol. 68, No. 9, 5416-9.

Shimada Y, Komatsu Y, Ikezawa-Suzuki I, Tai H, Noriko Sugita & Yoshie H. (2010) The Effect of Periodontal Treatment on Serum Leptin, Interleukin-6, and C-Reactive Protein. *Journal of Periodontology*, Vol. 81, No. 8, 1118-1123.

Offenbacher S. (2003). Relationship between periodontal disease and C-reactive protein among adults in the Atherosclerosis Risk in Communities study. *Archives of Internal Medicine*, Vol. 163, No. 10, 1172-9.

Sonnenfeld G, Aviles H, Belay T, Vance M, Fountain K. (2002). Stress, suspension and resistance to infection. *Journal of Gravitational Physiology*, Vol. 9, No. 1, 199–200.

Sonoki K, Nakashima S, Takata Y Naito T, Fujisawa K, Ootsubo T, Wakisaka M, Iwase M, Iida M & Yokota M. (2006). Decreased lipid peroxidation following periodontal therapy in type 2 diabetic patients. *Journal of Periodontology*, Vol. 77, No. 11, 1907–1913.

Soory, M. (2009). Redox status in periodontal and systemic inflammatory conditions including associated neoplasias: Antioxidants as adjunctive therapy? Infectious Disorders -Drug Targets (supplement), Vol. 9, No. 4, 415-27.

Soory M. (2010a). Chronic periodontitis as a risk marker for systemic diseases with reference to cardiometabolic disorders: Common pathways in their progression. *Immunology and Immunogenetic Insights*, Vol. 2, 7-21.

Soory M. (2010b). Association of periodontitis with rheumatoid arthritis and atherosclerosis: Novel paradigms in etiopathogeneses and management? *Rheumatology: Research and Reviews*, Vol. 2, 1–16.

Sorensen LK, Havemose-Poulsen A, Bendtzen K & Holmstrup P. (2009). Aggressive periodontitis and chronic arthritis: blood mononuclear cell gene expression and plasma protein levels of cytokines and cytokine inhibitors. *Journal of Periodontology*, Vol. 80, No. 2, 282–9.

Steel DM & Whitehead AS. (1994). The major acute phase reactants: C-reactive protein, serum amyloid P component and serum amyloid A protein. *Immunology Today*, Vol. 15, No. 2, 81–88.

Takeda M, Ojima M, Yoshioka H, Inaba H, Kogo M, Shizukuishi S, Nomura M & Amano A. (2006). Relation of serum advanced glycation end products with deterioration of periodontitis in type 2 diabetic patients. *Journal of Periodontology, Vol.* 77, No. 1, 15–20.

Taylor GW, Burt BA, Becker MP Genco RJ, Shlossman M, Knowler WC & Pettitt DJ. (1996). Severe periodontitis and risk for poor glycemic control in patients with noninsulin-dependent diabetes mellitus. *Journal of Periodontology*, Vol. 67, (Supplement 10),1085–1093.

Teng HC, Lee CH, Hung HC, Tsai CC, Chang YY, Yang YH, Lu CT, Yen YY & Wu YM. (2003). Lifestyle and psychosocial factors associated with chronic periodontitis in Taiwanese adults. *Journal of Periodontology, Vol.* 74, No. 8, 1169-1175.

Tilg H & Moschen AR. (2008). Inflammatory mechanisms in the regulation of insulin resistance. *Molecular Medicine*, Vol. 14, No. 3-4, 222-231.

Torzewski M, Rist C, Mortensen RF Zwaka TP, Bienek M, Waltenberger J, Koenig W, Schmitz G, Hombach V & Torzewski J. (2000). C-reactive protein in the arterial intima: role of C-reactive protein receptor-dependent monocyte recruitment in atherogenesis. *Arteriosclerosis, Thrombosis and Vascular Biology*, Vol. 20, No. 9, 2094–2099.

Van Dyke TE. (2005). Risk Factors for Periodontitis. *Journal of the International Academy of Periodontology*, Vol. 7, No. 1, 3-7.

Von Schacky C & Harris WS. (2007). Cardiovascular benefits of omega-3 fatty acids. *Cardiovascular Research*, Vol. 73, No. 2, 310-5.

Vozarova B, Weyer C, Hanson K, Tataranni PA, Bogardus C & Pratley RE. (2001). Circulating interleukin-6 in relation to adiposity, insulin action, and insulin secretion. *Obesity Research*, Vol. 9, No. 7, 414–417.

Welsh P, Polisecki E, Robertson M, Jahn S, Buckley BM, de Craen AJ, Ford I, Jukema JW, Macfarlane PW, Packard CJ, Stott DJ, Westendorp RG, Shepherd J, Hingorani AD, Smith GD, Schaefer E & Sattar N. (2010). Unravelling the directional link between adiposity and inflammation: a bidirectional Mendelian randomization approach. *Journal of Clinical Endocrinology and metabolism*, Vol. 95, No, 1, 93-9.

Wimmer G, Janda M, Wieselmann-Penkner K, Jakse N, Polansky R, Pertl C. (2002). Coping with stress: its influence on periodontal disease. *Journal of Periodontology*, Vol. 73, No. 11, 1343–1351.

Yamagishi SI, Edelstein D, Du XL, Kaneda Y, Guzman M & Brownlee M. (2001). Leptin induces mitochondrial superoxide production and monocyte chemoattractant protein-1 expression in aortic endothelial cells by increasing fatty acid oxidation via protein kinase A. *Journal of Biological Chemistry*, Vol. 276, No. 27, 25096-25100.

Yamaguchi R, Yoshimura A, Yoshioka H, Kaneko T & Hara Y. (2009). Ability of supragingival plaque to induce toll-like receptor 4- mediated stimulation is associated with cytokine production by peripheral blood mononuclear cells. *Journal of Periodontology*, Vol. 80, No. 3, 512–20.

Yamazaki K, Honda T, Domon H, Okui T, Kajita K, Amanuma R, Kudoh C, Takashiba S, Kokeguchi S, Nishimura F, Kodama M, Aizawa Y & Oda H. (2007). Relationship of periodontal infection to serum antibody levels to periodontopathic bacteria and inflammatory markers in periodontitis patients with coronary heart disease. *Clinical and Experimental Immunology*. Vol. 149, No. 3, 445–452.

Yamazaki K, Honda T, Oda T, Ueki-Maruyama K, Nakajima T, Yoshie H & Seymour GJ. (2005). Effect of periodontal treatment on the C-reactive protein and pro-inflammatory cytokine levels in Japanese periodontitis patients. *Journal of Periodontal Research*, Vol. 40, No. 1, 53-58.

Ziccardi P, Nappo F, Giugliano G, Esposito K, Marfella R, Cioffi M, D'Andrea F, Molinari AM & Giugliano D. (2002). Reduction of inflammatory cytokine concentrations and improvement of endothelial functions in obese women after weight loss over one year. *Circulation*, Vol. 105, No. 7, 804-809.

4

Salivary Acute Phase Proteins as Biomarker in Oral and Systemic Disease

Assya Krasteva and Angelina Kisselova
Medical University, Sofia
Bulgaria

1. Introduction

The purpose of this review is to present the latest research data regarding the physiological and diagnostic significance of acute phase proteins concentrations in saliva during oral and systemic diseases. We also show some interesting advantages in using saliva sample as a diagnostic fluid.

2. Saliva as diagnostic tool

Saliva is a unique biological fluid, with an important role in the oral physiology. It is a major player in the process of oral and general health maintenance (Humphrey, 2001). According to recent data it mirrors general health condition thus reflecting various systemic changes in the body (Chiappelli, 2006; Nagler, 2002, 2008).

Saliva is a colorless viscous liquid mixture of oral fluids which includes secretions from both the major and minor salivary glands. Additionally, it contains several constituents of non-salivary origin: gingival crevicular fluid, expectorated bronchial and nasal secretions, serum and blood derivates from oral wounds, bacteria and bacterial products, viruses and fungi, desquamated epithelial cells, leukocytes, electrolytes, immunoglobulins, proteins and enzymes, food debris and a small portion is gastro-esophageal reflux, etc. (Edgar, 1990; Nagler, 2002).

These facts motivate more extended use of saliva samples for diagnosis of different oral and systemic diseases.

2.1 Advantages of saliva as research material

Recently, saliva has been proven to be among credible diagnostic tools for detecting different biomarkers. Its promising future relies on two main reasons. Firstly, characteristic biomarkers for different diseases were found in significant concentrations among the components of the saliva. Second, the improvement of existing technologies and development of new, highly sensitive methods has succeeded to reveal the acceptable sensitivity and specificity of salivary biomarkers in term of different local and systemic conditions.

Additionally, the raised interest in saliva as a useful diagnostic fluid during last few decades is motivated by the proven ability to monitor the general health, to discover the disease onset and to follow up the progression to be used in large scale screening and epidemiologic studies (Irwin, 1990; Jentsch, 2004; Yu-Hsiang, 2009).

Compared to the other diagnostic media (such a tissue samples, serum, cerebrospinal fluid, etc.) saliva sampling is easy collectable, cost-effective, non-invasive diagnostic tool for research and often is preferred as an alternative diagnostic approach.

Advantages of saliva sampling are mostly seen in some patient's categories which are historically problematic to manage as children, IVDU or any other case when venepuncture is difficult to achieve. The saliva collection does not cause anxiety or discomfort and studies are reproducible (Hu, 2008). It could be performed by the individuals themselves after minimal training, without the help of medical staff. Furthermore it is relatively safe to obtain numerous samples during the course of the disease with minimal risk of contamination both for the patient and the healthcare staff.

2.2 Whole or gland-specific saliva?

Using the whole saliva and gland-specific saliva as objects of diagnostic investigations has some specific concerns. Most frequently whole saliva is examined mainly because of its simple and facile mode of collection. There are some difficulties to collect and separate the gland-specific saliva from individual salivary glands: parotid, submandibular, sublingual, and minor salivary glands. When gland-specific samples are compulsory needed, use of specific devices is advised (Navazesh, 1993). In case of inflammatory and obstructive diseases of the particular salivary gland, examination of gland-specific saliva is more accurate and thus is preferable.

Analysis of the saliva may be useful in increasing number of clinical situations, such as infectious diseases, hereditary disorders, autoimmune diseases, malignant and endocrine disorders. It is also beneficial in the assessment of therapeutic levels of drugs and the monitoring of illicit drug use (Yu-Hsiang, 2009). The list of the implicated clinical and research use of the saliva samples is kept growing.

Furthermore, the whole, unstimulated saliva contains serum and local constituents, which reliably reflect changes in the local immunity. These components are derived from the local vasculature of the salivary glands and also reach the oral cavity via the flow of gingival fluid.

2.3 The collection of saliva

The preanalitic stage is essential for obtaining reliable and reproducible study results. This is the reason many authors to focus particular attention to the prerequisites which patients and devices need to meet before collection of the saliva sample. Usually several conditions have to be fulfilled. Avoiding of any oral-hygienic procedures on the study day, restrain of food, liquids and smoking before sample collection are among most popular, but might vary according to the objectives of the study (Dawes, 1990, Jentisch, 2004). It is found that best approach is to obtain samples at the same time of the day, most often between 8 and 9 a.m. (Dawes, 1990).

Importantly, in healthy subjects, gingival crevicular fluid from the tooth/gum margin may constitute up to 0.5% of the volume of mixed saliva (Cimasoni, 1974). During the oral-hygiene procedures minor abrasions appear and plasma exudate from in the mouth increased. Therefore, it is usually recommended that subjects should not brush their teeth or practice any other methods of oral hygiene for several hours before collecting a saliva sample (Hold, 1999).

2.3.1 Collection time of saliva

From practical point of view, time for collection of the saliva is usually from 5 to 15 minutes. The necessary quantity is 2-10 ml according of the number of tested components (Dawes, 1990, Jentisch, 2004; Marton, 2004). The samples are gathered in special sterile containers, which might be plastic, glass, polypropylene, etc. However, small molecules tend to stick to the polyethylene container for collection. Therefore, the most suitable plastic material is polypropylene, but not if recycled (Hold, 1999).

2.3.2 Methods of saliva collection

Techniques for the collection of saliva

Several methods have been described for the collection of mixed saliva:

- Draining method - the patients are instructed to swallow before collecting saliva. The saliva is secreted in the collecting bottle using a funnel, held near the mouth (Navazesh, 1993).
- Spitting method - saliva is collected in the mouth while patient keeps lips closed. At the end of each minute the patient emerged oral samples in sterile bottles (Navazesh, 1993).
- Suction method - the procedure starts with swallowing, to release the mouth of available saliva. Special devices are placed under the tongue and attached to the suction pump that drains saliva. At the end of the procedure the suction tube is placed in the vestibulum and in the floor of mouth and, likewise, is collecting residual saliva (Navazesh, 1993).
- Absorbent method - absorbent tampons or sponges (0.2 x 0.6 cm) are placed under the tongue near the exit channels of the sublingual and submandibular glands. Two other sponges are placed between the gingiva and cheek at the exit channel of the parotid gland (Navazesh, 1993).

2.4 Stimulated and unstimulated saliva

Although most patients prefer donating saliva rather than blood, a substantial social barrier exists to "spitting". For this and other reasons, subjects often experience decreased salivary secretion (dry mouth) if asked to provide a sample. Many researchers have found it advantageous to further stimulate salivation and a number of stimuli have been used: mechanical with inert material - paraffin wax, parafilm, rubber bands, pieces of teflon, polytetrafluoroethylene (PTFE), chewing gum or chemical stimulation with 2% citric acid, acid lemon drops or a few drops of 0.5 mol/l citric acid are among the most potent of taste stimuli and will generally induce a maximal secretion of 5 to 10 ml/min (Dawes, 1992; Hold, 1999; Ruhl, 2004).

Some authors recommend that, when these types of stimuli are used, the subject should allow saliva to accumulate in the mouth until the desire to swallow occurs, at which time the fluid can be expelled smoothly into a vessel. Repeated expectorations should be avoided since this introduces bubbles, which may result in changes in pH leading to errors in interpretation of the saliva/plasma concentration ratio (S/P ratio) (Hold, 1999).

There are several advantages of stimulating salivary flow. Firstly, large volumes of saliva can be obtained within a short time. Secondly, the pH of stimulated saliva mostly lies within a narrow range around the value of 7.4, whereas the pH of unstimulated saliva shows a larger variability. It may be of importance for the salivary secretion of weak acidic and basic compounds (Feller, 1977; Ritschel, 1983). The last, but not at least the intersubject variability in the S/P ratio may be diminished when stimulated saliva is used, as has been reported for digoxin (Hold, 1999).

2.5 Storage of saliva

Some authors believe that saliva rest stable at room temperature for several days (George, 1997; Schramm, 1991, Wade, 1991). Other recommend elimination of bacteria and enzymes prior to storage or otherwise stabilizers might need to be added stabilizers (Frerichs, 1992). Most authors suggest freezing the material immediately after collecting, especially when evaluating levels of hormones, immunoglobulins and interleukins (Zapryanova, 1989). Further processing of collecting saliva depends on the methods of study that will be used, but most usually saliva is centrifuged at 15 000G 4 $^{\circ}$ C for 10 minutes (Jentisch, 2004; Rohan, 2000; Ruhl, 2004; Zapryanova, 1989).

2.6 Diagnostic features of saliva

Currently, three major restrictions limit the development of clinical diagnostics:

- The lack of definitive molecular biomarkers for specific diseases;
- The lack of easy and inexpensive method of sampling with minimal discomfort;
- The lack of accurate, easy to use and portable platform to facilitate early detection disease (Yu-Hsiang, 2009).

Since 2002, the National Institute of Dental and Craniofacial Research (NIDCR) has created opportunities to overcome these limitations by exploring oral fluids as a diagnostic tool for assessment of health and disease status. Through the visionary investment by the NIDCR, the discovery of salivary biomarkers and ongoing development of salivary diagnostics technologies now provide promising solutions for the rest (Yu-Hsiang, 2009).

2.6.1 Tested substances in saliva

Like blood, saliva is a complex fluid containing a variety of numerous organic and inorganic constituents, of which the most frequent subject of investigations is: proteins, enzymes, hormones, carbohydrates, calcium, sodium, magnesium, copper and others.

Also it is important that saliva is a biologic medium for the study of genomic DNA (Ng, 2004). Therefore it is a unique fluid for the development of molecular diagnostics. Unfortunately its potential seems to be frequently underestimated due to technological barriers. Further studies are awaited to prove if it meets the requirements necessary to screen saliva containing complex constituents with low concentration (Yu-Hsiang, 2009).

Some of the components exert similar concentrations in blood and saliva and it is possible to easily move from their determination in serum to saliva. It is supposed that the saliva is functionally equivalent to serum in reflecting the physiological state of the body, including emotional, hormonal, nutritional, and metabolic variations (Ivanova, 2009). Others substances (like cholesterol, creatinine, uric acid etc) have very low concentration making their determination with the available techniques in saliva unreliable and clinically unfeasible (Ivanova, 2009).

2.6.2 Techniques for investigating saliva

The concentration of many substances in saliva was significantly lower than in blood plasma and this requires the use of highly sensitive tests and methods designed for saliva, and the proper collection of material.

At this level of knowledge the researchers aim to improve the sensitivity of the different methods that is believe to help further implementation of saliva sampling in diagnostic process in various disease processes. The low concentration of different substances compared with levels in the blood may prevent salivary diagnostics from being clinically practical. However this limitation was recently overcome as new and highly sensitive techniques (e.g., molecular diagnostics, nanotechnology) were developed. Unfortunately, they are still available only in a limited number of specifically equipped labs (Yu-Hsiang, 2009).

Most commonly radial immunodiffusion, immunoelectrophoresis, turbidimetry, nephelometry are used for determining salivary protein levels. For detecting cytokines levels ELISA, flowcytometry, ELISPOT, RT-PCR are preferred. The most common ELISA method is characterized with quite low sensitivity. The ELISPOT assays surpass ELISA techniques in terms of higher sensitivity achieved, but the proceeding times are usually longer. Compared to precipitation methods, ELISA essays are more sensitive thanks to the use of monoclonal antibodies (Altankova, 2001).

Based on currently emerging biotechnology in salivary diagnostics became possible to determine the number of biomarkers for various diseases. The list includes malignancies (Kaufman, 2000), hereditary, autoimmune, viral and bacterial infections, cardiovascular diseases, HIV related conditions. We cannot miss the convenient use of saliva diagnostics in therapeutic drug monitoring, measurement of hormone levels, and of course diagnosis of local oral disease. These developments have extended the range of saliva-based diagnostics from the simple oral cavity to the whole physiological system. Thus, saliva-based diagnostics is on the cutting edge of diagnostic technology, and may offer a robust alternative for clinicians to use in the near future to make clinical decisions and predict post-treatment outcomes (Yu-Hsiang, 2009).

For the past two decades, salivary diagnostic approaches have been focused on the oral diseases. Interest represents a concentration of proven proteins in saliva, on the other hand their attitude to medical conditions and diseases affecting not only the oral cavity and the body. Therefore we would like to direct the focus of this review on determination the positive and negative acute phase protein in saliva in oral and systemic diseases.

3. Acute phase proteins in saliva

3.1 Origin of acute phase proteins in saliva

The serum concentration of the most acute phase proteins increases in response to tissue injury, inflammation or infection. The changes in serum/plasma concentrations correlate with increased hepatic synthesis (Fournier, 2000). The majority of acute phase proteins are synthesized in the liver and some of them diffuse or are actively transported into saliva from the blood. Others are locally produced, including into the salivary glands.

Although haptoglobin is mainly produced in the liver, some other organ may contribute: skin, lungs, kidneys, adipose tissue (Li, 2005). A local synthesis in oral cavity of transferrin, alpha 1-acid glycoprotein, alpha 1-antitrypsin and haptoglobin was observed in infants (Szabo, 1988). Increased CRP mRNA expression in the submandibular glands of rats with experimentally induced inflammation was recently reported (Dillon, 2010). It is now widely accepted that acute phase protein synthesis may take place in extra-hepatic cell types. Presumably, the same inflammatory mediators as observed in hepatocytes regulate the process (Fournier, 2000). Depending on the quantity of measured level, acute phase

response might be positive or negative. Some protein levels are found elevated during the acute phase (positive acute phase proteins), while the production of other proteins is decreased (negative acute phase proteins).
When the concentration of specific component in saliva strongly correlates the serum one, a serum source is accepted (Nagler, 2008). However, the lack of a high correlation between concentrations of a component in saliva and in serum does not necessarily reject the serum origin. It may simply reflect variability in the diffusion process or local synthesis for the component (Nagler, 2008).
The determination of the salivary acute phase proteins' concentration is an object of many studies. Basically it is not a routine practice in the daily dentistry, but we hope it would be soon.

3.2 Positive acute-phase proteins in saliva (positive app)

Abnormal serum levels of positive acute phase proteins have been reported in various studies on myocardial infarction, Inflammatory bowel disease psoriasis, and malignancy. Some oral diseases as parodontitis, oral lichen planus, oral levkoplakia, oral squamous cell carcinoma etc. are also characterized with increased positive APP.

3.2.1 Haptoglobin

The diagnostic and prognostic value of haptoglobin and CRP in different diseases motivates further interest of their salivary concentrations and dynamics (Rocha-Pereira, 2004; Chen, 1989; Clayman, 1992).
There are a limited number of studies regarding the salivary haptoglobin (Backhausz, 1975; Grimoud, 1998; Katnik, 1990). This might be at least partially explained by the difficulties in determination of the acute phase protein in the oral cavity due to their low concentrations (Backhausz, 1975; Grimoud, 1998; Katnik, 1990; Keur, 1994).
Some authors reported immunoenzyme method to determine haptoglobin in different biofluids, including saliva, which ranged 5 to 150 μg/l (Katnik, 1990). The salivary haptoglobin measurement is commonly used in the veterinary practice (Hiss, 2003; Parra, 2005).
Human studies show that saliva haptoglobin increases in patients with parodontitis (Backhausz, 1975). Bell's palsy (Keur, 1994) and in oral manifestation of AIDS (Grimoud, 1998).
Backhausz et al. investigated salivary samples from 60 individuals by immuno-electrophoresis. Transferrin and haptoglobin levels in subjects with periodontal inflammation were found twice as frequent as in control individuals, which is indicative of a correlation with the inflammatory process (Backhausz, 1975).
Keur et al. evaluated the flow rate of extra-parotid and parotid saliva in patients with Bell's palsy compared to healthy volunteers. Concentration of total protein and seven acute-phase proteins were measured. Either extra-parotid or parotid saliva APP levels do not differ by means of patient's age. Interestingly, an elevated concentration of haptoglobin, alfa2-macroglobulin and ceruloplasmin were found in extra-parotid saliva, while only haptoglobin and ceruloplasmin were increased into saliva from parotid gland (Keur, 1994). This study demonstrates that haptoglobin presence in parotid and extraparotid saliva might serve as a reliable marker and it is worth to determine it in whole as well as in gland-specific saliva.

In HIV positive patients presented with typical oral mucosal manifestations a correlation between salivary and serum concentrations of IgA, haptoglobin and alpha1-protease inhibitor were observed (Grimoud, 1998). This is additional confirmation of reliability of saliva sampling for studying the diseases natural history and may successfully replace or at least add value to serum samples.
There is a number of data confirming that haptoglobin levels can predict the clinical outcome. In 2003 S. Hiss et al. created an immune-enzyme technique to determine haptoglobin in different swine fluids with sensitivity threshold of 0.02 mg/l. haptoglobin concentrations in swine's saliva were found between 0.3 and 3.0 microg/ml and correlated poor with serum levels (n=93, r=0.35, p<0.001) (Hiss, 2003). Parra et al. reported highly sensitive immunofluorimetric method for evaluation of dog serum and saliva haptoglobin. The detection level was 0.002 microg/ml. Saliva haptoglobin levels in diseased dogs were found significantly higher than in healthy ones (Parra, 2005).

3.2.2 CRP (C-reactive protein)

CRP serum concentration usually increases in case of systemic inflammation. Explicably CRP is the most commonly used acute phase protein in clinical practice. Few studies evaluated the CRP levels in oral cavity. It was detected in whole saliva in study which included 45 adults. The concentrations (range from 0 to 472 pg/ml) were found higher in patients with gingivitis, moderate and severe periodontitis (Pederson, 1995). Additionally, edentulous volunteers showed lower levels than healthy subjects (Pederson, 1995, Sibraa, 1991). Some authors used monoclonal antibodies and a radioisotope assay to measure CRP levels in gingival crevicular fluid (GCF) from 24 periodontitis patients. CRP did not differ significantly between diseased and healthy sites in same patients (Sibraa, 1991).

Salivary haptoglobin and CRP in oral neoplasm

The serum levels of C-reactive protein and haptoglobin have prognostic and diagnostic value in patients with oral cancer, inflammatory bowel disease and psoriasis (Vucelić, 1990, Florin, 2006; Solem, 2005; Landowski, 2007; Koelewijn, 2008).
It is known that serum levels of both proteins reflect disease activity and treatment outcome and might challenge the prognosis. Lead by the question if these changes are also observed in saliva, we conducted prospective study to evaluate if the saliva concentrations followed the same trend. We prospectively studied the haptoglobin and CRP levels in saliva samples from 16 patients with parotid tumors and 35 treatment-naïve oral squamous cell carcinoma. Thirty-one healthy subjects served as matched controls. The results clearly showed elevated CRP and haptoglobin levels in both study subgroups as compared to the controls (Table 1).

Groups	CRP (mg/1)	Haptoglobin (mg/l)
Healthy subjects (n=31)	0,105 ± 0,115	15 ± 12,9
Patients with parotid tumors (n=16)	0,185 ± 0,89*	38 ± 58*
Patients with oral squamous cell carcinoma (n=35)	0,346 ± 0,602*	45 ± 61*

*p<0.05 versus healthy subjects

Table 1. Saliva CRP and haptoglobin levels in patients with parotid tumors and oral squamous cell carcinoma

Three months even insignificant decrease of CRP and haptoglobin was found (Krasteva, 2009).

As discussed above, the haptoglobin is found in the cytoplasm of epidermal Langerhans cells (Li, 2005). Basically, we believe that that increased levels found in squamous cell carcinomas patients are related to local production and in oral mucosa. Possibility of systemic/serum origin however could not be overlooked. The levels of CRP in untreated oncology patients were almost three times higher than in control subjects almost 25% of the untreated cancer patients had levels above the established highest value in controls.

Following appropriate treatment (chemotherapy, radiotherapy, surgery) 15 patients had salivary haptoglobin and CRP which were not different from the control subjects (mean 17 ± 36 mg/l and 0,136 ± 0,72 mg/l respectively). Salivary haptoglobin and CRP levels decreased after treatment as expected due to the removal of tumor and subsiding of the inflammatory process (Krasteva, 2009).

We found moderate correlation between CRP and haptoglobin (r = 0,502, p = 0,008) which provides additional evidence to confirm the same trend of elevation of both APP the parallel movement (increase) of two acute phase proteins (Krasteva, 2009).

Salivary haptoglobin and CRP in systemic disease

In 32 currently untreated psoriatic patients with PASI >10 we observed increased salivary CRP and haptoglobin levels (Table 2).

Groups	CRP (mg/l)	Haptoglobin (mg/l)
Healthy subjects (n=31)	0,10 ± 0,115	15 ± 12,9
Patients with psoriasis (n=32)	0,166 ± 0,55	26,9 ± 24,6

*p<0.05 versus healthy subjects

Table 2. Saliva level of CRP and haptoglobin in psoriatic patients

We suggest that elevated salivary haptoglobin levels may be due to transudation or local production in Langerhans cells and keratinocytes of oral mucosa. This could reflect a kind of local defense mechanisms involving systemic inflammatory process, which underline the basis of psoriasis.

Furthermore the salivary levels of haptoglobin and CRP in 31 patients with inflammatory bowel disease (IBD) under immunosuppressive therapy were also examined. No significant difference in the salivary concentrations as compared with healthy individuals was found (Table 3).

Groups	CRP (mg/l)	Haptoglobin (mg/l)
Healthy subjects (n=31)	0,105 ± 0,115	15 ± 12,9
IBD (n=31)	0,175 ±0 ,246	20,6 ± 28,8

Table 3. Saliva level of CRP and haptoglobin in psoriatic patients

This could be partially explained by the lack of oral inflammation or might reflect the treatment-induced control of the disease. In patients with more active disease we observed slight increase of CRP values (slight elevation of Mayo index and CDAI index) (Krasteva, 2009).

Published data and our results has driven the conclusion that routine determination of CRP and haptoglobin in saliva in oral diseases as well as in systemic disorders. They could be

used as biomarkers in addition to diagnostic and prognostic value in patients. It would be most useful if they could be determined at the baseline and during the treatment with a regular follow up at first, third, sixth and twelfth month.
There are just a few data for the presence of the other positive acute phase proteins in saliva.

3.2.3 Alpha 2-macroglobulin

Alpha-2-macroglobulin is a large plasma protein produced by the liver. It is able to inactivate an enormous variety of proteinases (including serine-, cysteine-, aspartic- and metalloproteinases).

Alpha 2-macroglobulin was studied in patients with oral diseases (Sengupta, 1988; Pederson, 2005, Rao, 1995). Alpha 2-macroglobulin levels in whole saliva were found between 0 and 4941 ng/ml using ELISA (Pederson, 2005). It has been often studied in patients with gingivitis and periodontitis (Sengupta, 1988; Pederson, 2005, Rao, 1995).and the salivary levels was found even higher in severe disease (Pederson, 2005).

The concentration of alpha 2-macroglobulin in human gingival sulci has been investigated in gingival washings of experimental gingivitis and in crevicular fluid before and after initial periodontal therapy (Condacci, 1982). The alpha 2-M was found elevated in the washings. The absolute amount of alpha 2-M in the crevicular fluid showed a significant decrease and ever reached undetectable levels after treatment (Condacci, 1982).

In opposite of the above studies, Sibraa et al. found in gingival crevicular fluid lower levels of alpha-2-macroglobulin in periodontally diseased than healthy sites ($p < 0.001$) (Sibraa, 1991). Gautam et al. found lower concentrations both in the serum and saliva in phenytoin treated patients with varying grades of gingival enlargement compared to phenytoin-naïve subjects with normal gingiva. The mean serum and salivary concentrations increased after the fading the inflammatory process (Gautam, 2009).

Recently, Chen et al. both alpha-2-macroglobulin and alpha-2-macroglobulin-like protein are essential components of the salivary innate immunity acting like a natural inhibitor against swine origin influenza A virus (Chen, 2010). Additionally, alpha 2-macroglobulin was reported between salivary biomarkers of type-2 diabetes (Rao, 1995).

3.2.4 Alpha 1-antitrypsin (A1AT)

Alpha 1-antitrypsin inhibits a wide variety of proteases. It protects tissues from enzymes of inflammatory cells, especially neutrophil elastase.

There is very few data for alpha 1-antitrypsin in saliva. Alpha 1-antitrypsin was measured in whole saliva between 2-2271 ng/ml by ELISA (Pederson, 1995). In contrast to alpha-2-macroglobulin, A1AT was not found to increase in case with gingivitis (Pederson, 1995). However, similarly to alpha-2-macroglobulin it was lower in phenytoin gingival enlargement compared to normal gingival (Gautam, 2009). Smokers have also low levels of A1AT in crevicular fluid (Persson, 2001).

3.2.5 Alpha-1-acid glycoprotein (A1AG)

Alpha-1-acid glycoprotein or orosomucoid is a 41-43-kDa glycoprotein, one of the major acute phase proteins in humans, rats, mice and other species (Fournier, 2000). A1AG is synthesized primarily in hepatocytes, but mild production was also found in the salivary glands and spleen. Minor expression is detected in all other tissues, including lung, lymph nodes, uterus, ovary, kidney and tongue (Lecchi, 2009). In the setting of established

immunomodulatory and direct antibacterial activity of A1AG, its expression in the salivary glands might be explained with local immunity, even in healthy condition (Lecchi, 2009).
In pre-matured infants the salivary A1AG and albumin concentration were found higher than in controls, due to the increase of the protein transudation. The last is a late consequence of intrauterine malnutrition (Szabó S, 1988).

3.2.6 Fibrinogen

Fibrinogen is a soluble plasma glycoprotein, synthesised by the liver, that is converted by thrombin into fibrin during blood coagulation. It may be elevated in any form of inflammation, it is especially apparent in human gingival tissue during the initial phase of periodontal disease (Page, 1976)
One of the first, but unfortunately unsuccessful attempts for fibrinogen determination in saliva was made in 1965 (Brandtzaeg, 1965). Almost three decades later, Sukharev et al. succeeded to determine salivary lactoferrin and fibrinogen levels in 1205 salivary samples using an agar immunodiffusion test (Sukharev, 1991). Salivary fibrinogen degradation products and lactoferrin detection rates do not depend on the subject's gender but increases with age and intensity of the aggressive admixture effects in inhaled air. These are also related to the intensity of the inflammatory and proliferative processes in the oral cavity and bronchopulmonary system (Sukharev, 1991).

3.2.7 Ferritin

Ferritin is a ubiquitous intracellular protein that stores iron and releases it in a controlled fashion. In humans, it acts as a buffer against iron deficiency and iron overload.
Inflammation induces the hepatic synthesis of the apo-ferritin, which is released into the circulation, and behaves as an acute phase protein.
Very recent study revealed corresponding salivary and serum ferritin levels in 33 children suffering from protein-energy malnutrition – PEM. The salivary ferritin was measured very low both in serum and saliva in children with PEM even in grade I, as compared to normal children. In PEM grade III the mean ferritin value was reported 3.28 +/- 0.75 µg/l versus 169.3 +/- 21.9 µg/l in normally nourished children. The salivary ferritin levels in PEM may be used to distinguish the early stage of the disease and to estimate the disease severity (Agarwal, 1984).

3.3 Negative acute phase proteins

3.3.1 Albumin

Albumin is the main protein of plasma; it binds water, cations, fatty acids, hormones, bilirubin and drugs - its main function is to regulate the colloidal osmotic pressure of blood.
Common saliva albumin concentration usually is not found decreased in inflammation and is often used as a marker for the degree of mucositis or inflammation in the oral cavity (Izutsu, 1981). Whole saliva albumin as an indicator of stomatitis in cancer therapy patients. On the contrary, albumin is substantially increased, like lactoferrine, in case of acute inflammation of the salivary glands (Dodds, 2000).
in saliva arises from contamination by either traces of blood or gingival fluids. Normal range of albumin in saliva is still issue of debate. Different concentrations of salivary albumin in healthy adults were reported (Ruhl, 2004 - S 38.5 µg/ml and Vaziri, 2009 - 64.50 ± 38.40 µg/ml).

Almost all samples obtained after stimulation of the major salivary glands contain albumin in concentration about r below the detection limit of 18.9 μg/ml (Ruhl, 2004).
Salivary albumin was evaluated in early childhood. High levels of albumin are found in saliva of 63 newborn infants, as early as within the first 10 days of life (Bastian Manfred Seidel) (Selner, 1968).
The median concentrations of serum albumin in whole saliva increased from 1 to 12 μg/ml during the first year of infancy, within an intra-individual range from 10.4 to 105 μg/ml. A shift in median concentrations was observed prior to the eruption of the first teeth. In individual infants, the albumin concentration started to rise about a month before eruption of the first tooth (Ruhl, 2005).
The concentration and the within-child variability of albumin increased with age (from 6 months to 5 years). Between-child variances were greater than the within-child variances by a factor of 1.3 for log (albumin). There were no changes in albumin levels between infection and non-infection periods, suggesting a local immune response rather than serum leakage. (Gleeson, 1991).
There was not any difference in the concentration of salivary albumin depending on pregnancy, as the same levels were measured in pregnant and non-pregnant women (Selby, 1988).
Salivary albumin concentration in subjects with gingivitis or perodontitis is caused by leakage of plasma proteins (Henskens, 1993). The increase in the concentration of albumin in whole saliva was always detected prior to the clinical appearance of stomatitis, suggesting that albumin in whole saliva may be a marker and predictor of this complication. Therefore, the monitoring of salivary albumin can assist in the identification of stomatitis at a pre-clinical stage and enable the chemotherapy dosage to be adjusted or treatment for the stomatitis to be initiated at an early stage (Izutsu, 1981)
Differences between glandular and gingival contributions to the composition of saliva were explored in patients medicated with cyclosporin who exhibited gingival overgrowth (responders), those without gingival overgrowth (non-responders). In responders the albumin level was 88 μg/ml and in non-responders 52 μg/ml (Ruhl, 2004).
Unfortunately, measurement of the salivary albumin failed to predict microvascular impairment in diabetic patients (Fisher, 1991). Twenty years later Vaziri et al. found adults with type 2 diabetes mellitus have higher concentration of salivary albumin (73.47 ± 31.35 μg/ml versus 64.50 ± 38.40 μg/ml in controls). It is discussed it may play a diagnostic role in oral health and disease in diabetic patients (Vaziri, 2009).
Importantly, the saliva albumin and prealbumin concentrations in elderly are correlated with serum ones (albumin: $R^2 = 0.308$, $p = 0.0010$, prealbumin: $R^2 = 0.433$, $p<0.0001$). Thus salivary determination of these markers might facilitate the evaluation of protein nutritional status in this specific group (Murayama, 1999).

3.3.2 Transcortin

Transcortin, also corticosteroid-binding globulin officially called serpin peptidase inhibitor is an alpha-globulin and binds several steroid hormones: Cortisol, Progesterone, Aldosterone, 11-Deoxycorticosterone.
Early reports failed to detect transcortin in saliva (Riad-Fahmy, 1982), but low transcortin's concentration (about 25 pg/l), was detected some years later in saliva (Hammond, 1986; Chu, 1988). About 15% of salivary cortisol is bound to transcortin, which is a normal

component of uncontaminated parotid saliva. The cortisol in saliva being mainly free, implying that the elevation of the salivary cortisol concentration is not due to higher concentrations of transcortin (Umeda, 1981; Hammond, 1986; Chu, 1988).

One of the first reports regarding detection of salivary transferrin was published by Gugler et al. (Gugler, 1968). The study demonstrated the presence of pre-albumin, albumin, alpha-1-antitrypsin and transferrin in submaxillary saliva. Retinol (pre-albumin) could not be detected in parotid saliva (Gugler, 1968). The salivary transferrin is supposed to be a marker of blood contamination (Schwartz, 2004). This underlies its suggestive use as a biomarker for early detection of oral cancer (Jou, 2010).

It is quite important to known if the blood components are present in the oral mucosa as the quantitative estimates of different salivary tests may be compromised. To provide a quantitative measure of blood contamination in saliva, Schwartz et al. developed an enzyme immunoassay for transferrin, which is usually present in very small amounts (<5 mg/l) in saliva and in high concentration in whole blood (Schwartz, 2004). Transferrin saliva concentration was found below 4.0 mg/l in healthy volunteers. These results suggest that salivary transferrin can serve as a marker for quantification of blood contamination in saliva in the absence of visual evidence of blood contamination (Schwartz, 2004), especially in the absence of oral abnormalities. Further more than three hundreds and sixty children's saliva samples were studied to reveal if blood contamination could influence the measurement of salivary cortisol, testosterone, and dehydroepiandrosterone. Transferrin levels averaged 0.37 mg/dl (3,7 mg/l) that in fact supported previously mentioned results and clearly demonstrated that blood contamination in children saliva samples is quite rare.

Studies, which involved oncology patients, are important as most of them aim to provide new serum or other body fluids biomarkers for early detection of cancer. Very recently Jou et al. studied saliva samples from patients diagnosed with oral cancer patients aiming to identify salivary markers for early cancer detection. In neck squamous cell carcinoma patients the transferrin levels in the saliva were found increased more than 3 times than normal values. Additionally, the increased salivary transferrin levels strongly correlated with the size and stage of the tumor (Jou, 2010). As the saliva biologically is within an immediate surrounding of the developing tumor the detection of Transferrin might be useful. Many experts thus agreed that it is worth to include Transferrin in a panel of biomarkers for therapeutic monitoring and for early detection of HNSCC (Dowling, 2008).

Similarly the iron binding proteins, lactoferrin and transferrin were measured higher in patients with periodontitis, partial dentures and edentulous patients as well as those wearing complete dentures. A probable explanation is their bacteriostatic effect on salivary gram-positive and negative bacteria (Emiko, 2000).

The future

Human saliva proteomics is a novel approach in the search of protein biomarkers for detection of different local and systemic diseases. Currently more than 1400 salivary proteins have been identified (Scarano, 2010). Proteomics is the large-scale study of proteins, particularly their structures and functions. After genomics, proteomics is considered the next step in the study of biological systems. It is much more complicated than genomics mostly because while an organism's genome is more or less constant, the proteome differs from cell to cell and from time to time (Wilkins, 2009; Wasinger, 1995). Understanding the proteome, the structure and function of each protein and the complexities of protein-protein interactions will be critical for developing the most effective diagnostic techniques and disease treatments in the future. CH Chen using a proteomic approach describes the immune properties of alpha-2-macroglobulin in saliva (Chen, 2010). The emerging proteomic technologies aim to identify biomarkers for head and neck squamous cell carcinoma diagnostics (Drake, 2005).

4. Conclusion

Assess the health in the oral cavity requires specific tests and non-invasive approach to detect and monitor the diseases are preferred.Saliva is a unique clear fluid, composed of electrolytes, immunoglobulins, proteins and enzymes. The basic role of saliva is to assure the integrity of the upper part of the alimentary tract, through: lubrication; buffering action and clearance; maintaining tooth and mucosal integrity; antibacterial and antiviral activity as well as taste and digestion. In the last 10 years, saliva has become the object of various studies. Curiously, there are most of the papers on saliva samples are used for analysing drug abuse individuals as well as detection of various oral and systemic diseases. The most important advantage in collecting saliva samples is that an easy access and non-invasive nature of this approach is permitted. Furthermore, the possibility to measure a wide range of molecules both in saliva and serum allows evaluating microbiological, immunological, hormonal, pharmacological and oncological biomarkers. The FDA defines a biomarker as, "A characteristic that is objectively measured and evaluated as an indicator of normal biologic processes, pathogenic processes, or pharmacologic responses to a therapeutic intervention".Historically the blood levels of the acute phase proteins are used as biomarkers in physiology and disease. Haptoglobin might serve as a simple example. Its serum levels increases during acute conditions such as infection, injury, tissue destruction, some cancers, burns, surgery, or trauma. Levels are low in some diseases and hemolysis is a classic example of a dramatic decrease. Haptoglobin binds the free hemoglobin released from erythrocytes. Haptoglobin also contributes in the regulation of the host immunity (Huntoon, 2008). There are enough data to support the acute phase proteins determination in saliva. In contrast to the serum levels the negative acute phase proteins are found in higher concentration in saliva in oral diseases. Elevation of albumin in gingivitis and paradontitis as well as those of transferrin in blood contamination has been already discussed above.

However, we still need larger and logtidinal studies to define the normal limits of the salivary concentration of different proteins. Table 4 summarizes the reported levels in healthy subjects. Comparability of the different studies however is still controversial deopending on different non standardized methods used.

Determination of the concentrations of the APP in paired serum (plasma) and saliva samples allow easy to calculate "serum-salivary gradient". Table 5 summarizes a proposed relative gradient, calculated from the published serum and saliva upper limits of normal in healthy controls for every of the evaluated proteins. The salivary concentration of the acute phase proteins usually is about 1 - 2% from the plasma (serum) levels. The lower values are difficult to be explained.

Most of the discussed data were obtained from small number of observational studies. We do believe that large, prospective, controlled and longitudinal studies are needed to confirm the range of saliva APP and its correlation with serum levels. This seems to be mandatory before using the saliva APP evaluation routinely in the setting of sepsis, malignancy, inflammation, autoimmune diseases and transplantation.

Protein	Salivary level	Author
Albumin	38.5 µg/ml	Ruhl, 2004
Albumin	64.50 ± 38.40 µg/ml	Vaziri, 2009
Alpha 1-antitrypsin	2-2271 ng/ml	Pederson, 1995
Alpha 2-macroglobulin	0 - 4941 ng/ml	Pederson, 1995
CRP	0 - 472 pg/ml	Pederson, 1995
CRP	0,105 ± 0,115 mg/l	Krasteva, 2009
Ferritin	169.3 ± 21.9 µg/l	Agarwal, 1984
Haptoglobin (in animals)	0.3 - 3.0 µg/ml	Hiss, 2003
Haptoglobin	15 ± 12,9 mg/l	Krasteva, 2009
Transcortin	25 pg/l	Hammond, 1986; Chu, 1988
Transferrin	< 5 mg/l	Schwartz, 2004

Table 4. Salivary level of acute phase proteins in controls

Parameter	Saliva level (%)	Author
Alpha-1 antitrypsin	0,2	Gautam, 2009
Alpha-2 macroglobulin	1	Gautam, 2009
Haptoglobin	1,7	Krasteva, 2009
Transcortin	0,1	Hammond, 1986; Chu, 1988
Transferrin	0,5	Schwartz, 2004
CRP	1,2	Krasteva, 2009

Table 5. Saliva/serum concentration ratio of acute phase protein in controls

5. References

Agarwal, P.; Agarwal, K. & Agarwal, D. (1984). Biochemical changes in saliva of malnourished children. *American Society for Clinical Nutrition*, Vol. 39, No 2, February 1984, pp. 181-184, ISSN 0002-9165

Altankova, I. & Naumova, E. (2008). *Clinical Immunology*. Publisher "Lice", IBSN 9789549426212, Sofia

Backhausz, V.; Torteli, A., & Bruder, S. (1975). Immunoelectrophoretic study of salivary proteins. *Gesellschaft für Stomatologie der DDR*, Vol. 25, No 4, April 1975, pp. 256–229, ISSN 0302-4725

Brandtzaeg, P. Immunochemical comparison ofproteins in human gingival pocket fluid, serum and saliva. *Archives of Oral Biology*, Vol. 10, No 5, September-October 1965, pp. 795-802, ISSN 0003-9969

Chiappelli, F.; Iribarren, F. & Prolo, P. (2006). Salivary biomarkers in psychobiological medicine. *Bioinformation*, Vol. 8, No 1, December 2006, pp. 331–334, ISSN 0973-2063

Chen, P., Zhonghua, E., Yan, Bi et al. (1989). Serum acute phase proteins in nasopharyngeal carcinoma and laryngeal cancers. *Zhonghua yi xue hui*, Vol. 24, No 3, 1989, pp. 174–6, 190, ISSN: 0412-3948

Chen, C., Zhang, X., Lo, C., et al. (2010). The essentiality of alpha-2-macroglobulin in human salivary innate immunity against new H1N1 swine origin influenza A virus. *Proteomics*, Vol. 12, No 10, June 2010, pp. 2396-2401, ISSN 1615-9853

Chu, F., Ekins, R. (1988). Detection of corticosteroid-binding-globulin in parotid fluids: evidence for the presence of both protein and non-protein-bound steroids in uncontaminated saliva. *Acta endocrinologica,* Vol 119, No 1, 1988, pp.56-60, ISSN 0001-5598

Cimasoni, G. (Ed.). (1974). *Monographs in oral science. The crevicular fluid,* Vol. 3, Karger, ISBN: 978-3-8055-1699-0, Basel, Switzerland

Clayman, G., Liu, F., Savage, H. et al. Acute-phase proteins in patients with head and neck cancer treated with interleukin 2/interferon alfa. *Archives of otolaryngology-head & neck surgery,* Vol. 118, No 1, January 1992, pp. 1366–1367, ISSN 0886-4470

Condacci, I., Cimasoni, G., Ahmad-Zadeh, C. (1982). Alpha 2-macroglobulin in sulci from healthy and inflamed human gingiva. *Infection and immunity,* Vol. 36, No 1, April 1982, pp. 66–71, ISSN 0019-9567

Dawes, C., Weatherell, J. (1990). Kinetics of fluoride in the oral fluids. *Journal of dental research,* Vol. 69, February 1990, pp. 638–644, ISSN 0022-0345

Dillon, M., Opris, D., Kopanczyk, R., et al. (2010). Detection of Homocysteine and C-Reactive Protein in the Saliva of Healthy Adults: Comparison with Blood Levels. *Biomarker insights,* Vol. 5, No 20 , July 2010; pp. 57–61, ISSN 1177-2719

Dodds, M., Yeh, C., Johnson, D. (2000). Salivary alterations in type2 (non-insulin dependent) diabetes mellitus and hypertension. *Community dentistry and oral epidemiology,* Vol. 28, No 5, October 2000, pp. 373-381, ISSN 0301-5661

Dowling, P., Wormaldb, R., Meleadya, P., Henrya, M., et al. (2008). Aongus Curranb and Martin ClynesAnalysis of the saliva proteome from patients with head and neck squamous cell carcinoma reveals differences in abundance levels of proteins associated with tumour progression and metastasis. *Journal of Proteomics,* Vol. 71, No 2, July 2008, pp. 168-175, ISSN 1874-3919

Drake, R., Cazare, L., Semmes, O., Wadsworth, J. (2005). Serum, salivary and tissue proteomics for discovery of biomarkers for head and neck cancers. *Expert review of molecular diagnostics,* Vol. 5, No 1, January 2005, pp. 93-100, ISSN 1473-7159

Edgar, W., Mullane, D. (1990). Saliva and oral health. Vol. 1, *British dental Association* , ISBN 0 9045 88 47 5, London

Emiko, K., Yukie, S., Akihiko, S., Shintaro, M., Kiyoshi S., et al. (2000). Assay of the iron-binding proteins, lactoferrin and transferrin, in the saliva of patients wearing complete and partial dentures. *Journal of the Japan Salivary Gland Society,* Vol. 15, No 10, October 1977, pp. 468-469, ISSN 0916-1104

Fisher, B.,Lameyc, P-J., Sweeneyc, D. et al. (1991). Salivary secretion of albumin in type 1 (insulin-dependent) diabetes. *Diabetes Research and Clinical Practice,*Vol. 11, No 2, February 1991, pp. 117-119, ISSN 0168-8227

Florin, T., Paterson, E., Fowler, E., et al. (2006). Clinically active Crohn's disease in the presence of a low C-reactive protein. *Scandinavian journal of gastroenterology,* Vol. 41, No 3, March 2006, pp. 306-311, ISSN 0036-5521

Fournier, T., Medjoubi-N, N., Porquet, D. (2000). Alpha-1-acid glycoprotein. *Biochimica et biophysica acta,* Vol. 1482, No 1-2, October 2000, pp. 157-171, ISSN 0006-3002

Frerichs, R., Htoon, M., Eskes N. et al. (1992). Comparison of saliva and serum for HIV surveillance in developing countries. *Lancet,* Vol. 19, No 340, December 1992, pp. 1496-1499, ISSN 0140-6736

Gautam, D. (2009). Comparative evaluation of alpha-2 macroglobulin and alpha-1 antitrypsin in serum and saliva of phenytoin patients with varying grades of gingival enlargement. A biochemical study. *Indian Journal of Dental sciences*, Vol. 1, No 2, November 2009, pp. 52-58, ISSN 0975-1475

George, J., Fitchen, J. (1997). Future applications of oral fluid specimen technology. *The American journal of medicine*, Vol. 102, No 4A, April 1997, pp. 21–25, ISSN 0002-9343

Gleeson, M., Dobson, A., Firman D., Cripps, A., et al. (1991). The Variability of Immunoglobulins and Albumin in Salivary Secretions of Children. *Scandinavian Journal of Immunology*, Vol. 33, No 5, May 1991, pp. 533–541, ISSN 0300-9475

Grimoud, A., Arnaud, C., Dellamonica, P. et al. (1988). Salivary defence factor concentrations in relation to oral and general parameters in HIV positive patients. *European journal of oral sciences*, Vol. 106, No 6, December 1998, pp. 979–985, ISSN 0909-8836

Gugler, E., Pallavicini, J., Swerdlow, H., Zipkin, I. (1968). Immunological studies of submaxillary saliva from patients with cystic fibrosis and from normal children. *The Journal of Pediatrics*, Vol. 73, No 4, October 1968, pp. 548-559, ISSN 0022-3476

Hammond, G., Langley, M. (1986). Identification and measurement of sex hormone binding globuline (SHBG) and corticosteroid binding globuline (CBG) in human saliva. *Acta endocrinologica (Copenhagen)*, Vol. 112, No 4, August 1986, pp. 603-608, ISSN 0001-5598

Henskens, Y., van der Velden, U., Veerman, E., Nieuw Amerongen, A. (1993). Protein, albumin and cystatin concentrations in saliva of healthy subjects and of patients with gingivitis periodonitis. *Journal of periodontal research*, Vol. 28, No 1, January 1993, pp. 43–48, ISSN 0022-3484

Hiss, S., Knura-Deszczka, S., Regula, G., et al. (2003). Development of an enzyme immuno assay for the determination of porcine haptoglobin in various body fluids: testing the significance of meat juice measurements for quality monitoring programs. *Veterinary immunology and immunopathology*, Vol. 96, No. 1-2, November 2003, pp. 73–82, ISSN 0165-2427

Hold K., M., Douwe de Boer, Zuidema J. et al. (1991). Saliva as an analytical tool in toxicology. *International Journals of Drug Testing*, Vol. 1, No 1, 1999, pp. 1–36

Hu, S., Arellano, M., Boontheung, P., et al. (2008). Salivary proteomics for oral cancer biomarker discovery. *Clinical cancer research: an official journal of the American Association for Cancer Research*, Vol. 14, No 19, October 2008, pp. 6246–6252, ISSN 1078-0432

Humphrey, S., Williamson, R. (2001). A review of saliva: normal composistion, flow and function. *The Journal of prosthetic dentistry*, Vol. 85, No 2, February 2001,pp. 162–168, ISSN: 0022-3913

Huntoon, K., Wang, Y., Eppolito, C., Barbour, K., et al. (2008). The acute phase protein haptoglobin regulates host immunity. *Journal of Leukocyte Biology*, Vol. 84, No 1, July 2008, pp. 170-181, ISSN 0741-5400

Irwin, D. (1990). The diagnostic uses of saliva. *Journal of Oral Pathology & Medicine*, Vol. 19, No 3, March 1990, pp. 119–125, ISSN 0904-2512

Izutsu, K., Truelove, E., Bleyer, W., Anderson, W., et al. (1981). Whole saliva albumin as an indicator of stomatitis in cancer therapy patients. *Cancer*, Vol. 48, No 6, September 1981, pp. 1450-1454, ISSN 0008-543X

Jentisch, H., Beetke, E., Göche, R. (2004). Salivary analyses and caries increment over 4 years an approach by cluster analysis. *Clinical oral investigations*, Vol, 8, No 3, September 2004, pp. 156-160, ISSN 1432-6981

Jou, Y-J., Chia-Der, L., Chih-Ho, L., Chao-Hsien, C., Jung-Yie, K., Shih-Yin C., et al. (2010). Proteomic identification of salivary transferrin as a biomarker for early detection of oral cancer. *Analytica chimica acta*, Vol. 681, No 1-2, November 2010, pp. 41-48, ISSN 0003-2670

Katnik, I., Dobryszycka, W. (1990). Enzyme immunoassay to measure low levels of haptoglobin in biological fluids. *Journal of immunoassay*, Vol. 11, No 4, 1990, pp. 503-517, ISSN 0197-1522

Kaufman, E., Lamster, I. (2000). Analysis of saliva for periodontal diagnosis—a review. *Journal of clinical periodontology*, Vol. 27, No 7, July 2000, pp. 453-465, ISSN 0303-6979

Keur, I., Abraham-Inpijn, L., Nieuw Amerongen, A. (1994). Salivary flow rate and acute-phase proteins in Bell's palsy. *Clinical otolaryngology and allied sciences*, Vol. 19, No 5, October 1994, pp. 415-421, ISSN 0307-7772

Krastev, Z., Kisselova, A., Kolarov, R. (2009). *Oral medicine*. Publisher Ivan Sapundjiev EOOD, ISBN 978 954 9971 48-4, Sofia

Krasteva, A. (2009). The whole unstimulated saliva as diagnostic tool in some systemic disease and oral neoplasm. *PhD work*, Sofia

Landowski, P., Liberek, A., Szlagatys-Sidorkiewicz, A., et al. (2007). Inflammatory bowel disease in children - an analysis of the clinical symptoms and selected biochemical parameters. *M Medycyna wieku rozwojowego*, Vol. 11,No 4, October - December 2007, pp. 401–407, ISSN 1428-345X

Lecchi, C., Avallone, G., Giurovicha, M., Roccabiancaa, P., Ceciliania, F. (2209). Extra hepatic expression of the acute phase protein alpha 1-acid glycoprotein in normal bovine tissues. *The Veterinary Journal*, Vol. 180, No 2, May 2009, pp. 256-258, ISSN 1090-0233

Li, P., Gao, X., Chen, H., et al. (2005). Localization of haptoglobin in normal human skin and some skin diseases. *International journal of dermatology*, Vol. 44, No 4, April 2005, pp. 280–284, ISSN 0011-9059

Marton, K., Boros, I., Fejerdy, P., et al. (2004). Evaluation of unstimulated flow rates of whole and palatal saliva in healthy patients wearing complete dentures and in patients with Sjogren's syndrome. *The Journal of prosthetic dentistry*, Vol. 91, No 6, June 2004, pp. 577–581, ISSN 0022-3913

Murayama, N.,Hirota, K., Sugiyama, M., Amamoto, H., Totani, M. (1999). Salivary indicators of protein nutritional status in the elderly. *Nutrition Research*, Vol. 19, No 7, July 1999, pp. 979-988, ISSN 0271-5317

Nagler, R., Hershkovich, O., Lischinski, S., et al. (2002). Saliva analysis in clinical setting: revisiting an underused diagnostic tool. *Journal of investigative medicine: the official publication of the American Federation for Clinical Research*, Vol. 50, No 2, May 2002, pp. 214–225, ISSN 1081-5589

Nagler, R. (2008). Saliva Analysis for Monitoring Dialysis and Renal Function. *Clinical Chemistry*, Vol. 54, No 9, September 2008, pp. 1415-1417, ISSN 0009-9147

Navazesh, M. (1993). Methods for collecting saliva. *Annals of the New York Academy of Sciences*, Vol. 20, No 694, 1993, pp. 72–77, ISSN 0077-8923

Ng, D., Koh, D., Choo, S., et al. (2004). Effect of strage conditions on the extraction of PCR-quality genomic DNA from saliva. *Clinica chimica acta; international journal of clinical chemistry*, Vol. 343, No 1-2, May 2004, pp.191–194, ISSN 0009-8981

Page, R., Schroeder, H. (1976). Pathogenesis of inflammatory periodontal disease. A summary of current work. Laboratory investigation; a journal of technical methods and pathology, Vol. 34, No 3, March 1976, pp. 235–249, ISSN 0023-6837

Parra, M., Tecles, F., Martinez-Subiela, S., et al. (2005). C-reactive protein measurement in canine saliva. *Journal of veterinary diagnostic investigation: official publication of the American Association of Veterinary Laboratory Diagnosticians*, Inc, Vol. 17,No 2, March 2005, pp. 139–144, ISSN 1040-6387

Parra, M., Väisänen, V., Cerón, J,. (2005). Development of a time-resolved fluorometry based immunoassay for the determination of canine haptoglobin in various body fluids. *Veterinary research*, Vol. 36, No 1, January-February 2005, pp. 117–129, ISSN 0928-4249

Pederson, E., Stanke, S., Whitener, S., et al. (1995). Salivary levels of 2-macroglobulin, alpha-1-antitrypsin, C-reactive protein, cathepsin G and elastase in humans with or without destructive periodontal disease. *Archives of oral biology*, Vol. 40, No 12, December 1995, pp. 1151–1155, ISSN 0003-9969

Persson, L., Bergström, J., Ito, H., Gustafsson, A. (2001). Tobacco smoking and neutrophil activity in patients with periodontal disease. *Journal of periodontology*, Vol, 72, No 1, January 2001, pp. 90–95, ISSN 0022-3492

Rao, R., Balamuralikrishnan, K., Vasantkumar, A., Karanth, K., Bhat, M., Aroor, A. (1995). A study of antitrypsin and macroglobulin levels in serum and saliva of patients with gingivitis. *Indian journal of dental research : official publication of Indian Society for Dental Research*, Vol. 6, No 2, April-June 1995, pp. 41-46, ISSN 0970-9290

Riad-Fahmy, D., Read, G., Walker, R., Griffiths, K. (1982). Steroids in saliva for assessing endocrine function, *Endocrine reviews*, Vol. 3, No 4, Fall 1982, pp. 367-395.

Ritschel, W., Thompson, G. (1983). Monitoring of drug concentrations in saliva: a non-invasive pharmacokinetic procedure. *Methods and Findings in Experimental and Clinical Pharmacology*, Vol. 5, No 8, October 1983, pp. 511-525, ISSN 0379-0355

Rocha-Pereira, P., Santos-Silva, A., Rebelo, I., et al. (1976). Immunological aspects of psoriasis. I. Immunoglobulins and anti-IgG factors. *The British journal of dermatology*, Vol. 94, No 5, May 1976, pp.501–507, ISSN 0007-0963

Rocha-Pereira, P., Santos-Silva, A., Rebelo, I., et al. (2004). The inflammatory response in mild and in severe psoriasis. *The British journal of dermatology*, Vol. 150, No 5, May 2004, pp. 917–928, ISSN 0007-0963

Ruhl, S., Rayment, S., Schmalz, G., Hiller, K. Troxler, R. (2005). Proteins in Whole Saliva during the First Year of Infancy. *Journal of dental research*, Vol. 84, No 1, January 2005, pp. 29-34, ISSN 0022-0345

Ruhl, S., Hamberger, S., Betz, R., et al. (2004). Salivary proteins and cytokines in drug-induced gingival overgrowth. *Journal of dental research*, Vol. 83, No 4, April 2004, pp. 322–326, ISSN 0022-0345

Scarano, E., Fiorita, A., Picciotti, P., Passali, G., Calò, L., Cabras, T., et al. (2010). Proteomics of saliva: personal experience. *Acta otorhinolaryngologica Italica: organo ufficiale della Società italiana di otorinolaringologia e chirurgia cervico-facciale*, Vol. 30, No 3, June 2010, pp. 125-130, ISSN 0392-100X

Schramm, W., Smith, R. (1991). An ultrafiltrate of saliva collected in situ as a biological sample for diagnostic evaluation. *Clinical chemistry,* Vol. 37, No 1, January 1991, pp.114–115, ISSN 0009-9147

Schwartz, E., Granger, D. (2004). Transferrin enzyme immunoassay for quantitative monitoring of blood contamination in saliva. *Clinical Chemistry,* Vol. 50, No 3, March 2004, pp.654-656, ISSN 0009-9147

Selby, C., Lobby, P., Jeffcoate, W. (1988). Sex hormone binding globulin in saliva. Clinical Endocrinology, Vol. 28, No 1, January 1988, pp. 19–24, ISSN 0300-0664

Selner, J., Merrill, D., Claman, H. (1968). Salivary immunoglobulinand albumin: Development during the newborn period. *The Journal of Pediatrics,* Vol. 72, No 5, May 1968, pp. 685-689, ISSN 0022-3476

Senguptaa, S., Lamster, I., Khochta, A., Duffya, T., Gordon, J. (1988). The effect of treatment on IgG, IgA, IgM and α-2-macroglobulin in gingival crevicular fluid from patients with chronic adult periodontitisa. *Archives of Oral Biology,* Vol. 33, No 6, 1988, pp. 425-431, ISSN 0003-9969

Sibraa, P., Reinhardt, R., Dyer, J., DuBois, L. (1991). Acute-phase protein detection and quantification in gingival crevicular fluid by direct and indirect immunodot. *Journal of Clinical Periodontology,* Vol, 18, No 2, February 1991, pp. 101-106, ISSN 0303-6979

Solem, C., Loftus, E., Tremaine, W., et al. (2005). Correlation of C-reactive protein with clinical, endoscopic, histologic, and radiographic activity in inflammatory bowel disease. *Inflammatory bowel diseases,* Vol. 11, No 8, August 2005, pp. 707–712, ISSN 1078-0998

Sukharev, A., Nikolaev, A., Nikolaeva, N., Sukhareva, N. (1991). Lactoferrin and fibrinogen degradation products in saliva. *Laboratornoe delo,* Vol. 5, 1991, pp. 20-24, ISSN 0023-6748

Szabó, S., Száva Szabó, A., Nagy, V., Vargancsik-Mosoni, M. (1988). Serum and salivary proteins in dysmature infants. *Physiologie,* Vol. 25, No 4, October-December 1988, pp. 169-176, ISSN 1011-6206

Umeda, T., Hiromatsu, R., Iwaoka, T., Shimada, T., et al. (1981). Use of saliva for monitoring unbound free cortisol levels in serum. *Clinica chimica acta; international journal of clinical chemistry,* Vol. 110, No 2-3, March 1981, pp. 245-253, ISSN 0009-8981

Vaziri, P., Vahedi, M., Abdollahzadeh, S., Abdolsamadi, H., et al. (2009). Evaluation of Salivary Albumin in Diabetic Patients. *Iranian Journal of Public Health,* Vol. 38, No. 3, 2009, pp.54-59, ISSN 0304-4556

Vucelić, B., Krznarić, Z., Sentić, M., et al. (1990). Value of C-reactive protein in the evaluation of activity in ulcerative colitis and Crohn's disease. *Liječnički vjesnik,* Vol. 112, No 9-10, September-October 1990, pp. 281–284, ISSN 0024-3477

Wade, S., Haegele, A. (1991). Time-integrated measurement of corticosteroids in saliva by oral diffusion sink technology. *Clinical chemistry,* Vol. 37, No 7, July 1991, pp. 1166–1172, ISSN 0009-9147

Wasinger, V., Cordwell, S., Cerpa-Poljak, A., Yan, J., Gooley, A., et al. (1995). Progress with gene-product mapping of the Mollicutes: Mycoplasma genitalium. *Electrophoresis,* Vol. 7, No 7, July 1995, pp. 1090–1094, ISSN 0173-0835

Wilkins, M. (2009). Proteomics data mining. Expert review of proteomics. *Expert Reviews,* IBSN 1478-9450, England

Yu- Hsiang, L., Wong, D. (2009). Saliva: An emerging biofluid for early detection of diseases. *American Journal of Dentistry*, Vol. 22, No. 4, August 2009, pp. 241-248, ISSN 0894-8275

Zaprjanova, M. (1989). *Laboratory tests in dentistry*. Publisher: Medicine and sport, Sofia

5

Acute Phase Protein's Levels as Potential Biomarkers for Early Diagnosis of Neurodegenerative Diseases

De Pablos V, Barcia C, Yuste-Jiménez JE, Ros-Bernal F, Carrillo-de Sauvage MA, Fernández-Villalba E and Herrero MT
Clinical and Experimental Neuroscience and Centro de Investigación Biomedica en Red de Enfermedades Neurodegenerativas (CIBERNED) School of Medicine, University of Murcia, Campus de Espinardo, Murcia Spain

1. Introduction

1.1 Inflammation

Inflammation is a response of the organism that facilitates the immune response and/or repair after a harmful stimulus, such as pathogens, damaged cells, or irritants. The inflammatory process is necessary for the healing of the tissues. However, the uncontrolled chronic inflammation can also lead to harmful diseases, such as atherosclerosis or rheumatoid arthritis, among others (Eming et al., 2007; Tabas, 2010; Libby, 2008).

The cause of inflammation may be of different origin. An inflammatory response could be stimulated by chemical or physical damages, but also by pathogens or immune reactions (Moore et al., 2010).

The cardinal signs of inflammation in the majority of the tissues include pain, redness, immobility, swelling and heat. These signs usually encompass the increase of blood flow in the inflamed area and the accumulation of fluids that help to increase the possibilities of tissue repair. However, inflammation of particular tissues, such as in the central nervous system (CNS), those characteristics are not fully applicable (Carson et al., 2006).

Many cells are implicated in the inflammatory process. One of the initial players is the resident macrophages, that are able to respond rapidly to damage. Particularly in the CNS, the macrophage-analogue cells are the resident microglia but their role is not fully understood and it is some how different from macrophages (Schwartz, 2003). Other tissue resident cells, like Dendritic cells or Kupfer cells, not present in the CNS, may also be initial responders to inflammation but other cells, entering in the CNS and coming from the systemic circulation, such as natural killer (NK) cells, leukocytes, and lymphocytes are also implicated in the inflammatory response (McMahon et al., 2006; Haskill et al., 1992).

Inflammation also comprises a complex biological response implicating vascular tissues and the activation of the endothelium to facilitate the specific entrance of blood cells (Trepels et al., 2006).

After a specific insult, several cascades of factors are activated. The plasma derived inflammatory mediators such as the complement and the coagulation system, together with the cell-derived inflammatory mediators (Pesce and Dosekun, 1983). In the latter case, resident inflammatory cells start to release different factors that trigger and amplify the local inflammatory response. Among these factors, the cytokines and chemokines are the crucial players in the inflammation cascade (Luster, 1998) and, as we describe in depth in following sections of this chapter, are important mediators of the Acute Phase Protein (APP) response.

Pro-inflammatory cytokines are proteins able to induce specific inflammatory responses in the tissue. Each type of cytokine participates in a particular function and it is specifically stimulated in particular scenarios and pathologies (Kopf et al., 2010). In the CNS, the cytokines play very important roles and their deregulation may result in neurological disorders. In fact, cytokines has been many times proposed as biomarkers for neurodegenerative diseases (Reale et al., 2009). The most studied cytokines, with clear effects in the CNS are the tumor necrosis factor alpha (TNF-α), the interferon gamma (IFN-γ), interleukin (IL)-6, IL-1β IL-17, and transforming growth factor beta (TGF-β) among many others.

TNF-α is a cytokine involved in many inflammatory processes, with fundamental roles in inflammation and lymphoid organogenesis as well as in neuro-degenerative diseases (Idriss and Naismith, 2000). It is expressed by several cell-types including macrophages, lymphocytes and NK cells. Its deficiency or exacerbation may cause inflammatory and autoimmune diseases. The blockade of TNF-α with specific antibodies has been largely developed with therapeutic purposes as for example anti tumor activity, but also it has been developed for brain disorders.

IFN-γ is produced mainly in lymphocytes and NK cells and its expression by macrophages is still controversial. It has a crucial role in maintaining the host defense against pathogens and has been linked with the progression of many autoimmune diseases including those in the brain. Surprisingly, mice lacking IFN-γ or IFN-γ receptor (IFN-γR) develop an exacerbated inflammation in models autoimmune diseases, which suggest that Th1 T cells, that produce IFN-γ, may be indirectly involved in these diseases (Jacob, 1992; Olsson, 1992).

IL-1 is produced by several types of cells and it is involved in many inflammatory responses (Dinarello, 2006). The overproduction of IL-1β has been associated with a group of inflammatory disorders. Mice lacking the receptor for IL-1 or lacking both IL-1α and IL-1β are protected from the development of autoimmune alterations. IL-1β promotes dendritic cell maturation and Th-17 cell clonal expansion, contributing to autoimmunity in brain diseases. The blockade of IL-1β has also been developed as a possible anti-cancer treatment (Dinarello, 2010; Curti et al., 1995) and may be beneficial to treat some brain degenerative disorders.

IL-6 is produced by various cell types in response to infection or tissue alteration. Importantly, it is a crucial mediator of the immune system inducing a liver APP response and the B cell and T cell effector responses to pathogens (Hirano, 1992). Its target has therapeutic potential, since it is directly involved in some inflammatory diseases such as arthritis or colitis (Dayer and Choy, 2009; Atreya et al, 2000). As we describe below IL-6 is critically involved in the APP regulation.

Chemokines also contribute to the specific inflammatory responses in the tissue. There are many types of chemokines involved in particular scenarios and pathologies similarly to cytokines. Importantly, chemokines play crucial roles in recruiting factors and cells into the parenchyma, contributing to enhance the local inflammatory response (Semple et al., 2010). Chemokines also may be considered biomarkers for tissue alteration. One of the most important subfamily of chemokines is the subgroup so called CC chemokine ligand (CCL). Examples of CC chemokine include the CCL2, formerly called monocyte chemoattractant protein-1 (MCP-1), which is involved in the extravasation and recruitment of macrophages and lymphocytes into the tissue. CCL5 or RANTES also contributes to the entrance of T cells, basophils and eosinophils (Ge et al., 2008). In the CNS, CCL2 seems to play a key role in some neurodegenerative diseases. Accordingly, in other neuro-inflammatory processes, such as acute brain trauma, stroke, as well as during chronic affections like multiple sclerosis or Alzheimer´s Disease (AD), prolonged and sustained inflammation mediated by CCL2 may have cytotoxic effects, aggravating the incidence and the severity of the disease (Conductier *et al*, 2010). Therefore, the CCL2 modulation may be considered as an interesting potential therapeutic target to control local inflammatory responses.

This complex inflammatory response, driven by cytokines and chemokines, and consequently by APP, although it is necessary for the repair of the tissue, if is not controlled may contribute to the development of pathological conditions. Particularly in the CNS, increasing evidences show that the inflammatory response may be a crucial contributor to the neurodegenerative process.

1.2 Inflammation and neurodegenerative diseases

The inflammatory response in the CNS is very different from the rest of the systems. The particular anatomical location, inside the cranium, and the crucial importance of the brain function has shaped the need for a particular immune response. These characteristics have lead many scientists to think that the brain is an immune privileged tissue. The special brain blood barrier (BBB) and the absence of dendritic cells, or clear analogous cells, makes difficult to understand the mechanisms of the immune responses in the brain keeping in mind the standards of other tissues (Yong and Rivest, 2009). Glial cells, and in particular microglial cells, has been widely known as the initial responders of the immune response in the brain, however, there are many questions that remain unanswered regarding their function in neurodegenerative diseases (Henkel et al, 2009).

The glial activation is a histological hallmark in many neurodegenerative diseases. *Post mortem* histopathology of brains from patients with Parkinson's disease (PD) and AD show activation of microglial cells and astrocytes, which suggests that the neuronal degeneration is associated with inflammatory response (McGeer et al., 1988). However, it is still unclear whether glial activation precedes or is secondary to the neuro-degeneration. Previous studies in experimental Parkinsonism have shown that exacerbated microglial activation lead to the degeneration of dopaminergic neurons (Mount et al., 2007, Barcia et al., 2004). In line with this, when the microglial cells are activated locally with lipopolysaccharide (LPS), a large molecule found in the outer membrane of Gram-negative bacteria that elicits a strong immune response in animals, the local dopaminergic neuronal loss is exacerbated (Saijo et al., 2009). However, the endogenous and constitutive factors responsible of the local glial activation that may lead to degeneration in neurodegenerative disorders are still uncertain. Cytokines and chemokines are clear candidates to be directly involved in the activation of glial cells in the brain. Recent studies performed in our laboratory have shown in experimental models of PD that cytokines, specifically IFN-γ and TNF-α, are responsible of the local glial activation in the brain parenchyma. Importantly, the levels of cytokines in the brain correlates with the neuronal degeneration and are persistently increased along the years, which suggest that the perpetuation of the neuronal loss may be mediated by certain cytokines (Barcia et al., 2011). Moreover, and most importantly for this review, the cytokines are also increased in the circulating plasma demonstrating that the inflammatory response goes beyond the brain parenchyma in neurodegenerative processes. In addition, other studies have demonstrated that the artificial induction of increasing circulating levels of specific cytokines in the blood exacerbates the neuronal death in experimental models of neuro-degeneration *in vivo* (Pott Godoy et al., 2008). Coherently with this evidences, patients with neurodegenerative disorders also show increased levels of cytokines in the blood and cerebrospinal fluid (CSF), which suggests a general and systemic inflammatory response involving the whole organism (Reale et al., 2009). This generalized inflammatory response could certainly activate many other inflammatory cascades in other organs. One of the general responses that may be activated is the APP reaction. However, there are many proteins that are included in the APPs, and each disorder may have a particular response involving different proteins. Unfortunately, one of the caveats to keep in mind for this kind of measurements is the putative variation of these proteins that individuals may have when they are under pharmacological treatment. Nevertheless, the clinical significance of specific APP levels in serum or plasma of patients for specific neurological symptoms may be crucial in order to find biomarkers that may help for the early and accurate diagnosis of neurodegenerative diseases.

1.3 Acute phase response and acute phase proteins

The first reaction of the body to immunological stress is the innate, non-specific response preceding specific immune reactions. The acute phase response (APR) is a prominent systemic reaction of the organism as a result of this innate response to local or systemic disturbances in its homeostasis and may be caused by infection, tissue injury, trauma or surgery, neoplastic growth or immunological disorders (Gordon and Koy, 1985; Gruys et al., 1999).

This response takes place at the very beginning of the inflammatory process and lasts for 1-2 days. After that, the host returns to normal functions. However, the systemic response can also be prolonged, if acute inflammation becomes chronic (Kushner et al., 1981).

The purpose of acute-phase reaction is to counteract the underlying challenge in order to restore rapidly the homeostasis. This phenomenon is accomplished by isolating and destroying the infective organisms, or removing the harmful molecules, and activating the process of repair. Their function in neurodegenerative disorders is unclear but there are evidences that suggest their involvement and may be important for diagnosis. Acute-phase reaction includes a wide range of neuroendocrine (Fever, anorexia, decrease of thyroxine, increase of cortisol), hematopoietic (Anemia, leukocytosis, thrombocytosis), and metabolic changes (muscle atrophy, increase of lipolysis) that can be reflected systemically (Woo and Gorman, 1992; Whicher and Westacott, 1992).

Precisely, one of the most interesting features of the acute-phase is the change in the concentrations of many plasma proteins, known as the acute-phase proteins, which can be easily detected in the blood. The APP has been defined as one whose plasma concentration increases (positive acute-phase proteins) or decreases (negative acute-phase proteins) by at least 25 percent during inflammatory reactions (Gabay and Kushner, 1999). The very first APP to be described, C-reactive protein (CRP), was discovered in 1930 in the plasma of patients during the acute phase of pneumococcal infection. In some pathologies CRP may even increase more than 1000 times (Gabay and Kushner, 2001) being an excellent marker for diagnosis.

1.4 The regulation of the acute-phase expression and activation

The synthesis and release of plasma APP takes place in the liver and it is regulated by inflammatory mediators. These mediators fall into four major categories: IL-6-type cytokines, IL-1-type cytokines, glucocorticoids, and growth factors. Cytokines mainly stimulate the APP gene-expression, while glucocorticoids and growth factors modulate the cytokine activity (**Figure 1**). Binding of the inflammatory mediators to their respective receptors on hepatocytes and the transduction of this signal induce changes in APP gene expression that are primarily regulated at transcriptional level (Gauldie et al., 1987).

As we stated above, cytokines are a group of proteins acting as extracellular and intercellular signaling molecules. The role of cytokines during inflammation is both initiation and fine-tuning of the whole process: some cytokines initiate and amplify the response, others sustain or attenuate it, and some of them cause it to resolve (Martínez-Subiela, 2001, Heinrich et al., 1990).

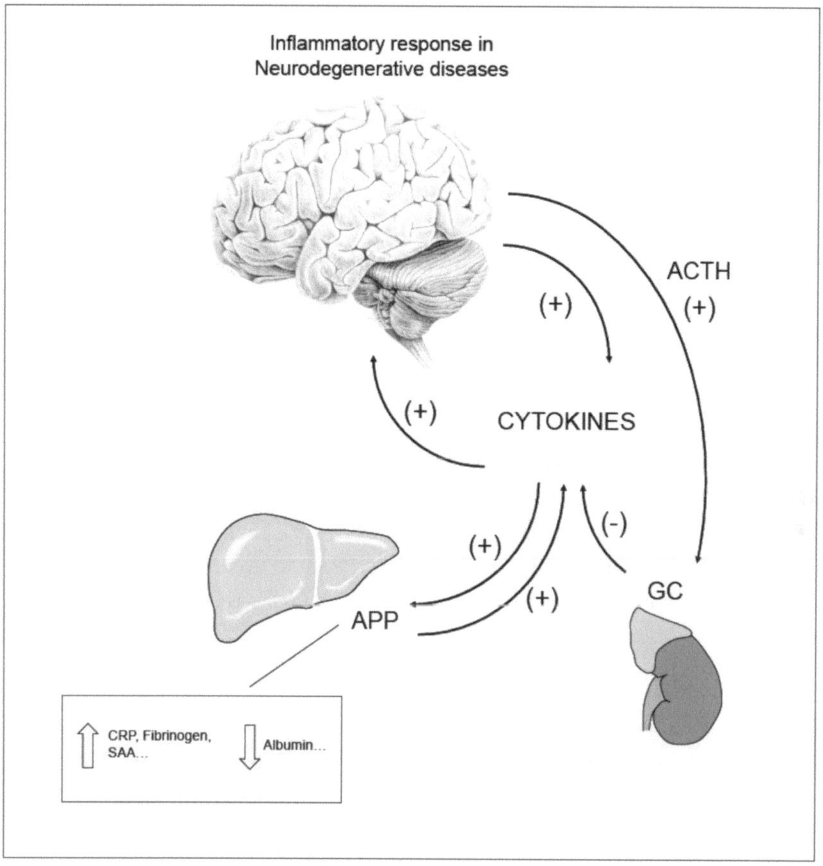

Fig. 1. Local inflammation in neurodegenerative diseases induces a Serum amyloid A (SAA) APP peripheral inflammatory responses in a cytokine-dependent fashion. This APP response is orchestrated in the liver, and it is characterized by the increase of some factors such as CRP, fibrinogen or SAA and the reduction of some others like albumin. Furthermore, this response may contribute to the general inflammatory response and may exacerbate the local neuro-degeneration.

During inflammation, inflammatory cells, mainly macrophages and neutrophils that assemble at the site of challenge, together with endothelial cells, secrete the so-called pro-inflammatory cytokines TNF-α, IL-1β, and IL-6, in that order. This order is important, since each cytokine fulfills a precise role in up-regulating or down-regulating the expression of the others. TNF-α released by T cells and macrophages precedes the release of IL-1β and both stimulate the anti-inflammatory or proinflammatory cytokines (Feldmann, 2002).
Pro-inflammatory cytokines induce a number of local and systemic responses like: a) the expression of selectins on local endothelial cells, that recruit inflammatory cells from the bloodstream; b) the activation of recruited cells in developing their optimal defensive activity, i.e. increased expression of receptors (Complement receptors), or cell metabolism, such as oxidative burst, and c) expression of other cytokines, such as chemokines, that recruit more and more defensive cells to the inflammation site (Richards *et al.*; 1992) and importantly d) the production of APPs.
Then, cytokines are clear inducers of the APP response and both, cytokines and APP, may vary by the same pattern. However, changes in cytokines are less evident and more difficult to be measured while APPs changes are usually higher and clearly identifiable, which makes them suitable for early diagnosis.

1.5 Classification of APP

Since their discovery several classifications of acute phase proteins have been proposed. All the up-regulated proteins have been called "positive APP", in order to differentiate them from the so-called "negative APP", that are down regulated. Importantly, the most physiologically expressed proteins, albumin and several other proteins, usually present in blood, belong to the latter group, which makes the positive ones suitable for diagnosis.
Another interesting classification differentiates the APPs for the rate of their expression. For example, the apolipoproteins serum amyloid SAA1 and SAA2 (commonly called SAA) are considered "major acute-phase proteins" and their concentration, as we have stated above, can increase as much as 1000-fold. Other major APPs are CRP and Alpha-1-acid glycoprotein (AGP) (Gabay and Kushner, 2001) which are important for degenerative disorders.

Relevant APPs for CNS disorders

C-Reactive Protein (CRP)

CRP is an acute phase protein that circulates as a pentamer (pentameric CRP) in plasma and with serum levels rising as much as 1000-fold following injury or infection. It is increased by bacterial infections and generally less elevated in viral infections (Jaye and Waites, 1997).
The name derives from its ability to react with the C polysaccharide of *Streptococcus pneumoniae,* but it may also bind to chromatin in nuclear DNA-histone complexes. Once bound, it is able to activate the classical complement pathway (Woo and Gorman, 1992).
An increased CRP may be due to: (i) inflammatory disorders, e.g. inflammatory arthritis, vasculitis, Crohn's disease, (ii) tissue injury or necrosis, e.g. burns, necrosis, myocardial infarction, pulmonary embolus, (iii) Infections, especially bacterial, (iv) malignancy, and (v) tissue rejection.

CRP concentrations typically return to normal level after 7 days of appropriated treatment for bacterial meningitis, if no complications are developed. Thus, serial monitoring of CRP concentrations in serum and CSF concentrations may be clinically useful.

However, CRP is non-specific and its clinical usefulness is therefore limited, especially in diagnosis. CRP is useful in monitoring inflammatory disease activity, including rheumatoid arthritis, infections or malignancy and can also be useful as a prognostic marker for some conditions (e.g. acute pancreatitis). There is also evidence that CRP has a stronger predictive value for the risk of coronary heart disease and stroke events than low-density lipoprotein (LDL) cholesterol (Ridker *et al.*, 2002), in contrast its predictive value for neurodegenerative diseases is still under development.

Homocysteine

Homocysteine (Hcy) is an amino acid formed from the metabolism of the essential amino acid, methionine. It is a homologue of the amino acid cysteine, differing by an additional methylene (-CH2-) group. It is biosynthesized from methionine by the removal of its terminal C methyl group. Homocysteine can be recycled into methionine or converted into cysteine with the aid of B-vitamins (Selhub, 1999).

High dietary consumption of methionine, which can be found in meats and dairy products, can result in the overproduction of homocysteine. Once homocysteine is produced it is metabolized in the body through one of two possible pathways - remethylation or trans-sulfuration. Re-methylation is a process that utilizes folate, vitamin B12 or betaine (trimethylglycine) to convert homocysteine back to methionine. Alternately, trans-sulfuration utilizes vitamin B6, pyridoxal-5-phosphate, to catabolize excess homocysteine into a number of metabolites for eventual excretion from the body (Graham et al., 1997) and it can be increased in some neurodegenerative diseases, as we will describe below.

Plasma homocysteine concentrations may differ, depending on which metabolic homocysteine pathway is defective. An abundance of research indicates that an increased homocysteine level may indicate an increased risk of cardiovascular disease like coronary heart disease, stroke and peripheral vascular disease (Boushey et al., 1995)

Fibrinogen

Fibrinogen is a soluble plasma glycoprotein, with high molecular weight of 340 kDa, synthesised by the liver that is converted by thrombin into fibrin during blood coagulation. This is achieved through a process in the coagulation cascade that activates the zymogen prothrombin to the serine protease thrombin, which is responsible for converting fibrinogen into fibrin. Fibrin is then cross-linked by factor XIII to form a clot (Weisel, 2005).

Fibrinogen normal plasma levels are between 150 and 450 mg/dl. More than 300 mg/dl are related with the risk of heart attack. It is still controversial the role of fibrinogen as an atherosclerotic vascular disease risk factor; epidemiological evidences seem to be coincident about its role as a marker or predictor of new or reiterated atherothrombotic events (Paterno, 2000).

The reasons by which fibrinogen is elevated in cardiovascular disease and atherosclerosis are, in general, only incompletely understood; but all cells involved in the atherogenetic process are able to produce cytokines, which induce an acute phase reaction that increases fibrinogen levels in plasma (Canseco-Ávila et al., 2006).

Recent research has also shown that fibrin also plays a key role in the inflammatory response and the development of rheumatoid arthritis. In addition, it has been related with AD as we will discuss in following sections.

Serum amyloid A proteins (SAA)

SAA constitutes a protein family related to the A proteins of secondary amyloidosis (Bausserman et al, 1980, 1982; Betts et al, 1991; Strachan et al, 1989).
SAA is one of the major APPs (encoded by SAA1 and SAA2; collectively referred to also as A-SAA (acute phase serum amyloid A). Its level in the blood increases dramatically (up to 1 000-fold; 1 000 micrograms/mL) in response to various stimuli, which suggests an important short-term beneficial role in responses to tissue injury and inflammation. Although the liver is the primary site of synthesis of both A-SAA and C-SAA, extrahepatic production has also been reported for most family members in most of the mammalian species studied. Bacterial lipopolysaccharides and several cytokines (mainly IL-1β, IL-6 and TNF-α but also LIF, CNTF, oncostatin M, IL-11, and cardiotrophin-1) are involved in the induction of SAA synthesis and some of these cytokines act synergistically (Benigni et al, 1996).
Although the precise role of A-SAA in host defense during inflammation has not been defined, many potential clinically important functions have been proposed for individual SAA family members. These include involvement in lipid metabolism/transport, induction of extracellular-matrix-degrading enzymes, and chemotactic recruitment of inflammatory cells to sites of inflammation. A-SAA is potentially involved in the pathogenesis of several chronic inflammatory diseases: it is the precursor of the amyloid A protein deposited in amyloid A amyloidosis, and it has also been implicated in the pathogenesis of atheroscelerosis, rheumatoid arthritis and, importantly, PD.

2. Neurodegenerative diseases and Acute Phase Protein

2.1 Alzheimer's disease and APP

AD is a complex neurodegenerative disorder characterized by progressive loss of cognitive function and subsequent death. Since the first case of this disease was diagnosed one century ago, much effort has been dedicated to find a cure. However, even though progress has been made in the knowledge of the pathogenesis of this disease, its ultimate cause remains unknown. An effective treatment has not yet been found and the efforts to prevent the neuronal death are crucial. Therefore, new approaches are urgently needed regarding the early diagnosis.
The relevance of APP measurements in the diagnosis of neurodegenerative diseases like AD is actually under evaluation. Obviously, the inflammatory response generated in these kinds of illnesses is less noteworthy than the inflammatory response that may be observed in other pathological conditions such as viral or bacterial infections.
A large number of proteins, peptides and aminoacids, other than β-amyloid, have been examined in plasma, based on their putative role in AD pathology. Perhaps the two most consistent findings are the increase in total Homocystein (tHcy) and CRP seen in AD. First reported by Clarke and colleagues, an increase of tHcy in plasma has been widely reported and a recent systematic review of large and prospective studies, found a relative risk of AD in individuals with elevated tHcy. Increased tHcy and CRP are both associated with a risk of cardiovascular disease but it is worth noting that neither contributes to risk estimation, even in cardiovascular disease, enough to warrant recommendation for use in clinical practice. Given that the association with AD may well be weaker than

cardiovascular disease, this emphasizes the gap between finding an association with disease and proof of utility as a biomarker. Nonetheless, CRP and tHcy may have independent effects on the risk of developing AD. Regarding CRP, the studies are some how controversial and complex. Some studies reported that an elevation in CRP has been associated the rate of progression of AD but also with MCI and Down's syndrome. However, other large longitudinal studies found that markers of inflammation, such as TNF-α but not CRP, were associated with the risk of dementia while others found an association between CRP and vascular dementia (VD).

Accordingly, a recent study by O'Bryant and colleagues (2010) analyzing a combined pool of 192 patients diagnosed with probable AD and 174 non-demented controls show that mean CRP levels were found to be significantly decreased in AD (2.9 mg/mL) versus controls (4.9 mg/mL; $P<.003$). These findings, together with previously published results, are consistent with the hypothesis that these changes in CRP may be time-dependent, therefore, midlife elevations in CRP may be associated with increased risk of AD development, although elevated CRP levels may not be useful for prediction in the immediate prodrome years before AD becomes clinically expressed.

There is significant evidence that AD patients suffer from inadequate circulation and cerebrovascular pathology, and one theory that is gaining evidence is the importance of vascular factors in the onset and progression of this disease (Farkas et al., 2001; Iadecola C, 2004; de la Torre 2004). In line with this, AD patients have an abnormal cerebral vasculature and brain hypoperfusion, and a large body of research, implicates cerebrovascular dysfunction as a contributing factor to AD. Some recent studies show how reducing fibrinogen, a circulating protein critical in hemostasis, provides a significant decrease in the neurovascular damage, blood–brain barrier permeability and neuroinflammation present in AD. These studies involve fibrinogen as a possible contributor to AD (Cortes-Canteli and Strickland, 2009).

On the other hand, some other studies show increased levels of tHcy in patients with probable AD and established negative correlation between serum tHcy concentrations and cognitive damage tested By Mini-Mental State Examination (MMSE) scores, suggesting a potential role for tHcy in the pathogenesis of AD and cognitive impairment (Lepara et al., 2009).

These findings imply that the serum tHcy level may be a potential biomarker for AD, as well as a marker of cognitive damage associated with this disease.

2.2 Parkinson's disease and APP

PD is a neurodegenerative disorder characterized by the loss of dopaminergic neurons of the Substantia Nigra *pars compacta* (SNpc). A big problem with this particular disease is that the neurological symptoms only appear when more than 60% of the neurons are already lost. For this reason the early diagnosis is crucial to prevent the neuronal degeneration. The areas of neurodegeneration are accompanied by local inflammation characterized by a strong glial response mediated by cytokines. These proinflammatory compounds also travel outside the brain and can be detected in the blood.

It is known that some cytokines, such as IL1-β, TNF-α and IFN-γ, are increased in the blood and cerebrospinal fluid (CSF) of patients with PD. These cytokines are able to reactivate the local inflammation in the CNS but they are also able to induce the activation of other peripheral inflammatory pathways such as the activation of APP. Then, the measurement of blood APP levels may be a valuable tool for assessing and confirming the early diagnosis in Parkinsonism, and the secretion of these anti-inflammatory markers such as cytokines or APPs could be utilized to help the diagnose of the disease (de Pablos et al., 2009).

There are very few studies regarding the levels of APP in PD and some of the results are apparently in conflict. Dufek and coworkers (2009) only found sporadic and slight abnormalities in the concentration of CRP and SAA in the serum of PD patients but McGeer and coworkers (2004), however, observed an increase of CRP in the affected dopaminergic areas of the brain. This apparent contradiction may be explained since the patients studied by Dufek and colleagues were moderately impaired and were all taking antiparkinsonian drugs, which may interfere in the peripheral APP measurements. In fact, a study of our laboratory shows that tHyc is increased in PD patients under L-dopa treatment (Martín-Fernández et al., 2010). On the other hand, other study regarding the APP levels in the blood of PD patients show an increase of CRP in the plasma according with the Hoehn-Yahr stages of PD severity (Seet et al., 2009). Importantly, in the study of Seet and coworkers the patients were advised to refrain from consuming their anti-parkinsonian medications 4 h before collection of the samples suggesting that a previous wash out of drugs may be needed in order to detect changes in these proteins. These results suggest that the dopaminergic loss in the brain is able to induce an increase of the peripheral APP that can be detected in the serum. In line with this, previous studies of our group have demonstrated that the specific degeneration of dopaminergic neurons induced by MPTP administration in non-human primate, stimulates an increase of CRP, SAA and Haptoglobin (HP) in plasma (de Pablos et al., 2009). This increase is very fast and transient, except for HP, which suggest that this response is related with the immediate effect of the toxin. On the other hand, a persistent increase of APP in the plasma suggests a persistent damage, which can be related with chronic degeneration.

The role of APP in PD is still unclear but increasing evidences show that the local inflammatory response in the brain is also reflected by several markers systemically and may be easily detected in the blood by well-established techniques. CRP seems to be a clear candidate as a PD biomarker but further studies are needed to soundly determine the specific factors that are increased in PD, which APPs are particularly increased and how are they correlated with the dopaminergic degeneration and the level of Parkinsonism.

2.3 Vascular dementia and APP

Several inflammatory proteins, such as cytokines are linked with AD and some APP, such as tHcy and CRP, has been associated with the disease (Clarke et al., 1998). However, the relation between the APP and the presence of absence of dementia is still unclear. Very few studies report changes in the APP levels in VD and some of them present inconclusive results. Mancinella and coworkers (Mancinella et al., 2009) described that CRP levels are elevated in patients with VD respect to controls but still they show lower levels than patients with AD, which makes difficult to distinguish both disorders based in the peripheral biomarkers. Other authors did not find any differences in the CRP levels in VD but they however found an increase in tHcy (Davis et al., 2009). Importantly, high blood levels of tHcy have been related with cardiovascular diseases and may be also related with similar alterations in the VD (Lepara et al., 2009).

A. Proteins whose plasma concentrations increase
Complement system
C3
C4
C9
Factor B
C1 inhibitor
C4b-binding protein
Mannose-binding lectin
Coagulation and fibrinolytic system
Fibrinogen
Plasminogen
Tissue plasminogen activator
Urokinase
Protein S
Vitronectin
Plasminogen-activator inhibitor 1
Antiproteases
α-1 -Protease inhibitor
α–1 -Antichymotrypsin
Pancreatic secretory trypsin inhibitor
Inter α-trypsin inhibitors
Transport proteins
Ceruloplasmin
Haptoglobin
Hemopexin
Participants in inflammatory responses
Secreted phospholipase A2
Lipopolysaccharide-binding protein
Interleukin-1-receptor antagonist
Granulocyte colony-stimulating factor
Others
C-reactive protein
Serum amyloid A
α–1 -Acid glycoprotein
Fibronectin
Ferritin
Angiotensinogen
B. Proteins whose plasma concentrations decrease
Albumin
Transferrin
Transthyretin
Alpha-2-HS glycoprotein
Alpha-fetoprotein
Thyroxine-binding globulin
Insulin-like growth factor I
Factor XII

Table 1. Human Acute-Phase proteins.

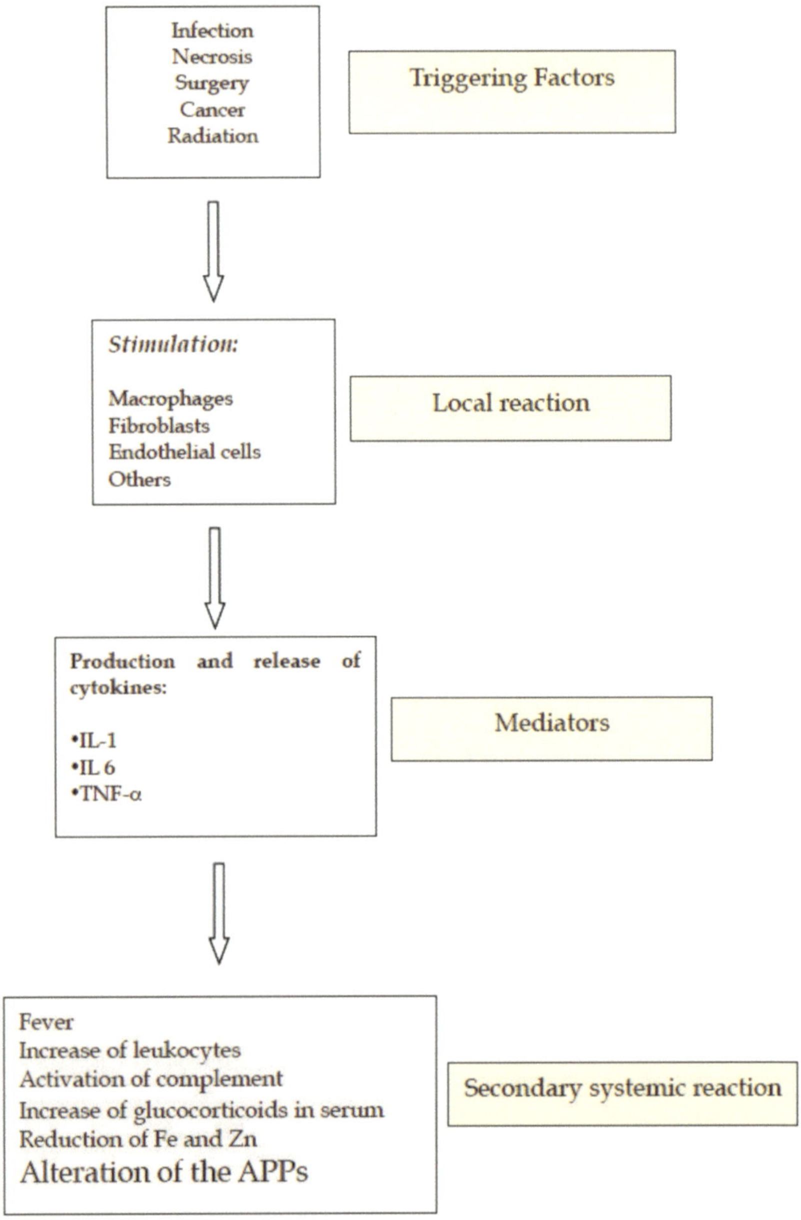

Fig. 2. Different inflammatory triggering factors activate cells to stimulate local reactions. This response is mediated by different cytokines that are able to provoke a secondary systemic reaction characterized by the increase of leukocytes, activation of complement, increase of glucocorticoids in serum, reduction of Fe^{++} and Zn^{+} and the cascade of APPs.

Acute Phase Protein	Normal concentration in plasma (mg/l)
GROUP 1 (50% increase)	
Ceruloplasmin	150-600
C3-Complement	800-1700
C4-Complement	150-650
GROUP 2 (2-5-fold increase)	
Haptoglobin	400-1800
α1-glycoprotein	550-1400
α1 antichemotrypsin	300-1600
α1 protease inhibitor protease	2000-4000
Fibrinogen	2000-4500
GROUP 3 (1000 -fold increase)	
C-Reactive Protein	< 5.0
Serum Amyloid A	<10.0

Table 2. APP Classification production depending on the rate of their expression and normal concentration in human.

3. Conclusions and therapeutic perspectives

In neurodegenerative diseases changes observed blood parameters could be considered as putative hallmark of diseases evolution that might be helpful for personalized diagnosis, prognostic and/or progression diseases monitoring.

Obviously, the inflammatory response triggered in neurodegenerative diseases such as PD or AD is less easily detectable than those observed in other pathological conditions such as viral or bacterial infections. Accordingly, the APPs increase observed in neurodegenerative diseases is of less extent than the increase observed in infectious pathologies. Therefore, it is to be expected that the increase in APPs in patients exhibiting neurodegenerative diseases will be low as compared with other diseases. Although the relevance of APP measurements in the diagnosis of neurodegenerative diseases should need further evaluations, we believe that the prospects for blood-based biomarkers may be useful in the near future. We suggest that blood-based APP markers, perhaps in association with other biomarkers, will be useful tools for diagnosis of neurodegenerative diseases such as AD or PD and it is very likely that plasma markers will become part of the armamentarium for the investigation of CNS disorders.

The measurement of blood APP levels will be a safe and valuable tool for assessing and confirming the diagnosis of some disorders; the secretion of anti-inflammatory markers such as cytokines or APPs could be used to help to diagnose and evaluate the progression of the neurodegenerative process. However, more sensitive techniques of APP detection are needed, in particular to be used as putative diagnosis marker of neurodegenerative disorders.

4. Acknowledgements

This work was supported by grants from: the Spanish Ministry of Science & Innovation (SAF 2007-62262; FIS P10/02827), *Fundación Séneca* (FS/07/05662; FS/10/15329) and CIBERNED (*Centro de Investigación Biomédica en Red sobre Enfermedades Neurodegenerativas*) to MTH. The authors would also like to thank Mr. P. Thomas for comments and language suggestions on this manuscript. Finally, the authors declare that there is no conflict of interest in the present work.

5. References

Atreya R, Mudter J, Finotto S, Müllberg J, Jostock T, Wirtz S, Schütz M, Bartsch B, Holtmann M, Becker C, Strand D, Czaja J, Schlaak JF, Lehr HA, Autschbach F, Schürmann G, Nishimoto N, Yoshizaki K, Ito H, Kishimoto T, Galle PR, Rose-John S, Neurath MF. Blockade of interleukin 6 trans signaling suppresses T-cell resistance against apoptosis in chronic intestinal inflammation: evidence in crohn disease and experimental colitis in vivo. Nat Med. 2000 May;6(5):583-8. Erratum in: Nat Med. 2010 Nov;16(11):1341.

Barcia C, Ros CM, Annese V, Gomez A, Ros-Bernal F, Aguado-Yera D, Martínez-Pagán ME, de Pablos V, Fernández-Villalba E, Herrero MT. IFN-γ signaling, with the synergistic contribution of TNF-α mediates cell specific microglial and astroglial activation in experimental models of Parkinson's disease. Cell Death & Disease. 2011. Apr 7;2:e142.

Barcia C, Sánchez Bahillo A, Fernández-Villalba E, Bautista V, Poza Y Poza M, Fernández-Barreiro A, Hirsch EC, Herrero MT. Evidence of active microglia in substantia nigra pars compacta of parkinsonian monkeys 1 year after MPTP exposure. Glia. 2004;46(4):402-9.

Bausserman LL, Herbert PN, McAdam KP. Heterogeneity of human serum amyloid A proteins. J Exp Med. 1980 Sep 1;152(3):641-56.

Benigni F, Fantuzzi G, Sacco S, Sironi M, Pozzi P, Dinarello CA, Sipe JD, Poli V, Cappelletti M, Paonessa G, Pennica D, Panayotatos N, Ghezzi P. Six different cytokines that share GP130 as a receptor subunit, induce serum amyloid A and potentiate the induction of interleukin-6 and the activation of the hypothalamus-pituitary-adrenal axis by interleukin-1. Blood. 1996 Mar 1;87(5):1851-4.

Betts JC, Edbrooke MR, Thakker RV, Woo P. The human acute-phase serum amyloid A gene family: structure, evolution and expression in hepatoma cells. Scand J Immunol. 1991 Oct;34(4):471-82.

Boushey CJ, Beresford SA, Omenn GS, Motulsky AG. A quantitative assessment of plasma homocysteine as a risk factor for vascular disease. Probable benefits of increasing folic acid intakes. JAMA. 1995; 274:1049-57.

Canseco-Ávila LM, Jerjes-Sánchez Carlos, Ortiz-López Rocío, Rojas- Martínez Augusto, Guzmán-Ramírez Denisse. Fibrinogen. Cardiovascular risk factor or maker? Arch. Cardiol. Mex. 76:S4. 158-172, 2006

Carson MJ, Doose JM, Melchior B, Schmid CD, Ploix CC. CNS immune privilege: hiding in plain sight. Immunol Rev. 2006 Oct;213:48-65.

Clarke R, Smith AD, Jobst KA, Refsum H, Sutton L, Ueland PM. Folate, vitamin B12, and serum total homocysteine levels in confirmed Alzheimer disease. Arch Neurol 1998;55(11):1449–1455.

Conductier G, Blondeau N, Guyon A, Nahon JL, Rovère C.The role of monocyte chemoattractant protein MCP1/CCL2 in neuroinflammatory diseases. J Neuroimmunol. 2010;224(1-2):93-100.

Cortes-Canteli M, Strickland S.Fibrinogen, a possible key player in Alzheimer's disease. J Thromb Haemost. 2009;7 Suppl 1:146-50

Curti BD, Smith JW 2nd. Interleukin-1 in the treatment of cancer. Pharmacol Ther. 1995 Mar;65(3):291-302.

Dayer JM, Choy E. Therapeutic targets in rheumatoid arthritis: the interleukin-6 receptor. Rheumatology (Oxford). 2010 Jan;49(1):15-24.

De la Torre JC. Is Alzheimer s disease a neurodegenerative or a vascular disorder? Data, dogma, and dialectics. Lancet Neurol 2004; 3: 184–90

De Pablos, V, Barcia C, Martínez S, Gomez A, Ros-Bernal F, Zamarro-Parra J, Soria-Torrecillas J, Hernández J, Ceron JJ, Herrero MT. MPTP administration increases plasma levels of acute phase proteins in non-human primates (Macaca fascicularis) Neuroscience Letters 463 (2009) 37–39

Dinarello CA. Interleukin 1 and interleukin 18 as mediators of inflammation and the aging process. Am J Clin Nutr. 2006 Feb;83(2):447S-455S.

Dinarello CA. Why not treat human cancer with interleukin-1 blockade? Cancer Metastasis Rev. 2010 Jun;29(2):317-29.

Dufek M, Hamanová M, Lokaj J, Goldemund D, Rektorová I, Michálková Z, Sheardová K, Rektor I.Serum inflammatory biomarkers in Parkinson's disease. Parkinsonism Relat Disord. 2009;15(4):318-20.

Eming SA, Krieg T, Davidson JM. Inflammation in wound repair: molecular and cellular mechanisms. J Invest Dermatol. 2007 Mar;127(3):514-25.

Farkas E, Luiten PG. Cerebral microvascular pathology in aging and Alzheimers disease. Prog Neurobiol 2001; 64: 575–611.

Feldmann M. Development of anti-TNF therapy for rheumatoid arthritis. Nat Rev Immunol 2002 May; 364-371.

Gabay C, Kushner I. Acute-phase proteins and other systemic responses to inflammation. N Engl J Med. 1999 Feb 11;340(6):448-54.

Gabay C, Kushner I: Acute Pase Proteins. Encyclopedia of Life Sciences. Nature Puplishing Group, 2001.

Gauldie J, Richards C, Harnish D, Lansdorf P y Baumann H: Interferon β2/B-cell stimulary factor type 2 shares identity with monocite-derived hepatocite-stimulating factor and regulates the major acute phase protein response in liver cells. Proceedings of the National Academy of Sciences of the USA 84: 7251-7255, 1987.

Ge S, Song L, Serwanski DR, Kuziel WA, Pachter JS. Transcellular transport of CCL2 across brain microvascular endothelial cells. J Neurochem. 2008 Mar;104(5):1219-32.

Gordon AH, Koy A. The Acute Phase Response to Injury and Infection. The Roles of Interleukin 1 and Other Mediators. Amsterdam: Elsevier; 1985. ISBN: 0444-80648-2

Graham IM, Daly LE, Refsum HM, Robinson K, Brattstrom LE, Ueland PM, Palma-Reis RJ, et al. Plasma homocysteine as a risk factor for vascular disease. The European Concerted Action Project. JAMA. 1997; 277(22):1775-81.

Gruys E, Toussaint MJM, Landman WJM, et al. Infection, Inflammation and Stress Inhibit Growth. Mechanisms and Non-specific Assessment of the Processes by Acute Phase Proteins. In: Wensing T, editor. Production Diseases in Farm Animals. 10th International Conference, 1998. Wageningen: Wageningen Press; 1999. pp. 72–87. ISBN: 90-74134-60-

Haskill S, Yurochko AD, Isaacs KL. Regulation of macrophage infiltration and activation in sites of chronic inflammation. Ann N Y Acad Sci. 1992;664:93-102.

Heinrich PC, Castell JV Andus T: Interleukin-6 and the acute phase response. Biochem. J. 265: 621-636, 1990.

Henkel JS, Beers DR, Zhao W, Appel SH. Microglia in ALS: the good, the bad, and the resting. J Neuroimmune Pharmacol. 2009 Dec;4(4):389-98.

Hirano T. Interleukin-6 and its relation to inflammation and disease. Clin Immunol Immunopathol. 1992 Jan;62(1 Pt 2):S60-5.

Iadecola C. Neurovascular regulation in the normal brain and in Alzheimer s disease. Nat Rev Neurosci 2004; 5: 347–60

Idriss HT, Naismith JH. TNF alpha and the TNF receptor superfamily: structure-function relationship(s). Microsc Res Tech. 2000 Aug 1;50(3):184-95.

Jacob CO. Tumor necrosis factor and interferon gamma: relevance for immune regulation and genetic predisposition to autoimmune disease. Semin Immunol. 1992 Jun;4(3):147-54.

Jaye DL y Waites KB: Clinical applications of C-reactive protein in pediatrics. Pediatr. Infect Dis J: 16:735-747, 1997.

Kopf M, Bachmann MF, Marsland BJ. Averting inflammation by targeting the cytokine environment. Nat Rev Drug Discov. 2010 Sep;9(9):703-18.

Kushner I, Gewurtz H, Benson MD: C-Reactive Protein and the acute phase response. J. Lab. Clin. Med. 97: 739-749. 1981.

Lepara O, Alajbegovic A, Zaciragic A, et al. Elevated serum homocysteine level is not associated with serum C-reactive protein in patients with probable Alzheimer's disease. J Neural Transm 2009;116(12):1651–1656.

Libby P. Role of inflammation in atherosclerosis associated with rheumatoid arthritis. Am J Med. 2008 Oct;121(10 Suppl 1):S21-31.

Luster AD. Chemokines--chemotactic cytokines that mediate inflammation. N Engl J Med. 1998 Feb 12;338(7):436-45.

Mancinella A, Mancinella M, Carpinteri G, Bellomo A, Fossati C, Gianturco V, Iori A, Ettorre E, Troisi G, Marigliano V. s there a relationship between high C-reactive protein (CRP) levels and dementia? Arch Gerontol Geriatr. 2009;49 Suppl 1:185-94.

Martín-Fernández JJ, Carles-Díes R, Cañizares F, Parra S, Avilés F, Villegas I, Morsi-Hassan O, Fernández-Barreiro A, Herrero MT. Homocysteine and cognitive impairment in Parkinson's disease. Rev Neurol. 2010 Feb 1-15;50(3):145-51.

Martínez-Subiela S, Tecles F, Parra MD y Cerón JJ: Proteínas de fase Aguda: Conceptos básicos y principales aplicaciones clínicas en medicina veterinaria. Anales de Veterinaria 17:99-116, 2001.

McGeer PL, Itagaki S, Boyes BE, McGeer EG. Reactive microglia are positive for HLA-DR in the substantia nigra of Parkinson's and Alzheimer's disease brains. Neurology. 1988 Aug;38(8):1285-91.

McGeer PL, McGeer EG. Inflammation and the degenerative diseases of aging. Ann N Y Acad Sci. 2004;1035:104-16.

McMahon EJ, Bailey SL, Miller SD. CNS dendritic cells: critical participants in CNS inflammation? Neurochem Int. 2006 Jul;49(2):195-203. Epub 2006 May 30.

Moore MM, Chua W, Charles KA, Clarke SJ. Inflammation and cancer: causes and consequences. Clin Pharmacol Ther. 2010 Apr;87(4):504-8. Epub 2010 Feb 10.

Mount MP, Lira A, Grimes D, Smith PD, Faucher S, Slack R, Anisman H, Hayley S, Park DS. Involvement of interferon-gamma in microglial-mediated loss of dopaminergic neurons. J Neurosci. 2007 Mar 21;27(12):3328-37.

O'Bryant SE, Waring SC, Hobson V, Hall JR, Moore CB, Bottiglieri T, Massman P, Diaz-Arrastia R. Decreased C-reactive protein levels in Alzheimer disease. J Geriatr Psychiatry Neurol. 2010;23(1):49-53.

Olsson T. Cytokines in neuroinflammatory disease: role of myelin autoreactive T cell production of interferon-gamma. J Neuroimmunol. 1992 Oct;40(2-3):211-8.

Orhan Lepara, Azra Alajbegovic, Asija Zaciragic, Emina Nakas-Icindic, Amina Valjevac, Dzenana Lepara, Almira Hadzovic-Dzuvo, Almir Fajkic, Aida Kulo, Emin Sofic. Elevated serum homocysteine level is not associated with serum C-reactive protein in patients with probable Alzheimer's disease. Neural Transm (2009) 116:1651–1656

Paterno CA. Los enigmas del fibrinogeno y la enfermedad coronaria. Rev Fed Arg Cardiol 29: 515-517, 2000

Pesce AJ, Dosekun AK. Interrelationships between the immune systems, complement, coagulation and inflammation. Clin Physiol Biochem. 1983;1(2-5):92-116.

Pott Godoy MC, Tarelli R, Ferrari CC, Sarchi MI, Pitossi FJ. Central and systemic IL-1 exacerbates neurodegeneration and motor symptoms in a model of Parkinson's disease. Brain. 2008 Jul;131(Pt 7):1880-94. Epub 2008 May 26.

Reale M, Greig NH, Kamal MA. Peripheral chemo-cytokine profiles in Alzheimer's and Parkinson's diseases. Mini Rev Med Chem. 2009 Sep;9(10):1229-41.

Richards CD, Brown TJ, Shoyab M, Baumann H y Gauldie J: Recombinant oncostatin M stimulates the production of acute phase proteins in Hep G2 cells and rat primary hepatocytes in vitro. Journal of Inmunology., 148, 1731, 1992.

Ridker PM, Rifai N, Rose L, et al; Comparison of C-reactive protein and low-density lipoprotein cholesterol levels in the prediction of first cardiovascular events. N Engl J Med. 2002 Nov 14;347(20):1557-65.

Saijo K, Winner B, Carson CT, Collier JG, Boyer L, Rosenfeld MG, Gage FH, Glass CK. A Nurr1/CoREST pathway in microglia and astrocytes protects dopaminergic neurons from inflammation-induced death. Cell. 2009 Apr 3;137(1):47-59.

Schwartz M. Macrophages and microglia in central nervous system injury: are they helpful or harmful? J Cereb Blood Flow Metab. 2003 Apr;23(4):385-94.

Seet RC, Lee CY, Lim EC, Tan JJ, Quek AM, Chong WL, Looi WF, Huang SH, Wang H, Chan YH, Halliwell B. Oxidative damage in Parkinson disease: Measurement using accurate biomarkers. Free Radic Biol Med. 2010 Feb 15;48(4):560-6.

Selhub J. Homocysteine metabolism. Annu Rev Nutr. 1999; 19:217-46.

Semple BD, Bye N, Rancan M, Ziebell JM, Morganti-Kossmann MC. Role of CCL2 (MCP-1) in traumatic brain injury (TBI): evidence from severe TBI patients and CCL2-/- mice. J Cereb Blood Flow Metab. 2010 Apr;30(4):769-82.

Strachan AF, Brandt WF, Woo P, van der Westhuyzen DR, Coetzee GA, de Beer MC, Shephard EG, de Beer FC. Human serum amyloid A protein. The assignment of the six major isoforms to three published gene sequences and evidence for two genetic loci. J Biol Chem. 1989 Nov 5;264(31):18368-73.

Tabas I. Macrophage death and defective inflammation resolution in atherosclerosis. Nat Rev Immunol. 2010 Jan;10(1):36-46.

Trepels T, Zeiher AM, Fichtlscherer S. The endothelium and inflammation. Endothelium. 2006 Nov-Dec;13(6):423-9.

Weisel JW. Fibrinogen and fibrin. Adv Protein Chem 2005; 70: 247–99.

Whicher JT y Westacott CI The acute phase response. En Biochemestry of inflammation. Pp 243-271. Eds:

Wicher JT y Evans SW. Kluwer Academic Londres. 1992.

Woo P y Gorman NT: Respuesta de proteínas de fase aguda y amiloidosis. Inmunología clínica Veterinaria. Rew Halliwell y NT Gorman. Editorial Acribia, Zaragoza, 1992.

Yong VW, Rivest S. Taking advantage of the systemic immune system to cure brain diseases. Neuron. 2009 Oct 15;64(1):55-60.

6

The Role of the Acute-Phase Proteins in the Development and Progression of Liver Diseases

Méndez Sánchez Nahum, Kobashi Margáin Ramón Arturo, Gavilanes Espinar Juan, Gutiérrez Grobe Ylse, Gutiérrez Jiménez Ángel and Uribe Misael
Liver Research Unit, Medica Sur Clinic & Foundation
Mexico City
Mexico

1. Introduction

The liver is a unique organ that is rich in cellular effectors for diverse systems, including the innate immune system, which plays a central role in hepatocellular injury (Gabay & Kushner, 1999). The innate immune system is based on broadly specific antigen recognition and does not rely on the more specialized antigen recognition pathways of the adaptive immune system. Although the innate immune response has broad specificity and is complex, acute-phase proteins (APPs) have been identified as biomarkers of the innate response (Table 1).

APPs are mostly synthesized in the liver. Their concentrations in plasma increase (positive APPs) or decrease (negative APPs) by at least 25% during inflammatory disorders. Most changes in APP concentration are due to infection, trauma, surgery, burns, tissue infarction, immunologically mediated or crystal-induced inflammation, and advanced cancer. Exercise, heatstroke, childbirth, or even psychological stress and some psychiatric disorders may also affect concentrations of these proteins. Cytokines are the chief stimulators and regulators of the production of these proteins. Interleukin (IL)-6 is the principal stimulator of APPs but other proinflammatory cytokines such as IL-1β, tumor necrosis factor alpha (TNF-α), interferon gamma (INF-γ), and transforming growth factor beta (TGF-β), and chemokines such as IL-8 are also involved.

In the liver, the Janus kinase signal transducer and activator of transcription (STAT) pathway has been implicated in the action of cytokines. STAT 1 and STAT 2, which are activated by INF-α/β, are involved in antiviral defense and the former is involved in liver inflammation and injury. STAT 3 has been implicated in the acute-phase response as well as in hepatoprotective effects and liver regeneration. This pathway is mostly activated by IL-6. STAT 4 and STAT 6 are associated with the ischemia/reperfusion cycle as promoters of and protectors against injury, respectively, and STAT 5 plays an important role in the regulation of hepatic genes and growth factors. Several studies have confirmed that IL-6 and IL-22 (a related cytokine) are responsible for important liver functions such as liver regeneration, glucose and lipid metabolism, and induction of antiapoptotic proteins (Gao, 2005).

ACUTE PHASE PROTEINS	
POSITIVE	**NEGATIVE**
Complement system	Albumin
C3, C4, C9, Factor B, C1 INH, C4b-binding protein, Mannose binding lectin	Transferrin
Coagulation and fibrinolytic system	Transthyretin
Fibrinogen, Plasminogen, Tissue plasminogen activator, Urokinase, Protein S, Vitronectin, Plasminogen activator inhibitor-1	A2-HS glycoprotein
Antiproteases	Alpha-fetoprotein
α1-Protease inhibitor, α1-Antichymotrypsin, Pancreatic secretory trypsin inhibitor, Inter- α -trypsin inhibitors	Thyroxin-binding globulin
Transport proteins	Insulin-like growth factor-1
Ceruloplasmin, Haptoglobin, Hemopexin	Factor XII
Inflammation responders	Antithrombin
Phospholipase A2, Lipopolysaccharide-binding protein, IL-1R antagonist, Granulocyte colony-stimulating factor	Retinol-binding protein
Others	α1-Acid glycoprotein
C-reactive protein, Serum amyloid A and P, Fibronectin, Ferritin, Angiotensinogen, α2-Macroglobulin	

Table 1. Descriptive table of some of the positive and negative acute-phase proteins.

Many clinical applications are based on these proteins. The most widely used indicators of the APP response are erythrocyte sedimentation rate (ESR) and plasma C-reactive protein (CRP) concentration. The latter is considered more reliable because ESR changes slowly, whereas CRP concentration changes rapidly.

2. Acute-phase proteins and the liver

The synthesis of these proteins takes place, as mentioned before, in the liver, which is an organ with multiple implications for the metabolism of many compounds in the organism. It is logical to believe that any impairment in the functioning of this organ would affect the concentrations of and, therefore, the function of these proteins. In this chapter, the pathophysiology of these changes and the clinical repercussions thereof are discussed.

To begin this chapter, it is important to review information on one of the APPs that has been most associated with the liver. It is well known that albumin is the most abundant protein in the body and albumin concentration is often used to assess liver function as well as the nutritional state of the patient because a decrease in the level of this protein is often associated with liver dysfunction. As such, it is an important component in several scales of dysfunction and prognosis. Albumin level is a component of the Child–Turcotte–Pugh scale, the Model of End-stage Liver Disease scale (specifically designed for the liver), and global scales such as the Sepsis-related Organ Failure scale and the Acute Physiology and Chronic Health Evaluation scale. Some authors (Chan, 2010) have detected albumin mRNA in the blood, indicating that cell death could occur in liver impairment, which would release this element to the blood. Unlike albumin, the albumin mRNA level increases at an early stage of liver impairment.

Research is needed to confirm this finding, but analysis of levels of circulating nucleic acids may be an interesting option for opportune detection of liver damage. Furthermore, in acute liver failure, the reduction in the production of albumin and α1-acid-glycoprotein alters the protein-bound fraction of many drugs, resulting in higher levels of the free and active forms of drugs and their associated effects. Nevertheless, albumin is not entirely specific for liver function impairment or injury; therefore, several other biomarkers have been investigated. These will be discussed in relation to the various liver pathologies.

2.1 Alcoholic liver disease

Although liver disease may have many etiologies, alcohol is still the most frequent cause of liver deterioration, whether acute or chronic. The hepatotoxic threshold at which alcoholic liver disease (ALD) develops is 40 g of ethanol per day (about four drinks) for men and 20 g of ethanol per day (about two drinks) for women and it has been estimated that 7.4% of the adult population of the USA and 20–30% of the adult population of Europe consume high quantities of alcohol. It is alarming that, in these locations and in many developing countries, the increase in alcohol consumption has been continuous and is predicted to continue during the next decade. Figure 1 shows worldwide mortality due to alcoholic liver disease.

	Country	Description	Amount
1.	Hungary	496.89 deaths per 1 million people	
2.	Denmark	132.26 deaths per 1 million people	
3.	Finland	130.78 deaths per 1 million people	
4.	Mexico	129.39 deaths per 1 million people	
5.	Germany	126.91 deaths per 1 million people	
6.	Estonia	120.00 deaths per 1 million people	
7.	Lithuania	108.37 deaths per 1 million people	
8.	Bahamas, The	96.76 deaths per 1 million people	
9.	Czech Republic	86.86 deaths per 1 million people	
10.	Croatia	82.72 deaths per 1 million people	
11.	Chile	81.33 deaths per 1 million people	
12.	Luxembourg	77.80 deaths per 1 million people	
13.	Romania	50.59 deaths per 1 million people	
14.	Puerto Rico	46.17 deaths per 1 million people	
15.	Austria	40.49 deaths per 1 million people	
16.	Korea, South	37.67 deaths per 1 million people	
17.	Costa Rica	36.14 deaths per 1 million people	
18.	Brazil	34.86 deaths per 1 million people	
19.	Canada	33.96 deaths per 1 million people	
20.	Norway	32.57 deaths per 1 million people	
21.	Australia	32.24 deaths per 1 million people	
22.	Netherlands	30.39 deaths per 1 million people	
23.	Malta	30.23 deaths per 1 million people	
24.	Nicaragua	28.73 deaths per 1 million people	

Fig. 1. Annual mortality from alcoholic liver disease. The countries with the highest mortality rates are shown.

Nevertheless, alcohol consumption is considered by many people to be normal and customary; this and the fact that patients usually do not seek medical assistance until the damage is well established (it is usually asymptomatic in the early stages) suggests that the prevalence of ALD is underestimated.

Several studies have proven that activation of Kupffer cells increases TNF-α secretion, and therefore the immune response. Su and colleagues (Su et al., 1998) found in rat models that lipopolysaccharide, an endotoxin usually present in Gram-negative bacteria, is responsible for the activation of Kupffer cells. Lipopolysaccharide binding protein (LBP) opsonizes cells and presents the endotoxin to CD14, a membrane-bound glycoprotein that activates macrophages. Alcohol is one of the stimuli necessary to increase the level of LBP-1 and, therefore, mediates liver damage. Until recently, IL-17 was thought to play an important role in alcohol-induced liver damage by activating T-helper cells, which maintain and increase inflammatory damage.

Another APP that has been associated with alcohol is alpha-fetoprotein (AFP). Although AFP has been considered a biomarker for hepatocellular carcinoma (see later in this chapter), this can be misleading because AFP is also present in ALD.

2.2 Liver steatosis

Nonalcoholic fatty liver disease (NAFLD) is the most common metabolic cause of liver dysfunction worldwide. It is believed that 10–24% of the general population has NAFLD, most cases of which are asymptomatic. It is a form of chronic liver disease that encompasses a wide spectrum of conditions that range from deposits of lipids (liver steatosis) to liver damage caused by proinflammatory compounds (nonalcoholic steatohepatitis, NASH). The natural history of this pathology has been thoroughly studied and it has been reported that NAFLD represents the first step in a progression to NASH (10–20% of cases develop NASH), liver cirrhosis (3–5% of cases develop liver cirrhosis), and hepatocellular carcinoma (Figure 2).

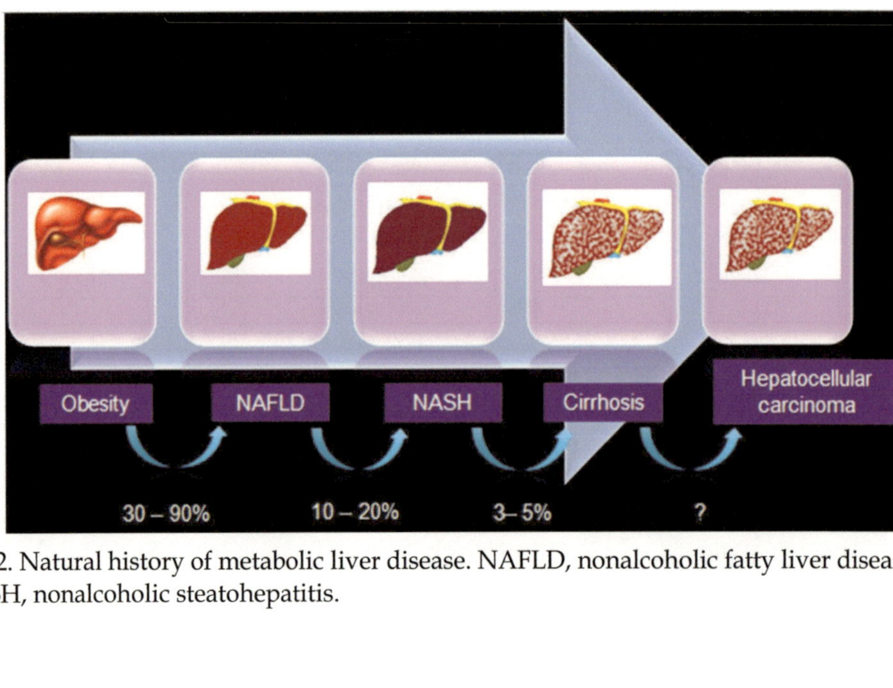

Fig. 2. Natural history of metabolic liver disease. NAFLD, nonalcoholic fatty liver disease; NASH, nonalcoholic steatohepatitis.

Under normal conditions, the liver is often exposed to endo- and exotoxins, which initiate the innate immune response. TNF-α target genes are normally expressed at minimal levels, preventing damage to the organ. Furthermore, it has been demonstrated that TNF-α is responsible for promoting liver regeneration. NAFLD and NASH are characterized by an increase in free fatty acid levels and NASH is also accompanied by an increase in lipid peroxidation and high concentrations of TNF-α, which cause mitochondrial dysfunction. Mitochondrial impairment renders the cell susceptible to TNF-α-induced cytotoxic damage.

Obesity has been considered a major risk factor for the development of NAFLD because it produces a proinflammatory state that gradually injures the liver. Nevertheless, authors such as Crespo and colleagues found that TNF-α levels are significantly higher in patients with NASH than in obese patients without NAFLD, suggesting that the former patients have increased susceptibility to TNF-α-mediated injury, rather than there being a cause-effect relationship between the cytokine and NASH.

Although several biomarkers of hepatic fibrosis have been identified (as is discussed later in this chapter), there are no reliable markers for NAFLD or NASH. Alanine aminotransferase is considered a marker for liver injury, but obesity may reduce the level of alanine aminotransferase, rendering it misleading in patients with NASH. Another issue is that identification of alcoholic and nonalcoholic liver damage is difficult. Gamma-glutamyl transpeptidase (GGT) levels are commonly used for this purpose but, in cases of NASH, they have also led to uncertain conclusions. Another report (Ohtsuka, 2005) suggested that carbohydrate-deficient transferrin could be a marker for differentiating between NAFLD and NASH. Nevertheless, Yoneda and colleagues (Yoneda et al., 2008) found that, although CRP and amyloid A levels are often used to assess inflammatory injury to the liver in clinical practice, these APPs are members of the short pentrexin family, the levels of which are only elevated as a systemic response to inflammation, whereas the long pentrexin, PTX3, is rapidly induced in damaged tissue in a tissue-specific manner. Thus, they concluded that PTX3 could be a more important biomarker for NASH than for non-NASH cases of liver damage.

2.3 Viral hepatitis

Infection with the hepatitis C virus (HCV) is a leading cause of chronic liver disease. According to the World Health Organization, over 3% of the world's population (about 180 million people) is infected and about 130 million are at risk of developing cirrhosis. The majority of those infected with HCV (60–80%) develop chronic hepatitis, which is associated with progressive fibrosis. Of chronic hepatitis patients, 3–9% develop cirrhosis within 20 years. El-Serag and colleagues (El-Serag et al., 2003) found that HCV-infected patients are more frequently coinfected with viral or bacterial entities than are patients with other liver diseases. Few studies have been performed to explain this finding, but Wegert and colleagues (Wegert, 2009) found that CRP, SAA, haptoglobin, and fibrinogen levels are diminished secondary to an impairment caused by an HCV core protein that inhibits activation of transcription factors for protein production and disrupts TNF-α and IL-6 signaling, affecting the whole immune response, at least in mice. Complement activity has also been suggested as an inducer of fibrosis and, therefore, of progression to cirrhosis in HCV-infected patients. It was reported that C5 is associated with this progression (Hillebrandt, 2005), but subsequent studies have failed to demonstrate this relationship; thus, it is unclear if this component is relevant to the induction of fibrosis in humans (Halangk, 2008). Despite this, the involvement of complement in the progression of fibrosis is still a topic of research. Interestingly, HCV-infected patients also have significantly lower

cholesterol levels than normal subjects. This may be associated with APP level, which, as mentioned before, is reduced, as in the proinflammatory and proatherogenic states.
On the other hand, even though vaccination has considerably diminished the number of cases of HBV infection, the prevalence of this disease is high. About 350 million people worldwide are infected and are at risk of progression to a worse state (Te, 2002). Some authors have found that the response to the vaccine is closely related to complement activity. C4, a crucial protein for the classical complement pathway, links innate immunity with adaptive immunity by targeting the antigen to follicular dendritic cells and B cells through the specific receptors, CD21 and CD35. It has been shown that patients who do not show the expected response to the vaccine have human leukocyte antigen class-II alleles, which impair C4 activity. Vaccines should be linked to complement fragments to avoid this problem.
Both HCV and HBV infections are considered chronic. This characteristic enables a proinflammatory state to exist, which will eventually affect the synthesis of APP in the liver. Although other hepatotropic infections may also produce an acute state, it is usually self-limited and therefore the levels of APP do not change markedly.

2.4 Liver cirrhosis

Fibrosis is a type of tissue repair that is characterized by the replacement of normal parenchyma with connective tissue (collagen) and is mainly secondary to chronic inflammation. Fibroblasts and myofibroblasts are partly responsible for this process, and it is important to note that the principal stimulus for these cells is IL-6, which is initially secreted by macrophages and subsequently secreted by B cells at the site of the lesion. When inflammation is chronic, the stimulus is persistent; thus, abundant amounts of collagen are synthesized, resulting in abnormal accumulation of connective tissue. The gold standard for the diagnosis of cirrhosis is still the liver biopsy. Several scoring systems have been developed to stage cirrhosis. The Metavir scoring scale is most commonly used to indicate the grade of inflammation and scarring on the liver and was first developed for HCV-infected patients. The Knodell score is a histological staging system that assesses the extent of inflammation: a score of 0–10 is allocated to periportal or bridging necrosis and a score of 0–4 is allocated to intralobular degeneration and portal inflammation. The various grades used in these two scoring systems are shown in tables 2 and 3.

Grade	Description
0	No scarring
1	Minimal scarring
2	Scarring has occurred and extends to blood vessels
3	Bridging fibrosis
4	Advanced scarring, cirrhosis

Table 2. The METAVIR scoring system for cirrhosis.

Score	Description
0	No inflammation
1–4	Minimal inflammation
5–8	Mild inflammation
9–12	Moderate inflammation
13–18	Marked inflammation

Table 3. The Knodell scoring system for cirrhosis.

Although the gold standard for the diagnosis of cirrhosis is the liver biopsy, the invasive nature of this procedure makes it difficult to perform with every patient. Although noninvasive methods such as the FibroScan and FibroTest are available, they may result in false-negative results in obese patients or patients with ascites. Although CRP and serum amyloid A (SAA) levels are biomarkers for liver injury and inflammation, it has been demonstrated that they are not correlated with fibrosis. Fortunately, there are other biomarkers that have been validated in several studies. Alpha-2 macroglobulin (A2M) is a protein that inactivates proteinases and inhibits fibrinolysis by reducing plasmin and kallikrein expression; thus, it inhibits the catabolism of matrix proteins, facilitating the development of fibrosis. The FibroTest involves this biomarker (Franciscus, 2010). The level of apolipoprotein A1 (ApoA1), a structural component of high-density lipoprotein cholesterol, is also correlated with the advanced stages of fibrosis (F3–F4). Other authors (Ho et al., 2010) described a novel biomarker: vitamin D binding protein (VDBP). Although A2M expression is upregulated in fibrotic livers, both ApoA1 and VDBP are negative APPs and are downregulated in fibrotic livers.

As mentioned in the introduction, there are several signaling pathways that control diverse functions. In the case of fibrosis, the STAT 3 family has the greatest impact. Activation and high activity of this signaling pathway have been implicated in the genesis of cirrhosis as well as in its evolution to HCC. Under normal circumstances, insulin-like growth factor-1 (IGF-1) maintains the activity of the STAT 5 signaling pathway; nevertheless, when liver damage occurs, growth hormone is released, with consequent lowering of IGF-1 level (therefore, it is known as a negative APP), which stops the activation of the STAT 5 pathway and the phosphorylation of STAT 3. TGF-β is a closely related cytokine because it is also secreted when liver damage occurs and it activates the STAT 3 pathway as well as the expansion of T-helper cells, which increases fibrosis.

It has also been reported (Parsian et al., 2010) that expression of other components such as hyaluronic acid, alpha glycosaminoglycan distributed in extracellular spaces and synthesized by hepatic stellate cells in the liver, and laminin, a basal membrane glycoprotein synthesized in hepatocytes, also increase in the early stages of fibrosis in chronic liver diseases. These serum parameters have been compared with APP-based indices such as A1-apolipoprotein level and prothrombin time, and it was found that hyaluronic acid is the most strongly correlated with liver fibrosis.

2.5 Hepatocellular carcinoma and other liver tumors

As mentioned in the discussion of cirrhosis, downregulation of the STAT 5 signaling pathway and activation of the STAT 3 pathway increase fibrosis. Practically all chronic liver diseases result in fibrosis and, if not controlled, in malignant transformation of hepatocytes, and HCC (figure 3).

HCC accounts for 5.6% of all human cancers, more so among men than women (7.5% and 3.5%, respectively), and its prevalence increases with age. It has a 5-year survival rate of 6.5% and is considered responsible for 660,000 deaths per year worldwide. Viral hepatitis, alcohol, oral contraceptives, and aflatoxins are the most important risk factors for its development and its prevalence is expected to increase in the future.

HCV and HBV infection are the main causes of HCC; they are responsible for 80% of HCC cases (96% in HBV endemic regions). It has been established that 10–40% of all chronic HBV patients will develop this entity. The progression to liver cancer is monitored using serum levels of alpha-fetoprotein (AFP), an oncofetal glycoprotein that serves as an APP for several

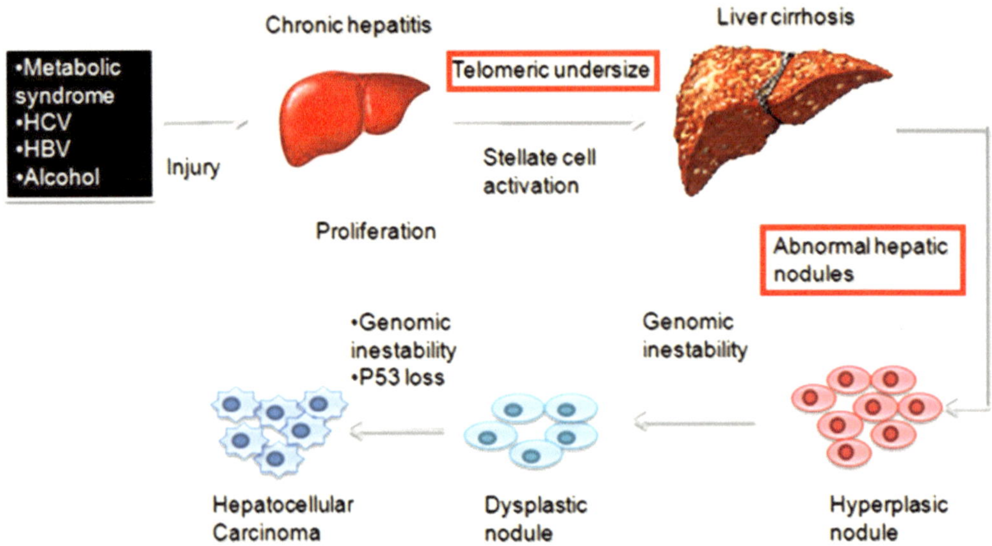

Fig. 3. Evolution and risk factors for the development of hepatocellular carcinoma.

liver diseases; nevertheless, it is not cancer specific. Comunale and colleagues (Comunale et al., 2010) identified more than 100 glycoproteins that are elevated in cirrhotic and HCC patients and that may serve as markers of the early development of HCC, and they suggested that alpha-1-antitrypsin was the most promising.

CRP and SAA levels are correlated with tumor activity (Jong, 2001), i.e., with increasing tumor load, necrotic tumors, and tissue destruction. Levels of these proteins are even increased by gastric and colorectal metastases. It has also been suggested that APPs provide an ideal environment for tumor recurrence or growth (Harimoto et al., 2009). It is also accepted that CRP-positivity in HCC patients often indicates a poor prognosis and portal vein invasion.

As mentioned earlier in the chapter, hypoalbuminemia was considered a marker of liver impairment. For a long time, it was thought that tumor activity was responsible for the decrease in albumin level; however, recent studies (Al-Shaiba et al., 2004) have demonstrated that the reduction in serum albumin level is related to the inflammatory response rather than to nutritional depletion caused by the tumor.

2.6 Autoimmune hepatitis

Autoimmunity is also an important cause of liver disease. It encompasses a broad spectrum of diseases, including autoimmune hepatitis (AIH), primary biliary cirrhosis (PBC), primary sclerosing cholangitis (PSC), and autoimmune cholangitis. The most common are AIH and PBC. Clinical, biochemical, histopathological, and cholangiographic criteria are used for differential diagnosis (Table 4).

AIH is characterized by severe liver damage with a modest or low elevation of alkaline phosphatase level (Oo, 2010). It is classed into three types according to the autoantibodies expressed: type 1, smooth muscle antibodies (SMA) or anti-nuclear antibodies (ANA) are present; type 2, anti-liver kidney microsomal antibodies (LKM) are present; and type 3, soluble liver antibodies (SLA) or liver/pancreas antigens are present. All of these antibodies induce proinflammatory cells that mostly activate T-helper cells, which cause liver damage.

Parameter	AIH	PBC	PSC	AIC
Female:male	4:1	9:1	1:2	9:1
Liver test elevation	ALT, AST	AP, GGT	AP, GGT	AP, GGT
Ig elevation	IgG	IgM	IgG, IgM	IgM
Autoantibodies	ANA, ASMA, LKM, SLA, p-ANCA	AMA, AMA-M2	p-ANCA	ANA, ASMA
HLA association	A3, B8, DR3, DR4	DR8	DR52	B8, DR3, DR4
Histology	Lymphocyte interface hepatitis	Florid bile duct lesion	Fibrosing bile duct lesion	Florid bile duct lesion

Table 4. Comparative table for the differential diagnosis of autoimmune liver diseases. AIH, autoimmune hepatitis; PBC, primary biliary cirrhosis; PSC, primary sclerosing cholangitis; AIC, autoimmune cholangitis; ALT, alanine aminotransferase; AST, aspartate aminotransferase; AP, alkaline phosphatase; GGT, gamma-glutamyl transpeptidase; Ig, immunoglobin; ANA, anti-nuclear antibodies; ASMA, anti-smooth muscle antibodies; LKM, anti-liver kidney microsomal; SLA, anti-soluble liver antigen; p-ANCA, perinuclear anti-neutrophil cytoplasmic antibodies; AMA, anti-mitochondrial antibodies; UDCA, ursodeoxycholic acid.

In PBC (Poupon, 2010), inflammation is associated with similar rates of apoptosis and proliferation of biliary cells. Cytolytic T cells are attracted to autoantibody-marked cells by cytokines and chemokines, which also induce the killing of cells via TNF-α, CD-40, and Fas receptors. It is under this pressure that cholangiocytes proliferate to compensate for cell death. It has been suggested that the cholinergic pathway, the IGF-1 system, and estrogens (through alpha receptors) are possible mediators of this process.

Takahashi and colleagues (Takahasi et al., 2010) found that ALT and transferrin levels are correlated in autoimmune diseases and in other collagen-related diseases. CRP and AP levels are also correlated, at least in vasculitis syndrome. The explanation for these results is that, because the immunological response is increased in all these diseases, APPs are induced. IL-17 is a new cytokine that has been suggested to play an important role in the pathogenesis of AIH, as it is a strong neutrophil recruiter and, importantly, is also associated with the pathogenesis of ALD.

Furthermore, several authors have described "overlap syndromes". These entities are characterized by clinical or biochemical features common to two or more autoimmune diseases affecting the liver. In overlap syndromes, the magnitude of the immunological response in the early stage is elevated in that APP levels are altered to a greater extent. Comorbidities are not considered overlap syndromes. Kessel and colleagues (Kessel et al., 2007) reported that HCV-infected patients have a high titer of CRP antibodies, which is correlated with the level of rheumatoid factor, cryoglobulinemia, and the severity of liver disease, suggesting that it facilitates autoimmune liver disorders. This is important because it has been shown that 65% of patients infected with HCV have low titers of ANA, SMA, and anti-thyroid antibodies, and 7% have anti-LKM-1 antibodies. Some authors suggest that, if titers of these antibodies are >1:320, and/or hypergammaglobulinemia, and other risk factors (female gender, young age, and other autoimmune disorders) are present, it should be considered as a co-morbidity between HCV and AIH (Beuers, 2005).

3. Clinical repercussions

Clinically, insulin resistance (IR) and cardiovascular disease (CVD) have been suggested to arise from a common basis, i.e., chronic inflammation. As mentioned before, chronic liver diseases are important sources of a proinflammatory state and, therefore, several studies have tried to link liver impairment with the development of IR, type 2 diabetes mellitus (T2DM), and CVD. It is important to comment on this situation because several reports have suggested that the prevalence of chronic liver diseases will increase in the next few years and have shown that chronic liver diseases are currently among the leading causes of mortality in all parts of the world.

3.1 Liver-related insulin resistance (IR)

One of the manifestations of liver impairment is IR. IR is defined as an increased need for insulin in the peripheral tissues (muscle and adipose tissue) to achieve normal cellular glucose uptake and to reduce glucose output from the liver. The incidence of T2DM is increasing worldwide. IR is considered the pathophysiological basis of T2DM and is responsible for micro- and macrovascular complications associated with this condition. Some studies have associated IR with other deleterious effects on the biliary tract and liver such as the induction of gallstones and NAFLD, considered the most common chronic liver disease in Western countries and the liver manifestation of metabolic syndrome (MS), a pathology proven to be intrinsically related to IR. Some studies have even found that IR tends to favor the progression of NAFLD to NASH, cirrhosis, and HCC.

To comprehend the entire pathophysiology of IR, it is important to understand the normal physiology of insulin signaling. The main signaling pathway begins with the binding of insulin to its receptor, which activates insulin receptor substrates (ISR-1 or ISR-2), which activate phosphatidylinositol-3 kinase (PI3K). The subsequent cascade results in the production of protein kinase Cξ or λ, which promotes translocation of the glucose transporter, GLUT 4, and activation of Akt, facilitating glucose uptake, gluconeogenesis, and protein synthesis through the production of GSK-3, FOXO-1, and mTOR, respectively. The last-mentioned mediator also exerts negative feedback on insulin signaling by phosphorylating IRS-1 (Méndez et al., 2005) (figure 4).

Two main pathways are involved in liver-related IR. One path is through the production of free fatty acids, an increased level of which inhibits insulin-induced suppression of endogenous glucose production, and the other is through stimulation of gluconeogenesis, associated with activation of protein kinase Cδ.

Nevertheless, there are other factors associated with IR, such as a mutation of 2,6 fructose bisphosphonatase that causes an alteration in the fructose 2,6-bisphosphonate, which causes three results: a lower efficiency of suppression of hepatic glucose production (increased gluconeogenesis); a disruption of glucose flux, and a decrease in insulin-induced Akt phosphorylation in the liver. Furthermore, phosphorylation of ISR-2 in the cascade of activation of insulin also has an important impact on glycogen synthesis. It has been demonstrated that ISR-2 phosphorylation inhibits glycogen synthetase-3-kinase, which, in normal situations, induces glycogen synthesis and increases the use of plasma glucose. In pathological cases, synthesis is interrupted and glucose is not taken up by cells, promoting the progression of IR.

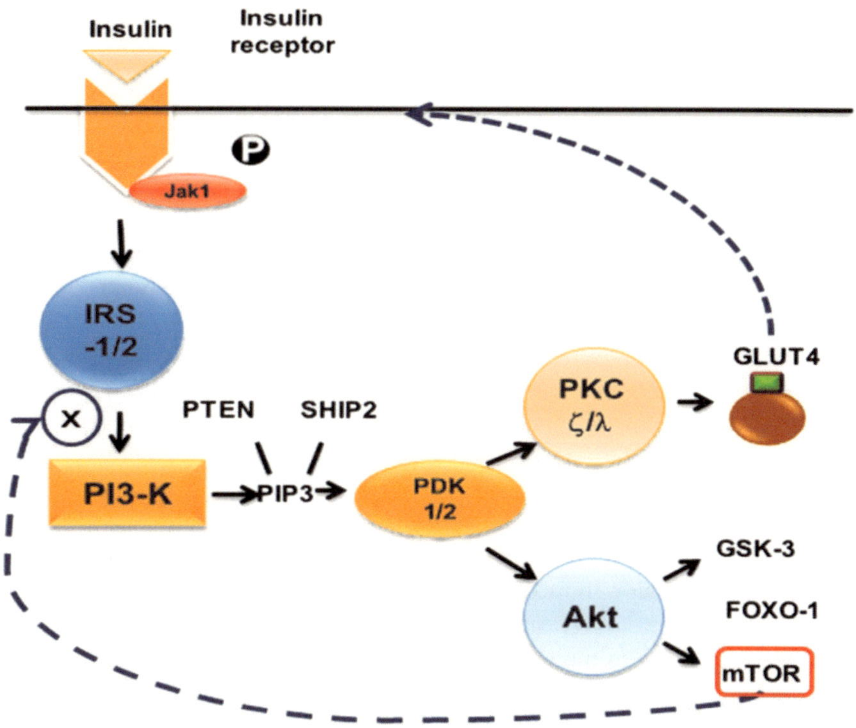

Fig. 4. Mechanisms involved in insulin signaling. Under normal circumstances, insulin binds to its receptor, which activates IRS 1/2, which then initiates a cascade of reactions that activate PKC, inducing the synthesis and migration of GLUT4 to the cell membrane, and Akt, which promotes glucose uptake, gluconeogenesis, and protein synthesis. mTOR also exerts negative feedback on the activation of IRS. IRS, insulin receptor substrate; PI3K, phosphatidylinositol-3 kinase; PKC, protein kinase C.

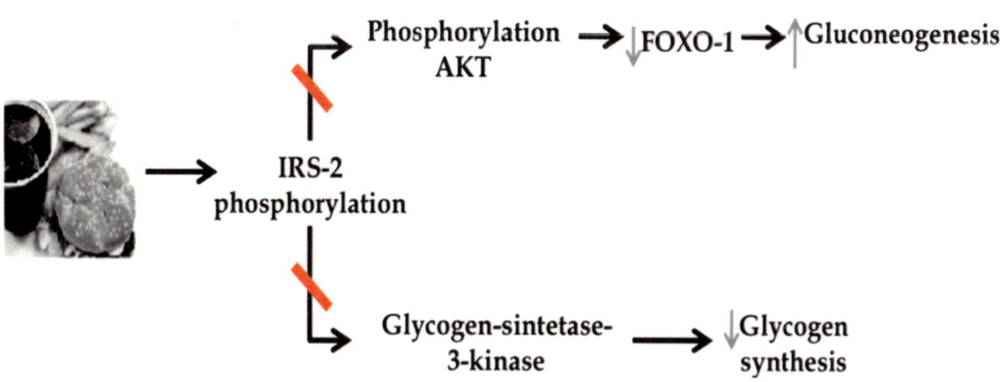

Fig. 5. Liver-related insulin resistance. FFA, free fatty acids; IRS, insulin receptor substrate.

As mentioned before, TNF-α concentrations are elevated in liver diseases and, through the activation of inhibitory κB, which enables activation of nuclear factor-κB, cause upregulation of IL-6. IL-6 induces the suppressor of cytokine signaling (SOCS), which induces IR through a specific inhibitor of IRS-2 (SOCS-1) or by competition for the docking sites of SOCS-3 (Méndez et al., 2005).

Festa and colleagues (Festa et al., 2002) reported that APPs are not only impaired in cases of T2DM but proposed that they serve as early biomarkers of T2DM. CRP and fibrinogen were related to IR, but several studies have related them to adipose tissue secretion, and therefore to body mass index. Nevertheless, they also found that PAI-1 was independently related to the development of T2DM when compared with BMI and other risk factors, even IR, suggesting that this APP is suitable for early screening of people who are predisposed to T2DM.

Recent studies have also confirmed a close relationship between IR and liver diseases such as chronic hepatitis caused by HBV and HCV, hemochromatosis, cirrhosis, and HCC. Some authors have even reported so-called "hepatogenous diabetes", which is recognized by the World Health Organization as an independent entity that refers to the development of the T2DM due to cirrhosis.

It is important to note that the incidence of viral hepatitis has increased worldwide, especially the types that produce a chronic state. In regards to these, some studies have reported that HCV infection induces degradation of IRS-1 through activation of the mTOR pathway (genotype 1) or SOCS-7 and PPAR-γ (genotype 3). In either eventuality, the result is IR. It is also important to mention that these two genotypes have been related to IR in HCV infection.

Several studies have been performed to analyze the relationships of IR and T2DM with liver disease. Although the prevalence of liver diseases varies between countries, it has been noted that liver cirrhosis and viral hepatitis C infection have the strongest relationship with T2DM; nevertheless, other liver diseases have also been correlated with T2DM. Table 5 shows the prevalence of these diseases.

3.2 Relationship between cardiovascular risk and liver impairment

Metabolic syndrome is the pandemic of the new millennium and is considered a major risk factor for CVD. NAFLD is now considered a liver manifestation of this syndrome. As mentioned before, IR is the pathophysiological basis of metabolic syndrome and is therefore closely linked to both CVD and liver diseases.

As also mentioned above, CRP is considered the most important APP correlated with IR and CVD; nevertheless, there are some studies that have shown that CRP has anti-inflammatory properties and is involved in the reduction of the development of atherosclerosis in mouse models with hypercholesterolemia. This is most probably due to CRP-mediated upregulation of the IL-1 receptor antagonist and upregulation of serum leptin-interacting protein activity.

NASH, as also mentioned before, characteristically elevates CRP, PAI-1, and fibrinogen activities (more so than NAFLD), which are also correlated with CVD and could be considered markers for this entity because these APPs have been demonstrated to be related to cardiovascular events independently of other risk factors such as age, visceral adiposity, and metabolic abnormalities. As such, patients with viral hepatitis also have a markedly greater carotid artery intimae medial thickness. Figure 6 shows the physiopathology of this interaction.

Study	Country	Prevalence of T2DM (%)
Hepatitis B virus		
Arao M et al., 2003	Japan	11.9
Knobler H et al., 2000	USA	12
Kobashi R et al., 2010	Mexico	16.7
Hepatitis C virus		
Moucari R et al., 2008	USA	33
Mangia A et al., 1998	Italy	23
Lecube A et al., 2004	Spain	
Arao M et al., 2003	Japan	20
Singal AK et al., 2008	Saudi Arabia	22
Fraser GM et al., 1996	Israel	39
Kobashi R et al., 2010	Mexico	22.7
Nonalcoholic fatty liver disease		
Dixon JB et al., 2001	USA	20–45
Gaiani S et al., 2009	Italy	80
Bellentani S et al., 2007		30–50
Targher G et al., 2007		
Mendez N et al., 2007	Mexico	15.9–45
DeLusong MAA et al., 2008	Philippines	60
Kobashi R et al., 2010	Mexico	17.6
Nonalcoholic steatohepatitis		
Nugent C et al., 2007	USA	25–45
Harrison SA et al., 2006		
Prashanth M et al., 2009	India	25
Amarapurkar DN et al., 2008		27
Kobashi R et al., 2010	Mexico	25
Cirrhosis		
Tolman KG et al., 2007	USA	25–30
Hickman IJ et al., 2007		
Zeinn NN et al., 2000		34
Arao M et al., 2003	Japan	30.8
Costa-Braganca et al., 2010	Brazil	64.5
Kobashi R et al., 2010	Mexico	34.4
Hepatocellular carcinoma		
Davila JA et al., 2010	USA	9.7
Donadon V et al., 2008	Italy	31.2
Lagiou P et al., 2000	Greece	18
Kobashi R et al., 2010	Mexico	35.7
Hemochromatosis		
Sampson MJ et al., 2000	USA	0.4
Conte D et al., 1998		1.34
Adams PC et al., 1991		50–85 (hereditary)
Kobashi R et al., 2010	Mexico	0.77 (general)
Autoimmune hepatitis		
Jalihal A et al., 2009	Brunei	21
Choudohuri G et al., 2003	India	39.5
Kobashi R et al., 2010	Mexico	25

Table 5. Prevalence of type 2 diabetes mellitus (T2DM) and liver diseases reported from several studies worldwide (from Kobashi et al., 2010).

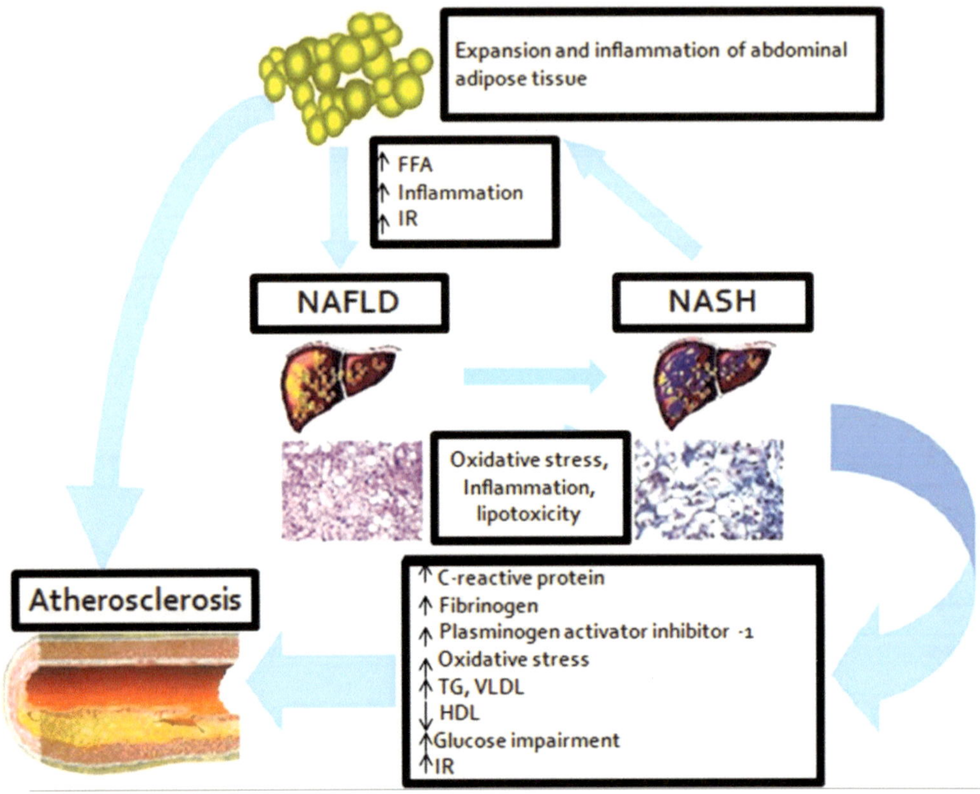

Fig. 6. Relationship between liver steatosis and cardiovascular events (atherosclerosis). Several APPs are elevated in NASH, which may directly injure the endothelium, but adipose tissue alone may also produce the same alteration. FFA, free fatty acids; IR, insulin resistance; NAFLD, nonalcoholic fatty liver disease; NASH, nonalcoholic steatohepatitis; TG, triglyceride; VLDL, very low density lipoprotein; HDL, high density lipoprotein.

It is important to mention that several risk factors for the development of CVD are also important risk factors for diabetes and some liver diseases. The transport of cholesterol is intrinsically related to these pathologies. Recently, studies have focused on the ATP binding cassette, A-1 (ABCA-1), an ATP-binding membrane transporter that plays an important role in cholesterol efflux from tissues and interacts directly with apolipoprotein A1, which is a structural component of high density lipoprotein cholesterol (HDL-c) and therefore plays a crucial role in lipid transportation. Because ABCA-1 and Apo-A1 have been demonstrated to be reduced in some liver diseases, it is comprehensible that liver impairment could be reflected in decreased HDL-c levels through this mechanism (Figure 7). HDL-c plays a protective role in cardiovascular events because it transports cholesterol from peripheral tissues to the liver where lipid is metabolized. The metabolism and transport of cholesterol demonstrates the close relationship between liver diseases and cardiovascular events.

Several studies have also pointed out that adiponectin, an adipocyte-derived enzyme, plays a protective role in the pathogenesis of liver impairment (induction of NAFLD) and therefore, in the increase in cardiovascular risk. Acetyl-CoA carboxylase (ACC) and fatty acid synthase (FAS) are important rate-limiting enzymes for fatty acid synthesis. The

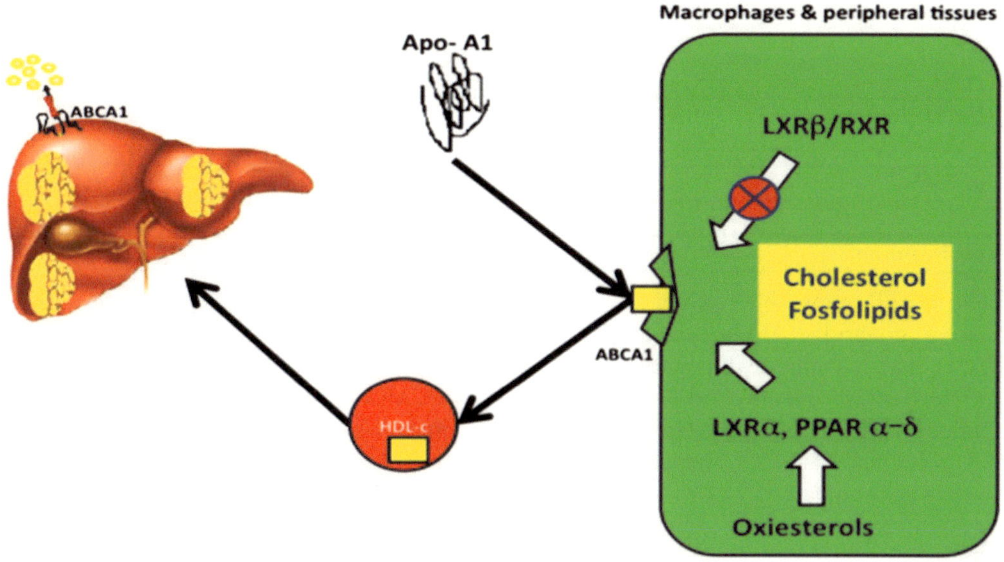

Fig. 7. Cholesterol reverse transport metabolism. Oxysterols (ligands for LXR receptors) and activators of PPARα–δ induce the production of ABC-A1, which transports molecules of cholesterol from inside the cell to the outer cell membrane. Once presented, the structural molecule, ApoA1, of HDL-c attaches to the molecules of cholesterol and they are transported to the liver where they can be metabolized and excreted from the organism. In the absence of HDL-c stimulation (i.e., in liver diseases), the LXR-β receptor and RXR are activated and inhibit ABC-A1, maintaining cholesterol accumulation within tissues. LXR, liver X receptor; RXR, retinoid X receptor.

activity of these enzymes and that of carnitine palmitoyl transferase I (CPT-I), which mediates fatty acid entry to the mitochondrion, where the fatty acids are degraded, are regulated by adiponectin. This enzyme promotes CPT-I expression and inhibits ACC and FAS expression, reducing serum and hepatic lipid concentrations and, thus, the activity of TNF-α. Uribe and colleagues (Uribe et al., 2008) have shown that adiponectin expression is reduced in metabolic liver diseases and in obesity.

4. Conclusions

Although albumin level is generally correlated with liver disease, it is not specific for the various liver diseases. Consequently, several studies have been conducted to identify biomarkers specific for each liver disease. Table 6 lists APPs associated with various liver diseases.

It is important to mention that although chemical analysis has improved over the years, the clinical status of the patient is the most important and reliable factor in the approach of the patient. APPs measurement gives the clinician, the proper guidance and orientation of the problems, that usually are subclinical, but they are not the gold standard for any liver disease; therefore, they all need a confirmation with some other studies.

Liver disease	Positive APP	Negative APP
Alcoholic disease	AFP, LBP-1	
NAFLD	ALT	
NASH	GGT, CRP, SAA, PTX3	
Viral hepatitis		CRP, SAA, Fibrinogen, Complement activity (C4, C5)
Cirrhosis	A2MG	ApoA1, VDBP, HA, IGF-1
HCC	AFP, A1AT, CRP, SAA	
Autoimmune	CRP, ALT, AP	

Table 6. APP, acute-phase protein; AFP, alpha-fetoprotein; LBP-1, lipopolysaccharide binding protein 1; NAFLD, nonalcoholic fatty liver disease; ALT, alanine aminotransferase; NASH, nonalcoholic steatohepatitis; GGT, gamma-glutamyl transpeptidase; CRP, c-reactive protein; SAA, serum amyloid A; PTX3, pentrexin 3; A2MG, alpha-2 macroglobulin; ApoA1, apolipoprotein A1; VDBP, vitamin D binding protein; HA, hyaluronic acid; IGF-1, insulin-like growth factor-1; HCC, hepatocellular carcinoma; A1AT, alpha-1 antitrypsin; AP, alkaline phosphatase.

5. References

Gabay C & Kushner I.(1999). Acute Phase proteins and other systemic responses to inflammation. *New England Journal of Medicine*. Vol. 340, No. 6,(February, 1999), pp. 448-54

Gao B (2005). Cytokines, STATs and Liver Disease. *Cellular and Molecular Immunology*. 2005. Vol. 2. No. 2,(April, 2005), pp. 92-100

Farnsworth N, Fagan SP, Berger DH & Awad SS (2004). Child-Turcotte-Pugh versus MELD score as predictor of outcome after elective emergent surgery in cirrhotic patients. *American journal of Surgery*. 2004. Vol. 188. No. 5, (November, 2004), pp. 580-3

Vincent JL, Moreno R, Takala J, Willatts S, De Medonca A, et al. (1996). The SOFA (Sepsis-related Organ Failure Assessment) score to describe organ dysfunction/failure. On behalf of the Working Group on Sepsis-Related Problems of the European Society of Intensive Care Medicine.. Intensive Care Medicine. Vol. 22, No. 7, (July, 1996), pp. 07-10

Knaus WA, Wagner DP, Draper EA, Zimmerman JE, Bergner M, et al (1991). The APACHE III prognostic system. Risk prediction of hospital mortality for critically ill hospitalized adults. *Chest*. Vol. 100, No.6, (December, 1991), pp. 1619-36

Chan RWY, Wong J, Chan HL, Mok TS, Lo WY, et al (2010). Aberrant concentrations of liver-derived plasma albumin mRNA in liver pathologies. *Clinical Chemistry*. Vol. 56, No. 1, (January, 2010), pp. 82-9

Crone CC, Gabriel GM & DiMartini A (2006). An overview of psychiatric issues in liver disease for the consultation-liason psychiatrist. *Psychosomatics*. Vol. 47, No. 3, (May-June, 2006), pp. 188-205

Méndez-Sánchez N, Almeda-Valdés P & Uribe M (2005). Alcoholic liver disease. An update. *Annals of Hepatology*. Vol 4, No. 1, (January-March, 2005), pp. 32-42

Méndez-Sánchez N, Villa AR, Chávez-Tapia NC, Ponciano-Rodriguez G, Almeda-Valdés P, et al (2005). Trends in liver disease prevalence in Mexico from 2005 to 2050 through mortality data. *Annals of Hepatology*. Vol. 4, No. 1, (January-March, 2005), pp. 52-5

Méndez-Sánchez N, García-Villegas E, Merino-Zeferino B, Ochoa-Cruz S, Villa AR, et al (2010). Liver disease in Mexico and their associated mortality trends form 2000 to 2007: A retrospective study of the nation and federal states. *Annals of Hepatology*. Vol. 9, No. 4, (October-December, 2010), pp. 428-38

Su GL, Rahemtulla A, Thomas P, Klein RD, Wang SC, et al (1998). CD14 and lipopolysaccharide binding protein expression in a rat model of alcoholic liver disease. *American Journal of Pathology*. Vol. 152, No. 3, (March, 1998), pp. 841-9

Lemmer A, Moreno C, Gustot T, Maréchal R, Degré D, et al (2009). The interleukin-17 pathway is involved in human alcoholic liver disease. Hepatol. Vol. 49, No. 2, (February, 2009), pp. 646-57

Miller AI, Moral MD & Schiff ER (1975). Presence of serum alpha-1-fetoprotein in alcoholic hepatitis. *Gastroenterology*. Vol. 68, No. 2, (February, 1975), pp. 381-3

Mohamed HA (2007). The road map for the diagnosis of nonalcoholic fatty liver disease. *American Journal of Clinical Pathology*. Vol. 127, No. 1, (January, 2007), pp. 20-2

Feldstein AE (2010). Novel insights into the pathophysiology of nonalcoholic fatty liver disease. *Seminar of Liver Diseases*. Vol. 30, No. 4, (November, 2010), pp. 391-401

Méndez-Sánchez N, Chávez-Tapia NC, Zamora-Valdés D, Medina-Santillán R & Uribe M (2007). Hepatobilliary diseases and insulin resistance. *Current Medicine and Chemistry*. Vol. 14, No. 18, (January, 2007), pp. 1988-1999

Méndez Sánchez N, Arrese M, Zamora-Valdés D & Uribe M (2007). Current concepts in the pathogenesis of nonalcoholic fatty liver disease. *Liver International*. Vol. 27, No. 4, (May, 2007), pp. 423-33

Mohamed HA (2007). The road map for the diagnosis of nonalcoholic fatty liver disease. *American Journal of Clinical Pathology*. Vol. 127, No. 1, (January, 2007), pp. 20-2

Ohtsuka T, Tsutsumi M, Fukumura A, Tsuchishuma M & Takase S (2005). Use of serum carbohydrate-deficient transferring values to exclude alcoholic hepatitis from non alcoholic steatohepatitis: a pilot study. *Alcoholism: Clinical and Experimental Research*. Vol. 29, No. 12 (Suppl), (December, 2005), pp. 236S-9S

Yoneda M, Uchiyama T, Kato S, Endo H, Fujita K, et al (2008). Plasma pentraxin3 is a novel marker for nonalcoholic steatohepatitis (NASH). *BMC Gastroenterology*. Vol. 8, No. 53, (November, 2008) pp. 1-9

Barnes E, (2010). Hepatitis C virus, viral cancers. In *World Health Organization*. Date of access: January, 24th, 2011, Available from http://www.who.int/vaccine_research /diseases/viral_cancers/en/index2.html

El-Serag HB, Anand B, Richardson P & Rabenek L (2003). Association between hepatitis C infection and other infectious diseases: a case for targeted screening?. *American Journal of Gastroenterology*. Vol. 98, No. 167, (January, 2003), pp. 167-74

Wegert M, La Monica N, Tripodi M, Adler G & Dikopoulos N (2009). Impaired interferon type I signalling in the liver modulates the hepatic acute phase response in hepatitis C virus transgenic mice. *Jorunal of Hepatology*. Vol. 51, No. 2, (August, 2009), pp. 271-8

Hillebrandt S, Wasmuth HE, Weiskirchen R, Hellerbrand C, Keppeler H, et al (2005). Complement factor is a quantitative trait gene that modifies liver fibrogenesis in mice and humans. *Nature Genetics*. Vol. 37, No. 8, (August, 2005), pp. 835-43

Halangk J, Sarrazin C, Neumann K, Puhl G, Mueller T, et al (2008) . Evaluation of complement factor 5 variants as genetic risk factors for the development of advanced fibrosis in chronic hepatitis C infection. *Journal of Hepatology*. Vol. 49, No. 3, (September, 2008), pp. 339-45

Ali-Goughoulte M, Banerjee A, Meyer K, Mazumdar B, Saito K, et al (2010). Hepatitis C virus core protein interacts with fibrinogen-beta and attenuates cytokine stimulated acute-phase proteins. *Hepatology*. Vol. 51, No. 5, (May, 2010), pp. 1505-13

Te H & Jensen DM (2010). Epidemiology of Hepatitis B and C viruses: A Global Overview. *Clinics in Liver Disease.* Vol. 14, No. 1, (February, 2010), pp. 1-21

Höhler T, Stradmann-Bellinghausen B, Starke R, Sänger R, Victor A, et al (2002). C4A deficiency and nonresponse to hepatitis B vaccination. *Journal of Hepatology*. Vol. 37, No. 3, (September, 2002), pp. 387-92

Wynn TA. Cellular and molecular mechanisms of fibrosis. *Journal of Pathology*. Vol. 214, No. 2, (January, 2008), pp. 199-210

Franciscus A. (2010). HCV diagnostic tools: grading & staging a liver biopsy. In *hcspFACTsheet*. January 5th, 2011. Available in http://www.hcvadvocate.org/hepatitis/factsheets_pdf/grade_stage_biopsy_2010.pdf

Ho AS, Cheng CC, Lee SC, Liu ML, Wang WM, et al (2010). Novel biomarkers predict liver fibrosis in hepatitis C patients: alpha 2 macroglobulin, vitamin D binding protein and apolipoprotein A1. *Journal of Biomedical Science.* Vol.17, No. 58, (July, 2010), pp. 58-65

Hosui A, Kimura A, Yamaji D, Zhu BM, Na R, et al (2009). Loss of STAT5 causes liver fibrosis and cancer development through increased TGF-b and STAT 3 activation. *Journal of Experimental Medicine*. Vol. 206, No. 4, (April, 2009), pp. 819-31

Parsian H, Rahimipour A, Nouri M, Hossein-Somi M, Qujeq D, et al (2010). Serum hyaluronic acid and laminin as biomarkers in liver fibrosis. *Journal of Gastrointestinal and Liver Diseases*. Vol. 19, No. 2, (June, 2010), pp. 169-74.

Bosch FX, Ribes J, Cléries R & Díaz M (2009). Epidemiology of hepatocellular carcinoma. Clinics in Liver Disease. Vol. 9, No. 2, (May, 2009), pp. 191-211

Comunale MA, Rodemich-Betesch L, Hafner J, Wang M, Norton P, et al (2010). Linkage specific flucosylation of alpha-2-antitrypsin in liver cirrhosis and cancer patients: implications for a biomarker of hepatocellular carcinoma. *Plos One*. Vol. 5, No. 8, (August, 2010), pp. 1-9

Jong KP, von Geusau BA, Rottier CA, Bijzet J, Limburg PC, et al. Serum response of hepatocyte growth factor, insulin-like growth factor-1, interleukine-6, and acute phase proteins in patients with colorectal liver metastases treated with partial hepatectomy or cryosurgery. *Journal of Hepatology*. Vol. 34, No. 3, (March, 2001), pp 422-7

Harimoto N, Shirabe K & Abe T (2005). Interleukine-8 producing hepatocellular carcinoma with pyrexia. *HPB Surgery*. Vol. 23, No. 2, (September, 2009), pp. 1-5

Beuers, U (2005). Hepatic overlap syndromes. *Journal Hepatology*. Vol. 42, No. 1 (Suppl), (September, 2005), pp. S93-S99

Oo YH, Hubscher SG & Adams DH (2010). Autoimmune hepatitis: new paradigms in the pathogenesis, diagnosis, and management. *Hepatology International*. Vol. 4, No. 2, (May, 2010), pp. 475-93

Poupon R (2010). Primary biliary cirrhosis: A 2010 update. *Journal of Hepatology*. Vol. 52, No. 5, (May, 2010), pp. 745-58

Takahashi A, Abe K, Yokokawa J, Iwadate H, Kobayashi H, et al (2010). Clinical features of liver dysfunction in collagen diseases. Hepatology Research. Vol 40, No. 11, (November, 2010), pp. 1092-7

Kessel A, Elias G, Pavlotzky E, Zuckerman E, Rosner I, et al (2007). Anti-C-reactive protein antibodies in chronic hepatitis C infection: correlation with severity and autoimmunity. *Human Immunology*. Vol. 68, No. 10, (October, 2007), pp. 844-8

Douglas MW & George J (2009). Molecular mechanisms of insulin resistance in chronic hepatitis C. *World Journal of Gastroenteroogy*. Vol. 15, No. 35, (September, 2009), pp. 4356-64

Sindelar DK, Chu CA, Rohlie M, Neal DW, Swift LL, et al (1997). The role of fatty acids in mediating the effects of peripheral insulin on hepatic glucose production in the conscious dog. *Diabetes*. Vol. 46, No 2, (February, 1997), pp. 187-96

Boden G, Chen X, Capulong E & Mozzoli M (2001). Effects of free fatty acids on gluconeogenesis and autoregulation of glucose production in type 2 diabetes. *Diabetes*. Vol. 50, No. 6, (April, 2001), pp. 810-6

Lam TK, Yoshii H, Haber CA, Bogdanovic E, Lam L, et al (2002). Free fatty acid-induced hepatic insulin resistance: a potential role for protein kinase C-delta. *American Journal of Physiology, Edocrinology and Metabolism*. Vol. 283, No. 4, (October, 2002), pp.E682-91

Wu C, Khan SA, Peng LJ, I H, Carmella SG et al (2006). Perturbation of glucose flux in the liver by decreasing F26P2 levels causes hepatic insulin resistance and hyperglycemia. *American Journal of Physiology, Endocrinology and Metabolism*. Vol. 291, No. 3, (September, 2006), pp. E536-43

Festa A, DÁgostino Jr. R, Tracy RP & Haffner SM (2002). Elevated levels of acute-phase proteins and plasminogen activator inhibitor-1 predict the development of type 2 diabetes. The insulin resistance atherosclerosis study. *Diabetes*. Vol. 51, No. 4, (April, 2002), pp. 1131-7

Almeda-Valdés P, Cuevas-Ramos D & Aguilar-Salinas CA (2009). Metabolic syndrome and non-alcoholic fatty liver disease. *Annals of Hepatology*. Vol. 8, No. 1 (Suppl), (January-March, 2009), pp. S18-S24

Kovacs A, Tornvall P, Nilsson R, Tegner J, Hamsten A, et al (2007). Human C-reactive protein slows atherosclerosis development in a mouse model with human-like hypercholesterolemia. *Proceedings of the National Academy of Science*. Vol. 104, No. 34, (August, 2007), pp. 13768-73

Tilg H & Moschen AR (2008). Inflammatory mechanisms in the regulation of Insulin resistance. *Molecular Medicine*. Vol. 14, No. 3-4, (March-April, 2008), pp. 222-31

Chen K, Li F, Li J, Cai H, Strom S, et al (2006). Induction of leptin resistance through direct interaction of C-reactive protein with leptin. *Nature Medicine*. Vol. 12, No. 4, (April, 2006), pp. 425-32

Targher G, Day CP & Bonora E. Risk of cardiovascular disease in patients with nonalcoholic fatty liver disease. *New England Journal of Medicine*. Vol. 363, No. 14, (September, 2010), pp. 1341-50

Freeman AJ, Dore GJ, Law MG, Thorpe M, Von Overbeck J, et al (2001). Estimating progression to cirrhosis in chronic hepatitis C virus infection. *Hepatology*. Vol. 34, No. 4 (pt 1), (October, 2001), pp. 809-16

Taniguchi CM, Ueki K & Kahn R. Complementary roles of IRS-1 and IRS-2 in the hepatic regulation metabolism. *Journal of Clinical Investigation*. Vol. 115, No. 3, (March, 2005), pp. 718-27

Kobashi-Margáin RA, Gutiérrez-Grobe Y, Ponciano-Rodríguez G, Uribe M, Méndez-Sánchez N (2010). Prevalence of type 2 diabetes mellitus and chronic liver disease: a retrospective study of the association of two increasingly common diseases in Mexico. *Annals of Hepatology*. Vol. 9, No. 3, (July-September, 2010), pp.282-8

Uribe M, Zamora-Valdés D, Moreno-Portillo M, Bermejo-Martínez L, Pichardo-Bahena R, et al (2008). Hepatic expression of ghrelin and adiponectin and their receptors in patients with nonalcoholic fatty liver disease. *Annals of Hepatology*. Vol. 7, No. 1, (January-March, 2008), pp.67-71.

Harring TR, Guiteau JJ, Nguyen NT, Cotton RT, Gingras MC, et al (2011). Building a comprehensive genomic program for hepatocellular carcinoma. *World Journal of Surgery*. Epub ahead of print.

7

Acute Phase Proteins as Biomarkers of Disease: From Bench to Clinical Practice

Francisco J. Salgado, Pilar Arias,
Ana Canda-Sánchez and Montserrat Nogueira
University of Santiago de Compostela
Spain

1. Introduction

The term acute phase response (APR) refers to the inflammatory response of the host occurring shortly after the tissue injury. It comprises a wide variety of reactions started by different causes, like infection, tissue injury, burn, trauma, surgery, cancer or immunological disorders. These reactions aim to prevent ongoing tissue damage, isolate and eliminate the cause of the inflammation, and begin the repair process necessary to restore the normal function. Usually, the local response is accompanied by a systemic reaction characterized by the fast alteration of the concentrations of several plasmatic proteins, the APPs (Acute Phase Proteins) produced by the liver (Baumann & Gauldie, 1994). In some diseases, the persistent immunological activation can cause chronic inflammation, often with pathological consequences. In other words, APR is a physiological condition occurring at the beginning of the inflammatory process and it is independent of the inflammation origin.

1.1 The inflammatory response

The inflammation is the ordered process mediated by the appearance of intercellular adhesion molecules on endothelia, and various inflammatory mediators released by tissue cells and leucocytes in response to tissue aggression; it is a protective response to injury or destruction of tissues, which serves to destroy, dilute, or wall off both the injurious agent and the injured tissues. It is the first reaction of the body under a situation of immunological stress: the innate non-specific response preceding specific immune reactions.

The term inflammation is purely descriptive and originally defined by the four Latin words dolor, rubor, calor and tumor (meaning pain, redness, warmth and swelling); these are the result of changes in the local blood vessels which in turn, lead to their dilatation and increased stickiness and permeability for passing leukocytes. Combined, the cell and fluid leakage into the tissue, as well as their local activities, account for the pain and swelling. The function of this inflammatory response is to bring serum molecules and immune cells to the damaged zone. In this response three principal components can be considered: i) increased blood supply, ii) increased capillary permeability and, iii) migration of cells out of the vessels and into the tissues.

In an inflammatory reaction there are implicated several cells of the immunological system and a great variety of response mediators. The uncontrolled migration of different leukocytes populations would make impossible the generation and control of the immune response. In this setting, the endothelium plays a key role. Endothelial cells are multifunctional cells that form a thin layer in the interior surface of blood vessels (Cines et al., 1998). They are responsible for maintaining the vascular homeostasis but, also, they are capable of secreting biologically active mediators when affected by infection, stress, hypertension, dyslipidemia or high homocysteine levels. The primary essential function of these endothelial cells is to regulate the permeability of the blood vessel and the exchange of fluids and cells between the blood and the surrounding tissue. In the inflammatory response they raise the expression of cell adhesion molecules that, therefore, increments the number of leukocytes binding endothelium (Pate et al., 2010). The increased permeability of the endothelium allows the migration of these cells, a process called extravasation, where they will exert its function. That is why they are so important for the recruitment and orchestration of an acute inflammatory response.

The role of the different cells and different interactions has been extensively described (Imhof & Aurrand-Lions, 2004; Langer & Chavakis, 2009; Ley et al., 2007; Schenkel et al., 2004; Vestweber, 2007), but briefly we are going to comment those. Normally, neutrophils are the first cells to appear at acute phase response, followed by macrophages (monocytes), lymphocytes (if there is an immunological challenge) and a small amount of basophils and eosinophils; if an extreme vascular leakage occurs, red blood cells may also be found. We can distinguish three steps for the migration of cell to the tissue during the inflammatory response (Butcher, 1991):

1-Receptor-mediated recruitment and adhesion to the endothelial cells: the regulation of the expression of selectin-P and selectin-E by the endothelium is key in this process (Lasky, 1995; Lawrence & Springer, 1991). The expression of P-selectin is increased by inflammatory molecules such as histamine and thrombine, it is a weak binder to the leukocytes but causes them to "slow" their movement in the vessel. Selectin-E expression, on the other hand, it is upregulated by cytokines produced by injured cells, such as IL-1 and TNF-α; these cytokines also activate and increase the expression of integrins on the circulating leukocytes. Activated leukocytes, therefore, increase the affinity of their integrins for certain ligands on the endothelial surface, attaching them firmly to the endothelium.

2- Transmigration, or the movement of the activated leukocytes through the endothelium to reach the damaged tissue: the leukocytes adhered to the endothelium are stimulated by the chemokine gradient to move between the endothelial cells and across the basal membrane to the damaged area. Among the chemotactic factors we can find: i) products of the complement like C3a, C4a, C5a (Hartmann et al., 1997; Okusawa et al., 1988), ii) fibrin degradation products (FDPs) like the D-dimer (Gross et al., 1997), iii) prostaglandins (PGD2, PGE2) (Konya et al., 2010; Kuehn et al., 2011), iv) leukotrienes (LTB4) (Aked & Foster, 1987) and chemokines like CCL5 (Kawai et al., 1999; Murooka et al., 2008) and IL-8 (Huber et al., 1991).

3- Movement of the activated leukocytes through the tissue: the binding to extracellular matrix proteins through the integrins and the CD44 protein allows these cells to arrive to the origin of the inflammation following the chemokine gradient (Kinashi, 2005).

1.1.1 The Pro-inflammatory cytokines

But in this local inflammatory process, activated leukocytes are not passive: in turn, they release cytokines and other mediators like glucocorticoids into the bloodstream, thus eliciting a widespread reaction in the organism. There are at least 15 cytokines known to be

involved in this process. Some of them are positive/negative regulators of cell growth (IL-2, IL-3, IL-4, IL-7, IL-10, IL-11, IL-12 and GM-CSF), while others have got pro-inflammatory (TNF-α/β, IL-1α/β, IL-6, IFN-α/γ, IL-8) or anti-inflammatory activities (IL-1 antagonists, soluble IL-1R, IL-1 and TNF-α binding protein)(van Miert, 1995).
Proinflammatory cytokines, released mainly by activated macrophages, are crucial for the induction of other cytokines (IL-6, IL-8), while agents such as platelet activating factor, prostaglandins, leukotrienes and nitric oxide increase the chemotactic gradient and therefore the leukocyte recruitment to the inflammation site. They are also responsible for the fever and catabolism of muscle proteins through their action at the CNS level: We will briefly comment some carachteristics of the proinflammatory cytokines involved in the acute phase reaction and the production of APPs:

- Tumor necrosis factor-alpha (TNF-α)

TNF-α is the main cytokine that mediates acute inflammation. TNF is produced by monocytes, macrophages, dendritic cells, Th1 cells, and other cells. Some of its functions include: to stimulate the cells from the endothelium to produce selectins and the leukocytes to express integrins, to activate the coagulation pathway, to increase the production of chemokines in endothelial cells and macrophages, to activate neutrophils and their killer activity, etc (Baud & Karin, 2001). It is also responsible for stimulating the liver to produce APPs (Xanthoulea et al., 2004), and acting on muscles (Collins & Grounds, 2001) and fat (Lu et al., 2006; Plomgaard et al., 2008; Rydén et al., 2002) to stimulate catabolism for energy conversion. In addition, it interacts with the hypothalamus to induce lack of appetite (Tracey et al., 1990), fever (Rothwell & Hopkins, 1995; Stefferl et al., 1996) and sleep (Deboer et al., 2002; Fang et al., 1997). It also participates in the cicatrization process through the stimulation of collagen and collagenase synthesis (Theiss et al., 2005).

-Interleukin-1 (IL-1)

IL-1 function is similar to TNF-α as it also mediates acute inflammatory responses, and together they enhance the inflammatory response (Dinarello & Wolff, 1993; Vassalli, 1992). Monocytes, macrophages, dendritic cells and endothelial cells are the main sources of IL-1. Functions of IL-1 include the promotion of the inflammation through the activation of the coagulation pathway and the synthesis of adhesion factors on endothelial cells and leukocytes (Bevilacqua et al., 1984; Nawroth et al., 1986) and the activation of macrophages (Dinarello, 1988). It is also responsible for stimulating the liver to produce APPs (Baumann & Gauldie, 1994; Mortensen et al., 1988; Prowse & Baumann, 1989), for activating the catabolism of the fat tissue for energy conversion (Feingold et al., 1992; Tocco-Bradley et al., 1987); and for regulating the synthesis of collagen and collagenase for scar tissue formation (Duncan & Berman, 1989; Mizel et al., 1981).
It is also noteworthy the role that IL-1 plays in the induction of the fever and sleep (Krueger et al., 1984; Opp & Krueger, 1991), as well as the stimulatory effect of IL-1 on the pituitary-adrenal axis in the CNS (Besedovsky et al., 1986; Sapolsky et al., 1987), thus making it responsible for the control of food intake (Luheshi et al., 1999) during the acute phase response.
Interleukin-1 and TNF-α have also being linked to the depression and sickness behaviour associated to the inflammatory response (Dantzer, 2001; Konsman et al., 2002). One theory behind this effect it is the role of IL-1 over serotoninergic neurons, where IL-1 could activate the serotonin transporter directly. This could lead to the removal of serotonin from the synaptic cleft, thus generating a serotoninergic deprivation signal together with the tryptophan deprivation derived from the APPs production (Leonard & Song, 1999).

- Interleukin-6 (IL-6)

IL-6 stimulates the liver to produce APPs and it is released by many cells including T-lymphocytes, macrophages, monocytes, endothelial cells, and fibroblasts (Prowse & Baumann, 1989). It is also responsible for the proliferation stimulation of B-lymphocytes (Muraguchi et al., 1988; Taga et al., 1987) and increases the neutrophil activity (Brom & König, 1992).

The outcome of the inflammation will depend on the tissue as well as the extent of injury and the injurious agent that has caused it. Usually, the resolution will bring the inflamed tissue to its status prior to the injury but, some times, the inflammation is not resolved properly. Sometimes a persistent damage or an incomplete resolution process can produce a chronic inflammation due to the continuous production of pro-inflammatory cytokines. Often, the reason behind the abnormal inflammatory response is not known, and it is the reason behind many human diseases. Some of them have got an immunological origin like the allergic reactions or myopathies (Lundberg & Grundtman, 2008); but sometimes the origin is non-immunological like in rheumatoid arthritis, cancer (Coussens & Werb, 2002), atherosclerosis (Libby, 2002), ischaemic heart disease (Maseri et al., 1996), inflammatory bowel diseases (Fiocchi, 1998), etc (many articles, reviews and books cover these topics, so this is not an extensive list). In all of the above mentioned disorders we can also see alterations in the levels of different APPs produced by the liver; the next section will present an extensive list of these proteins, where the main characteristics of the different groups will be commented briefly.

2. Acute phase proteins

APPs is a group of plasma proteins whose concentration varies in response to inflammation (Baumann & Gauldie, 1994). They are synthesized mainly by the liver but also by other cell types (monocytes, endothelial cells, fibroblasts and adipocytes). According to the variations in the concentration of these proteins they can be classified in positive APPs, those that increase the concentration, and negative APPs, those that show decreased concentrations upon the inflammatory response. There are also other sub-classifications for the positive APPs, according to the variation in concentration: Group I positive APPs increase up to 50% (ceruloplasmin and complement factor-3 (C3)), Group II from 2 to 5 times (haptoglobin, fibrinogen, α-globulins with antiprotease-activity and lipopolysaccharide binding protein), and Group III from 5 to more than 1000 times (CRP and SAA) (Dowton & Colten, 1988).

There is a lot of diversity regarding the timings that each of these proteins show any variation on its levels. Some proteins alter their levels as soon as 4 h, while others can take up to 24 h or even days. CRP (C-reactive protein) and SAA (serum amyloid A) are some of these very rapidly increasing proteins: they elevate their levels within the first 4 h after tissue injury, opposite to the lipopolysaccharide binding protein, that requires at least 8 h, or the serum alpha-l-acid glycoprotein, that needs 48 h. Some of these proteins remain elevated for various days, while other only for few hours. The origin behind the inflammation is also important: the plasma fibrinogen shows a peak in the concentration at 24 h-48 h or at 96 h, depending on the inflammatory stimulus (Colley et al., 1983; Gruys et al., 2005)

As commented before TNF-α, IL-1, and IL-6 are the main cytokines involved in the hepatocytic secretion of APPs, but there are many others. Indeed, all type of combinatorial effects can regulate the hepatocytic secretion of an APP (addition, synergy, antagonism). IL-1 and IL-6 have been used to classify APPs into two subgroups: Type 1 requires the

synergistic effect of both interleukins for maximum synthesis (examples: CRP, SAA, Alpha-1-acid glycoprotein 1); type 2 are those that only require IL-6 and usually IL-1 acts suppressing more than enhancing its production (examples: fibrinogen chains, haptoglobin, alpha-2-Macroglobulin (Ramadori & Christ, 1999)). There are some cytokines that regulate the expression of one or two APPs, like Activin A, a cytokine related with the superfamily of TGF-β. On the other hand, other APPs are the result of a wider combination of cytokines. That is the case of SAA that requires the synergitic effect of bacterial LPS and several cytokines (mainly IL-1, IL-6, and TNF, but also LIF, CNTF, oncostatin M, IL-11, and cardiotrophin-1) to be produced (Benigni et al., 1996).
The main structural characteristics of APPs can be found in Table 1. Regarding their functions, summarized in Table 2, they are opsonisation and elimination of microorganisms and their products (CPR), activation of the complement system (complement C4a, C4b) and the lectin complement pathway (manan-binding lectin), inhibition of certain enzymes (alpha-1-antitrypsin, alpha-2-antiplasmin) or interleukins (interleukin-1 receptor antagonist protein), blockade of free radicals and/or elimination of haemoglobin residues (haptoglobin, serotransferrin, hemopexin), regulation of the immune response (serum amyloid P), coagulation and tissue repair/remodelling (fibrinogen, plasminogen), transport of ions (apolipoproteins, calcitonin precursor) and hormones (serum albumin), etc. Others, like alpha 2-macroglobulin and the coagulation factors, also play an important role in wound healing, because they collaborate with the immune system by increasing the vascular permeability, because they have chemotactic properties, or even because they are able of trapping pathogens in local blood clots.

3. Acute phase proteins currently used in routine clinical practice

As compared with cytokine and other short distance mediators of cellular responses production, which occurs in pulsed patterns cleared from the circulation within a few hours due to their small size, the native molecular mass of APPs secreted by the liver is larger than the kidney filtration cutoff (about 45 kDa). An example is albumin, which is just larger and has a lifetime of about 21 days. This fact, together with their large half-life, ensures an extended residence time in plasma, which means that levels of some APPs may remain unchanged for days and may be useful for diagnostic purposes. Currently, alterations in levels of some APPs are used to assess either the health/nutritional status of an individual or, mainly, to check for the presence of reactive processes, which has more advantages than measuring IL-6, a sensitive indicator of inflammation or infection but with a normal range of 0-5 pg/ml and short plasma clearing times. An analysis of US Food and Drug Administration (FDA) approvals for IVD assays aimed to the quantitative detection of acute phase reactants reveals about 80 companies involved (Table 3), of which 15 dominate the market: Abbott Laboratories, Beckman Coulter, Dade Behring, Diasorin, Globalemed, Kamiya Biomedical, Kent Laboratories, Nitto Boseki, Olympus Life Science Research, Ortho-Clinical Diagnostics, Polymedco, Randox Laboratories, Roche Diagnostics, Siemens Medical Solutions Diagnostics, and The Binding Site.
About 51% of FDA-cleared or approved IVD assays are aimed to the detection of unique plasma or serum proteins that carry out their normal function in plasma. Most of these proteins are negative or positive acute phase reactants, like albumin, C-reactive protein, α 1 antitrypsin, transferrin, ceruloplasmin, or fibrinogen. Table 4 summarizes different tests from the companies listed in Table 3 intended to the detection of APPs in clinical practice.

Recommended name	Short name	n° aa/Mr (d)	Post-translational modification (nª)	FAMILY/DOMAIN	Gen name (synonyms)	Polimorfismo/ Natural variations	Uniprot
Alpha-1-acid glycoprotein	AGP, (OMD) (1, 2)	201/23512 (1) 201/23603 (2)	Glycosylation: N-linked (5). Mod- Res: Pyrrolidone carboxylic acid (1). -S-S- (2)	Calycin superfamily. Lipocalin family.	ORM1(AGP1) ORM2(AGP2)	Allele AGP1(3). Nat-Var AGP1(3), AGP2(5)	P02763 (1) P19652 (2)
Alpha-1-anti chimotrypsin	ACT	423/47651	Glycosylation: N-linked (6)	Serpin family.	SERPINA3 (AACT)	3 Isoforms. 4 Alt-Seq. 7 Nat-Var.	P01011
Alpha-2-antiplasmin	Alpha-2-AP	491/54566	Cross-link: Isoglutamyl Lys isopeptide interchain (1). Glycosylation: N-linked (4). Mod-Res: PTyr (1). -S-S- (1).	Serpin family.	SERPINF2 (AAP, PLI)	8 Nat-Var.	P08697
Antithrombin-3	ATIII	464/52602	Glycosylation: N-linked (4). Mod-Res: PSer (1). -S-S- (3)	Serpin family.	SERPINC1 (AT3)	91 Nat-Var .	P01008
Alpha-1-antitrypsin	AAT	418/46737	Glycosylation: N-linked (3) Mod-Res: S-cysteinyl Cys	Serpin family.	SERPINA1 (AAT, PI)	4 Allele. 3 Isoforms. 2 Alt-Seq. 38 Nat-Var.	P01009
Alpha-1B-glycoprotein	ABG	495/54254	Glycosylation: N-linked (4). -S-S- (5)	5 Ig-like V-type (Ig-like) domains.	A1BG	2 Isoforms. 1 Alt-Seq. 2 Nat-Var.	P04217
Alpha-2-HS-glycoprotein	AHSG	367/39325	Glycosylation: N-linked (2), O-linked (3). Mod-Res: PSer (6). -S-S- (6, 1 inter chain)	Fetuin family. 2 Cystatin domains.	AHSG FETUA	5 Nat-Var.	P02765
Alpha-2-macroglobulin	A2M	1474/ 163291	Cross-link: Isoglutamyl Lys isopeptide (Gln-Lys) inter- (2). Cross-link: Isoglutamyl Cys thioester (Cys-Gln) (1). Glycosylation: N-linked (8). -S-S- intra- (11), inter- (2).	Protease inhibitor I39 (alpha-2-macroglobulin).	A2M (CPAMD5)	5 Nat-Var.	P01023

Recommended name	Short name	nº aa/Mr (d)	Post-translational modification (nª)	FAMILY/DOMAIN	Gen name (synonyms)	Polimorfismo/ Natural variations	Uniprot
Apolipoprotein AI	ApoAI	267/30778	Glycosylation: N-linked (1). Mod-Res: PSer (1)	Apolipoprotein A1/A4/E family.	APOA1	26 Nat-Var.	P02647
Apolipoprotein B-100	Apo-B100	4563/ 515605	Lipidation: S-palmitoyl Cys (1). Glycosylation: N-linked (19). Mod-Res: PSer (2), N6-acetyl Lys (1). -S-S- (8)	1 Vitellogenin domain.	APOB	56 Nat-Var.	P04114
Apolipoprotein E	Apo-E	317/36154	Glycosyla tion: O-linked (3), N-linked (1). Mod-Res: PSer (1).	Apolipoprotein A1/A4/E family.	APOE	3 Allele. 33 Nat-Var.	P02649
Beta-2-glicoproteina1	B2GPI	345/38298	Glycosylation: O-linked (1), N-linked (4). -S-S- (11)		APOH	6 Nat-Var.	P02749
Beta-2-microglobulin	B2M	119/13715	Glycosylation: N-linked (7). Mod-Res: Pyrrolidone carboxylic acid. -S-S- (1)	Beta-2-microglobulin family. 1 Ig-like C1-type domain.	B2M	1 Nat-Var.	P61769
Calcitonin precursor	CCP, PDN-21	141/15466	Glycosylation: N-linked (6). Metal binding: Copper (6). Mod-Res: Pro amide (1). -S-S-(1)	Calcitonin family.	CALCA (CALC1)	3 Isoforms. 1-Alt-Seq. 6 Nat-Var.	P01258
Ceruloplasmin	CER, EC=1.1 6.3.1	1065/ 122205	-S-S- (5). Mod-Res: PTyr (2), PSer (1).	Multicopper oxidase family.	CP	7 Nat-Var.	P00450
Coagulation factor VIII,	AHF	2351/2670 09	Glycosylation N-linked (22). Mod-Res: SulfoTyr (6). -S-S- (8)	Multicopper oxidase family, contains 3 F5/8 type A, 2 F5/8 type C and 6 plastocyanin-like domains.	F8, (F8C)	465 Nat-Var.	P00451

Recommended name	Short name	n° aa/Mr (d)	Post-translational modification (n[a])	FAMILY/DOMAIN	Gen name (synonyms)	Polimorfismo/ Natural variations	Uniprot
Complement C2	EC=3.4.21.43	752/83268	Glycosylation: N-linked (8) -S-S- (8)	Peptidase S1 family. 1 Peptidase S1, 3 Sushi (CCP/SCR), and 1 VWFA domains.	C2	6 Nat-Var.	P06681
Complement C3	C3	1663/ 187148	Cross-link: Isoglutamyl Cys thioester (Cys-Gln). Glycosylation: N-linked (3). Mod-Res: PSer (3), P Tyr (1). -S-S- (13, 1 interchain).	1 Anaphylatoxin-like and 1 NTR domains.	C3, CPAMD1	2 Allele. 22 Nat-Var.	P01024
Complement C4A	C4A	1744/ 192771	Cross-link: Isoglutamyl Cys thioester (Cys-Gln) (1). Glycosylation: N-linked (4). Mod-Res: SulfoTyr (3). -S-S- (5).	1 Anaphylatoxin-like and 1 NTR domains.	A-C4A (CO4, CPAMD2)	13 Allele of C4A. 11 Nat-Var.	P0C0L4
Complement C4B	C4B	1744/ 192793	Cross-link: Iso glutamyl Cys thioester (Cys-Gln) (1). Glycosylation N-linked (4). Mod-Res: SulfoTyr (3).-S-S- (5).	1 Anaphylatoxin-like and 1 NTR domains.	C4B (CO4, CPAMD3)	22 Allele of C4B. 8 Nat-Var.	P0C0L5
Complement C5,	C5	1676/ 188305	Glycosylation: N-linked (4) -S-S- (14)	1 Anaphylatoxin-like and 1 NTR domains.	C5, CPAMD4	16 Nat-Var.	P01031
Complement C9,	C9	559/63173	Glycosylation: C-linked (2), N-linked (2). Mod-Res: PSer (1). -S-S- (12)	C6/C7/C8/C9 family. 1EGF-like, 1 LDL-receptor class A, 1 MACPF and 1 TSP type-1 domains.	C9	6 Nat-Var.	P02748

Recommended name	Short name	nº aa/Mr (d)	Post-translational modification (nª)	FAMILY/DOMAIN	Gen name (synonyms)	Polimorfismo/ Natural variations	Uniprot
C4 binding protein,	C4BPA C4BPB	597/67033 (A) 252/28357 (B)	Glycosylation: N-linked a (3), b(5). –S-S-: A(18, 2 interchain), B(8, 2 interchain)	Sushi (CCP/SCR) domain: A(8), B(3).	a-C4BPA (C4BP) b-C4BPB	Isoforms B(2). Alt-Seq B(1). Nat-Var: A(6), B(2).	P04003 (A) P20851 (B)
Corticosteroid-binding globulin	CBG	405/45141	Binding site: corticosteroid (3). Glycosylation: N-linked (6).	Serpin family	SERPINA 6, (CBG)	3 Nat-Var.	P08185
C-reactive protein	CRP	224/25039	Metal binding: calcium (2), Pyrrolidone carboxylic acid. -S-S- (1)	Pentaxin family. 1 Pentaxin domain.	CRP, (PTX1)	2 isoforms. 1 Alt-Seq.	P02741
Factor B	GBG, EC=3.4. 21.47	764/85533	Glycosylation: N-linked (5) -S-S-: (11)	Peptidase S1 family. 1 Peptidase S1, 3 Sushi (CCP /SCR) , and 1 VWFA domains.	CFB (BF, BFD)	2 isoforms. 2 Alt-Seq. 17 Nat-Var.	P00751
Ferritin	Subunits: L, H (EC1.16 .3.1)	175/20020 183/21226	Metal binding: L[Iron (1)], H[Iron, (2)]. Mod-Res: L[N-acetyl Ser(1), N6-acetylLys (1)], H [(PThr(1), PSer (2)]	Ferritin family. Ferritin-like Diiron domain (L and H).	FTL FTH1 (FTH1, FTHL6)	L: 1 Nat-Var.	P02792 (L) P02794 (H)
Fibrinogen,	FGA(α) FGB(β) FGG(γ)	866/94973 (A) 491/55928 (B) 453/51512 (G)	Cross-link: Isoglutamyl Lys isopeptide interchain A(8), G(2). Glycosylation: N-linked A(2), B(1), G(2). Mod-Res: B(Pyrrolidone carboxylic acid), A[PSer (6), PThr (1), PTyr (1)] G[Sulfo Tyr (2)]. -S-S- A (7, 6-interchain), B (8, 5-interchain), G (8, 6-interchain).	Fibrinogen C-terminal domain (a, B, G).	FGA(α) FGB(β) FGG(γ)	Isoforms A(2), G(2). Alt-Seq: A(2), G(1). Nat-Var: A(19), B(14), G(19).	P02671 (α) P02675(β) P02679 (γ)

Recommended name	Short name	nº aa/Mr (d)	Post-translational modification (nª)	FAMILY/DOMAIN	Gen name (synonyms)	Polimorfismo/ Natural variations	Uniprot
Fibronectin,	FN	2386/ 262625	Cross-link: Isoglutamyl Lys isopeptide (Gln-Lys) (3). Glycosylation: N-linked (6), O-linked (2). Mod-Res: Pyrrolidone carboxylic acid, SulfoTyr (2), PSer (4). -S-S- (30, 2 interchain).	12 Fibronectin type-I, 2 Fibronectin type-II and 16 Fibronectin type-III domains.	FN1 (FN)	15 isoforms. 14 Alt-Seq. 12 Nat-Var.	P02751
Haptoglobin	Hp (α, β)	406/45205	Glycosylation: N-linked (4) -S-S- (8, 3 interchain)	Peptidase S1, 1 Peptidase S1 and 2 Sushi (CCP/SCR) domains.	HP	2 Allele. 4 Nat-Var.	P00738
Heme oxigenase 2	HO-2, EC=1.1 4.99.3	316/36033	Metal binding: Iron (1). Mod-Res: N-acetylSer (1)	Heme oxygenase family. 2 HRM (heme regulatory motif) repeats.	HMOX2 (HO2)	2 Nat-Var.	P30519
Hemopexin	HPX	462/51676	Glycosylation: N-linked (5), O-linked (1). Metal binding: Iron (1). -S-S- (6)	Hemopexin family. 5 Hemopexin-like domains.	HPX	2 Nat-Var.	P02790
Heparin cofactor 2	HC-II, HLSII	499/57071	Glycosylation: N-linked (3).Mod-Res: PSer (1), SulfoTyr (2).	Serpin family.	SERPIND1, (HCF2)	9 Nat-Var.	P05546
Hepcidin	LEAP-1, PLTR	84/9408	-S-S- (4)	Hepcidin family.	HAMP (HEPC, LEAP1)	4 Nat-Var.	P81172
Histidine-rich glycoprotein	HPRG	525/59578	Glycosylation N-linked (4). -S-S- (5)	2 Cystatin domains.	HRG	10 Nat-Var.	P04196

Recommended name	Short name	n° aa/Mr (d)	Post-translational modification (n[a])	FAMILY/DOMAIN	Gen name (synonyms)	Polimorfismo/ Natural variations	Uniprot
Inter-alpha-trypsin inhibitor	ITI-HC1 ITI-HC2 ITI-HC3 ITIH4	911/101389 (HC1) 946/106463 (HC2) 890/99849 (HC3)	Glycosylation: N-linked HC1(3), HC2(3), HC3(2), O-linked HC1(1), HC2(4), S-linked HC1(1). Mod-Res: PThr HC1(2), PTyr HC1(1), PSer HC2(1), 4-carboxyGlu HC2(2), Asp 1-(chondroitin 4-sulfate)-ester HC1(1), HC2(1), HC3(1).-S-S- HC1(2), HC2(2)	ITIH family. 1 VIT and 1 VWFA domains.	ITIH1 (IGHEP1) ITIH2 (IGHEP2) ITIH3 ITIH4	Isoforms (CH3(2). Alt-Seq (CH3(1). Nat-Var HC1(5), HC2(3), HC3(6).	P19827 (HC1) P19823 (HC2) Q06033 (HC3) Entrez 3700
Interleukin-1 receptor antagonist protein	IL-1RN IL-1ra IRAP	177/20055 (1) 159/17888 (2) 180/19897 (3) 143/16142 (4)	Glycosylation: N-linked (1) -S-S- (1)	Interleukin 1 cytokine family.	IL1RN (IL1F3, IL1RA)	Isoforms 1,2,3,4(4). Alt-seq 1(1). Nat-Var 1(1).	P18510
Kallikrein-1	KLK1	262(1)/	Glycosylation: O-linked (3),N-linked (3). -S-S- (5).	Peptidase S1 family. Kallikrein subfamily.		2 Isoforms. 1 Alt-Seq. 4 Nat-Var.	P06870
Leucine-rich alpha-2-glycoprotein	LRG	347/38178	Glycosylation: N-linked (4), O-linked (1). -S-S- (2)	8 LRR (leucine-rich) repeats.	LRG1 (LRG)	2 Nat-Var.	P02750
Lipopolysaccharide binding protein	LBP	481/53384	Glycosylation: N-linked (4)	BPI/LBP/Plunc superfamily. BPI/LBP family.	LBP	14 Nat-Var.	P18428
Superoxide dismutase [Mn], mitochondrial	E.C.1.1 5.1.1	222/24722	Binding manganese (4) Nitrated Tyr, N6-acetylLys (2)	Iron/manganese superoxide dismutase family.	SOD2	6 Nat-Var.	P04179

Recommended name	Short name	n° aa/Mr (d)	Post-translational modification (nª)	FAMILY/DOMAIN	Gen name (synonyms)	Polimorfismo/ Natural variations	Uniprot
Mannose-bin ding protein C	MBP-C	248/26144	Mod-Res: HydroxyPro (5), -S-S-(2)	C-type lectin, Collagen-like domains.	MBL2 (COLEC1, MBL)	5 Nat-Var.	P11226
Annexin A5	CBP-I, PAP-1, VAC-a, PP4,	320/35937	Mod-Res: N-acetylAla (1), N6-acetylLys (5), PTyr(1)	Annexin family. Contains 4 Annexin repeats.	ANXA5 (ANX5, ENX2, PP4)		P08758
Plasma protease C1 inhibitor	C1 Inh,	500/55154	Glycosylation: N-linked (7), O-linked (7). -S-S- (2)	Serpin family.	SERPING1 (C1IN, C1NH)	31 Nat-Var.	P05155
Plasminogen	PLA EC=3.4. 21.7	810/90569	Binding sites: Fibrin (2), Omega-amino carboxylic acids (5). Glycosylation: O-linked (2), N-linked (1). Mod-Res: PSer (1). -S-S- (24, 2 interchain)	Peptidase S1 family. Plasminogen subfamily. 5 Kringle, 1 PAN and 1 Peptidase S1 domains.	PLG	19 Nat-Var.	P00747
Plasminogen activador inhibitor I	PAI, PAI-1	402/45060	Glycosylation: N-linked (3)	Serpin family.	SERPINE1, (PAI1, LANH1)	5 Nat-Var.	P05121
Properdin	CFP	469/51276	Glycosylation: O-linked (4), N-linked (1), C-linked (14). -S-S- (12)	6 TSP type-1 domains.	CFP (PFC)	8 Nat-Var.	P27918
Protein AMBP	Protein HC	352/38999	Binding site: Multimeric 3-hydroxykynure nine chromophore (covalent) (4). Glycosyla tion: O-linked (2), N-linked (3). –S-S- (7)	Calycin superfamily. Lipocalin family. BPTI/Kunitz inhibitor domain.	AMBP, (HCP, ITIL)		P02760

Recommended name	Short name	n° aa/Mr (d)	Post-translational modification (nª)	FAMILY/DOMAIN	Gen name (synonyms)	Polimorfismo/ Natural variations	Uniprot
Prothrombin,	PTR EC=3.4. 21.5	622/70037	Glycosylation: N-linked (3). Mod-Res: 4-carboxyglutamate (10). -S-S- (12, 1-interchain).	Peptidase S1 family. 1 Gla (gamma-carboxi-Glu), 2 Kringle and 1 Peptidase S1 domains.	F2	12 Nat-Var.	P00734
Retinol-binding protein 4	RBP, PRBP	201/23010	-S-S- (3)	Calycin superfamily. Lipocalin family.	RBP4	2 Nat-Var.	P02753
Serotransferrin	Transfe rrin	698/77064	Glycosylation: N-linked (2), O-linked (1). Binding site: carbonate (2). Metal binding: Iron (2). Mod-Res: Omega-N-methylated Arg(1), PTyr(1), -S-S- (19)	Transferrin family. 2 Transferrin-like domains.	TF	16 Nat-Var.	P02787
Serum albumin	ALB	609/69367 (1) 417/47360 (2)	Glycosylation: N-linked (24). Metal binding: copper (1), Zinc(4). Binding site: bilirubin(1). Mod-Res: PThr(2), PSer(4), PTyr(2). -S-S- (17)	ALB/AFP/VDB family. 3 Albumin domains.	ALB	2 isoform. 1 Alt-Seq. 66 Nat-Var.	P02768
Serum amyloid A protein	SAA1 SAA2 SAA3P SAA4 (C-SAA)	122/13532 122/13532 122/13440 130/14747	Glicosilation: N-linked A4 (1). Mod-Res: N4,N4-dimethylAsn A1(1), A2(1)	SAA family.	SAA 1 SAA2 SAA3 SAA4 (CSAA)	Isoforms. Nat-Var A1(10), A2(10), A4(1).	P02735 (A1, A2) P22614 (A3) P35542 (A4)

Recommended name	Short name	n° aa/Mr (d)	Post-translational modification (nª)	FAMILY/DOMAIN	Gen name (synonyms)	Polimorfismo/ Natural variations	Uniprot
Serum amyloid P component	SAP	223/25387	Glycosylation: N-linked (1). Metal binding: Calcium (2). Mod-Res: PThr (2), Pser (1), N-acetylMet (1). -S-S- (1),	Pentaxin family. 1 Pentaxin domain.	APCS (PTX2)	3 Nat-Var.	P02743
Tetranectin	TN	202/22537	Glycosylation O-linked (1) -S-S- (3)	1 C-type lectin domain.	CLEC3B, (TNA)	3 Nat-Var.	P05452
Transthyretin	TTR	147/15887	Binding site: Thyroid hormones (2). Glycosylation: N-linked (1). Mod-Res: 4-carboxyGlu (1)	Transthyretin family.	TTR, (PALB)	87 Nat-Var.	P02766
Vitamin D-binding protein	DBP VDB	474/52964 (1) 352/39542 (2)	Glycosylation: N-linked (1). -S-S- (14)	ALB/AFP/VDB family. 3 Albumin domains.	GC	2 Isoforms. 1 Alt -Seq. 4 Nat-Var.	P02774
Von Willebrand factor	vWF	2813/309265	Cross-link: Glycyl Lys isopeptide (Lys-Gly) (interchain). Glycosylation: N-linked (16), O-linked (10). -S-S- (29).	Inhibitor family I8. 1 CTCK (C-terminal cystine knot-like, 4 TIL (Trypsin inhibitory-like), 3 VWFA, 3 VWFC, 4 VWFD domains.	VWF (F8VWF)	58 Nat-Var.	P04275
Zinc-alpha-2-glycoprotein	Zn-alpha-2-GP	298/34259	Glycosylation: N-linked (4). Mod-Res: Pyrrolidone carboxylic acid. -S-S- (2)	MHC class I family. 1 Ig-like C1-type domain.	AZGP1 (ZAG, ZNGP1)		P25311

Table 1. Main characteristics of APPs. There are represented the classical APPs and other proteins that have been reported as inflammation related proteins, and cited as putative APPs. Abbreviatures: Alternative Sequence, Alt-Seq; Disulfide Bond, -S-S-; Immunoglobulin, Ig; Interleukin, IL; Major Histocompatibility Complex, MHC; Modified residue, Mod-Res; Natural variants, Nat-Var; Phosphoserine, PSer; Phosphothreonine, PThr; Phosphotyrosine, PTyr; other abbreviatures are specified in the text.

Protein	Alternative names	Function
Alpha-1-acid glycoprotein	•Orosomucoid	Acts as a carrier of basic and neutrally charged lipophilic compounds (interaction with collagen promotion of growth of fibroblasts binding of certain steroids)
Alpha-1-antichymotrypsin	•Cell growth-inhibiting gene 24/25 protein •Serpin A3	Physiological function unclear, it can inhibit neutrophil cathepsin G and mast cell chymase, both of which can convert angiotensin-1 to active angiotensin-2.
Alpha-2-antiplasmin	• 2-plasmin inhibitor •Serpin F2	The major targets of this inhibitor are plasmin and trypsin, but it also inactivates chymotrypsin.
Alpha-1-antitrypsin	•Alpha-1 protease inhibitor •Alpha-1 antiproteinase •Serpin A1	Inhibitor of serine proteases. Acts mainly in the protection of the lower respiratory tract against proteolytic destruction by human leukocyte elastase (HLE). The aberrant form inhibits insulin-induced NO synthesis in platelets, decreases coagulation time and has proteolytic activity. Short peptide from AAT (SPAAT) is a reversible chymotrypsin inhibitor.
Alpha-2-HS-glycoprotein	•Alpha-2Z-globulin •FetuinA •Ba-alpha-2-glycoprotein	Promotes endocytosis, possesses opsonic properties and influences the mineral phase of bone. Shows affinity for calcium and barium ions.
Alpha-2-macroglobulin	•C3-PZP-like 2-macroglobulin domain-containing protein 5	Inhibitor of four classes of proteinases by a unique 'trapping' mechanism which contains specific cleavage sites for different proteinases. After the cleavage, a thioester bond is hydrolyzed and mediates the covalent protein-proteinase bond.
Alpha-1B-glycoprotein	•Alpha-1-B glycoprotein	Specific and high-affinity ligand of CRISP3 that in human is present in exocrine secretions and in secretory granules of neutrophilic granulocytes and is believed to play a role in innate immunity.
Antithrombin-3	•Serpin C1	Most important serine protease inhibitor in plasma that regulates the blood coagulation cascade. AT-III inhibits thrombin as well as factors IXa, Xa and XIa. Its inhibitory activity is greatly enhanced in the presence of heparin.
Apolipoprotein AI	•Apolipoprotein A1	Participates in the reverse transport of cholesterol from tissues to the liver for excretion by promoting its efflux and as cofactor for the lecithin cholesterol acyltransferase (LCAT). As part of the SPAP complex, activates spermatozoa motility.

Protein	Alternative names	Function
Apolipoprotein B-100		Major protein constituent of chylomicrons (apo B-48), LDL (apo B-100) and VLDL (apo B-100). Apo B-100 functions as a recognition signal for the cellular binding and internalization of LDL particles by the apoB/E receptor.
Apolipoprotein E		Mediates the binding, internalization, and catabolism of lipoprotein particles. It can serve as a ligand for the LDL (apo B/E) receptor and for the specific apo-E receptor (chylomicron remnant) of hepatic tissues.
Beta-2-glicoproteina 1	• Apolipoprotein H • Activated C binding protein • APCinhibitor	Binds to various kinds of negatively charged substances such as heparin, phospholipids, and dextran sulfate. It can prevent activation of the intrinsic blood coagulation cascade by binding to phospholipids on the surface of damaged cells.
Beta-2-microglobulin		Component of the Class I Major Histocompatibility Complex (MHC).
Calcitonin precursor	•Calcitonin carboxyl-terminal peptide	Causes a rapid but short-lived drop in the level of Ca^{+2} and phosphate in blood by promoting the incorporation of those ions in the bones. Katacalcin is a potent plasma calcium-lowering peptide.
Ceruloplasmin	•Ferroxidase	A blue copper-binding (6-7 atoms per molecule) glycoprotein. It has ferroxidase activity oxidizing Fe^{2+} to Fe^{3+} without releasing radical oxygen species. It is involved in iron transport across the cell membrane.
Coagulation factorVIII	• Antihemophilic factor	Along with Ca^{+2} and phospholipid, acts as a cofactor for factor IXa when it converts factor X to Xa, the activated form.
Complement C2	•C3/C5 convertase	Is part of the classical complement pathway and cleaved by activated factor C1 into two fragments: C2b and C2a. C2a, a serine protease, then combines with C4b to generate the C3 or C5 convertase.
Complement C3	•C3 and PZP-like alpha-2-macroglobulin domain-containing protein 1.	Its processing by C3 convertase is the central reaction in both classical and alternative complement pathways. Activated C3b can bind covalently to cell surface carbohydrates or immune aggregates. The anaphylatoxin C3a is a mediator of local inflammation, induces the contraction of smooth muscle, increases vascular permeability and causes histamine release.

Protein	Alternative names	Function
Complement C4a	•Acidic complement C4-C3 and PZP-like alpha-2-macroglobulin domain-containing protein 2.	Plays a central role in the activation of the classical complement pathway. It is processed by activated C1 which removes from the chain the C4a anaphylatoxin. C4a-anaphylatoxin is a mediator of local inflammation that induces the contraction of smooth muscle and increases vascular permeability.
Complement C4b	•Basic complement C4-C3 and PZP-like alpha-2-macroglobulin domain-containing protein 3	Plays a central role in the activation of the classical complement pathway. The C4b fragment is the major activation product and is an essential subunit of the C3 and the C5 convertases.
Complement C5	•C3 and PZP-like alpha-2-macroglobulin domain-containing protein 4	C5 convertase initiates the spontaneous assembly of the late complement components, C5-C9, into the MAC. The C5b-C6 complex is the base upon which the lytic complex is assembled. The C5a anaphylatoxin, produced by proteolysis, is a mediator of local inflammation and stimulates the migration of leukocytes.
Complement C9		Constituent of the membrane attack complex (MAC) that plays a key role in the innate and adaptive immune response by forming pores in the plasma membrane of target cells. C9 is the pore-forming subunit of the MAC.
C4 binding protein	•Proline-rich protein (a)	Controls the classical pathway of complement activation. It binds as a cofactor to C3b/C4b inactivator (C3bINA), which then hydrolyzes C4b. It accelerates the degradation of the C4bC2a complex (C3 convertase) by dissociating the C2a. It also interacts with anticoagulant protein S and with serum amyloid P component.
C-reactive protein		Displays functions associated with host defense: promotes agglutination, bacterial capsular swelling, phagocytosis and complement fixation, and interacts with DNA and histones to scavenge particles released from damaged circulating cells.
Corticosteroid-binding globulin	•Transcortin, Serpin A6	Major transport protein for glucocorticoids and progestins in the blood of almost all vertebrate species.
Factor B	•C3/C5 convertase •Glycine-rich beta glycoprotein •Properdin	Factor B, from the alternate complement pathway, is cleaved by factor D into 2 fragments: Ba and Bb. Bb, a serine protease, binds to C3b to generate the C3 convertase; and it has been implicated in the proliferation and differentiation

Protein	Alternative names	Function
	factor B	of preactivated B-cells, rapid spreading of monocytes and lysis of erythrocytes. Ba inhibits the proliferation of preactivated B-cells.
Ferritin		Stores iron in a soluble, non-toxic, readily available form. Iron is taken up in the ferrous form and deposited as ferric hydroxides after oxidation. It also plays a role in delivery of iron to cells.
Fibrinogen		Has a double function, yielding monomers that polymerize into fibrin and acting as a cofactor in platelet aggregation.
Fibronectin	•Cold-insoluble globulin	Bind cell surfaces and various compounds including collagen, fibrin, heparin, DNA, and actin. It also is involved in cell adhesion, cell motility, opsonization, etc. Both anastellin (a fragment of fibronectin) and superfibronectin inhibit tumor growth, angiogenesis and metastasis. Anastellin also activates p38 MAPK and inhibits lysophospholipid signalling.
Haptoglobin		Combines with free plasma hemoglobin, preventing the loss of iron through the kidneys and protecting them from hemoglobin damage, while making the hemoglobin accessible to degradative enzymes.
Heme oxigenase		Cleaves heme ring to form biliverdin that is subsequently converted to bilirubin. Its activity is highest in the spleen, where senescent erythrocytes are destroyed. Also seems to be involved in the production of carbon monoxide in brain.
Hemopexin	•Beta-1B-glycoprotein	Binds heme and transports it to liver for breakdown and iron recovery, after free hemopexin returns to the circulation.
Hepcidin	•Liver-expressed antimi crobial peptide 1, •Putative liver tumor regressor	Seems to act as a signalling molecule involved in the iron homeostasis and to be required in conjunction with HFE to regulate both intestinal iron absorption and iron storage in macrophages. It has strong antimicrobial activity against several types of bacterias (E.coli, S.aureus, etc) and fungus (C.albicans).
Heparin cofactor 2	•Heparin cofactor II, •Protease inhibitor leuserpin-2, •Serpin D1	Thrombin inhibitor activated by the glycosaminoglycans, heparin or dermatan sulfate. In the presence of the latter, HC-II is the predominant thrombin inhibitor instead of AT-III. Inhibits chymotrypsin in a glycosaminoglycan-independent manner. Peptides at the N-terminal of HC-

Protein	Alternative names	Function
		II have chemotactic activity for both monocytes and neutrophils.
Histidine-rich glycoprotein	•Histidine-proline-rich glycoprotein	Function not yet known. It binds heme and divalent metal ions. Interact with heparin and the lysine-binding site of plasminogen. On the basis of its His-rich region may mediate the activation phase of intrinsic blood coagulation cascade
Inter-alpha-trypsin inhibitor	•Inter- -trypsin inhibitor complex component •Serum-derived hyaluronan-associated protein.	May act as a carrier of hyaluronan in serum or as a binding protein between hyaluronan and other matrix protein, including cell surfaces, to regulate its localization, synthesis and degradation. ITI-HC1 contains a peptide which could stimulate a broad spectrum of phagocytotic cells. ITIH4 is secreted into the blood, where it is cleaved by plasma kallikrein.
Interleukin 1 receptor antagonist protein	•ICIL-1RA, IL1 inhibitor •INN=Anakinra	Inhibits the activity of IL-1 by binding to its receptor, but no IL-1 like activity.
Kallikreins	•Kidney/pancreas/salivary gland kallikrein. •Tissue kallikrein	Diverse physiologic functions in many tissues. Contact of human plasma with a negatively charged surface such as dextran sulfate activates prekallikrein to kallikrein, which releases the peptide bradykinin from high-molecular-weight kininogen. Kallikreins are involved in the posttranslational modification of polypeptide hormones precursors and growth factors.
Leucine-rich alpha-2-glycoprotein		Family of proteins, including LRG1 that have been shown to be involved in protein-protein interaction, signal transduction, and cell adhesion and development. LRG1 is expressed during granulocyte differentiation.
LPS binding protein	•Lipopolysaccharide-binding protein	Binds to the lipid A moiety of bacterial lipopolysaccharides (LPS), a glycolipid present in the outer membrane of all Gram-negative bacteria. The LBP/LPS complex seems to interact with the CD14 receptor.
Manganese-superoxide dismutase		Destroys radicals which are normally produced within the cells and which are toxic to biological systems.
Manan-binding lectin	•Collectin-1 •MBP1 •Mannan-binding protein •Mannose-binding lectin	Calcium-dependent lectin involved in innate immune defense. Binds mannose, fucose and N-acetylglucosamine of different microorganisms and activates the lectin complement pathway. Binds to late apoptotic cells, as well as to apoptotic blebs and to necrotic cells, facilitating their uptake by macrophages. May bind DNA.

Protein	Alternative names	Function
PAP-1	•Anchorin CII •Annexin V •Calphobindin I •etc.	Anticoagulant protein that acts as an indirect inhibitor of the thromboplastin-specific complex, which is involved in the blood coagulation cascade.
Plasma protease C1 inhibitor	•C1 esterase inhibitor •C1-inhibiting factor •Serpin G1.	Controls the activation of the C1 complex. It forms a proteolytically inactive stoichiometric complex with the C1r or C1s proteases. May play a role in regulating important physiological pathways including complement activation, blood coagulation, fibrinolysis and the generation of kinins. Efficient inhibitor of FXIIa. Inhibits chymotrypsin and kallikrein.
Plasminogen	•Plasmin heavy chain A •Activation peptide •Angiostatin •Plasmin heavy chain A short form •Plasmin light chain B.	Dissolves the fibrin of blood clots and acts as a proteolytic factor in various processes: embryonic development, tissue remodeling, tumor invasion, and inflammation, and may be modulated by CSPG4. It activates the urokinase-type plasminogen activator, collagenases and several complement factors (C1, C5) and cleaves fibrin, fibronectin, thrombospondin, laminin and von Willebrand factor. Angiostatin is an angiogenesis inhibitor that blocks vascularization and growth of experimental primary and metastatic tumors *in vivo*.
Plasminogen activador inhibitor-1	•Endothelial plasminogen activator inhibitor •Serpin E1	This inhibitor acts as 'bait' for tissue plasminogen activator, urokinase, and protein C. Its rapid interaction with TPA may function as a major control point in the regulation of fibrinolysis.
Protein AMBP	• -1 microglycoprotein •Complex-forming glycoprotein •Bikunin •etc.	Inter-alpha-trypsin inhibitor inhibits trypsin, plasmin, lysosomal granulocytic elastase, and calcium oxalate crystallization. Alpha-1-microglobulin occurs as a monomer and also in complexes with IgA and albumin and interacts with FN1.
Prothrombin	•Coagulation factor II	Thrombin, which cleaves bonds after Arg and Lys, converts fibrinogen to fibrin and activates factors V, VII, VIII, XIII, and, in complex with thrombomodulin, protein C. Functions in blood homeostasis, inflammation and wound healing
Retinol-binding protein	•Plasma retinol-binding protein	Delivers retinol from the liver stores to the peripheral tissues. In plasma, the RBP-retinol complex interacts with transthyretin, this prevents its loss by filtration through the kidney glomeruli.
Serum amyloid A protein	•Amyloid protein A •Amyloid fibril protein A	Major acute phase reactant. Apolipoprotein of the HDL complex.

Protein	Alternative names	Function
Serum amyloid P component	•9.5S alpha-1-glycoprotein	Can interact with DNA and histones and may scavenge nuclear material released from damaged circulating cells. May also function as a calcium-dependent lectin.
Serum albumin		Serum albumin, the main protein of plasma, has a good binding capacity for water, Ca^{2+}, Na^{+}, K^{+}, fatty acids, hormones, bilirubin and drugs. Its main function is the regulation of the colloidal osmotic pressure of blood. Major zinc transporter in plasma, typically binds about 80% of all plasma zinc.
Serotransferrin	•Beta-1 metal-binding globulin, •Siderophilin	Iron binding transport proteins which can bind two Fe^{3+} ions in association with the binding of an anion, usually bicarbonate. Responsible for the transport of iron from sites of absorption and heme degradation to those of storage and utilization. It may also have a further role in stimulating cell proliferation.
Tetranectin	•C-type lectin domain family 3 member B •etc.	Tetranectin binds to plasminogen and to isolated kringle 4. May be involved in the packaging of molecules destined for exocytosis.
Transthyretin	•ATTR •Prealbumin •TBPA	Thyroid hormone-binding protein. Probably transports thyroxine from the bloodstream to the brain.
Properdin	•Complement factor P	Positive regulator of the complement alternate pathway. Binds to and stabilizes the C3- and C5-convertase complexes.
Vitamin D-binding protein	•Gc-globulin •Group-specific component	Multifunctional protein found in plasma, ascitic fluid, cerebrospinal fluid, urine and on the surface of many cell types. In plasma, it carries the vitamin D and prevents polymerization of actin. Associates to membrane- bound Ig on the surface of B-lymphocytes and with IgG Fc receptor on the membranes of T-lymphocytes.
Von Willebrand factor	•Von Willebrand antigen II	Important in the maintenance of hemostasis, it promotes adhesion of platelets to the sites of vascular injury by forming a molecular bridge between sub-endothelial collagen matrix and platelet-surface receptor complex GPIb-IX-V. It also acts as a chaperone for coagulation factor VIII, delivering it to the site of injury, stabilizing its heterodimeric structure and protecting it from premature clearance from plasma.
Zinc-alpha-2-glycoprotein		Stimulates lipid degradation in adipocytes and causes the extensive fat losses associated with some advanced cancers. May bind polyunsaturated fatty acids.

Table 2. Main functions of Acute Phase Proteins.

Existing APPs test provide a spectrum of clinical information, including definitive diagnosis of acute events (e.g. CRP), prediction of disease risk (CRP increases in coronary disease) or detection of disease recurrence. Thus, if we check the clinical diagnostic catalog at the Beckman Coulter home page, one of the companies with the broader list of IVD tests for APPs (Table 3), we will find that those tests have the following intended uses https://www.beckmancoulter.com/eCatalog/Catalog/Disease_Management): albumin, to evaluate the hepatic/renal function, infectious diseases, inflammatory responses or nutritional assesment; alpha 1 acid glycoprotein, to assess the existence of infectious diseases or inflammation; alpha 1 antitrypsin, to check the presence of infectious diseases or inflammation; alpha 2 macroglobulin and antithrombin III, to detect anemia, thrombofilia or to assay the hepatic function; ApoA1 and ApoB, to measure the cardiovascular risk; ceruloplasmin, for the evaluation of the hepatic function or the detection of infection/inflammation; complement factors (C3 and C4), to evaluate the liver function or unmask autoimmune or inflammatory processes; fibrinogen, for thrombofilia and bledding disorders detection; haptoglobin, to uncover infectious diseases, inflammation, and anemia; plasminogen, to assess fibrinolysis; transferrin, to value the presence of anemia, the nutritional status, the presence of infectious diseases, or the renal function; and finally transthyretin/prealbumin, for hepatic function and nutritional assesment. In addition, detection of beta 2 microglobulin (e.g. Quantikine® IVD® Human β_2M Immunoassay, R&D) is an aid in the diagnosis of autoimmune diseases (rheumatoid arthritis, systemic lupus erithematosus), viral infections or reduced glomerular filtration rates (kidney diseases). On the other hand, low levels of plasminogen activator inhibitor 1 (PAI-1) are linked to bleeding, while its elevation is related with an increased number of blood clots (surgery, infection, diabetes) and elevated risk of heart attack or coronary artery disease (CAD).

	Company name			Company name	
1	Abaxis, Inc	ABX	40	Health Chem Diagnostics, Llc	**HCD**
2	Abbott Laboratories	ABL	41	Horiba Abx	**HOR**
3	Access Bio, Inc	ACC	42	Human Diagnostics Worldwide	**HDW**
4	Affinity Biologicals, Inc	AFF	43	Ibl, Gmbh	**IBL**
5	Alfa Wassermann Diagnostic Technologies, Inc	AWDT	44	Immunostics, Inc	**IMMTICS**
6	American Diagnostica, Inc	AMER	45	Immuno, Gmbh	**IMM**
7	Amico Lab, Inc	AMI	46	Instrumentation Laboratory, Co	**ILAB**
8	Arkray, Inc	ARK	47	Jas Diagnostics Systems, Gmbh	**JAS**
9	Arlington Scientific, Inc	ARL	48	Kamiya Biomedical, Co	**KB**
10	Axes-Shield Diagnostics, Ltd	AS	49	Kent Laboratories, Inc	**KL**
11	Bacton Assay Systems	BAS	50	Medical Diagnostic	**MDT**

				Technologies	
12	Baxter Diagnostics, Inc	BAX	51	Medical Laboratory Automation Systems, Inc	MLAS
13	Beckman Coulter, Inc	BC	52	Nitto Boseki Co., Ltd (Medical Division)	NB
14	Biocheck, Inc	BCK	53	Novamed, Ltd	NVM
15	Bio/Data, Corp	BIODT	54	Olympus Life Science Research Europa, Gmbh (Europa)	OLSR
16	Biokit, S.A.	BK	55	Ortho-Clinical Diagnostics, Inc	OCD
17	Bio-Medical Products, Corp	BMP	56	Polymedco, Inc	POL
18	Biopool AB	BAB	57	Precisa Intl Corp	PREC
19	Boditech Dioagnostics, Inc	BODIT	58	Quidel Corp	QUID
20	Brahms AG	BAG	59	R2 Diagnostics, Inc	R2
21	Carolina Liquid Chemistries, Corp	CLC	60	Randox Laboratories, Ltd	RDXL
22	Cenogenetics, Corp	CNG	61	Reagents Applications, Inc	RA
23	Cezanne SAS	CSAS	62	Remel, Inc	REM
24	Cliniqa, Corp	CLINQ	63	R&D Systems	R&D
25	Covance Research Products, Inc	CRP	64	Roche Diagnostics, Gmbh	ROD
26	Dade Behring, Inc	DB	65	Rowley Biochemical Institute, Inc	ROW
27	Dako Denmark A/S	DAK	66	Seradyn, Inc	SER
28	Dexall Biomedical Labs, Inc	DEX	67	Shanghai Shenfeng Biochemistry Reagent Co, Ltd	SSBR
29	Diagnostica-Stago	DS	68	Siemens Medical Solutions Diagnostics	SMSD
30	Diagnostix Technology, Inc	DT	69	Stago R&D	STG
31	Diamedix Corp	DIAMED	70	Sterling Diagnostics, Inc	SD
32	Diasorin, Inc	DIA	71	Teco Diagnostics	TECO
33	Diasys Diagnostics Systems, Gmbh	DSYS	72	Texas Immunology	TEXAS
34	Dominion Biologicals, Ltd	DOM	73	The Binding Site, Inc	TBS
35	DRG Instruments, Gmbh	DRGI	74	Tosoh Bioscience, Inc	TOS
36	Eucardio Laboratory, Inc	EUL	75	Trinity Biotech, Plc	TB
37	Fisher Diagnostics	FISH	76	Ventana Medical Systems, Inc	VMS
38	Genetic Technologies, Inc	GEN	77	Wako Pure Chemicals, Inc	WAKO
39	**Globalemed, Llc**	**GBL**	**78**	**YK & E Advance Trading, Inc**	YK&EAT

Table 3. Some companies developing *in vitro* diagnostics (IVD) tests for clinical use.

This table is not expected to be a comprehensive summary of all existing IVD companies. Mainly, data have been collected from different sources, like the US Food and Drug Administration Home Page (http://www.fda.gov), ZapConnect.com, or the home page of each company.

Amongst this first group of IVD tests for APPs, C-reactive protein/CRP is, by far, the most frequent offered by different companies (Table 4). That is due to a dual use: On the one hand, a low sensitivity test for inflammation or infectious/autoimmune diseases. On the other hand, systemic inflammation and CRP levels increase as the amount of visceral adipose tissue and the waist circumference become excessive, and that is because CRP (as well as the fibrinolysis inhibitor PAI-1) are not only produced by liver but also by adipocytes (Libby et al., 2010). Based on that, a high-sensitivity assay for cardiovascular risk (denoted hs-CRP) has been developed to predict future clinical cardiovascular events. Elevation of average hs-CRP level is linked to atheroesclerosis, and therefore point to a higher potential of stroke, myocardial infarction or severe peripheral vascular disease development. Thus, apparently healthy people with some inflammation (above median hsCRP) but below median levels of low-density lipoprotein (LDL) could nonetheless benefit from statin therapy (Libby et al., 2010).

Moreover, these companies are continuosly adding new products to their growing portfolio of IVD assays, as it is the case for some acute phase reactants (Table 4). For example, tests for factor VIII (hemophilia A) and von Willebrand (von Willebrand disease) are included within the pannels of reagents to check hemostasis, and alpha 1 microglobulin is been introduced in market for the functional evaluation of liver and kidney, diabetes and stroke. As well, elevation of calcitonin precursor levels in plasma represent a high risk for progression to severe sepsis if the measurement of this acute phase reactant is done shortly after the systemic infection process has started (on the first day). Still, there are other IVD tests that have not been included in Table 4, like properdin Factor B (autoimmune diseases) or apolipoprotein (a)(cardiovascular risk), that are also manufactured by some companies.

A large majority of APPs are typically measured by enzyme immunoassays (EIA, ELISA), but also by immunoturbidimetric or nephelometric technologies through chemistry analyzers such as Alfa Wassermann Alera/ACE, Roche/Hitachi, Roche/Cobas, Beckman Synchron®, Beckman/Olympus, Abbot Aeroset, Siemens/Bayer Advia or Siemens/Dade Dimension. There are some radioimmuno- (RIA) (e.g., Abbott Beta-2-Microglobulin RIA) and chromogenic assays too (e.g., BCG method for albumin), and some of these analytes have waived versions (simple and accurate, according to the CLIA complexity classification; e.g., Abaxis, Inc).

4. New methods and technologies for the quantification of acute phase proteins: APPs as disease biomarkers

The high-throughput genomic and proteomic technologies, combined with bioinformatics, give the most recent approaches to the study and analysis of APPs in human body fluids (plasma, serum). There are different methods that permit the simultaneous qualitative/quantitative analysis of several APPs from small volume of samples: 2-DE/MS, 2-DE-DIGE/MS, MALDI-TOF-MS, SELDI-TOF-MS, label-free LC-MS profiling, CE-ESI-MS, isotope tagging/MS/MS, or antibody arrays for serum profiling. Proteomic methods can now detect more than 1000 proteins in plasma at the same time. However, the comprehensive analysis of the proteome of any body fluid is still beyond our reach, despite great methodological advances in recent years. Several major challenges must be faced by researchers. For instance, proteomics of body fluids is limited to a ~μg/L (ng/mL)

	Acute phase proteins																								
Company name	ALB	AGP	AAT	Alpha-2-	A1M	A2M	ATIII	APOLIPOP	B2M	CER	COMPLE	CCP	CRP	AHF	FG	HP	HPX	PAI-1	PLA	PTR	RBP	Transferrin	TTR	vWF	
	11	11	18	2	2	8	8	21	15	7	24	3	34	4	8	14	2	5	10	2	3	18	18	1	N[er]
ABX	X																								
ABL	X	X	X					X	X	X	X		X			X						X	X		←
ACC													X												
AFF														X											
AMI											X														
AWDT	X							X														X			
AMER																		X							
ARK	X																								
ARL													X												
AS									X																
BAS								X																	
BAX																		X							
BC	X	X	X		X	X	X	X	X	X	X		X			X			X			X	X		←
BCK									X				X												
BIODT															X										
BK		X	X						X				X											X	
BMP													X												
BAB																		X							
BODIT													X												
BAG												X													
CLC	X										X					X						X			
CNG													X												
CSAS												X													
CLINQ																X							X		
CRP			X																						
DB	X	X	X	X		X	X	X	X	X	X		X	X		X	X		X		X	X	X		←
DAK									X																
DEX													X												
DS			X	X		X	X				X				X				X	X					
DT													X												
DIA		X	X			X	X		X	X	X		X			X			X			X	X		←
DIAMED											X														
DSYS								X															X		
DOM													X												
DRGI								X																	
EUL								X																	
FIS															X										
GEN													X												
GBL			X			X		X	X		X		X						X		X	X			←
HCD			X																						

HOR																							X		
HDW	X							X			X		X		X							X			
IBL											X														
IMMTICS													X												
IMM								X																	
ILAB														X	X										
JAS																							X		
KB		X	X		X		X	X			X		X	X	X	X			X			X	X		←
KL		X	X			X				X	X		X			X	X					X	X		←
MDT																		X							
MLAS																		X							
NB		X	X				X				X					X			X			X	X		←
NVM								X																	
OLSR		X	X					X	X	X	X		X			X						X			←
OCD			X					X			X		X			X						X	X		←
POL	X							X			X		X									X	X		←
PREC													X												
QUID											X														
R2																									
RDXL	X							X			X		X									X	X		←
RA		X									X		X			X									
REM													X												
R&D									X																
ROD			X						X		X		X			X						X	X		←
ROW															X										
SER													X												
SSBR								X															X		
SMSD	X		X			X		X	X		X	X	X									X			←
STG											X								X						
SD													X												
TECO													X												
TEXAS													X												
TBS		X	X			X	X		X	X	X					X			X		X	X	X		←
TB							X								X				X	X					
TOS									X																
VMS			X																						
WAKO								X					X										X		
YK&EAT								X																	

Table 4. *In vitro* diagnostic (IVD) tests for the quantitative determination of acute phase proteins in serum or plasma.

This table is not intended to be a comprehensive summary. Data come from different sources, like the US Food and Drug Administration Home Page (http://www.fda.gov), ZapConnect.com, or the home page of each company. Sometimes this one does not offer directly IVD tests for some APPs, but can do it through strategic alliances that are not reflected in Table 3 (e.g., Beckman Coulter and Instrumentation Laboratory and the HemosIL® Fibrinogen-C kit). Abbreviations used for the name of the companies are the same as in Table 3. Abbreviations for APPs are the same as in Table 1.

sensitivity, which is roughly 1000-fold less sensitive than the most specific immunoassays. Another additional problem is the range of protein concentrations in body fluids. The dynamic range of plasma proteins concentrations spams from that much as 40 mg/mL for albumin (50% of the total mass of plasma proteins) to less than 4 pg/mL; i.e., the concentration of many cytokines. Therefore, we are talking about 10-12 orders of magnitude, which means that disease-mediated alterations in soluble mediators (e.g., cytokines), or modifications in those released into the circulation through cell-leaking processes during normal cell turnover (apoptosis) or specific injuries (e.g., myocardial infarction), are hardly detectable. For example, the most common technology for fractionating and identifying proteins, 2-DE, has a range of detection of no more than 3-4 orders of magnitude with differential gel electrophoresis (DIGE). About 99% of total protein mass in plasma depends on only 22 abundant species, like albumin (35-45 mg/mL), IgG, IgA, IgM (12-18 mg/mL), α2 and β-lipoproteins (LDL; 4-7 mg/mL), fibrinogen (2-6 mg/mL), α1-antitrypsin (2-5 mg/mL), α2-macroglobulin (2-4 mg/mL), transferrin (2-3 mg/mL), α1-acid-glycoprotein (1 mg/mL), hemopexin (1 mg/mL), α-lipoproteins (HDL, 0.6-1.5 mg/mL), haptoglobin (0.3-2 mg/mL), prealbumin (0.3-0.4 mg/mL) or ceruloplasmin (0.3 mg/ml). Most of them are acute phase reactants; i.e., plasma resident proteins with a molecular mass larger than the kidney filtration cutoff and large half-lives, both characteristics ensuring an extended residence time and high protein concentrations (45 mg/mL-0.001 mg/mL). Thus, this high abundance makes them easily accessible to proteomic technologies, although there are still a couple of questions to consider: complexity of this family of proteins and their time-dependent concentration modulation (kinetics).

Regarding complexity, the most important APPs are usually glycoproteins. This means that APPs, like immunoglobulins, are highly heterogeneous (Anderson and Anderson, 2002). The difficulty of their analysis is even enhanced by processing events, that lead to the generation of smaller proteins or peptides from larger precursors (both the plasma and cells contains numerous proteases), or the presence of genetic variants in acute phase reactants as apoE, apoH, transferrin or haptoglobin. Two-dimensional electrophoresis (2-DE) was the first used method in clinical biofluids proteomics, and still is one of the most used nowadays for different reasons. After the introduction of high resolution 2-DE in 1975 this technique was applied to the plasma proteins (Anderson & Anderson, 1977). These authors were able to resolve by 2-DE about 300 or more spots and a number of about 40 distinct plasma proteins. This initial amount has been extended to 626 identified spots, 1966 detected spots and 69 proteins in the current Swiss 2D-Page Web site (http://expasy.org/swiss-2dpage), which may represent the limit in terms of 2-DE analysis of unfractionated plasma. Therefore, it was clear very soon than 2-DE had limitations with respect to the resolution to cope with the extraordinary dynamic range of plasma proteins concentrations and the complexity issue, apart from additional problems: low and high molecular weight, hydrophobic, and very acid or basic proteins. Still, isolectric points of APPs are mostly between pH 5 and 6, and these proteins are originated mainly from liver secretion (not cell leakage; i.e., hydrophilic) and have a medium-high molecular size. In addition, there are means to reduce sample complexity and enhance the loading capacity of 2-DE (see below). Therefore, 2-DE is a technique specially suited to screen the acute phase response, and can be even essential to determine the post-translational and genetic modifications of APPs.

Nevertheless, and largely because of novel methods of serum fractionation and MS based protein identification, after the turn of the century the number of plasma proteins that could be identified increased over time. Thus, thanks to extensive fractionation serum fractionation and tandem mass spectrometry, Adkins et al. (2002) were able to identify 490 proteins. That number suffered a huge increase in 2004, to achieve an identification of 1,175 non-redundant plasma proteins, by using multidimensional chromatography and MS analysis (Anderson et al. 2004). At present, the Human Proteome Organization (HUPO) Plasma Proteome Project (PPP) has a list of 3020 plasma proteins (http://www.hupo.org/research/hppp/)

4.1 Quantitative proteomics technologies applied to the study of APPs

However, the elaboration of a detailed list of serum/plasma proteins provides relatively limited biological information. To understand the biology of any pathological process, quantitative analysis of these proteins is essential. Perhaps, 2-DE or 2-DE fluorescence differential gel electrophoresis (DIGE), followed by MS analysis, remains as the most commonly used method (see Table 5). DIGE is a quantitative technique that enhance the dynamic range of 2-DE up to four orders of magnitude. DIGE is commercially available from GE Healthcare, and allows the direct comparison of different samples at the same time on a single 2-DE gel. This technique involves the use of up to three different samples and three cyanide dyes (Cy2, Cy3, and Cy5). These dyes have an NHS-ester reactive group designed to covalently attach to the epsilon amino group of lysine of proteins via an amide linkage. In addition, dyes label 1-2% of all the available proteins (minimal labelling, about one dye molecule per protein), without changing their pI and adding only 0.5 kDa to the protein mass. Normally, a pooled sample, comprising equal amounts of each of the initial samples within the study, is labelled with Cy2 and used as internal control. This internal standard allows normalization and is an effective way to increase accuracy and reproducibility during quantification. On the contrary, one particular disadvantage of DIGE is the equipment required for visualization and spot excision, and another major problem with these 2-DE based methodologies is that they are labor intensive and difficult to automate. In addition, as we have just commented, they are not able to effectively mine the low abundance biofluids proteome (<100 ng/ml). Therefore, the detected proteins limit primarily to high (0.1–40 mg/ml) and medium abundance (0.1–100 μg/ml) species, which is enough to study the classical acute phase reactants (e.g., CRP <10 μg/ml), but does not allow to find new ones. All these limitations of 2-DE based methods are driving the development of new proteomic methodologies for serum/plasma profiling that seek to reduce the workload of 2-DE (since they use automated equipment), such as MALDI-TOF-MS, SELDI-TOF-MS, label-free LC-MS profiling, CE-ESI-MS, isotope tagging/MS/MS, or antibody arrays. Although it is outside the scope of this chapter to review comprehensively these techniques, we will go through a brief summary of some of them.

Simple adsorption/washing/desorption methods are fast, easily automated and have a widespread use (Table 5). In matrix-assisted laser desorption/ionization mass spectrometry (MALDI-TOF-MS) samples are digested with trypsin and deposited on the MALDI plate prior peptide mass fingerprinting (PMF) or partial sequencing of peptides (MS/MS; e.g., MALDI-TOF/TOF). In surface-enhanced laser desorption/ionization (SELDI) (e.g., ProteinChip®, Ciphergen Biosystems, Palo Alto, CA) different chromatographic surfaces (hydrophobic, hydrophilic, etc) are used on a metal array to bind a subset of proteins from a sample. The unbound proteins are washed away, the bound proteins are overlaid with an organic matrix, and finally this fraction is profiled by MS analysis (e.g., MALDI-TOF-MS), generating rather simple mass spectra which can be easily analyzed. SELDI is a very useful method for high throughput screening, although this approach is not very reproducible and quite cumbersome to identify detected proteins, since require mass spectrometers such as FT-ICR-MS instruments to get a direct fragmentation of high molecular weight ions. However, patterns of peaks are usually found to be useful for the classification of pathological samples (Table 5).

Combination of online sample preparation with liquid chromatography (LC) and mass spectrometry (MS; LC-MS) is a common practice. Leaving aside the peptidomics approach, which is perhaps less interesting to study acute phase reactants, these medium-high molecular weight proteins can be analyzed through shotgun proteomics (Murakoshi et al., 2011). During the shotgun proteomics approach the entire serum/plasma proteome is submitted to trypsin digestion followed by peptides separation through one or normally (due to the very complex mixture of peptides) several liquid chromatography steps prior to MS. Multidimensional protein identification technology (MudPIT), for example, consists of a 2D chromatography separation prior to electrospray (ESI)-MS. In MudPIT the first dimension is normally a high loading capacity strong cation exchange (SCX) column, while the second dimension is reverse phase chromatography. After this extensive peptide fractionation and MS, the fragmentation data are matched against sequence databases using different software (e.g., SEQUEST) in order to identify serum/plasma proteins. However, several runs are required to get a comprehensive analysis of the whole proteome and, as with 2-DE, there are problems to mine the low abundant subproteome. In addition, qualitative over quantitative data are obtained by LC-MS, although the use of label-free LC-MS profiling (Wesner et al., 2010) or techniques such as isotope-coded affinity tag (ICAT) (Lin et al., 2009), isobaric (iTRAQ) and MRM (multiple reaction monitoring; mTRAQ) tags for relative and absolute quantitation (Boylan et al., 2010; Kanq et al., 2010), or ^{18}O labelling (Qian et al., 2010) allows for quantitative comparisons between different samples. Finally, there are other high throughput methods to analyze the acute phase response in serum/plasma samples, such as capillary electrophoresis connected to electrospray ionization MS (CE-ESI-MS) or antibody arrays. Regarding antibody arrays, their main problem is that these methodologies are not discovery based; i.e., the only proteins that can be detected and quantitated are those targeted by the available antibodies. Moreover, several technological advances must be accomplished before truly high density antibody microarrays are readily available (Borrebaeck & Wingren, 2009)

4.2 Complexity and sensitivity: Strategies to enhance the detection of lower abundant APPs

The unmasking of low abundant proteins (protein depletion), together with new technologies with enhanced resolving power, will provide access to more sensitive and specific biomarkers, and it is likely that some of them will represent new acute phase reactants. One way to reduce sample complexity and enhance the capacity to detect proteins or peptides at lower concentrations is to remove high-abundance proteins selectively. Only albumin (3.4-5.4 g/L) and immunoglobulins (IgG, 7.2–15 g/L; IgA, 0.9–0.33 g/L; IgM, 0.5–2.5 g/L; IgD, 0–0.4 g/L; IgE, 100–200 μg/L) account for >70% of total serum proteins. Several affinity columns, based on dye ligands (e.g., Cibacron-blue) or specific antibodies (e.g., IgY, IgG), have been developed for albumin removal, while either thiophilic gels (Salgado, 2010) or resins with fixed antibodies (anti-IgG and, sometimes, even anti-IgA or anti-IgM) or immunoglobulin binding-proteins (protein A, protein G, protein A/G mixtures, protein L) have been used for immunoglobulins substraction methods (Fang & Zhang, 2008).

Although albumin is an acute phase reactant, removal of this abundant protein together with immunoglobulins facilitate the detection of less abundant or previously masked new acute phase reactants. A good example of this comes from our 2-DE analyses of human serum samples, where we were able to identify both leucine rich α2 glycoprotein (LRG) and apolipoprotein H (ApoH) (Salgado, 2010). LRG is a positive acute phase reactant whose concentration in serum (LRG; ~ 3 μg/ml) is close to the detection limit of 2-DE electrophoresis (μg/mL range), and therefore very difficult to show in order to measure quantitative differences. The second one, apolipoprotein H, has a position coincident with immunoglobulin G heavy chains in 2-DE maps, appearing fully hidden prior albumin/immunoglobulins depletion (Salgado et al., 2010).

Sometimes, methods to eliminate albumin or immunoglobulins can be rather inespecific. For example, dye-ligand affinity columns (e.g, Cibracron Blue-based kits), still used in proteomic studies due to its relatively low cost, show a low specific binding for albumin and causes retention of unwanted proteins (Bellei et al., 2011). Thus, to achieve deeper and more specific protein depletion, different companies have developed several alternatives, like antibody immunoaffinity media or combinatorial peptide libraries. An example is the MARS-Hu-14 column (Agilent Technologies, Santa Clara, California, USA), intended to deplete the 14 most abundant proteins from serum or plasma samples. Another one is the ProteoPrep® 20 Plasma Immunodepletion spin or LC-column from Sigma (St Louis, MO, USA), allowing the simultaneous depletion of 20 abundant proteins (97-98% of plasma/serum proteins) and up to 50-fold increased protein loads (according to the company data). However, despite these clear benefits, the use of these affinity chromatography technologies generates great losses of information about the acute phase response, since all the removed proteins are acute phase reactants themselves. For example, the ProteoPrep® 20 Plasma Immunodepletion column from Sigma eliminates albumin, IgG, transferrin, fibrinogen, IgA, α2- Macroglobulin, IgM, α1- Antitrypsin, complement C3, haptoglobin, apolipoprotein A1, A3 and B; α1-Acid Glycoprotein, ceruloplasmin, complement C4, C1q, IgD, transthyretin, and plasminogen.

Another choice to reduce sample complexity in order to study the acute phase response is to use ProteoMiner (Bio-Rad Laboratories) or ProSpectrum Libraries (Prolias). Both are approaches based upon a combinatorial peptide libraries displayed on beads. These beads are incubated with the starting material and are capable of interacting with most of proteins in serum/plasma proteome. Because the binding capacity of those beads is limited, and each peptide combination binds, in theory, to a unique protein sequence, the high-abundance proteins (e.g., albumin, immunoglobulins) quickly saturate the beads, so their excess can be washed away. Thus, low-abundance proteins are concentrated in the final sample, thereby decreasing the dynamic range of proteins and becoming a good alternative to immunoaffinity separation media. Using this technology, modification in APPs like apolipoprotein A1, apolipoprotein A4, antithrombin-III, C4a complement, vitamin D binding protein or apolipoprotein J can be easily traced (our unpublished data; Kolla et al., 2010).

Prefractionation is another choice to augment the depth of the analysis, even though at the expense of having to analyze multiple subsamples. One example is to select narrower pH ranges during the first dimension in 2-DE, to visualize only the part of the serum/plasma proteome we are interested in. Another way, perhaps not so popular, is to use preparative in-solution isoelectric focusing (e.g., Zoom IEF fractionator ®, Invitrogen) as the first step in body fluid analysis prior to 2-DE or, preferably, an automated method (e.g., LC-MS). Finally, the last strategy that we will mention to reduce sample complexity and cover more of the lower-abundance acute phase proteome is to enrich some protein families specifically. Thus, most of acute phase reactants are glycoproteins. Therefore, they can be enriched by a number of different techniques; one of the most commonly used is lectin affinity chromatography. More than 100 different lectins (concanavalin A, wheat germ agglutinin, peanut agglutinin, etc) are commercially available, which differ in specificity (a drawback of lectin chromatography). Glycoproteins are involved in many diseases (e.g., cancer), so the study of the O- and N-linked glycosilated APPs may therefore be particularly interesting (see below).

There is still another concern to address, which is associated with the removal of proteins like serum albumin or immunoglobulins. These high abundant proteins appear to fullfill the function of carriers for less abundant species, especially low molecular weight proteins (cytokines, growth factors, etc) that can only escape kidney clearance when bound to these high molecular weight carrier proteins. Moreover, some APPs, which are not so small, are also bound to these carrier proteins. Therefore, immunoaffinity subtraction may potentially remove non-targeted and potentially important APPs from serum/plasma samples, which may lead to unnoticed loses of information. In other words: what do we know about the interactome of APPs? For instance, it is known that transthyrretin binds another APP, the retinol binding protein (Folli et al., 2010), and the same happens with albumin (Gundry et al., 2007). In fact, almost every single APP has been described associated with albumin, like retinol-binding protein, α2-antiplasmin, complement factors, fibrinogen (α chain), histidine-rich glycoprotein, prothrombin, serum amyloid A4, α1-acid glycoproteins 1 and 2, α1-antichymotrypsin, α1-antitrypsin, α1B-glycoprotein, α2HS-glycoprotein, antithrombin III, apolipoproteins, ceruloplasmin, haptoglobin, hemopexin, inter-a-trypsin inhibitor (heavy chain H4), leucine-rich α2 glycoprotein, paraoxonase 1, plasminogen, transferrin, transthyretin, vitamin D-binding protein or zinc-α2-glycoprotein (Gundry et al., 2007; Salgado et al., 2010). Immunoglobulins are another example, since they fix complement factors. Immunoglobulins-complement factors interactions may cause unwanted loss of the second ones during the process of removing antibodies from biological fluids, which could account for the reduced levels of complement factors (C1, C3, C4) found in some clinic proteomic studies (Table 5). Finally, another good example comes from the association of haemoglobin and its scavenger protein haptoglobin with ApoA1 under an inflammatory context (Salvatore et al., 2007; Watanabe et al., 2009), so removal of haptoglobin can affect to ApoA1 detected levels, and vice versa. Despite these different setbacks, it can be stated that immunoaffinity depletion of just the two most abundant plasma proteins (i.e., albumin and immunoglobulins) still appears to be necessary, or at least beneficial, to enhance the resolving power (e.g., in 2-DE), reduce technical variation, detect or unmask lower abundant acute phase reactants (e.g, ceruloplasmin, C1q, ceruloplasmin, LRG) or reveal qualitative or quantitative differences in this group of plasma proteins more accurately. In any case, we always recommend analyze the retained fractions in order to extract more information from our clinical plasma/serum proteomic studies (Salgado et al., 2010).

Another problem of studying the APP is their modulation across the time. As commented in the introduction, the so-called negative acute phase reactants are highly abundant proteins which are rapidly down-regulated in response to a variety of stimuli, (e.g., transthyretin). The same "stressors", in turn, cause the up-regulation of another important subclass: the positive APPs. This last class may be divided into three subclasses (I-III), based on their normal plasma concentrations. Class I, like ceruloplasmin (0.3 mg/mL) or complement factors C3 (0.8-1.7 mg/mL) or C4 (0.15-0.65 mg/mL), whose concentration may increase by 50%; Class II (α1-acid glycoprotein, ~1 mg/mL; α1-antitrypsin, 2-5 mg/mL; α1-antichymotrypsin, 0.3-1.6 mg/mL; haptoglobin, 0.3-0.2 mg/mL; fibrinogen, 2-6 mg/mL) begin to increase 24 to 48 hours and reach to their maximum level (two to five fold enhancement) in about 7-10 days, and require about two weeks to return to their normal levels; and finally class III (e.g, C reactive protein/CRP < 5 μg/mL; serum amyloid A/SAA; < 10 μg/mL), whose concentrations rise as early as 4 hours after inflammatory stimulus and attain their maximum levels within 24 to 72 hours (concentration may increase up to 1000 fold) and also decline very rapidly. Thus, depending on the acute/chronic nature of the pathology or the sampling time, one may get different results.

4.3 Clinical proteomics

The field of clinical proteomics holds tremendous potential for discovery of noninvasive diagnostic and prognostic biomarkers or the identification of novel drugs targets, although there is a lack of approved IVD biomarkers (Table 4) based on clinical proteomics data (Anderson, 2010). However, scientists have accumulated during the last years a huge amount of high-throughput proteomic data with a true translational potential. Table 5 summarizes a literature review on different proteomics strategies used for the study of serum/plasma samples from several important diseases, as well as an overview on the major APPs alterations observed.

There are at least three sources of plasma/serum biomarkers: a) the primary diseased tissue, such as endothelial cells in atherosclerosis or neoplastic cells in cancer; b) the microenvironment around the primary cells; c) the systemic response to these local alterations, where APPs are involved. APPs are altered in bacterial infections, fractures, tumors, Crohn´s disease, surgery, rheumatoid arthritis,burns or systemic vasculitis; however, they remain unaltered in others. The use of this third source of biomarkers has a clear advantage, as the APR is a kind of "amplificated biological response" (Omenn et al., 2007). Maybe for that reason, most of candidate biomarkers discovered in clinical proteomic studies using biofluids (plasma, serum, urine, cerebrospinal fluid, pleural effusion, etc) are APPs, which are shared among different pathological situations, like different cancers or autoimmune diseases. Therefore, contrary to single proteins biomarkers like PSA (prostate cancer), CA 125 (ovarian cancer), CEA (pancreatic cancer or CA 19-9 (breast cancer), which show a low sensitivity and specificity during disease detection, acute phase reactants (for example, C-reactive protein and cardiovascular risk detection) are more sensitive, but lack specificity. For example, Table 5 shows that CRP is elevated in allogeneic hematopoietic stem cell transplantation/HSCT, Down syndrome (maternal plasma), or hepatocellular carcinoma. Similarly, alpha 1 acid glycoprotein, alpha 1-antichymotrypsin, α1- B-Glycoprotein, antithrombin III, apoA1, ceruloplasmin, leucine rich glycoprotein, prothrombin, serum amyloid A, serum amyloid P component, transferrin, transthyretin, vitamin D Binding Protein or zinc α2-glycoprotein are systematically either down- or up-regulated in different diseases (low specificity) (Table 5). This fact does not mean they are not useful as biomarkers. Rheumatoid arthritis (RA) is an autoimmune disease affecting 0.5-1% of adults characterized by persistent synovitis, systemic chronic inflammation and presence of autoantibodies. About 50-80% of RA patients are seropositive for rheumatoid factor (RF; IgM and IgA autoantibodies directed against the Fc region of IgG), antibodies against cyclic citrullinated peptides (anti-CCP), or both. Anti-CCP antibodies are more sensitive and specific for RA diagnosis than RF, which is present in up to 20% of elderly individuals, and also seem to be a better predictor of progressive joint destruction (Scott et al., 2010). Early diagnosis of RA is fundamental to achieve significantly better clinical outcomes, and acute-phase reactants can help to assess tha probability of developing RA once there are evidences of inflammatory arthritis. Indeed, the low specific C-reactive protein is part of the ACR (American College of Rheumatology)/EULAR (European League Against Rheumatism) 2010 criteria to classify both early and established disease. Also on this regard, in 2010 our group published a preliminary 2-DE study using Immunoglobulins/HSA-depleted serum samples from healthy individuals and recently diagnosed/untreated rheumatoid arthritis (RA) patients. This work found that leucine rich glycoprotein was significantly upregulated, while antithombin III was downmodulated (Salgado et al., 2010). Separately, Satoshi Serada (Serada et al., 2010), using iTRAQ, found that leucine rich glycoprotein is increased in RA patients before therapy. Like C-reactive protein, leucine rich glycoprotein is a low specific biomarker, as elevations of this APP are observed in bacterial (toxic shock syndrome) and viral (HIV) infections, autoimmune diseases (Crohn´s disease, Behcet´s disease) and some kind of cancers. However, this novel biomarker may be particularly useful to monitor disease activity in patients with active disease but normal C-reactive protein levels (Serada et al., 2010). In clear contrast (Table 5), other APPs, such as alpha 1 antitrypsin, hemopexin and, curiously, haptoglobin (considered a positive acute phase reactant), show a higher variability. Perhaps, such variability is rather due to genetic or posttranslational based changes more than simple augmented or reduced levels (see below), but there is not doubt that this kind of APPs may be more specific and therefore attractive from a diagnostic point of view.

Anyhow, the simple test paradigm, where one expects changes in the concentration of unique biomarkers linked to the diagnosis of single diseases, is gradually moving on to the use of multivariate tests. In classical clinical chemistry, a biomarker determination has diagnostic value only if compared with a reference interval including 95% (about 2 standard deviations above and below the mean value) of the reference values from the reference population (normally "healthy" people, but not always). Thus, plasma levels of a particular disease biomarker should lie within that reference interval, and values outside that reference range could point out (in theory) a pathological situation. However, this is not so straightforward. As mentioned above, it seems not likely to find a fully specific acute phase protein, since other diseases may alter the blood levels of this biomarker too (Table 5). What is more, acute phase protein concentrations within non-diseased subjects may vary substantially and overlap with those within diseased populations because: (A) genetic influences, like gender or race; (B) non genetic influences, like age, exercise, circadiam rhythm, season, smoking, diet or sleep; (C) medical treatment, such as drug therapy; and (D) pre-analytical phase variation, including sample drawing (body posture, time of venous occlusion by the tourniquet), transport and preparation. Indeed, there is a strong evidence of genetic control of plasma protein abundance: ~ 12-95% of the quantitative variation in specific plasma protein levels is genetic in origin (Anderson & Anderson, 2002). Therefore, it is important to control both the analytical and biological variation in any clinical proteomic study of the acute phase response in order to predict the number of samples and replicates that should be analyzed to find statistically significant differences (Hunt et al., 2005).

As we have just mentioned, most biomarker studies in scientific literature detecting acute phase response proteins are based on transversal/cross-sectional comparisons (e.g., healthy vs diseased group; Table 5). This approach suffers sometimes from large biological variation in the baseline values of APPs within the reference population, which, summed to the technical variation, generate a significant overlap with the concentration range of diseased populations. This overlap may mask the existence of significant changes and leads to low sensitivity (false negatives) and, especially for APPs, low specificity (false positives), once a cut-off value is set. ROC curves can help us to select such a discriminative value in order to maximize the specificity without renouncing to a good sensitivity level. Nonetheless, even if we find a sensitive and specific acute phase protein for a disease, the positive predictive value of that biomarker would depend, in the end, on the disease's prevalence, since even specificities as high as 99% will result in false positive results of low prevalent pathologies (Hoffman et al., 2007).

To solve these problems, two changes may help. The first one is the use of individual instead of population-based reference intervals for APPs (personalized medicine). Different authors have monitored the protein expression dynamics that take place within one individual to overcome all these limitations and to get more meaningful data; for example, to reveal serum/plasma biomarkers or to predict the recovery or treatment response during acute events such as trauma, infection or drug intervention. An example is the study of Han Roelofsen in 2007, who studied the kinetic of serum proteome before and after colon laparoscopic surgery (Roelofsen et al., 2007). Using SELDI-TOF-MS, this group could distinguish up to four groups of proteins based on their expression pattern kinetics. Thus, they identified serum amyloid protein and C-reactive protein as part of the positive slow response cluster, and transthyrretin as a negative reactant belonging to the fast response group. These authors were also able to observe serum amyloid protein differences between patients, related to their recovery from surgery (Roelofsen et al., 2007). Another interesting work was the recent study on the serum proteome changes produced during allo hematopoietic stem cell transplantation by Joohyun Ryu (Ryu et al., 2010). The aim of this work was to find biomarkers suited for the diagnosis and follow-up of patients who experience complications after allo-HSCT (Table 5). Using 2-DE analysis of HSA/IgG depleted sera obtained at different times (pretransplant, 7, 14 and 21 days), these authors found 14 differentially expressed APPs. They observed three different expression patterns: A) serum amyloid P, ApoE and C-reactive protein, elevated 14 or 21 days post-HSCT; B) haptoglobin, alpha 2 HS glycoprotein, decreased upon HSCT; C) and APPs with irregular patterns. Based on their data, this group has suggested CRP as a risk factor for the development of major transplant-related complications, and haptoglobin as a prognostic biomarker of relapses in underlying hematologic disease (Ryu et al., 2010). On the other hand, the second change consist in using multiplex panels of specific APPs (a proteome signature), which may improve diagnostic performance through the use of protein ratios (Gruys et al., 2006) or more sophisticated interpretive algorithms. In time, some of acute phase response biomarkers combinations might perhaps mature to FDA/EMEA-approvable IVD-tests, something costly and time-consuming (~10-20 years).

As commented above, 12-95% of the quantitative variation in specific plasma protein levels depends on genetic background. Thus, haptoglobin shows a 20% CV intraindividual, and 27.9% CV interindividual, and C-reactive protein 42.2% CV intraindividual and 92.5% CV interindividual (Anderson & Anderson, 2002). Polymorphic APPs, such as haptoglobin, alpha 2 HS glycoprotein, alpha 1 antitrypsin, vitamin D binding protein, and transferrin, have been detected by proteomic techniques (2-DE) since the seventies (Anderson & Anderson, 1977; Goldman et al., 1985; Salgado et al, 2010). Some of these variations have been associated with several pathological conditions. For example, schizophrenia shows enhanced levels of haptoglobin (Table 5) and a significant association with the HP 1-2 genotype (Wan et al., 2007), while the Hp 2-2 genotype seems rather linked to increased hemoglobin/haptoglobin/hemopexin content on HDL (ApoA1) particles and higher risk of coronary heart disease (Watanabe et al., 2009). It also has been found a higher susceptibility to chronic graft versus host disease (GVDH) after allogeneic hematopoietic cell transplantation (HSCT) in HP 2-2 patients (McGuirk et al., 2009). On the other hand, it was detected a higher incidence of myotrophic lateral sclerosis in vitamin D binding protein GC2 isoform carriers (Palma et al., 2008).

Post-translational modifications (PTMs) have also an important role in determining the function of proteins and come in a great degree of variation: citrullination, phosphorylation, proteolysis, glycosylation, oxidative modifications, etc. Many APPs show a complex combination of post-translational modifications, which may be disease- or inflammation-dependent. Thus, analysis of serum glycome in chronic inflammation associated to advanced ovarian cancer patients (Saldova et al., 2007) revealed sialyl Lewis x (SLe^x) structures in APPs that already had this marker: haptoglobin β-chain, alpha 1 acid glycoprotein, and alpha 1 antichymotrypsin. These glycosylation changes were parallel to the upregulation of these proteins (Amon et al., 2010; Lin et al, 2009) (Table 5), and could be tumour specific (Saldova et al., 2007). In addition, PTMs may have an impact on 2-DE patterns (Butler et al., 2003; Saldova et al., 2007), and application of lectin affinity chromatography prior 2-DE (or other proteomic techniques) could sometimes unmask previously unnoted expression changes (Seriramalu et al., 2010). Some of those pathological-dependent post-translational modifications in APPs may result in the generation of new antigens (neo-antigenicity), and hence autoantibodies against them (autoimmune diseases). Two good examples to illustrate this point are autoantibodies specific for citrullinated proteins in rheumatoid arthritis/multiple sclerosis and autoantibodies recognizing oxidatively modified C1q in rheumatoid arthritis and systemic erythematosus lupus (Eggleton, 2008). Similarly, phospholipids and apolipoproteins (e.g., ApoB100) of low-density lipoprotein (LDL) are also susceptible to oxidation, promoting chronic inflammation and the generation of autoantibodies against highly immunogenic oxidation-specific neoepitopes (Eggleton, 2008).

Disease	ALB	AAG	AAT	AAC	A1M	ABG	AHSG	A2M	ATIII	APOLIPO-PROTEINS	CER	COMPLEMENT FACTORS
CARDIOVASCULAR DISEASES: ATHEROSCLEROSIS, CORONARY RISK, MYOCARDIAL INFARCTION					↓					↑ Apo A1	↑	↓C1
TYPE 2 DIABETES	↑			↑				↑		↑ApoA1, ApoA2, ApoC2, ApoC3, ApoE	↑	↑ C3, C4, ↑C4A, C4B, ↑CFH, C1q, ↑C8
RHEUMATOID ARTHRITIS	↓		↓	↑		↓	↓	↓	↓	↓ApoA1 ↓ApoA4		↑ C3
SCHIZOPHRENIA			↑		↑				↑	↓Apo A1		
BIPOLAR DESORDER										↓Apo A1		
CYSTIC FIBROSIS			↓							↓Apo A1		↑ C4
WILSON DISEASE								↓				↓CFB, C3
SEVERE ACUTE RESPIRATORY SYNDROME		↑	↑	↑			↑		↑	↓↑ApoA1 ↑ApoE		↑C3, C4

Disease	CRP	FBR	HP	HPX	HRG	ITI	LRG	PLA	PON1	PTR	RBP	SAA	SAP	TN	TRF	TTR	VDBP	ZAG
CARDIOVASCULAR DISEASES: ATHEROSCLEROSIS, CORONARY RISK, MYOCARDIAL INFARCTION			↓	↓							↑		↓			↑↓	↑	
TYPE 2 DIABETES			↑	↑								↑						
RHEUMATOID ARTHRITIS			↑	↓			↑				↓	↑		↓		↓	↓	
SCHIZOPHRENIA			↑										↑				↑	
BIPOLAR DESORDER																		
CYSTIC FIBROSIS																		
WILSON DISEASE			↓															
SEVERE ACUTE RESPIRATORY SYNDROME			↑			↑	↑				↑	↑		↑	↓	↓↑	↑	

Disease	ALB	AAG	AAT	AAC	A1M	ABG	AHSG	A2M	ATIII	APOLIPO-PROTEINS
ALLOGENEIC HSCT			↑				↓			↑ApoAII, ApoE ↓ApoJ
DOWN SYNDROME (MATERNAL PLASMA)	↓		↓					↓		↓ ApoM, ApoA1, ApoA4, ApoB100, Lp(a)
ENDOMETRIAL ADENOCARCINOMA			↓			↑			↑	↑ Apo J
SQUAMOUS CELL CERVICAL CARCINOMA			↓			↑			↑	
CERVICAL ADENOCARCINOMA			↓			↑			↑	
OVARIAN CANCER	↓	↑	↑	↑						
BREAST CANCER	↑							↓↑	↑	↑ ApoA2 ↑ Apo D
HEPATOCELLULAR CARCINOMA	↑	↑	↑			↑		↓		↓Apo J
LUNG ADENOCARCINOMA			↑	↑				↑	↑	↑ Apo A1

Disease	CER	COMPLEMENT FACTORS	CRP	FBR	HP	HPX	HRG	ITI	LRG	PLA
ALLOGENEIC HSCT			↑		↓↑					
DOWN SYNDROME (MATERNAL PLASMA)		↑ CFH, CFB ↑C5, C8 ↓ C3	↑	↓	↑	↑		↑		
ENDOMETRIAL ADENOCARCINOMA									↑	
SQUAMOUS CELL CERVICAL CARCINOMA										
CERVICAL ADENOCARCINOMA										
OVARIAN CANCER		↑C4bp, C9 ↓ C2			↑	↑	↑	↑	↑	
BREAST CANCER		↑ C1, CFB, C8β ↓ C3, C4A, C8β			↑			↑↓		↓
HEPATOCELLULAR CARCINOMA	↑	↑C4A, CFH, C1r, C1q, CFB, C9	↑		↑					
LUNG ADENOCARCINOMA	↑			↑				↓		

Disease	PON1	PTR	RBP	SAA	SAP	TN	TRF	TTR	VDBP	ZAG
ALLOGENEIC HSCT	↑			↓	↑					↑
DOWN SYNDROME (MATERNAL PLASMA)		↑			↑		↓			
ENDOMETRIAL ADENOCARCINOMA										
SQUAMOUS CELL CERVICAL CARCINOMA										↑
CERVICAL ADENOCARCINOMA										↑
OVARIAN CANCER				↑				↓		
BREAST CANCER										
HEPATOCELLULAR CARCINOMA	↓	↑		↑	↑		↑	↓		
LUNG ADENOCARCINOMA									↑	

Table 5. Acute phase protein patterns revealed by proteomic studies in different diseases.

Sometimes, different studies on a particular disease yield opposite data regarding the same acute phase reactant, and there are examples even within the same paper: e.g., alpha 2 macroglobulin, inter-α-trypsin inhibitor in breast cancer, and transthyretin in severe acute respiratory syndrome. In the last case, this is due to different modulation of low a high molecular weight forms. Abbreviations are the same as in Table 1. Blue colour indicates prototypical positive acute phase proteins, while yellow colour points out characteristic negative acute phase reactants. Proteomic methodologies used: **Cardiovascular disease** (Kim et al., 2011) 2-DE. Silver staining. MS/MS. Western blot. ELISA. **Type 2 diabetes** (Li et al., 2008) 1-DE/Coomassie. **Rheumatoid arthritis** (Salgado et al., 2010) HSA/Ig depleted sera. 2-DE/Coomassie. MS/MS ; (Doherty et al., 1998) whole plasma. 2-DE/Coomassie. Immunoassays; (Serada et al., 2010) Sera were depleted with MARS-Hu-14 (14 abundant proteins removed, Agilent Technologies), iTRAQ labelling. nanoLC-MS/MS. ELISA. **Schizophrenia** (Wan et al. 2007) 2-DE/Coomassie. MALDI-MS (PMF). **Bipolar disorder** (Sussulini et al., 2011) SELDI-TOF. **Cystic fibrosis** (Charro et al., 2011) Pooled serum samples processed with Multiple Affinity Removal System (MARS) spin cartridges (6 abundant proteins removed ; Agilent Technologies). 2-DE/Coomassie. MALDI-TOF/TOF (MS/MS). Shotgun proteomics (nanoRPLC-MS/MS). **Wilson disease** (Park et al., 2009) Sera were depleted using MARS column (6 abundant proteins removed, Agilent Technologies). 2-DE/Coomassie. MALDI-TOF (MS), MS/MS and Western blot. **Severe acute respiratory syndrome** (Chen et al., 2004) Unfractionated plasma samples. 2-DE/Sypro Ruby. MALDI-TOF-MS and LC-MS/MS; (Wan et al., 2006) HSA/IgG depleted pooled plasma samples. 2-DE DIGE. MALDI-MS/MS and Western blot. **Allogeneic HSCT** (Ryu et al., 2010) HSA/IgG depleted sera. 2-DE/silver staining. L-MS/MS. (McGuirk et al., 2010) HSA depleted sera. 2-DE/Silver staining. LC-MS/MS. **Down syndrome** (Kolla et al., 2010) Plasma samples depleted with ProteoMiner Enrichment Kit (BioRad). Trypsin digestion, iTRAQ labelling, and SCX/Nano LC MALDI-TOF-TOF (MS/MS). **Endometrial adenocarcinome** (Abdul-Rahman et al., 2007). Unfractionated sera, 2-DE/ Silver Stain/Coomassie. MALDI-MS (PMF and MS/MS). Western blot. Competitive ELISA. **Squamous cell cervical carcinoma** (Abdul-Rahman et al., 2007). Unfractionated sera, 2-DE/ Silver Stain/Coomassie. MALDI-MS (PMF and MS/MS). Western blot. Competitive ELISA. **Cervical adenocarcinoma** (Abdul-Rahman et al., 2007). Unfractionated sera, 2-DE/ Silver Stain/Coomassie. MALDI-MS (PMF and MS/MS). Western blot. Competitive ELISA. **Ovarian cancer** (Amon et al., 2010) Serum samples were depleted using Multiple Affinity Removal System (MARS-7) columns (Agilent). 2D (Anion exchange/Reverse phase)-LC. MS/MS and ELISA. (Lin et al., 2009) Depleted sera (IgY12 columns). ICAT/μLC/MS/MS and ELISA. (Boylan et al., 2010) Depleted sera (MARS and IgY12 columns). Trypsin digestion, iTRAQ labelling, and SCX/reverse phase LC/MS/MS. Western blot. **Breast cancer** (Kadowaki et al., 2011) MARS-6 (Agilent) depleted sera. Reverse phase HPLC followed by 2-DE/Coomassie. Western blot and ELISA. **Hepatocellular carcinoma** (Yang et al., 2007) Serum samples. 2-DE/silver staining. Nano-HPLC-ESI-MS/MS. **Lung adenocarcinoma** (Hongsachart et al., 2009) Crude sera or WGA lectin-bound serum proteins. 2-DE/Sypro and 2-DE-DIGE. MALDI-TOF MS and MS/MS. Western blot.

5. Conclusion

The acute phase response is a highly conserved system that takes place during inflammation. During this response the serum levels of a continuously growing list of plasma proteins change, either up- (some of them even 1000 fold) or downwards, under the influence of cytokines like IL-1, IL-6 or TNFα. Some APPs have antiinflammatory effects (e.g., C-reactive protein, leptin), while others influence leukocyte activation/trafficking (e.g., serum amyloid A), modulate the coagulation/complement cascade (e.g., anti-thrombin 3, C-reactive protein) or work for example as scavenger proteins (e.g., haptoglobin, serum amyloid A). With such a variety of functions, it is not surprising to find that some of these APPs are useful for diagnosis and prognosis of different diseases, and for that reason different companies have developed a high number of IVD tests based on single acute phase reactants. For example, amongst others, APPs-based tests are being used nowadays in hepatic/kidney function or nutritional status evaluation, to check the presence of infectious diseases, inflammation or autoimmune diseases, or to detect anemia or thrombofilia/bledding disorders. Apart from the discovery of new APPs whose potential clinical interest awaits future studies, some older ones seem to have got a second life as biomarkers, like C-reactive protein and cardiovascular risk assesment. In addition, the role of many of these APPs has not been completely elucidated (e.g., leucine rich α2 glycoprotein, serum amyloid A), and experimental evidences also point out new associations of some of these proteins with different diseases, like for instance serum amyloid A and obesity-related disorders (e.g., cardiovascular diseases, atherosclerosis, diabetes, insulin resistence) (Zhao et al., 2010). Therefore, it can be said that much work remains to be done in the future around the acute phase reactants field. Actually, body fluid proteomics techniques have become promising tools to uncover new APPs and their associations with human disorders, and it is likely that some of these proteomic studies will finally reveal proteins within the expanding group of APPs with potential clinical interest. Moreover, these findings might even lead to the development and marketing of new IVD tests by the biotechnology industry. Nevertheless, according to data from different pathological scenarios, it is more likely that combinations of APPs will characterize disease states or predict disease outcomes better than single APPs. Thus, what the future may hold is the use of IVD assays with improved tests properties (e.g., sensitivity, specificity) based on disease-associated acute phase reactants patterns (or APPs "signatures").

6. References

Abdul-Rahman, P.S.; Lim, B.K. & Hashim, O.H. (2007). Expression of High-abundance Proteins in Sera of Patients with Endometrial and Cervical Cancers: Analysis Using 2-DE with Silver Staining and Lectin Detection Methods. *Electrophoresis*, Vol.28, No.12, (June 2007), pp. 1989-1996, ISSN 1522-2683

Adkins, J.N.; Varnum, S.M.; Auberry, K.J.; Moore, R.J.; Angell, N.H.; Smith, R.D.; Springer, D.L. & Pounds, J.G. (2002). Toward a Human Blood Serum Proteome: Analysis by Multidimensional Separation Coupled with Mass Spectrometry. *Molecular and Cell Proteomics*, Vol.1, No.12, (December 2002), pp. 947-955, ISSN 1535-9484

Aked, D.M., & Foster, S.J. (1987). Leukotriene B4 and Prostaglandin E2 Mediate the Inflammatory Response of Rabbit Skin to Intradermal Arachidonic Acid. *British Journal of Pharmacology*, Vol.92, No.3, (November 1987), pp. 545-552, ISSN 0007-118

Amon, L.M.; Law, W.; Fitzgibbon, M.P.; Gross, J.A.; O'Briant, K.; Peterson, A.; Drescher, C.; Martin, D.B. & McIntosh, M. (2010). Integrative Proteomic Analysis of Serum and Peritoneal Fluids Helps Identify Proteins that are Up-regulated in Serum of Women with Ovarian Cancer. *PLoS One*, Vol.5, No.6, (June 2010), e11137, ISSN 1932-6203

Anderson, L. & Anderson, N.G. (1977). High resolution Two-dimensional Electrophoresis of Human Plasma Proteins. *Proceedings of the National Academy of Sciences of the United States of America*, Vol.74, No.12, (December 1977), pp. 5421-5425, ISSN 0027-8424

Anderson, N.L. & Anderson, N.G. (2002). The Human Plasma Proteome. *Molecular and Cell Proteomics*, Vol.1, No.11, (November 2002), pp. 845-867, ISSN 1535-9484

Anderson, N.L.; Polanski, M.; Pieper, R.; Gatlin, T.; Tirumalai, R.S.; Conrads, T.P.; Veenstra, T.D.; Adkins, J.N.; Pounds, J.G.; Fagan, R. & Lobley, A (2004). The Human Plasma Proteome: a Nonredundant List Developed by Combination of Four Separate Sources. *Molecular and Cell Proteomics*, Vol.3, No.4, (April 2004), pp. 311-326, ISSN 1535-9484

Anderson, N.L. (2010). The Clinical Plasma Proteome: a Survey of Clinical Assays for Proteins in Plasma and Serum. *Clinical Chemistry*, Vol.56, No.2, (February 2010), pp. 177-185, ISSN 0009-9147

Baud, V. & Karin, M. (2001). Signal Transduction by Tumor Necrosis Factor and its Relatives. *Trends in Cell Biology* Vol.11, No.9, (September 2001), pp. 372-377, ISSN 0962-8924

Baumann, H & Gauldie, J. (1994). The Acute Phase Response. *Immunology Today*, Vol.15, No. 2, (February 1994), pp. 74-80, ISSN 0167-5699

Bellei, E.; Bergamini, S.; Monari, E.; Fantoni, L.I.; Cuoghi, A.; Ozben, T. & Tomasi, A. (2011). High-abundance Proteins Depletion for Serum Proteomic Analysis: Concomitant Removal of Non-targeted Proteins. *Amino Acids*, Vol.40, No.1, (January 2011), pp. 145-156, ISSN 1438-2199

Benigni, F.; Fantuzzi, G.; Sacco, S.; Sironi, M.; Pozzi, P.; Dinarello, C.A.; Sipe, J.D.; Poli, V.; Cappelletti, M.; Paonessa, G.; Pennica, D.; Panayotatos, N. & Ghezzi, P. (1996). Six Different Cytokines that Share GP130 as a Receptor Subunit, Induce Serum Amyloid A and Potentiate the Induction of Interleukin-6 and the Activation of the Hypothalamus-pituitary-adrenal Axis by Interleukin-1. *Blood*, Vol.87, No.5, (March 1996), pp. 1851-1854, ISSN 1528-0020

Besedovsky, H.; del Rey, A.; Sorkin, E. & Dinarello, C. (1986). Immunoregulatory Feedback between Interleukin-1 and Glucocorticoid Hormones. *Science*, Vol.233, No.4764, (August 1986), pp. 652-654, ISSN 1095-9203

Bevilacqua, M.P.; Pober, J.S.; Majeau, G.R.; Cotran, R.S. & Gimbrone, M.A. (1984). Interleukin 1 (IL-1) Induces Biosynthesis and Cell Surface Expression of Procoagulant Activity in Human Vascular Endothelial Cells. *The Journal of Experimental Medicine*, Vol.160, No.2, (August 1984), pp. 618 -623, ISSN 1540-9538

Borrebaeck, C.A. & Wingren, C. (2009). Design of High-density Antibody Microarrays for Disease Proteomics: Key Technological Issues. *Journal of Proteomics*, Vol.72, No.6, (August 2009), pp. 928-935, ISSN 1874-3919

Boylan, K.L.; Andersen, J.D.; Anderson, L.B.; Higgins, L. & Skubitz, A.P. (2010). Quantitative Proteomic Analysis by iTRAQ(R) for the Identification of Candidate Biomarkers in Ovarian Cancer Serum. *Proteome Science*, Vol.8, (June 2010), pp. 31, ISSN 1477-5956

Brom, J. & König, W. (1992). Cytokine-induced (Interleukins-3, -6 and -8 and Tumour Necrosis Factor-beta) Activation and Deactivation of Human Neutrophils. *Immunology*, Vol.75, No.2, (February 1992), pp. 281-285, ISSN 1365-2567

Butcher, E.C. (1991). Leukocyte-endothelial Cell Recognition: Three (or More) Steps to Specificity and Diversity. *Cell*, Vol.67, No.6, (December 1991), pp. 1033-1036, ISSN 0092-8674

Butler, M.; Quelhas, D.; Critchley, A.J.; Carchon, H.; Hebestreit, H.F.; Hibbert, R.G.; Vilarinho, L.; Teles, E.; Matthijs, G.; Schollen, E.; Argibay, P.; Harvey, D.J.; Dwek, R.A.; Jaeken, J. & Rudd, P.M. (2003). Detailed Glycan Analysis of Serum Glycoproteins of Patients with Congenital Disorders of Glycosylation Indicates the Specific Defective Glycan Processing Step and Provides an Insight into Pathogenesis. *Glycobiology*, Vol.13, No. 9, (September 2003), pp. 601-622, ISSN 0959-6658

Charro, N.; Hood, B.L.; Faria, D.; Pacheco, P.; Azevedo, P.; Lopes, C.; de Almeida, A.B.; Couto, F.M.; Conrads, T.P. & Penque, D. (2010). Serum Proteomics Signature of Cystic Fibrosis Patients: a Complementary 2-DE and LC-MS/MS Approach. *Journal of Proteomics*, Vol. 74, No.1, (January 2011), pp. 110-126, ISSN 1874-3919

Chen, J.H.; Chang, Y.W.; Yao, C.W.; Chiueh, T.S.; Huang, S.C.; Chien, K.Y.; Chen, A.; Chang, F.Y.; Wong, C.H. & Chen, Y.J. (2004). Plasma Proteome of Severe Acute Respiratory Syndrome Analyzed by Two-dimensional Gel Electrophoresis and Mass Spectrometry. *Proceedings of the National Academy of Sciences of the United States of America*, Vol.7, No.49, (December 2004), pp. 17039-17044, ISSN 0027-8424

Cines, D.B.; Pollak, E.S.; Buck C.A.; Loscalzo, J.; Zimmerman, G.A.; McEver, R.P.; Pober, J.S.; Wick, T.M.; Konkle, B.A.; Schwartz, B.S.; Barnathan, E.S.; McCrae, K.R.; Hug, B.A.; Schmidt, A.M. & Stern, D.M. (1998). Endothelial Cells in Physiology and in the Pathophysiology of Vascular Disorders. *Blood*, Vol.91, No.10, (May 1998), pp. 3527-3561, ISSN 1528-0020

Colley, C.M.; Fleck, A.; Goode, A.W.; Muller, B.R. & Myers, M.A. (1983). Early Time Course of the Acute Phase Protein Response in Man. *Journal of Clinical Pathology*, Vol.36, No. 2, (February 1983), pp. 203-207, ISSN 1472-4146

Collins, R.A. & Grounds, M.D. (2001). The Role of Tumor Necrosis Factor-alpha (TNF-α) in Skeletal Muscle Regeneration. Studies in TNF alpha(-/-) and TNF-alpha(-/-)/LT-alpha(-/-) mice. *Journal of Histochemistry & Cytochemistry*, Vol.49, No.8, (August 201), pp. 989-1001, ISSN 1551-5044

Coussens, L.M. & Werb, Z. (2002). Inflammation and Cancer. *Nature*, Vol.420, No.6917, (December 2002), pp. 860-867, ISSN 1476-4687

Dantzer, R. (2001). Cytokine-induced Sickness Behavior: Where do We Stand? *Brain, Behavior, and Immunity*, Vol.15, No.1 (March 2001), pp. 7-24, ISSN 0889-1591.

Deboer, T.; Fontana A. & Tobler I. (2002). Tumor Necrosis Factor (TNF) Ligand and TNF Receptor Deficiency Affects Sleep and the Sleep EEG. *Journal of Neurophysiology*, Vol.88, No.2, (August 2002), pp. 839-846, ISSN 1522-1598

Dinarello, C. (1988). Biology of Interleukin 1. *The FASEB Journal*, Vol.2, No.2 (February 1988), pp108-115, ISSN 1530-6860

Dinarello, C.A. & Wolff S.M. (1993). The Role of Interleukin-1 in Disease. *The New England Journal of Medicine*, Vol.328, No.2, (January 1993), pp. 106-113, ISSN 1533-4406

Doherty, N.S.; Littman, B.H.; Reilly, K.; Swindell, A.C.; Buss, J.M. & Anderson, N.L. (1998). Analysis of Changes in Acute-phase Plasma Proteins in an Acute Inflammatory Response and in Rheumatoid Arthritis using Two-dimensional Gel Electrophoresis. *Electrophoresis*, Vol.19, No.2, (February 1998), pp. 355-363, ISSN 1522-2683

Dowton, S.B. & Colten, H.R. (1988). Acute Phase Reactants in Inflammation and Infection. *Seminars in Hematology*, Vol.25, No.2, (April 1988), pp. 84-90, ISSN 1532-8686

Duncan, M.R. & Berman, B. (1989). Differential Regulation of Collagen, Glycosaminoglycan, Fibronectin, and Collagenase Activity Production in Cultured Human Adult Dermal Fibroblasts by Interleukin 1-Alpha and Beta and Tumor Necrosis Factor-Alpha and Beta. *Journal of Investigative Dermatol*, Vol.92, No.5 (May 1989), pp. 699-706, ISSN 1523-1747

Eggleton, P.; Haigh, R. & Winyard, P.G. (2008). Consequence of Neo-antigenicity of the "Altered Self". *Rheumatology*, Vol.47, No.5, (May 2008), pp. 567-571, ISSN 1462-0324

Fang, J.; Wang, Y. & Krueger, J.M. (1997). Mice Lacking the TNF 55 kDa Receptor Fail to Sleep More After TNFalpha Treatment. *The Journal of Neuroscience: The Official Journal of the Society for Neuroscience*, Vol.17, No.15, (August 1997), pp. 5949-5955.

Fang, X. & Zhang, W.W. (2008). Affinity Separation and Enrichment Methods in Proteomic Analysis. *Journal of Proteomics*, Vol.71, No.3, (August 2008), pp. 284-303, ISSN 1874-3919

Feingold, K.; Doerrler, W.; Dinarello, C.; Fiers, W., & Grunfeld, C. (1992). Stimulation of Lipolysis in Cultured Fat Cells by Tumor Necrosis Factor, Interleukin-1, and the Interferons is Blocked by Inhibition of Prostaglandin Synthesis. *Endocrinology*, Vol.130, No.1, (January 1992), pp. 10-16, ISSN 1945-7170

Fiocchi, C. (1998). Inflammatory Bowel Disease: Etiology and Pathogenesis. *Gastroenterology*, Vol.115, No.1, (July 1998), pp. 182-205, ISSN 0016-5085

Folli, C.; Favilla, R. & Berni, R. (2010). The Interaction between Retinol-binding Protein and Transthyretin Analyzed by Fluorescence Anisotropy. *Methods in Molecular Biology*, Vol.652, pp. 189-207, ISSN 1064-3745

Goldman, D.; Goldin, L.R.; Rathnagiri, P.; O'Brien, S.J.; Egeland, J.A. & Merril, C.R. (1985). Twenty-seven Protein Polymorphisms by Two-dimensional Electrophoresis of Serum, Erythrocytes, and Fibroblasts in Two Pedigrees. *The American Journal of Human Genetics*, Vol.37, No.5, (September 1985), pp. 898-911, ISSN 002-9297

Gross, T.J.; Leavell, K.J. & Peterson, M.W. (1997). CD11b/CD18 Mediates the Neutrophil Chemotactic Activity of Fibrin Degradation Product D Domain. *Thrombosis and Haemostasis*, Vol.77, No.5 (May 1997), pp. 894-900, ISSN 0340-6245

Gruys, E.; Toussaint, M.J.; Niewold, T.A.; Koopmans, S.J.; van Dijk, E. & Meloen, R.H. (2006). Monitoring Health by Values of Acute Phase Proteins. *Acta histochemica*, Vol.108, No.3, (May 2006), pp. 229-232, ISSN 0065-1281.

Gruys, E.; Toussaint, M.J.M.; Niewold, T.A., & Koopmans, S.J. (2005). Acute Phase Reaction and Acute Phase Proteins. *Journal of Zhejiang University Science B*, Vol.6, No.11, (November 2005), pp. 1045-1056, ISSN 1862-1783

Gundry, R.L.; Fu, Q.; Jelinek, C.K.; Van Eyk, J.E. & Cotter R.J. (2007). Investigation of an Albumin-enriched Fraction of Human Serum and its Albuminome. *Proteomics Clinical Applications*, Vol.1, No.1, (January 1), pp. 73-88, ISSN 1862-8354

Hartmann, K.; Henz, B.M.; Krüger-Krasagakes, S.; Köhl, J.; Burger, R.; Guhl, S.; Haase, I.; Lippert, U., & Zuberbier, T. (1997). C3a and C5a Stimulate Chemotaxis of Human Mast Cells. *Blood*, Vol.89, No.8, (April 15), pp. 2863-2870, ISSN 1528-0020

Hoffman, S.A.; Joo, W.A.; Echan, L.A. & Speicher, D.W. (2007). Higher Dimensional (Hi-D) Separation Atrategies Dramatically Improve the Potential for Cancer Biomarker Detection in Serum and Plasma. *Journal of Chromatography. B, Analytical Technologies in The Biomedical and Life Sciences*, Vol.849, No.1-2, (April 2007), pp. 43-52, ISSN 0021-9673

Hongsachart, P.; Huang-Liu, R.; Sinchaikul, S.; Pan, F.M.; Phutrakul, S.; Chuang, Y.M.; Yu, C.J. & Chen, S.T. (2009). Glycoproteomic Analysis of WGA-bound Glycoprotein Biomarkers in Sera from Patients with Lung Adenocarcinoma. *Electrophoresis*, Vol.30, No.7, (April 2009), pp. 1206-1220, ISSN 1522-2683

Huber, A.R.; Kunkel S.L.; Todd 3rd, R.F., & Weiss, S.J. (1991). Regulation of Transendothelial Neutrophil Migration by Endogenous Interleukin-8. *Science*, Vol.254, No.5028, (October 4), pp. 99-102, ISSN 1095-9203

Hunt, S.M.; Thomas, M.R.; Sebastian, L.T.; Pedersen, S.K.; Harcourt, R.L.; Sloane, A.J. & Wilkins, M.R. (2005). Optimal Replication and the Importance of Experimental Design for Gel-based Quantitative Proteomics. *Journal of Proteome Research*, Vol.4, No.3, (May-June 2005), pp. 809-819, ISSN 1535-3907

Imhof, B.A. & Aurrand-Lions, M. (2004). Adhesion Mechanisms Regulating the Migration of Monocytes. *Nature Reviews Immunology*, Vol.4, No.6, (June 2004), pp. 432-444, ISSN 1474-1741

Kadowaki, M.; Sangai, T.; Nagashima, T.; Sakakibara, M.; Yoshitomi, H.; Takano, S.; Sogawa, K.; Umemura, H.; Fushimi, K.; Nakatani, Y.; Nomura, F. & Miyazaki, M. (2011). Identification of Vitronectin as a Novel Serum Marker for Early Breast Cancer Detection Using a New Proteomic Approach. *Journal of Cancer Research and Clinical Oncology*, (January 2011), DOI: 10.1007/s00432-010-0974-9, ISSN 1432-1335

Kang, U.B.; Yeom, J.; Kim, H. & Lee, C. (2010). Quantitative Analysis of mTRAQ-labeled Proteome Using Full MS Scans. *Journal of Proteome Research*, Vol.9, No.7, (July 2010), pp. 3750-3758, ISSN 1535-3907

Kawai, T.; Seki, M.; Hiromatsu, K.; Eastcott, J.W.; Watts, G.F.; Sugai, M.; Smith, D.J.; Porcelli, S.A., & Taubman, M.A. (1999). Selective Diapedesis of Th1 Cells Induced by Endothelial Cell RANTES. *Journal of Immunology*, Vol.163, No.6, (September 1999), pp. 3269-3278, ISSN 1550- 6606

Kinashi, T. (2005). Intracellular Signalling Controlling Integrin Activation in Lymphocytes. *Nature Reviews Immunology*, Vol.5, No.7 (July 2005), pp. 546-559, ISSN 1474-1741

Kolla, V.; Jenö, P.; Moes, S.; Tercanli, S.; Lapaire, O.; Choolani, M. & Hahn, S. (2010). Quantitative Proteomics Analysis of Maternal Plasma in Down Syndrome Pregnancies Using Isobaric Tagging Reagent (iTRAQ). *Journal of Biomedicine and Biotechnology*, (November 2009), doi:10.1155/2010/952047, ISSN 1110-7251

Konsman, J.P.; Parnet, P. & Dantzer, R. (2002). Cytokine-induced Sickness Behaviour: Mechanisms and Implications. *Trends in Neurosciences*, Vol.25, No.3, (March 2002), pp. 154-159, ISSN 0166-2236

Konya, V.; Sturm, E.M.; Schratl, P.; Beubler, E.; Marsche, G.; Schuligoi, R.; Lippe, I.Th.; Peskar, B.A. & Heinemann, A. (2010). Endothelium-derived Prostaglandin I(2) Controls the Migration of Eosinophils. *The Journal of Allergy and Clinical Immunology*, Vol.125, No.5, (May 2010), pp. 1105-1113, ISSN 0091-6749

Krueger, J.M.; Walter, J.; Dinarello, C.A.; Wolff, S.M. & Chedid, L. (1984). Sleep-promoting Effects of Endogenous Pyrogen (Interleukin-1). *American Journal of Physiology - Regulatory, Integrative and Comparative Physiology*, Vol.246, No.6, (June 1984), pp. R994-R999, ISSN 1522-1490

Kuehn, H.S.; Jung, M.Y.; Beaven, M.A.; Metcalfe, D.D. & Gilfillan, A.M. (2011). Prostaglandin E2 Activates and Utilizes mTORC2 as a Central Signaling Locus for the Regulation of Mast Cell Chemotaxis and Mediator Release. *The Journal of Biological Chemistry*, Vol.286, No.1, (January 2011), pp. 391-402, ISSN 1083-351X

Langer, H.F. & Chavakis, T. (2009). Leukocyte-endothelial Interactions in Inflammation. *Journal of Cellular and Molecular Medicine*, Vol.13, No.7, (July 2009), pp. 1211-1220, ISSN 1582-1838

Lasky, L.A. (1995). Selectin-carbohydrate Interactions and the Initiation of the Inflammatory Response. *Annual Review of Biochemistry*, Vol.64, pp. 113-139, ISSN 0066-4154

Lawrence, M.B. & Springer, T.A. (1991). Leukocytes Roll on a Selectin at Physiologic Flow Rates: Distinction from and Prerequisite for Adhesion Through Integrins. *Cell* Vol.65, No.5, (May 1991), pp. 859-873, ISSN 0092-8674

Leonard, B.E. & Song, C. (1999). Stress, Depression, and the Role of Cytokines. *Advances in Experimental Medicine and Biology*, Vol.461, pp. 251-265, ISSN 0065-2598

Ley, K.; Laudanna, C.; Cybulsky, M.I. & Nourshargh, S. (2007). Getting to the Site of Inflammation: the Leukocyte Adhesion Cascade Updated. *Nature Reviews Immunology*, Vol.7, No.9, (September 2007), pp. 678-689, ISSN 1474-1741

Libby, P. (2002). Inflammation in Atherosclerosis. *Nature*, Vol.420, No.6917, (December 2002), pp. 868-874, ISSN 1476-4687

Libby, P.; Okamoto, Y.; Rocha, V.Z. & Folco, E. (2010) Inflammation in Atherosclerosis: Transition from Theory to Practice. *Circulation Journal*, Vol.74, No.2, (February 2010), pp. 213-220, ISSN 1347-4820

Lin, B.; White, J.T.; Wu, J.; Lele, S.; Old, L.J.; Hood, L. & Odunsi, K. (2009). Deep Depletion of Abundant Serum Proteins Reveals Low-abundant Proteins as Potential Biomarkers for Human Ovarian Cancer. *Proteomics Clinical Applications*, Vol.3, No.7, (July 2009), pp. 853-861, ISSN 1862-8354

Lu, B.; Moser, A.H.; Shigenaga, J.K.; Feingold, K.R. & Grunfeld, C. (2006). Type II Nuclear Hormone Receptors, Coactivator, and Target Gene Repression in Adipose Tissue in the Acute-phase Response. *Journal of Lipid Research*, Vol.47, No.10, (October 2006), pp. 2179-2190, ISSN 1539-7262

Luheshi, G.N.; Gardner, J.D.; Rushforth, D.A.; Loudon, A.S. & Rothwell N.J. (1999). Leptin Actions on Food Intake and Body Temperature Are Mediated by IL-1. *Proceedings of the National Academy of Sciences of the United States of America*, Vol.96, No.12, (June 8), pp. 7047-7052, ISSN 1091-6490

Lundberg, I.E. & Grundtman, C. (2008). Developments in the Scientific and Clinical Understanding of Inflammatory Myopathies. *Arthritis Research & Therapy*, Vol.10, No.5, (October 2008), pp. 220, ISSN 1478-6362

Maseri, A.; Biasucci, L.M. & Liuzzo, G. (1996). Inflammation in Ischaemic Heart Disease. *British Medical Journal*, Vol.312, No.7038, (April 1996), pp. 1049-1050, ISSN 1468-5833

McGuirk, J.; Hao, G.; Hou, W.; Abhyankar, S.; Williams, C.; Yan, W.; Yuan, J.; Guan, X.; Belt, R.; Dejarnette, S.; Wieman, J. & Yan, Y. (2009). Serum Proteomic Profiling and Haptoglobin Polymorphisms in Patients with GVHD after Allogeneic Hematopoietic Cell Transplantation. *Journal of Hematolology and Oncology*, Vol.2, No.17, (April 2009), doi:10.1186/1756-8722-2-17, ISSN: 1756-8722

Mizel, S.B.; Dayer, J.M.; Krane, S.M. & Mergenhagen S.E. (1981). Stimulation of Rheumatoid Synovial Cell Collagenase and Prostaglandin Production by Partially Purified Lymphocyte-activating Factor (Interleukin 1). *Proceedings of the National Academy of Sciences of the United States of America,* Vol.78, No.4, (April 1981), pp. 2474-2477, ISSN 1091-6490

Mortensen, R.F.; Shapiro, J.; Lin, B.F.; Douches, S. & Neta, R. (1988). Interaction of Recombinant IL-1 and Recombinant Tumor Necrosis Factor in the Induction of Mouse Acute Phase Proteins. *Journal of Immunology,* Vol.140, No.7, (April 1988), pp. 2260-2266, ISSN 1550-6606

Muraguchi, A.; Hirano, T.; Tang, B.; Matsuda, T.; Horii, Y.; Nakajima, K. & Kishimoto, T. (1988). The Essential Role of B cell Stimulatory Factor 2 (BSF-2/IL-6) for the Terminal Differentiation of B cells. *The Journal of Experimental Medicine,* Vol.167, No.2, (February 1988), pp. 332-344, ISSN 1540-9538

Murakoshi, Y.; Honda, K.; Sasazuki, S.; Ono, M.; Negishi, A.; Matsubara, J.; Sakuma, T.; Kuwabara, H.; Nakamori, S.; Sata, N.; Nagai, H.; Ioka, T.; Okusaka, T.; Kosuge, T.; Shimahara, M.; Yasunami, Y.; Ino, Y.; Tsuchida, A.; Aoki, T.; Tsugane, S. & Yamada, T. (2011). Plasma biomarker discovery and validation for colorectal cancer by quantitative shotgun mass spectrometry and protein microarray. *Cancer Science,* Vol.102, No.3, (March 2011), pp. 630-638, ISSN 1349-7006

Murooka, T.T.; Rahbar, R.; Platanias, L.C. & Fish, E.N. (2008). CCL5-mediated T-cell Chemotaxis Involves the Initiation of mRNA Translation Through mTOR/4E-BP1. *Blood,* Vol.111, No.10, (May 2008), pp. 4892-4901, ISSN 1528-0020

Nawroth, P.P.; Handley, D.A.; Esmon, C.T. & Stern, D.M. (1986). Interleukin 1 Induces Endothelial Cell Procoagulant while Suppressing Cell-surface Anticoagulant Activity. *Proceedings of the National Academy of Sciences of the United States of America,* Vol.83, No.10, (May 1986), pp. 3460-3464, ISSN 1091-6490

Okusawa, S.; Yancey, K.B.; van der Meer, J.W.; Endres, S.; Lonnemann, G.; Hefter, K.; Frank, M.M.; Burke, J.F.; Dinarello, C.A. & Gelfand, J.A. (1988). C5a Stimulates Secretion of Tumor Necrosis Factor from Human Mononuclear Cells In Vitro. Comparison with Secretion of Interleukin 1 Beta and Interleukin 1 Alpha. *The Journal of Experimental Medicine* 168, No.1, (July 1988), pp. 443-448, ISSN 1540-9538

Omenn, G.S.; Menon, R.; Adamski, M.; Blackwell, T.; Haab, B.B.; Gao, W. & States, D.J. (2007) The Human Plasma and Serum Proteome, In: *Proteomics of Human Body Fluids : Principles, Methods, and Applications,* V. Thongboonkerd., (Ed.),195-224, Humana Press Inc, ISBN 978-1-58829-657-3,Totowa, NJ.

Opp, M.R. & Krueger, J.M. (1991). Interleukin 1-receptor Antagonist Blocks Interleukin 1-Induced Sleep and Fever. *American Journal of Physiology - Regulatory, Integrative and Comparative Physiology,* Vol.260, No.2, (February 1991), pp. R453 -R457, ISSN 1522-1490

Palma, A.S.; De Carvalho, M.; Grammel, N.; Pinto, S.; Barata, N.; Conradt, H.S. & Costa, J. (2008). Proteomic Analysis of Plasma from Portuguese Patients with Familial Amyotrophic Lateral Sclerosis. *Amyotrophic Lateral Sclerosis,* Vol.9, No.6, (December 2008), pp. 339-349, ISSN 1748-2968

Park, J.Y.; Mun, J.H.; Lee, B.H.; Heo, S.H.; Kim, G.H. & Yoo, H.W. (2009). Proteomic Analysis of Sera of Asymptomatic, Early-stage Patients with Wilson's Disease.

Proteomics Clinical Applications, Vol.3, No.10, (October 2009), pp. 1185-1190, ISSN 1862-8354

Pate, M.; Damarla, V.; Chi, D.S.; Negi, S. & Krishnaswamy, G. (2010). Endothelial Cell Biology: Role in the Inflammatory Response. *Advances in Clinical Chemistry*, Vol.52, pp. 109-130, ISSN 0065-2423

Plomgaard, P.; Fischer, C.P.; Ibfelt, T.; Pedersen, B.K. & van Hall, G. (2008). Tumor Necrosis Factor-{alpha} Modulates Human in Vivo Lipolysis. *Journal of Clinical Endocrinolology & Metabolism*, Vol.93, No.2, (February 2008), pp. 543-549, ISSN 1945-7197

Prowse, K.R. & Baumann H. (1989). Interleukin-1 and Interleukin-6 Stimulate Acute-phase Protein Production in Primary Mouse Hepatocytes. *Journal of Leukocyte Biology*, Vol.45, No.1, (January 1989), pp. 55-61, ISSN 0741-5400

Qian, W.J.; Petritis, B.O.; Kaushal, A.; Finnerty, C.C.; Jeschke, M.G.; Monroe, M.E.; Moore, R.J.; Schepmoes, A.A.; Xiao, W.; Moldawer, L.L.; Davis, R.W.; Tompkins, R.G.; Herndon, D.N.; Camp, D.G. 2nd & Smith, R.D. (2010). Inflammation and the Host Response to Injury Large Scale Collaborative Research Program. Plasma Proteome Response to Severe Burn Injury Revealed by ^{18}O-labeled "Universal" Reference-Based Quantitative Proteomics. *Journal of Proteome Research*, Vol.9, No.9, (September 2010), pp. 4779-4789, ISSN 1535-3907

Ramadori, G. & Christ, B. (1999). Cytokines and the Hepatic Acute-phase Response. *Seminars in Liver Disease*, Vol.19, No.2, pp. 141-155, ISSN 0272-8087

Roelofsen, H.; Alvarez-Llamas, G.; Dijkstra, M.; Breitling, R.; Havenga, K.; Bijzet, J.; Zandbergen, W.; de Vries, M.P.; Ploeg, R.J. & Vonk, R.J. (2007). Analyses of Intricate Kinetics of the Serum Proteome During and After Colon Surgery by Protein Expression Time Series. *Proteomics*, Vol.7, No.17, (September 2007), pp. 3219-3228, ISSN 1615-9681

Rothwell, N.J. & Hopkins S.J. (1995). Cytokines and the Nervous System II: Actions and Mechanisms of Action. *Trends in Neurosciences*, Vol.18, No.3, (March 1995), pp. 130-136, ISSN 0166-2236

Rydén, M.; Dicker, A.; van Harmelen, V.; Hauner, H.; Brunnberg, M.; Perbeck, L.; Lönnqvist, F. & Arner P. (2002). Mapping of Early Signaling Events in Tumor Necrosis Factor-α-mediated Lipolysis in Human Fat Cells. *Journal of Biological Chemistry*, Vol.277, No.2, (January 2002), pp. 1085-1091, ISSN 1083-351X

Ryu, J.; Lee, S.R.; Park, S.G.; Kang, S.; Kim, H.J. & Park, B.C. (2010). Change in Serum Proteome During Allogeneic Hematopoietic Stem Cell Transplantation and Clinical Significance of Serum C-reactive Protein and Haptoglobin. *Experimental and Molecular Medicine*, Vol.42, No.9, (September 2010), pp. 651-661, ISSN 1226-3613

Saldova, R.; Royle, L.; Radcliffe, C.M.; Abd Hamid, U.M.; Evans, R.; Arnold, J.N.; Banks, R.E.; Hutson, R.; Harvey, D.J.; Antrobus, R.; Petrescu, S.M.; Dwek, R.A. & Rudd, P.M. (2007). Ovarian Cancer is Associated with Changes in Glycosylation in Both Acute-phase Proteins and IgG. *Glycobiology*, Vol.17, No.12, (December 2007), pp. 1344-1357, ISSN 1460-2423

Salgado, F.J.; Vázquez, S.; Iglesias, A.; Pérez-Díaz, A.; Mera-Varela, A.; Arias, P. & Nogueira, M. (2010). Application of Thiophilic Chromatography to Deplete Serum Immunoglobulins in Sample Preparation for Bidimensional Electrophoresis. *Analytica Chimica Acta*, Vol.658, No.1, (January 2010), pp. 18-31, ISSN 003-2670

Salvatore, A.; Cigliano, L.; Bucci, E.M.; Corpillo, D.; Velasco, S.; Carlucci, A.; Pedone, C. & Abrescia, P. (2007). Haptoglobin Binding to Apolipoprotein A-I Prevents Damage from Hydroxyl Radicals on its Stimulatory Activity of the Enzyme Lecithin-Cholesterol Acyl-transferase. *Biochemistry*, Vol.46, No.39, (October 2007), pp. 11158-11168, ISSN 0006-2960

Sapolsky, R.; Rivier, C.; Yamamoto, G.; Plotsky, P. & Vale, W. (1987). Interleukin-1 Stimulates the Secretion of Hypothalamic Corticotropin-releasing factor. *Science*, Vol.238, No.4826, (October 1987), pp. 522-524, ISSN 1095-9203

Schenkel, A.R., Mamdouh, Z. & Muller W.A. (2004). Locomotion of Monocytes on Endothelium is a Critical Step during Extravasation. *Nature Immunology*, Vol.5, No. 4, (April 2004), pp. 393-400, ISSN 1529-2916

Scott, D.L.; Wolfe, F. & Huizinga, T.W. (2010). Rheumatoid Arthritis. *Lancet*, Vol.376, No.9746, (September 2010), pp. 1094-108, ISSN 0140-6736

Serada, S.; Fujimoto, M.; Ogata, A.; Terabe, F.; Hirano, T.; Iijima, H.; Shinzaki, S.; Nishikawa, T.; Ohkawara, T.; Iwahori, K.; Ohguro, N.; Kishimoto, T. & Naka, T. iTRAQ-based Proteomic Identification of Leucine-rich Alpha-2 Glycoprotein as a Novel Inflammatory Biomarker in Autoimmune Diseases. *Annals of Rheumatic Diseases*, Vol.69, No.4, (April 2010), pp. 770-774, ISSN 1468-2060

Seriramalu, R.; Pang, W.W.; Jayapalan, J.J.; Mohamed, E.; Abdul-Rahman, P.S.; Bustam, A.Z.; Khoo, A.S. & Hashim, O.H. (2010). Application of Champedak Mannose-binding Lectin in the Glycoproteomic Profiling of Serum Samples Unmasks Reduced Expression of Alpha-2 Macroglobulin and Complement Factor B in Patients with Nasopharyngeal Carcinoma. *Electrophoresis*, Vol.31, No.14, (July 2010), pp. 2388-2395, ISSN 1522-2683

Stefferl, A.; Hopkins, S.J.; Rothwell, N.J. & Luheshi, G.N. (1996). The Role of TNF-alpha in Fever: Opposing Actions of Human and Murine TNF-alpha and Interactions with IL-beta in the Rat. *British Journal of Pharmacology*, Vol.118, No.8, (August 1996), pp. 1919-1924, ISSN 1476-5381

Sussulini, A.; Dihazi, H.; Banzato, C.E.; Arruda, M.A.; Stühmer, W.; Ehrenreich, H.; Jahn, O. & Kratzin, H.D. (2011). Apolipoprotein A-I as a Candidate Serum Marker for the Response to Lithium Treatment in Bipolar Disorder. *Proteomics*, Vol.11, No.2, (January 2011), pp. 261-269, ISSN 1615-9861

Taga, T.; Kawanishi, Y.; Hardy, R.R.; Hirano, T. & Kishimoto, T. (1987). Receptors for B Cell Stimulatory Factor 2. Quantitation, Specificity, Distribution, and Regulation of their Expression. *The Journal of Experimental Medicine*, Vol.166, No.4, (October 1987), pp. 967-981, ISSN 1540-9538

Theiss, A.L.; Simmons, J.G.; Jobin, C. & Lund P.K. (2005). Tumor Necrosis Factor (TNF) Alpha Increases Collagen Accumulation and Proliferation in Intestinal Myofibroblasts via TNF Receptor 2. *The Journal of Biological Chemistry*, Vol.280, No.43 (October 2005), pp. 36099-36109, ISSN 1083-351X

Tocco-Bradley, R.; Georgieff, M.; Jones, C.T.; Moldawer, L.L.; Dinarello, C.A.; Blackburn, G.L. & Bistrian B.R. (1987). Changes in Energy Expenditure and Fat Metabolism in Rats Infused with Interleukin-1. *European Journal of Clinical Investigation*, Vol.17, No.6, (December 1987), pp. 504-510, ISSN 1365-2362

Tracey, K.J.; Morgello, S.; Koplin, B.; Fahey 3rd, T.J.; Fox, J.; Aledo, A.; Manogue, K.R. & Cerami, A. (1990). Metabolic Effects of Cachectin/Tumor Necrosis Factor are

Modified by Site of Production. Cachectin/Tumor Necrosis Factor-secreting Tumor in Skeletal Muscle Induces Chronic Cachexia, while Implantation in Brain Induces Predominantly Acute Anorexia. *The Journal of Clinical Investigation*, Vol.86, No.6, (December 1990), pp. 2014-2024, ISSN 1558-8238

van Miert, A.S. (1995). Pro-inflammatory Cytokines in a Ruminant Model: Pathophysiological, Pharmacological, and Therapeutic Aspects. *The Veterinary Quarterly*, Vol.17, No.2, (June 1995), pp. 41-50, ISSN 0165-2176

Vassalli, P. (1992). The Pathophysiology of Tumor Necrosis Factors. *Annual Review of Immunology*, Vol.10, pp. 411-452, ISSN 0036-4665

Vestweber, D. (2007). Adhesion and Signaling Molecules Controlling the Transmigration of Leukocytes through Endothelium. *Immunological Reviews*, Vol.218, (August 2007), pp. 178-196, ISSN 1600-065X

Wan, C.; La, Y.; Zhu, H.; Yang, Y.; Jiang, L.; Chen, Y.; Feng, G.; Li, H.; Sang, H.; Hao, X.; Zhang, G. & He, L. (2007). Abnormal Changes of Plasma Acute Phase Proteins in Schizophrenia and the Relation between Schizophrenia and Haptoglobin (Hp) Gene. *Amino Acids*, Vol. 32, No.1, (January 2007), pp. 101-108, ISSN 1438-2199

Wan, J.; Sun, W.; Li, X.; Ying, W.; Dai, J.; Kuai, X.; Wei, H.; Gao, X.; Zhu, Y.; Jiang, Y.; Qian, X. & He, F. (2006). Inflammation Inhibitors were Remarkably Up-regulated in Plasma of Severe Acute Respiratory Syndrome Patients at Progressive Phase. *Proteomics*, Vol.6, No.9, (May 2006), pp. 2886-2894, ISSN 1615-9861

Watanabe, J.; Grijalva, V.; Hama, S.; Barbour, K.; Berger, F.G.; Navab, M.; Fogelman, A.M. & Reddy, S.T. (2009). Hemoglobin and Its Scavenger Protein Haptoglobin Associate with ApoA-1-containing Particles and Influence the Inflammatory Properties and Function of High Density Lipoprotein. *Journal of Biological Chemistry*, Vol.284, No.27, (July 2009), pp. 18292-18301, ISSN 0021-9258

Wiesner, C.; Hannum, C.; Reckamp, K.; Figlin, R.; Dubridge, R.; Roy, S.M.; Lin, S.; Becker, C.H.; Jones, T.; Hiller, J.; Cheville, J.C. & Wilson, K. (2010). Consistency of a two clinical site sample collection: a proteomics study. *Proteomics Clinical Applications*, Vol.4, No.8-9 (September 2010), pp. 726-738, ISSN 1862-8354

Xanthoulea, S.; Pasparakis, M.; Kousteni, S.; Brakebusch, C.; Wallach, D.; Bauer, J.; Lassmann, H. & Kollias, G. (2004). Tumor Necrosis Factor (TNF) Receptor Shedding Controls Thresholds of Innate Immune Activation that Balance Opposing TNF Functions in Infectious and Inflammatory Diseases. *The Journal of Experimental Medicine*, Vol.200, No.3, (August 2004), pp. 367-376, ISSN 1540-9538

Yang, M.H.; Tyan, Y.C.; Jong, S.B.; Huang, Y.F.; Liao, P.C. & Wang, M.C. (2007). Identification of Human Hepatocellular Carcinoma-related Proteins by Proteomic Approaches. *Analytical and Bioanalytical Chemistry*, Vol.388, No.3, (June 2007), pp. 637-643, ISSN 1618-2650

Zhao, Y.; He, X.; Shi, X.; Huang, C.; Liu, J.; Zhou, S. & Heng, C.K. (2010). Association between Serum Amyloid A and Obesity: a Meta-analysis and Systematic Review. *Inflammation Research*, Vol.59, No.5, (May 2010), pp. 323-334, ISSN 1420-908X

8

The Acute Phase Protein Complement 1 Inhibitor is an Indicator of Arterial Stiffness

Jong Kwon Park
Inje University College of Medicine, Haeundae Paik Hospital, Department of Surgery Busan Republic of Korea

1. Introduction

An acute phase protein has been defined as a protein whose plasma concentration increases (positive acute phase protein) or decreases (negative acute phase protein) by at least 25 percent during an inflammatory condition (Gabay & Kushner, 1999). The complement system is a biochemical cascade and major effecter mechanism of humoral or innate immunity. However, the complement system also has the potential to damage host tissues; thus, its activation must be tightly regulated (Zanker, 2008). Spontaneous complement activation continuously occurs at a low level, and if such activation is not appropriately controlled, damage to normal cells and tissues can occur.

Complement 1 (C1) inhibitor is a naturally occurring serine proteinase inhibitor that inhibits activated C1s and C1r, components of the classical complement pathway. It also inhibits other plasma serine proteinases, such as factors XIa and XIIa, plasmin, and kallikrein (Caliezi et al., 2000). C1 inhibitor is essentially an acute phase protein whose plasma level may increase 2- to 2.5-fold during an inflammatory episode (Kalter et al., 1985; Woo et al., 1985). Arteriosclerosis or arterial stiffness is hardening of the artery due to the loss of elasticity through any cause. On the other hand, atherosclerosis is a chronic inflammatory disease of the artery characterized by hardening of the artery specifically due to an atheromatous plaque or inflammation in the arterial wall (Kostner et al., 2006; Jani & Rajkumar, 2006; Ridker & Silvertown, 2008; Wykretowicz et al., 2009). Atherosclerosis is the most common form of arteriosclerosis, and is known to be positively correlated with brachial-ankle pulse wave velocity (baPWV), a parameter of arterial stiffness (Imanishi et al., 2004; Jani & Rajkumar, 2006; Nicoletti et al., 2000; van Popele et al., 2001; Wykretowicz et al., 2009; Yamashina et al., 2003). baPWV is a non-invasive test for arterial stiffness that has been used in large-scale population studies, and has become available in the clinical setting (Yamashina et al., 2002). Previous studies have shown that activation of the complement system is involved in the pathogenesis of atherosclerosis (Bhatia et al., 2007; Fosbrink et al., 2006; Niculescu & Rus, 2004; Oksjoki et al., 2003, 2007; Thorbjornsdottir et al., 2005; Yasojima et al., 2001). If atherosclerosis develops, inflammation of the arterial wall, increased arterial stiffness, and accompanying activation of the complement system simultaneously occur and progress. Production of the acute phase protein C1 inhibitor may also increase to regulate over-activation of the complement system. This chapter describes the role of the complement system in the development of atherosclerosis and the relationship between the acute phase protein C1 inhibitor and arterial stiffness.

2. Complement activation is involved in the development of atherosclerosis

The complement system was first identified by Bordet, who discovered serum factors that were inactivated by heat and assisted or complemented the lytic function of antibodies. The complement system is composed of plasma proteins that are normally inactive. However, under certain conditions, such as infection, trauma, surgery, burns, tissue infarction, various immunologically mediated and crystal-induced inflammatory conditions, and advanced cancer, they become activated and generate substances that mediate various effecter functions of the complement system. C3, C4, C9, Factor B, C1 inhibitor, C4b-binding protein (C4BP), and mannose-binding lectin are typical complements that are positive acute phase proteins (Gabay & Kushner, 1999). At the time of complement activation, regulators of complement activation are generated to limit over-activation of the complement system. C1 inhibitor, Factor I, Factor H, C4BP, membrane cofactor for protein (MCP CD46), decay-accelerating factor (DAF), and CD59 are well known regulators of complement activation (Abbas et al., 2010). Activation of the complement system has been suggested to be involved in the development of atherosclerosis, and there is extensive circumstantial evidence to support this hypothesis.

Vaccinia virus complement control protein (VCP) is a complement activation inhibitor. In an animal study of mice with diet-induced atherosclerosis, VCP was injected into the mice regularly once per week after 8 weeks of a high-fat diet. On microscopic examination, the atherosclerotic lesion at the aortic root exhibited a significant (50%) reduction in lesion size at 15 weeks (Thorbjornsdottir et al., 2005). This finding demonstrates that inhibition of complement activation slows the progression of atherosclerosis, and indicates the central role of the complement system in the pathogenesis of atherosclerotic disease. Atherosclerosis is essentially a chronic inflammatory disease of the arteries.

Inflammation and immunity, including the complement system, play important roles in the development of atherosclerosis. Activation of the complement system occurs in human atherosclerotic lesions and is regulated by local synthesis of complement components and accompanying complement regulatory proteins. It has been documented that potential triggers of complement activation in the arterial intima include immunocomplexes, C-reactive protein (CRP), modified lipoproteins, apoptotic cells, and cholesterol crystals (Oksjoki et al., 2003). Recently, it has been shown that enzymatically modified low-density lipoprotein (LDL) efficiently triggers C1 activation in the presence of excess C1 inhibitor (Biro et al., 2007). This result suggests that activation of the classical complement pathway by modified LDL may be important in the development of atherosclerosis. Clearance of apoptotic cells by phagocytes is important in the pathogenesis of atherosclerotic disease, and also plays a role in progression of atherosclerotic plaque (Seimon & Tabas, 2009).

In the early lesion, when apoptotic cells are present in atherosclerotic plaque, activation of C1 is important to prevent atherosclerotic plaque from progressing, likely through enhanced phagocytosis and subsequent removal of apoptotic cells. C1q has been found to be expressed on dendritic cells residing in the arterial wall (Cao et al., 2003). Professional phagocytes such as macrophages or dendritic cells expressing C1q are assumed to clear apoptotic cells from atherosclerotic lesions. In a recent study of C1q-deficient mice and normal C1q mice, the aortic roots were examined after feeding the mice a normal rodent diet for 22 weeks. In the aortic roots, apoptotic cells were detected in the C1q-deficient mice, but not in the normal-C1q mice; the C1q-deficient mice had 3-fold larger atherosclerotic lesions than the normal-C1q mice (Bhatia et al., 2007). This experiment suggests that activation of complement C1 in the early lesion reduces atherosclerotic plaque by enhancing the removal of apoptotic cells from the arterial wall, and that clearing apoptotic cells may be an important mechanism in preventing progression of the atherosclerotic lesion in the early stage of atherosclerosis. However, in the late stage of atherosclerosis, because phagocytosis of apoptotic cells by macrophages is significantly impaired, the detrimental effects of phagocytosis of lipoproteins, platelets, and erythrocytes outweigh the benefits of apoptotic cell uptake. Hence, atherosclerosis progresses despite phagocytosis of substances in the atherosclerotic lesion by macrophages (Schrijvers et al., 2007).

Recent studies have provided additional direct evidence that complement activation is crucial in the development of atherosclerosis. mRNA of C1r and C1s in atherosclerotic plaque has been shown to increase by 2.35- and 4.96-fold, respectively, compared to in normal arteries (Yasojima et al., 2001). These results indicate that C1 is locally synthesized in atherosclerotic lesions. C4BP is a major inhibitor of the classical complement pathway by interfering with the binding of C4b with C2b to form C4b2b, the C3 convertase of the classical complement pathway. Immunohistochemistry of human coronary arteries has shown C4BP to be virtually absent in normal arteries, but present in early and advanced atherosclerotic lesions (Oksjoki et al., 2007). This finding suggests that complement activation occurs in atherosclerotic lesions, and the accompanying regulator of complement activation C4BP actively participates in controlling complement activation.

The final step of complement activation is the formation of C5b-9, the membrane attack complex (MAC). In human and experimental atherosclerosis, C5b-9 deposition has been found in atherosclerotic lesions (Niculescu & Rus, 2004; Niculescu et al., 2004). Moreover, C5b-9 has been demonstrated to induce endothelial cell proliferation and migration in the aorta (Fosbrink et al., 2006). CD59 blocks C9 binding and inhibits formation of the MAC. Experiments with CD59 knockout mice showed that a CD59 deficiency accelerates development of atherosclerotic lesions and increases the plaque vascular smooth muscle cell composition (Wu et al., 2009; Yun et al., 2008). These results indicate that formation of the MAC is an important mechanism of atherogenesis. Activation of the complement 3 component is a key process in formation of the MAC. Complement 3 is the most abundant complement protein and plays a central role in the cascade of complement activation, classical, alternative, and lectin pathways.

Hepatocytes are the main source of C3; however, peripheral white blood cells (PWBCs) such as monocytes, macrophages, lymphocytes, and neutrophils also produce C3 in the blood stream (Einstein et al., 1977; Morgan & Gasque, 1997; Moshage, 1997). Previous studies have provided direct evidence that C3 is involved in the development of atherosclerotic lesions. In an animal study with mice, following intravenous injection of 20% Intralipid, C3 was observed to bind to albumin-encapsulated microbubbles and mediate microbubble adherence to the vascular endothelium during the atherosclerotic process (Anderson et al., 2007). In another mouse model animal study, in which a venous interposition was placed in the common carotid artery, interference with C3 activation resulted in a decrease in vein graft thickening (Schepers et al., 2006). DAF (CD 55) is a membrane protein that regulates complement pathway activity at the level of C3. An animal experiment with DAF knockout mice revealed that DAF deficiency increased deposition of C3d and C5b-9, and accelerated atherosclerotic lesion development (Leung et al., 2009). The results of these studies strongly suggest that activation of the complement system and induction of complement regulatory molecules are actively involved in the pathogenesis of atherosclerosis. High C3 is characteristic of progression of atherosclerosis. C3 has significant independent correlations with atherosclerotic risk factors, such as triglyceride, LDL, cholesterol, and cigarette smoking (Ajjan et al., 2005; Capuano et al., 2006). In women, C3 ≥ 1.8 g/L has been suggested as a value predictive of major complications of atherosclerosis (Szeplaki et al., 2004). The author has also shown that C3 has a strong positive correlation with baWPV, a measure of arterial stiffness (Table 1) (Chae & Park, 2009). In this study, C3 increased with baPWV, indicating that C3 has the potential to predict the extent and severity of atherosclerotic lesions.

Variables	Coefficient	*P*
Age	0.713	< 0.001*
BMI	0.362	< 0.001*
Total cholesterol	0.070	0.484*
LDL	0.037	0.710*
HDL	- 0.243	0.014†
TG	0.349	< 0.001†
HbA1C	0.414	< 0.001†
C1 inhibitor	0.329	< 0.001*
C3	0.329	< 0.001*
ESR	0.129	0.199†
CRP	0.324	< 0.001†

*Pearson correlation (variables with a normal distribution); †Spearman correlation (variables without a normal distribution); $P < 0.05$ was considered significant.

Table 1. Univariate correlations between brachial–ankle pulse wave velocity and patient characteristics

2.1 Complement 1 inhibitor

C1 inhibitor, a serine protease inhibitor, is one regulator of the complement system (Abbas et al., 2010). C1 inhibitor is a positive acute phase protein, and its blood level escalates under inflammatory conditions. Sixteen hours after acute myocardial infarction, plasma C1rC1s-C1 inhibitor complex increases 8-fold (Gabay & Kushner, 1999; Langlois & Gawryl, 1988). Increased production of C1 inhibitor in atherosclerosis is a systemic response to a local inflammatory condition in the atherosclerotic lesion. Although mRNA for C1r and C1s in atherosclerotic plaque increased by 2.35- and 4.96-fold compared to a normal artery, mRNA for C1 inhibitor did not show any significant difference between atherosclerotic plaque and a normal artery (Yasojima et al., 2001). These results suggest that the acute phase protein C1 inhibitor is not produced locally at the atherosclerotic lesion in the artery, but is synthesized in other cells or tissues as a systemic response. Although hepatocytes are the main source of C1 inhibitor, many other cells, including mononuclear phagocytes, microglial cells, fibroblasts, umbilical vein endothelial cells, the placenta, and megakaryocytes also synthesize and secrete C1 inhibitor into the blood stream (Carter et al., 1988; Lappin & Whaley, 1989; Prada et al., 1998; Zuraw & Lotz, 1990). The primary roles of C1 inhibitor are regulation of the activation of the classical complement pathway and of the contact system of kinin formation (Prada et al., 1998). The observed strong positive correlation between C1 inhibitor and C3 indicates that C1 inhibitor actively regulates the cascade of complement activation and coincides with the primary role of C1 inhibitor (Table 2) (Chae & Park, 2009). Moreover, the fact that C1 inhibitor also has significant correlation with the inflammatory marker CRP suggests that C1 inhibitor is another inflammatory marker which can reflect the inflammatory condition in atherosclerotic lesion (Table 2) (Chae & Park, 2009).

Inflammatory marker	Coefficient	*P*
C3	0.359	< 0.001
ESR	0.111	0.269
CRP	0.242	0.015

Spearman correlation; $P < 0.05$ was considered significant.

Table 2. Relationships between C1 inhibitor and inflammatory markers

The molecular weight of C1 inhibitor is 104 kD. C1 inhibitor interacts with C1r and C1s, subsequently dissociating them from C1q. The normal human serum concentration of C1 inhibitor is 200–230 µg/ml. In an experiment with C1 inhibitor-depleted serum, the minimum concentration of C1 inhibitor that limits spontaneous C1 activation was shown to be 55 µg/ml (22% of the normal concentration) (Windfuhr et al., 2005). C1 inhibitor exerts an anti-inflammatory and anti-apoptotic action on ischemic reperfusion injury, and it has been determined that the mechanism of the action is decreased mRNA expression of the adhesion molecules P-selectin and ICAM-1, induced by ischemic insult. C1 inhibitor also significantly downregulates the pro-inflammatory cytokines TNF-α and IL-18, although it increases protective cytokine IL-6 and IL-10 gene expression (Storini et al., 2005).

2.2 Brachial–ankle pulse wave velocity

baPWV is a noninvasive test for measuring arterial stiffness. In recent years, baPWV has become more widely available and used in clinical settings as a simple test for predicting the prognosis of patients (Farrar et al., 1978; Hung et al., 2009; Kim et al., 2008; Tomiyama et al., 2005; van Popele et al., 2001; Xu et al., 2008). Carotid femoral pulse wave velocity (cfPWV) and baPWV are frequently used clinical tests for measuring arterial stiffness, and both have clinical significance. In a multicenter study involving 2287 patients, there was a significant positive correlation between baPWV and cfPWV (Tanaka et al., 2009). baPWV is easy to conduct, and its clinical significance has been demonstrated in many studies. baPWV is measured in a stable environment (Chae & Park, 2009). The examination is performed in the morning after 10 minutes of rest in a temperature-controlled warm room (24 ± 1 °C). Measurements are performed in the supine position. Waveforms are obtained from volume plethysmographic sensors in cuffs on the right brachium and both ankles. The time interval (ΔT_{ba}) between the wave at the right brachium and at the ankles is recorded automatically by the machine. The distance between the sampling points is calculated using the following equations (Yamashina et al., 2002): L_b is the length from the suprasternal notch to the right brachium, and L_a is the length from the suprasternal notch to the ankle.

$$L_b = 0.2195 \times \text{height (cm)} - 2.0734 \quad (1)$$

$$L_a = 0.8129 \times \text{height (cm)} + 12.328 \quad (2)$$

$$\text{baPWV} = (L_a - L_b)/\Delta T_{ba} \quad (3)$$

The average values of the right and left baPWVs are used in the statistical analysis. The validity and reproducibility of baPWV measurements are high, and this method appears to be an acceptable indicator of vascular damage (Yamashina et al., 2002). In the author's study, using a volume plethysmographic apparatus (Vasoguard, model P84; Nicolet Vascular, Golden, CO, USA), inter-observer (reproducibility) and intra-observer reliability (repeatability), calculated using the intraclass correlation coefficient (ICC), were 0.8783 and 0.8927, respectively, indicating excellent reproducibility and repeatability (Fig. 1) (Chae & Park, 2009).

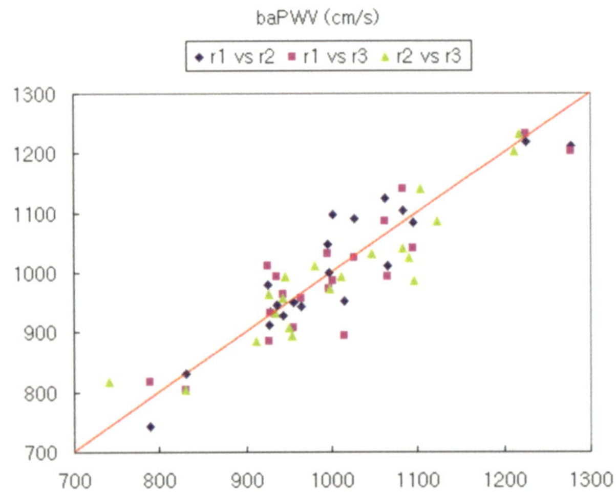

a)

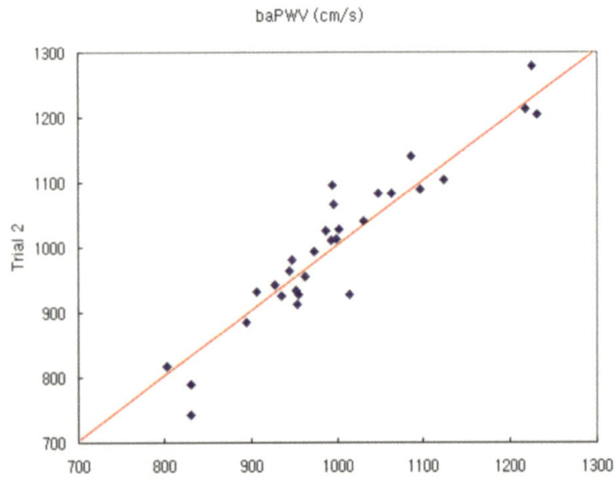

b)

Fig. 1. Inter-observer and intra-observer reliability of measurements of the brachial-ankle pulse wave velocity (cm/s). A) Inter-observer reliability (reproducibility) shows relationships for three independent measurements by three observers, r1 (observer 1), r2 (observer 2), and r3 (observer 3). The ICC value is 0.8783. B) Intra-observer reliability (repeatability) shows the relationship between two different measurement trials by one observer. The ICC value is 0.8927.

Vascular aging leads to loss of arterial elasticity and reduced arterial compliance. The single most important factor related to increased baPWV is age (Jani & Rajkumar, 2006; Tomiyama et al., 2003; Wykretowicz et al., 2009). Based on a study of 7881 healthy subjects (4488 males and 3393 females, 25–87 years old) without any atherogenic risk factors, it was determined that aging influences baPWV and its effect is more prominent in females (Tomiyama et al., 2003). The author has also demonstrated that baPWV increases in proportion to advancing age in both males and females, and that females had a stronger correlation between age and baPWV than males (Fig. 2) (Chae & Park, 2009).

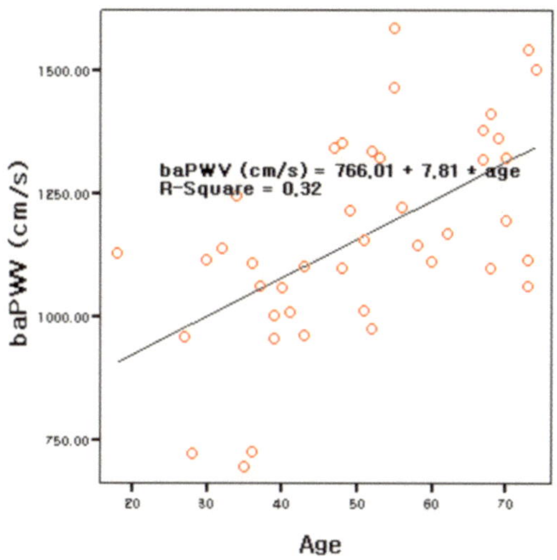

b)

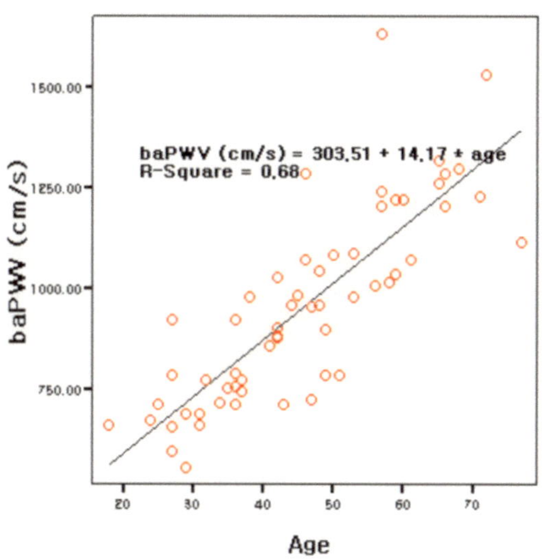

b)

Fig. 2. Linear regression graphs between baPWV and age in both males and females. A) male, B) female, baPWVs increase in proportion to the age in both males and females.

The mechanism of the more prominent relationship between age and baPWV in females compared to males is not clear; however, menopause appears to be a critical process that augments the increase in arterial stiffness with age in females, according to the author's and other reports (Tomiyama et al., 2003). Clinically, baPWV serves as an indicator of either atherosclerotic cardiovascular risk or the severity of atherosclerotic vascular damage (Imanishi et al., 2004; Yamashina et al., 2003).
Moreover, it has been shown that baPWV is also correlated with abdominal aortic calcification and long-term cardiovascular risk (Hung et al., 2009; Nakamura et al., 2003). baPWV > 14.0 m/sec has been suggested as a cutoff value for screening high-risk individuals for cardiovascular disease (Yamashina et al., 2003).

2.3 Complement 1 inhibitor has a strong positive correlation with brachial–ankle pulse wave velocity

Initially, C1 inhibitor was shown to be associated with angioedema, and its deficiency was identified as the cause of hereditary angioedema (Donaldson & Rosen, 1964; Johnson et al., 1971). However, C1 inhibitor belongs to a group of positive acute phase proteins whose production and release increase during inflammation (Gabay & Kushner, 1999; Kalter et al., 1985; Woo et al., 1985). C1 inhibitor has a tissue protection effect, and markedly inhibits activation and recruitment of macrophages (Storini et al., 2005). C1 inhibitor also limits neointimal plaque formation by blocking complement activation, inhibiting leukocyte recruitment, and reducing triglyceride levels (Shagdarsuren et al., 2008). Recently, it has been suggested that all of the risk factors for atherosclerosis contribute to its development by aggravating the underlying inflammatory process (Bisoendial et al., 2007; Buono et al., 2002; Kostner et al., 2006; Mallika et al., 2007; Natali et al., 2003; Nicoletti et al., 2000; Ridker & Silvertown, 2008; van Popele et al., 2001). The inflammatory cytokine interferon-γ (IFN-γ) has been demonstrated to be highly expressed in atherosclerotic lesions (McLaren & Ramji, 2008). IFN-γ enhances the expression of C1 inhibitor mRNA, primarily due to an increased transcription rate (Zahedi et al., 1994). Other cytokines, such as tumor necrosis factor-α, IFN-α, monocyte colony stimulating factor, and interleukin-6 have also been shown to stimulate the synthesis of C1 inhibitor (Caliezi et al., 2000; Gabay & Kushner, 1999). Clinically, C1 inhibitor is an independent predictor of cardiovascular disease (Kostner et al., 2006). In the author's study, the serum level of C1 inhibitor showed a positive correlation with baPWV (Fig. 3, Table 1, 3) (Chae & Park, 2009).

Variables	Regression Coefficient	*P*	R^2
Constant	657.06	< 0.001	
Age	7.365	< 0.001	
Gender	- 137.521	< 0.001	0.695
Hypertension	- 143.066	< 0.001	
Body mass index	14.605	0.006	
C1 inhibitor	6.367	0.025	

Multiple regression analysis (stepwise method); gender (male = 1, female = 2); hypertension (yes = 1, no = 2); P < 0.05 was considered significant.

Table 3. Predictors for brachial–ankle pulse wave velocity in multiple regression analysis

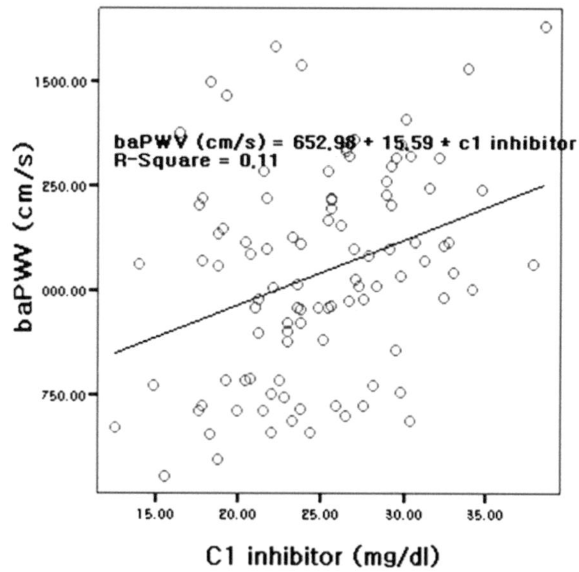

Fig. 3. Linear regression between baPWV and C1 inhibitor. baPWV showed a trend of positive relationship with the serum level of C1 inhibitor.

The results of the author's study suggest that the serum level of C1 inhibitor reflects the degree of arterial stiffness, thus having the potential to predict the severity of atherosclerosis.

3. Conclusion

Atherosclerosis is a chronic inflammatory disease of the artery, and activation of the complement system is an important underlying mechanism in atherosclerosis. Increased production of the acute phase protein C1 inhibitor is a systemic response to local inflammation of the atherosclerotic lesion in the artery. The serum level of C1 inhibitor has a positive correlation with baPWV, a measure of arterial stiffness. Based on this finding, it is suggested that C1 inhibitor is associated with atherosclerosis through its association with increased inflammation, and that the acute phase protein C1 inhibitor is a useful indicator of arterial stiffness. Future research should be directed toward the preventive or therapeutic use of C1 inhibitor, which will lead to progress in the treatment of atherosclerotic disease.

4. References

Abbas, A.K., Lichtman, A.H., & Pillai, S. (2010) *Cellular and Molecular Immunology* (international edition), Saunders, ISBN: 0808923587, Philadelphia, PA

Ajjan, R., Grant, P.J., Futers, T.S., Brown, J.M., Cymbalista, C.M., Boothby, M., & Carter, A.M. (2005) Complement C3 and C-reactive protein levels in patients with stable coronary artery disease. *Journal of Thrombosis and Haemostasis,* Vol. 94, Issue 5, pp. 1048-1053

Anderson, D.R., Tsutsui, J.M., Xie, F., Radio, S.J., & Porter, T.R. (2007) The role of complement in the adherence of microbubbles to dysfunctional arterial endothelium and atherosclerotic plaque. *Cardiovascular Research,* Vol. 73, Issue 3, pp. 597-606

Bhatia, V.K., Yun, S., Leung, V., Grimsditch, D.C., Benson, G.M., Botto, M.B., Boyle, J.J., & Haskard, D.O. (2007) Complement C1q reduces early atherosclerosis in low-density lipoprotein receptor-deficient mice. *American Journal of Pathology,* Vol. 170, Issue 1, pp. 416-426

Biro, A., Thielens, N.M., Cervenak, L., Prohaszka, Z., Fust, G., & Arlaud, G.J. (2007) Modified low density lipoproteins differentially bind and activate the C1 complex of complement. *Molecular Immunology,* Vol. 44, Issue 6, pp. 1169-1177

Bisoendial, R.J., Kastelein, J.J., & Stroes, E.S. (2007) C-reactive protein and atherogenesis: from fatty streak to clinical event. *Atherosclerosis,* Vol. 195, Issue 2 pp: e10-e18.

Buono, C., Come, C.E., Witztum, J.L., Maguire, G.F., Connelly, P.W., Carroll, M., & Lichtman, A.H. (2002) Influence of C3 deficiency on atherosclerosis. *Circulation,* Vol. 105, Issue 25, pp. 3025-3031

Caliezi, C., Wuillemin, W.A., Zeerleder, S., Redondo, M., Eisele, B., & Hack, C.E. (2000) C1-Esterase inhibitor: an anti-inflammatory agent and its potential use in the treatment of diseases other than hereditary angioedema. *Pharmacological Reviews,* Vol. 52, Issue 1, pp. 91-112

Cao, W., Bobryshev, Y.V., Lord, R.S., Oakley, R.E., Lee, S.H., & Lu, J. (2003) Dendritic cells in the arterial wall express C1q: potential significance in atherogenesis. *Cardiovascular Research,* Vol. 60, Issue 1, pp. 175-186

Capuano, V., D'Arminio, T., La Sala, G., & Mazzotta, G. (2006) The third component of the complement (C3) is a marker of the risk of atherogenesis. *European Journal of Cardiovascular Prevention and Rehabilitation,* Vol. 13, Issue 4, pp. 658-660

Carter, P.E., Dunbar, B., & Fothergill, J.E. (1988) Genomic and cDNA cloning of the human C1 inhibitor. Intron-exon junctions and comparison with other serpins. *European Journal of Biochemistry,* Vol. 173, Issue 1, pp. 163-169

Chae, Y.M. & Park, J.K. (2009) The relationship between brachial ankle pulse wave velocity and complement 1 inhibitor. *Journal of Korean Medical Science,* Vol. 24, Issue 5, pp. 831-836

Donaldson, V.H. & Rosen, F.S. (1964) Action of complement in hereditary angioneurotic edema: the role of C'1-esterase. *Journal of Clinical Investigation,* Vol. 43, pp. 2204-2213

Einstein, L.P., Hansen, P.J., Ballow, M., Davis, A.E. 3rd, Davis, J.S. 4th, Alper, C.A., Rosen, F.S., & Colten, H.R. (1977) Biosynthesis of the third component of complement (C3) in vitro by monocytes from both normal and homozygous C3-deficient humans. *Journal of Clinical Investigation,* Vol. 60, Issue 5, pp. 963-969

Farrar, D.J., Green, H.D., Bond, M.G., Wagner, W.D., & Gobbee, R.A. (1978) Aortic pulse wave velocity, elasticity, and composition in a nonhuman primate model of atherosclerosis. *Circulation Research,* Vol. 43, Issue 1, pp. 52-62

Fosbrink, M., Niculescu, F., Rus, V., Shin, M.L., & Rus, H. (2006) C5b-9-induced endothelial cell proliferation and migration are dependent on Akt inactivation of forkhead transcription factor FOXO1. *The Journal of Biological Chemistry,* Vol. 281, Issue 28, pp. 19009-19018

Gabay, C. & Kushner, I. (1999) Acute-phase proteins and other systemic responses to inflammation. *New England Journal of Medicine,* Vol. 340, Issue 6, pp. 448-454

Hung CS, Lin JW, Hsu CN, Chen, H.M., Tsai, R.Y., Chien, Y.F., & Hwang, J.J. (2009) Using brachial-ankle pulse wave velocity to associate arterial stiffness with cardiovascular risks. *Nutrition, Metabolism & Cardiovascular Diseases,* Vol. 19, Issue 4, 241-246

Imanishi, R., Seto, S., Toda, G., Yoshida, M., Ohtsuru, A., Koide, Y., Baba, T., & Yano, K. (2004) High brachial-ankle pulse wave velocity is an independent predictor of the presence of coronary artery disease in men. *Hypertension Research,* Vol. 27, Issue 2, pp. 71-78

Jani, B. & Rajkumar, C. (2006) Ageing and vascular ageing. *Postgraduate Medical Journal,* Vol. 82, Issue 968, pp. 357-362

Johnson, A.M., Alper, C.A., Rosen, F.S., & Craig, J.M. (1971) C1 inhibitor: evidence for decreased hepatic synthesis in hereditary angioneurotic edema. *Science,* Vol. 173, Issue 996, pp. 553-554

Kalter, E.S., Daha, M.R., ten Cate, J.W., Verhoef, J., & Bouma, B.N. (1985) Activation and inhibition of Hageman factor-dependent pathways and the complement system in uncomplicated bacteremia or bacterial shock. *Journal of Infectious Diseases,* Vol. 151, Issue 6, pp. 1019-1027

Kim, D.H., Kim, J., Kim, J.M., & Lee, A.Y. (2008) Increased brachial-ankle pulse wave velocity is independently associated with risk of cerebral ischemic small vessel disease in elderly hypertensive patients. *Clinical Neurology and Neurosurgery,* Vol. 110, Issue 6, pp. 599-604

Kostner, K.M., Fahti, R.B., Case, C., Hobson, P., Tate, J., & Marwick, T.H. (2006) Inflammation, complement activation and endothelial function in stable and unstable coronary artery disease. *Clinica Chimica Acta,* Vol. 365, Issue 1-2, pp. 129-134

Langlois, P.F. & Gawryl, M.S. (1988) Detection of the terminal complement complex in patient plasma following acute myocardial infarction. *Atherosclerosis,* Vol. 70, Issue 1-2, pp. 95-105

Lappin, D. & Whaley, K. (1989) Regulation of C1-inhibitor synthesis by interferons and other agents. *Behring Institute Mitteilungen,* Vol. 84, pp. 180-192

Leung, V.W., Yun, S., Botto, M., Boyle, J.J.; & Haskard, D.O. (2009) Decay-accelerating factor suppresses complement C3 activation and retards atherosclerosis in low-density lipoprotein receptor-deficient mice. *American Journal of Pathology,* Vol. 175, Issue 4, pp. 1757-1767

Mallika, V., Goswami, B., & Rajappa, M. (2007) Atherosclerosis pathophysiology and the role of novel risk factors: a clinicobiochemical perspective. *Angiology,* Vol. 58, Issue 5, pp. 513-522

McLaren, J.E. & Ramji, D.P. (2008) Interferon gamma: a master regulator of atherosclerosis. *Cytokine & Growth Factor Reviews,* Vol. 20, pp. 125-135

Morgan, B.P. & Gasque, P. (1997) Extrahepatic complement biosynthesis: where, when and why? *Clinical & Experimental Immunology,* Vol. 107, Issue 1, pp. 1-7

Moshage, H. (1997) Cytokines and the hepatic acute phase response. *The Journal of Pathology,* Vol. 181, Issue 3, pp. 257-266.

Nakamura, U., Iwase, M., Nohara, S., Kanai, H., Ichikawa, K., & Iida, M. (2003) Usefulness of brachial-ankle pulse wave velocity measurement: correlation with abdominal aortic calcification. *Hypertension Research,* Vol. 26, Issue 2, pp. 163-167

Natali, A., L'Abbate, A., & Ferrannini, E. (2003) Erythrocyte sedimentation rate, coronary atherosclerosis, and cardiac mortality. *European Heart Journal,* Vol. 24, Issue 7, pp. 639-648

Nicoletti, A., Caligiuri, G., & Hansson, G.K. (2000) Immunomodulation of atherosclerosis: myth and reality. *Journal of Internal Medicine,* Vol. 247, Issue 3, pp. 397-405

Niculescu, F., Niculescu, T., & Rus, H. (2004) C5b-9 terminal complement complex assembly on apoptotic cells in human arterial wall with atherosclerosis. *Experimental and Molecular Pathology,* Vol. 76, Issue 1, pp. 17-23

Niculescu, F. & Rus, H. (2004) The role of complement activation in atherosclerosis. *Immunologic Research,* Vol. 30, Issue 1, pp. 73-80

Oksjoki, R., Kovanen, P.T., & Pentikainen, M.O. (2003) Role of complement activation in atherosclerosis. *Current Opinion in Lipidology,* Vol. 14, Issue 5, pp. 477-482

Oksjoki, R., Kovanen, P.T., Mayranpaa, M.I., Laine, P., Blom, A.M., Meri, S., & Pentikainen, M.O. (2007) Complement regulation in human atherosclerotic coronary lesions. Immunohistochemical evidence that C4b-binding protein negatively regulates the classical complement pathway, and that C5b-9 is formed via the alternative complement pathway. *Atherosclerosis,* Vol. 192, Issue 1, pp. 40-48

Prada, A.E., Zahedi, K., & Davis, A.E. 3rd. (1998) Regulation of C1 inhibitor synthesis. *Immunobiology,* Vol. 199, Issue 2, pp. 377-388

Ridker, P.M. & Silvertown, J.D. (2008) Inflammation, C-reactive protein, and atherothrombosis. *Journal of Periodontology,* Vol. 79, Issue 8 Suppl, pp. 1544-1551

Schepers, A., de Vries, M.R., van Leuven, C.J., Grimbergen, J.M., Holers, V.M., Daha, M.R., van Bockel, J.H., & Quax, P.H.A. (2006) Inhibition of complement component C3 reduces vein graft atherosclerosis in apolipoprotein E3-Leiden transgenic mice. *Circulation,* Vol. 114, Issue 25, pp. 2831-2838

Schrijvers, D.M., De Meyer, G.R., Herman, A.G., & Martinet, W. (2007) Phagocytosis in atherosclerosis: molecular mechanisms and implications for plaque progression and stability. *Cardiovascular Research,* Vol. 73, Issue 3, pp. 470-480

Seimon, T. & Tabas, I. (2009) Mechanisms and consequences of macrophage apoptosis in atherosclerosis. *The Journal of Lipid Research,* Vol. 50 (Suppl), pp. S382-S387

Shagdarsuren, E., Bidzhekov, K., Djalali-Talab, Y., Liehn, E.A., Hristov, M., Matthijsen, R.A., Buurman, W.A., Zernecke, A., & Weber, C. (2008) C1-esterase inhibitor protects against neointima formation after arterial injury in atherosclerosis-prone mice. *Circulation,* Vol. 117, Issue 1, pp. 70-78

Storini, C., Rossi, E., Marrella, V., Distaso, M., Veerhuis, R., Vergani, C., Bergamaschini, L., & De Simoni, M.G. (2005) C1-inhibitor protects against brain ischemia-reperfusion injury via inhibition of cell recruitment and inflammation. *Neurobiology of Disease,* Vol. 19, Issue 1-2, pp. 10-17

Szeplaki, G., Prohaszka, Z., Duba, J., Rugonfalvi-Kiss, S., Karadi, I., Kokai, M., Kramer, J., Fust, G., Kleiber, M., Romics, L., & Varga, L. (2004) Association of high serum concentration of the third component of complement (C3) with pre-existing severe coronary artery disease and new vascular events in women. *Atherosclerosis,* Vol. 177, Issue 2, pp. 383-389

Tanaka, H., Munakata, M., Kawano, Y., Ohishi, M., Shoji, T., Sugawara, J., Tomiyama, H., Yamashina, A., Yasuda, H., Sawayama, T., & Ozawa, T. (2009) Comparison between carotid-femoral and brachial-ankle pulse wave velocity as measures of arterial stiffness. *Journal of Hypertension,* Vol. 27, Issue 10, pp. 2022-2027

Thorbjornsdottir, P., Kolka, R., Gunnarsson, E., Bambir, S.H., Thorgeirsson, G., Kotwal, G.J., & Arason, G. (2005) *Vaccinia virus* complement control protein diminishes formation of atherosclerotic lesions: complement is centrally involved in atherosclerotic disease. *Annals of the New York Academy of Sciences,* Vol. 1056, pp. 1-15

Tomiyama, H., Yamashina, A., Arai, T., Hirose, K., Koji, Y., Chikamori, T., Hori, S., Yamamoto, Y., Doba, N., & Hinohara, S. (2003) Influences of age and gender on results of noninvasive brachial-ankle pulse wave velocity measurement--a survey of 12517 subjects. *Atherosclerosis,* Vol. 166, Issue 2, pp. 303-309

Tomiyama, H., Koji, Y., Yambe, M., Shiina, K., Motobe, M., Yamada, J., Shido, N., Tanaka, N., Chikamori, T., & Yamashina, A. (2005) Brachial–ankle pulse wave velocity is a simple and independent predictor of prognosis in patients with acute coronary syndrome. *Circulation Journal,* Vol. 69, Issue 7, pp. 815-822

van Popele, N.M., Grobbee, D.E., Bots, M.L., Asmar, R., Topouchian, J., Reneman, R.S., Hoeks, A.P.G., van der Kuip, D.A.M., Hofman, A., & Witteman, J.C.M. (2001) Association between arterial stiffness and atherosclerosis: the Rotterdam Study. *Stroke,* Vol. 32, Issue 2, pp. 454-460

Windfuhr, J.P., Alsenz, J., & Loos, M. (2005) The critical concentration of C1-esterase inhibitor (C1-INH) in human serum preventing auto-activation of the first component of complement (C1). *Molecular Immunology,* Vol. 42, Issue 6, pp. 657-663

Woo, P., Lachmann, P.J., Harrison, R.A., Amos, N., Cooper, C., & Rosen, F.S. (1985) Simultaneous turnover of normal and dysfunctional C1 inhibitor as a probe of in vivo activation of C1 and contact activatable proteases. *Clinical & Experimental Immunology,* Vol. 61, Issue 1, pp. 1-8

Wu, G., Hu, W., Shahsafaei, A., Song, W., Dobarro, M., Sukhova, G.K., Bronson, R.R., Shi, G., Rother, R.P., Halperin, J.A., & Qin, X. (2009) Complement regulator CD59 protects against atherosclerosis by restricting the formation of complement membrane attack complex. *Circulation Research,* Vol. 104, Issue 4, pp. 550-558

Wykretowicz, A., Gerstenberger, P., Guzik, P., Milewska, A., Krauze, T., Adamska, K., Rutkowska, A., & Wysocki, H. (2009) Arterial stiffness in relation to subclinical atherosclerosis. *European Journal of Clinical Investigation,* Vol. 39, Issue 1, pp. 11-16

Xu, Y., Wu, Y., Li, J., Ma, W., Guo, X., Luo, Y., & Hu, D. (2008) The predictive value of brachial-ankle pulse wave velocity in coronary atherosclerosis and peripheral artery diseases in urban Chinese patients. *Hypertension Research,* Vol. 31, Issue 6, pp. 1079-1085

Yamashina, A., Tomiyama, H., Takeda, K., Tsuda, H., Arai, T., Hirose, K., Koji, Y., Hori, S., & Yamamoto, Y. (2002) Validity, reproducibility, and clinical significance of noninvasive brachial-ankle pulse wave velocity measurement. *Hypertension Research,* Vol. 25, Issue 3, pp. 359-364

Yamashina, A., Tomiyama, H., Arai, T., Hirose, K., Koji, Y., Hirayama, Y., Yamamoto, Y., & Hori, S. (2003) Brachial-ankle pulse wave velocity as a marker of atherosclerotic vascular damage and cardiovascular risk. *Hypertension Research,* Vol. 26, Issue 8, pp. 615-622

Yasojima, K., Schwab, C., McGeer, E.G., & McGeer, P.L. (2001) Complement components, but not complement inhibitors, are upregulated in atherosclerotic plaques. *Arteriosclerosis, Thrombosis, and Vascular Biology,* Vol. 21, Issue 7, pp. 1214-1219

Yun, S., Leung, V.W., Botto, M., Boyle, J.J., & Haskard, D.O. (2008) Brief report: accelerated atherosclerosis in low-density lipoprotein receptor-deficient mice lacking the membrane-bound complement regulator CD59. *Arteriosclerosis, Thrombosis, and Vascular Biology,* Vol. 28, Issue 10, pp. 1714-1716

Zahedi, K., Prada, A.E., & Davis, A.E. 3rd. (1994) Transcriptional regulation of the C1 inhibitor gene by gamma-interferon. *The Journal of Biological Chemistry,* Vol. 269, Issue 13, pp. 9669-9674

Zanker, K.S. (2008) General introduction to innate immunity: Dr. Jekyl/Mr. Hyde quality of the innate immune system. *Contributions to Microbiology,* Vol. 15, pp. 12-20

Zuraw, B.L. & Lotz, M. (1990) Regulation of the hepatic synthesis of C1 inhibitor by the hepatocyte stimulating factors interleukin 6 and interferon gamma. *The Journal of Biological Chemistry,* Vol. 265, Issue 21, pp. 12664-12670

9

Veterinary Biomarker Discovery: Proteomic Analysis of Acute Phase Proteins

Jamie L. Boehmer and Zohra Olumee-Shabon
U.S. Food and Drug Administration Center for Veterinary Medicine Office of Research
United States of America

1. Introduction

Modulation of acute phase protein (APP) expression in biological fluids and tissues during disease has emerged as a primary means of assessing both local and systemic innate immune responses. From a veterinary biomarker perspective, APPs are attractive candidates for the diagnosis of disease in food animals, as well as for differentiating between chronic and acute inflammation and for evaluating response to therapeutics (Horadagoda et al., 1999). Several diseases of economic importance in livestock, most notably respiratory disorders and mastitis in cattle, remain a primary focus of veterinary disease research, due to the lack of efficacious treatment options for the profound inflammation caused by exposure to causative bacterial agents. Additionally, inflammatory diseases are often accompanied by the widespread use of antibiotics for treatment and prevention; an aspect that causes concern for food safety, as well as for the emergence of resistant strains of bacteria. Accordingly, recent veterinary biomarker discovery initiatives have focused on the identification of sensitive and reliable indicators for use in evaluating the efficacy of adjunctive therapies for the treatment of inflammation associated with disease in food animal species. As a result, modulation in several APP, including haptoglobin (HPT), alpha-1-acid glycoprotein (AGP), bovine serum albumin (BSA), inter-alpha-trypsin inhibitor heavy chain-4 (ITIH4), and serum amyloid A (SAA), have been detected in the analyses of bovine milk, plasma, and broncheoalveolar lavage fluid (BALF) during both naturally occurring and experimentally induced disease (Boehmer et al., 2010; Danielsen et al., 2010; Mitchell et al., 2007; Eckersall et al., 2006).
Classic approaches to the characterization of protein changes in complex biological fluids have required the availability of species-specific antibodies for the detection and quantification of a given protein. Use of antibody-based strategies such as enzyme-linked immunosorbent assays (ELISA) in biomarker discovery analyses, however, limits the identification and characterization of novel candidates, as well as the detection of post-translational modifications (PTM) of target proteins. Previous research has established that APPs are subject to modifications, such as glycosylation, in altered physiological states (Gruys et al., 2005; Higai, et al., 2003; Anderssen et al., 2001). While APPs are thought to lack specificity as candidate biomarkers of disease because of their prominence during the innate immune response, there is evidence to suggest that the modification of certain APPs could be disease-specific. Thus, characterization of the post-translational modifications in APPs

during the inflammatory response in different diseases could aid in the establishment of the specificity of APPs as biomarkers.
Proteomics, defined as the identification of all proteins within a cell or tissue, involves the use of analytical methodologies such as liquid chromatography (LC) to separate proteins or peptides, and mass spectrometry (MS), to isolate, identify, and characterize proteins and their associated PTMs. An advantage of proteomics in biomarker discovery is the ability to detect a theoretically unlimited number of proteins in a given sample without the need for antibodies. Bottom-up proteomics including proteolytic digestion of proteins prior to the use of LC to separate peptides coupled with tandem MS (MS/MS) for peptide sequencing, a process commonly referred to as LC-MS/MS, has become the most widely used proteomic approach for the identification of individual proteins in complex mixtures. Additionally, advances in ion fragmentation strategies, including electron transfer dissociation (ETD), have provided superior tools for the characterization of modified peptides. Detection of disease-specific modifications of APP glycopeptides, however, is still an emerging aspect of veterinary biomarker discovery. The following chapter will discuss the role of APP as biomarkers of infection and inflammation in food animals, as well as proteomic strategies and the proteomic analyses of APPs during inflammatory disease in ruminant species. Strategies for characterizing modified glycopeptides will also be introduced, including the potential disease-specific modification of APPs.

2. Acute phase proteins: Biomarkers of infection and inflammation in food animals

Because APPs have demonstrated changes as great as 25% in serum concentrations during altered physiological states, APPs have garnered attention for use as potential biomarkers for diagnosing animal disease, monitoring health status, and evaluating responses to primary and adjunctive veterinary therapies (Eckersall and Bell, 2010). In particular, APPs have been investigated as potential biomarkers for inflammatory diseases in food animals, because the etiological agents are bacterial in origin, and the use of antibiotics for treatment and prevention is common. Antibiotic use in food animals, however, causes concern for food safety, and could increase selective pressures for the emergence of resistant strains of bacteria. Additionally, antibiotics are not always the appropriate treatment for diseases in food animals with affiliated inflammatory responses. Though APPs have been characterized as non-specific responders to pro-inflammatory signals, differences in APP expression during disease across species have been reported, and evidence exists that circulating concentrations of APPs in blood and other biological fluids are a direct indication of disease severity (Eckersall and Bell, 2010; Gruys et al., 2005; Murata et al., 2004). Additionally, more recent data based on the proteomic analyses of APPs during disease suggests that modification of glycoproteins could be disease specific (Wilson et al., 2008). The prospect of using APPs as biomarkers of inflammation and infection for veterinary applications has inspired a significant body of research, including the development of antibodies and other quantitative methods for analyzing APP expression during disease in food animal species (Murata et al., 2004). More recently, interest in APPs as potential veterinary biomarkers has led to the application of proteomic strategies for the evaluation of APPs and measures of the host response in complex biological samples (Bendixen et al., 2011; Boehmer et al., 2010; Danielsen et al., 2010; Smolenski et al., 2007).

2.1 Modulation of acute phase proteins during disease in swine

Alteration in APP expression has been associated with a number of food animal diseases (Table 1), including mastitis, metritis, and amyloidosis in lactating dairy cattle (Chan et al., 2010; Safi et al., 2009; Suojala et al., 2008; Eckersall et al., 2001, 2006; Takahashi et al., 2006; Grönlund et al., 2003, 2005); sepsis, trauma, and respiratory diseases in swine (Amory et al., 2007; Sorensen et al., 2006; Hultén et al., 2003; Heegaard et al., 1998; Eckersall et al., 1996); infectious bronchitis virus in chickens (Nazifi et al., 2011); respiratory diseases in beef cattle (Orro et al., 2011; Heegaard et al., 2000; Godson et al., 1996; Horadagoda et al., 1995); as well as pulmonary damage and caseous lymphadenitis in sheep (Eckersall et al., 2007; Pfeffer and Rogers, 1989).

Protein	Diseases	Species
Haptoglobin	Pneumonia, Sepsis, Inflammation	Swine
Serum amyloid A	Pneumonia, Sepsis	Swine
C-reactive rpotein	Sepsis, Inflammation	Swine
pig-MAP[1]	Sepsis	Swine
α-1-acid glycoprotein	Inflammation	Swine
Ceruloplasmin	Inflammation	Swine
Acid soluble glycoprotein	Inflammation	Swine
Haptoglobin	Infectious bronchitis	Chickens
Serum amyloid A	Infectious bronchitis	Chickens
Lipopolysaccharide binding protein	Mastitis, Respiratory Disease	Cattle
Serum Amyloid A	Mastitis, Respiratory Disease, Amyloidosis	Bovine
Haptoglobin	Mastitis, Respiratory Disease, Amyloidosis	Bovine
α-1-acid glycoprotein	Mastitis, Respiratory Disease	Bovine
Haptoglobin	Caseous lymphadenitis, Pulmonary damage	Sheep
Serum amyloid A	Caseous lymphadenitis	Sheep
α-1-acid glycoprotein	Caseous lymphadenitis	Sheep
Fibrinogen	Pulmonary damage	Sheep
Ceruloplasmin	Pulmonary damage	Sheep
Haptoglobin	Inflammation	Goat
Serum amyloid A	Inflammation	Goat
Fibrinogen	Inflammation	Goat
Acid soluble glycoprotein	Inflammation	Goat

pig-MAP[1] = pig major acute phase protein

Table 1. Acute phase proteins associated with disease in food animals

In swine, increased levels of serum HPT have been associated with pathological indications of *Mycoplasma hyopneumoniae*, a leading cause of porcine enzootic pneumonia (Amory et al., 2007). Similarly, serum concentrations of HPT and SAA were elevated in pigs with experimentally induced *Actinobacillus pleuropneumoniae* pneumonia (Hultén et al., 2003; Heegaard et al., 1998). Peak expression of HPT and SAA in pigs with *A.pleuropneumoniae* pneumonia was detected approximately 4 days following infection. However, serum HPT and SAA levels were lower in pigs treated with the antimicrobial enrofloxacin following experimental infection with *A.pleuropneumoniae*, which indicated the feasibility of using APPs to monitor response to therapeutic treatment (Hultén et al., 2003).

During experimental induction of sepsis, pigs infected with *Streptococcus suis* exhibited increases in serum concentrations of the APPs CRP, SAA, HPT, and pig-MAP (Sorensen et al., 2006). Both CRP and SAA peaked on day 1 following infection with *S. suis*, and returned to near baseline levels 5-12 days following infection, while HPT and pig-MAP peaked on days 5-8 following infection and remained elevated for the duration of the study (Sorensen et al., 2006). Conversely, serum levels of HPT and CRP peaked just 2 days after the experimental induction of inflammation in pigs, while ceruloplasmin levels did not reach peak concentrations until 4 days after experimental treatment with turpentine (Eckersall et al., 1996). Though the same positive APPs were detected in a variety of different experimental swine disease models, it should be noted that temporal expression patterns and peak serum concentrations of each APP varied for each disease, indicating some level of disease specificity.

2.2 Modulation of acute phase proteins during ruminant disease

Currently, only limited data is available regarding acute phase protein expression in small ruminants during disease. Experimental induction of inflammation in goats revealed increases in serum levels of HPT, SAA, fibrinogen, and acid soluble glycoprotein following injection with turpentine (González et al., 2008), while experimental-induction of caseous lymphadenitis in sheep revealed increases in serum levels of SAA, HPT, and AGP (Eckersall et al., 2007).

Conversely, there have been several investigations into the acute phase response during both naturally-occurring and experimentally-induced bovine diseases. In studies of bovine respiratory disease, peak levels of serum SAA and HPT were reported during week 3 of an outbreak of respiratory disease in calves caused by respiratory syncytial virus (Orro et al., 2011), while experimental infection with respiratory syncytial virus caused maximal increases in serum levels of HPT and SAA in cattle as early as 7-8 days following inoculation (Heegaard et al 2000). Of the bovine diseases studied, however, APP expression has been investigated most extensively during mastitis in lactating dairy animals (Safi et al., 2009; Suojala et al., 2008; Eckersall et al., 2006, 2001; Grönlund et al., 2003; Hirvonen et al., 1999). Mastitis is defined as an inflammation of the mammary gland, and is considered the most dominant and costly of diseases to affect lactating dairy cattle. *Staphylococcus aureus* and *Escherichia coli* are perhaps the most prevalent species of Gram-positive and Gram-negative bacteria, respectively, that cause clinical mastitis. Due to affiliated financial losses and food safety concerns, characterization of the innate immune response during clinical mastitis has remained a primary focus of veterinary research. Studies of the first line of defense against invading pathogens in the bovine mammary gland have provided valuable information on the expression of acute phase proteins during inflammation in dairy cattle, and have revealed differences in temporal expression of APPs dependent on the causative bacterial species (Bannerman et al., 2004). APPs have been the center of numerous studies of both naturally-occurring and experimentally-induced mastitis because of their ability to opsonize and trap microorganisms, activate complement, neutralize enzymes, and modulate the host response to infection (Gruys et al., 2005). Likewise, the bovine mammary gland is an established source of extra-hepatic APP production; thus the evaluation of APP expression in milk could aid in the early detection of mastitis (Hiss et al., 2004).

Studies directed at the innate immune response in the bovine mammary gland following challenge with either LPS or *Escherichia coli* (*E. coli*) have reported increases in the APPs SAA, HPT, AGP, and lipopolysaccharide binding protein (LBP) in milk and serum from cows during clinical mastitis (Suojala et al., 2008; Ceciliani et al., 2005; Hiss et al., 2004; Eckersall et al., 2001; Hirvonen et al., 1999). Increases in serum concentrations of both SAA and HPT following intra-mammary challenge with *E. coli* were reported 24 hours after experimental infection, with peak expression of both APPs apparent on day 3 after challenge (Suojala et al., 2008; Hirvonen et al., 1999). Intracisternal injection of lipopolysaccharide, however, caused elevations in serum HPT levels in infected cows as early as 9 hours following challenge (Hiss et al., 2004). Reports of serum HPT levels in cows with naturally occurring coliform mastitis were in accord with values detected following experimental challenge (Ohtsuka et al., 2001). LBP appeared to increase more rapidly than HPT and SAA in cows with experimentally-induced coliform mastitis, as peak expression was reported as early as 36 hours following challenge (Suojala et al., 2008). Conversely, reports of AGP indicate that peak expression was not detected in serum from cows with coliform mastitis until 9 days after the onset of clinical symptoms (Ohtsuka et al., 2001). The evaluation of APP expression in milk from cows with experimentally-induced coliform mastitis revealed increases in HPT, SAA, and LBP as early as 12 hours following challenge with peak expression at 44, 60, and 36 hours, respectively (Suojala et al., 2008). Increases in both milk and serum levels of HPT and SAA in cows experimentally infected with *Staphylococcus aureus* (*S. aureus*) have also been reported (Hiss et al., 2007; Eckersall et al., 2006; Grönlund et al., 2003). Evaluation of the acute phase response following experimental challenge with *S. aureus* revealed increases in HPT and the mammary isoform of SAA (M-SAA3) in both bovine serum and milk that were in accord with data from experimental challenge with *E. coli* (Eckersall et al., 2006; Grönlund et al., 2003).

While the primary source of APPs is the liver, local production of SAA, HPT, and AGP in the bovine mammary gland have also been demonstrated, which mark APPs as potential indicators of both systemic and local inflammation in cattle (Larson et al., 2006; Jacobsen et al., 2005; Ceciliani et al., 2005; Hiss et al., 2004). Additionally, aside from both local and hepatic production of AGP, the granules of bovine neutrophils are likewise a reported source of APPs (Rahman et al., 2008). Regardless of source of production, however, ruminant animals differ from other species in terms of APP expression during inflammation, in that HPT is the major APP in bovine innate immunity, whereas in other animal species CRP predominates the acute phase response (Ecksersall and Bell, 2010; Petersen et al., 2004).

2.3 Detection methods for acute phase proteins in biological samples

Most prior analyses of the acute phase response during bovine mastitis have utilized ELISAs, immunodiffusion, haemoglobin binding, or the evaluation of messenger RNA (mRNA) expression to evaluate changes in APP expression during disease (Hiss et al., 2007; Eckersall et al., 2006; 2005; 2001; Jacobsen et al., 2005; Grönlund et al., 2003). Use of such strategies in biomarker discovery analyses, however, limits the identification and characterization of novel protein candidates, as well as the detection of potential PTMs of APPs, due to a reliance on the availability of species-specific antibodies, and the ability to evaluate only one APP per assay. The most crucial element of the ELISA detection strategy is a highly specific antibody-antigen interaction. Thus, characterization of protein changes in complex biological fluids using ELISA requires the availability of species-specific antibodies for the detection and quantification of a given protein. Unfortunately, a very limited number of antibodies are commercially available for livestock species. Additionally, there is no practical protocol for the development of an immunoassay targeting a modified site if neither the site nor the modification is known.

Genomic methodologies, including gene arrays and the evaluation of mRNA expression can also limit biomarker discovery because of the demonstrated weak correlation that often exists between mRNA levels and actual protein concentration. Thus, quantitative mRNA data is often an inadequate indicator of protein expression (Gygi et al., 1999; Ideker et al., 2001; Griffin et al., 2002; Tian et al., 2004). However, advances in soft ionization techniques in mass spectrometry (MS), including electro-spray ionization (ESI), nano-spray ionization, and matrix-assisted laser desorption/ionization (MALDI), have broadened the applications of mass spectrometry to include the characterization of biopolymers such as intact proteins and peptides, and has given rise to a new field of protein study termed proteomics (reviewed in Mann et al., 2001). Proteomics, defined as a scientific approach used to elucidate all proteins within a cell or tissue (Colantonio and Chan, 2005) boasts a significant advantage over genomic and antibody-based analyses, because proteomics involves the use of analytical methodologies, such as LC and MS, to isolate, identify, and characterize proteins, and is not reliant on the use or availability of antibodies. Additionally, proteomic methodologies can detect a theoretically unlimited number of proteins in a given sample without the need for antibody or reagent development.

3. Proteomic strategies

Protein identification through the use of MS can be divided into two main categories, referred to as top-down and bottom-up. The primary distinguishing features between the two main proteomic approaches is the isolation and fragmentation of intact proteins using MS in a top-down approach, versus proteolytic digestion of mixtures of proteins, and the subsequent separation and fragmentation of peptides, in bottom-up proteomics. Identification of proteins in complex biological mixtures using bottom-up proteomics is reliant upon the measurement of the masses of the peptides that are generated following proteolytic cleavage of the proteins. The mass of a peptide is determined using MS, and is based upon a mass-to-charge ratio (m/z). Charged peptides are generated as a result of ionization, or the addition of a proton to the peptide, which results in the conversion of the peptide into an ion. The two most popular forms of ionization used in bottom-up proteomic analyses are ESI and MALDI.

3.1 Two-dimensional gels and MALDI-TOF mass spectrometry

Over the past two decades, two-dimensional gel electrophoresis (2D-GE) followed by MALDI time-of-flight (TOF) MS and LC-MS/MS have become the most widely used proteomic approaches in bottom-up proteomic analyses (Ferguson et al., 2003). Protein profiling by 2D-GE is characterized by a first dimension separation of proteins by charge (isoelectric point), followed by a second dimension separation by molecular weight. Advances in 2D-GE technology including gel strips with immobilized pH gradients have dramatically increased the resolving power of 2D-GE. Additionally, the development of radioactive and fluorescent labeling has improved the ability to visualize proteins in a 2D gel, as well as the detection of low-abundance and post-translationally modified proteins (Van den Bergh et al., 2005).

In a MALDI-TOF/MS experiment, the protein or peptide(s) of interest is mixed with a suitable energy-absorbing matrix and allowed to co-crystallize by air-drying on a stainless steel plate. Matrices used in MALDI-TOF/MS are typically small aromatic molecules capable of absorbing high levels of UV light at a specific wavelength, such as sinapinic acid (SPA) or alpha-cyano-4-hydroxycinnamic acid (CHCA). The generation of ions in MALDI-TOF/MS is initiated by short pulse irradiation with a laser (Karas and Krüger, 2003), typically nitrogen or neodymium-doped yttrium aluminum garnet (Nd:YAG), and occurs when the matrix becomes electronically excited following absorption of photons from the UV laser. Analytes in the sample accept a proton from the matrix and become singly charged positive ions as they are ejected from the matrix and converted into the gas phase. The ions are then directed into the TOF analyzer where they are separated based on their *m/z* and generate a mass spectrum. Separation of ions is based on the principle that ions with smaller *m/z* "fly" faster than larger ions. The subsequent protein identification is accomplished by peptide mass fingerprinting, which is the comparison of the set of peptide masses generated from a specific protein to a protein database containing theoretically calculated mass fingerprints of all known proteins. A process called post source decay (PSD) can be used on TOF instruments equipped with a reflectron to further enhance resolution of the MALDI peak separation. In this technique, the voltage on the reflectron is modulated during analysis to allow the detection of ion fragments formed during ionization or acceleration down the flight tube (Kaufmann et al., 1994).

3.2 LC-MS/MS

Despite the recent advancements in reproducibility and protein quantification, 2D-GE as a means of protein separation still suffers from issues including isolation of proteins with low abundance, high hydrophobicity, or extreme isolelectric points. Consequently, LC has emerged as the best alternative for the separation of proteins or peptides in solution prior to mass analysis using MS. Recently, the combination of two LC-based separation techniques coupled with MS was introduced, and has profoundly increased the ability to resolve and detect a greater number of peptides in LC-MS/MS-based proteomic experiments. Multidimensional protein identification technology (MudPIT), utilizes the combination of strong cation-exchange chromatography and reverse-phase chromatography followed by ESI-MS/MS for the characterization of proteins in a complex mixture (Washburn et al., 2001). Using the MudPIT approach, proteins are typically digested into peptides using a protease such as trypsin, which cleaves at every arginine and lysine residue, and separated online by 2-dimensional LC prior to introduction into the mass spectrometer for mass analysis. In 2-dimensional LC, peptides are separated in the first dimension by charge using ion exchange chromatography, and are then further separated in the second dimension by hydrophobicity using reversed-phase (RP) chromatography.

In a one-dimensional (1D) LC-MS/MS experiment, peptide mixtures are typically separated only by hydrophobicity by passage over a column packed with non-polar stationary phase. Thus, the number of proteins identified using 1D-LC-MS/MS is directly dependent on the efficiency of peptide separation prior to introduction into the mass spectrometer (Jensen et al., 1999). In LC-MS/MS experiments, ESI is the dominant method of ionization. Ionization occurs in ESI after the peptide solution is dispersed as a fine spray of charged droplets after passage through a heated metal capillary tube to which voltage is applied. The charged droplets get desolvated by a dry inert gas, and multiply charged ions are produced. Nano-spray ionization (NSI) functions in essentially the same manner as ESI, but flow rates from the LC instrument into the ionization source of the mass spectrometer are much lower with nano-spray than those used for ESI, and ionization efficiency is greatly improved (Wilm et al., 1996). Ions resulting from either ESI or NSI are then directed into the vacuum chamber of the MS instrument, and are resolved according to their *m/z* ratio to produce the first MS spectrum. While the first MS scan generates the mass of all peptides, peptide(s) of interest are subjected to further fragmentation by a process called collision-induced dissociation (CID) in the second MS scan. An inert gas such as argon (Ar) or helium (He) is introduced into the collision cell of the mass spectrometer which results in the production of a tandem or MS/MS spectrum. Peak lists generated from the fragment ion masses in tandem mass spectra are then searched against a protein database to determine the amino acid sequence of the peptides in the complex mixture. The assignment of the sequenced peptides to a given protein is the means by which protein identification is accomplished (Jensen et al., 1999).

3.3 Post-translational modifications

Comparative proteomic analyses are designed to elucidate changes in the relative abundance of proteins among different biological states, most commonly healthy versus diseased. Detection of the same peptides from a given protein is not always possible in comparative studies, however, because post-translational modification of peptides as a result of disease is expected. Characterization of PTMs is crucial for biomarker discovery, because much of the regulation of the biological activity of proteins is mediated by the modification of peptide amino acid residues, including the phosphorylation of serine and threonine, and the glycosylation of asparagine, arginine, or tyrosine. Identification of PTMs is especially useful for the detection and characterization of APPs during disease because APPs are glycoproteins and are subject to modification. Unfortunately characterization of PTM's has been hindered in past experiments due to the fact that modifications are labile and are often lost in a CID experiment. Electron-transfer dissociation (ETD), which is a superior fragmentation strategy for the analysis of PTMs, however, was recently introduced, and shows promise as a strategy for the characterization of APP modification during disease (Syka et al., 2004). The ETD technique uses electrons to promote fragmentation along the peptide backbone, which produces a series of c and z ions, instead of CID fragmentation, which produces a series of b and y ions. The fragmentation of the peptide backbone using ETD allows for amino acid side chains and modifications such as glycosylation and phosphorylation to remain intact, making it possible not only to deduce the amino acid sequence of a peptide, but also to detect any modified residues (Syka et al., 2004). Furthermore, the combination of CID and ETD has proven effective as well in the characterization of isolated glycopeptides, including modified peptides from HPT in human lung cancer patients (Wang et al., 2011).

4. Proteomic analysis of acute pphase proteins during animal disease

Proteomic approaches boast the capability to analyze an unlimited number of protein targets in a single experiment, independent of antibody availability. Proteomics is rapidly gaining popularity in veterinary biomarker studies, especially those aimed at the discovery of biomarkers of disease, productivity, product quality, and animal welfare in cattle and swine (Bendixen et al., 2010). Furthermore, compared to a recent review of the evaluation of

APP expression during disease in companion animals and cattle (Eckersall et al., 2010), a far greater overall number of APPs have been identified in biological fluids from food animals using proteomic strategies (Table 2) than have been detected using more traditional approaches.

The most widely studied biological fluids in proteomic-based biomarker discovery analyses in swine and cattle have been serum, plasma, and milk. To date, protein profiles have been generated for serum and plasma of both healthy cattle and pigs, using 2D-GE (Miller et al., 2009; Talamo et al., 2003; Wait et al., 2002). Comparative proteomic analyses have likewise been conducted using 2D-GE to profile differentially expressed proteins in plasma from pigs with peritonitis-induced sepsis, with findings that the APP inter-alpha trypsin inhibitor-heavy chain-4 (ITIH-4), HPT, hemopexin, alpha-2-HS-glycoprotein, albumin, and apolipoprotein-A1 all exhibited modulated expression levels as a result of disease (Thongboonkerd et al., 2009). Proteomics has also been applied to the study of the gastrointestinal tract in swine (Wang et al., 2009; Danielsen et al., 2007, 2006), as well as diet-induced fatty liver disease in Ossabaw pigs (Bell et al., 2010).

Studies aimed at the elucidation of potential biomarkers of bovine mastitis have specifically dominated veterinary biomarker initiatives in cattle, however, due in large part to affiliated inflammation, economic and food safety concerns, and the lack of efficacious treatment options (Boehmer et al., 2010; 2008; Danielsen et al., 2010; Smolenski et al., 2007; Hogarth et al., 2004). Several comparative proteomic studies have focused on the identification of diagnostic biomarkers of mastitis in bovine milk, though the proteomic analysis of mammary tissue from healthy cows and cows with clinical mastitis has also been conducted (Yang et al., 2009). Likewise, other diseases of economic importance to the cattle industry have been the focus of proteomic-based veterinary biomarkers studies, including the analysis of bronchoalveolar lavage fluid (BALF) from the bovine respiratory tract following administration of dexamethasone, as well as after the stress of transport (Mitchell et al., 2008, 2007).

The earliest comparative proteomic analyses of normal versus mastitic bovine milk were accomplished using 2D-GE followed by MALDI-TOF/MS (Smolenski et al., 2007; Hogarth et al., 2004), or MALDI-TOF/TOF PSD (Boehmer et al., 2008). Despite a limited number of proteins detected, promising discoveries that resulted from the 2D-GE- MALDI-TOF/MS of bovine milk included the identification of the APP α-1-acid glycoprotein (AGP) in both normal and mastitic whey samples, and the apparent higher relative abundance of AGP in mastitic milk as early as 18 hours following challenge (Boehmer et al., 2008). Previously, the analyses of APP expression in milk during bovine mastitis using more traditional quantitative strategies had only identified the APPs SAA, HPT, and LBP (Hiss et al., 2004; Bannerman et al., 2004; Eckersall et al., 2001). Similar to the 2D-GE- MALDI-TOF/MS of bovine milk, the proteomic analysis of changes in the bovine BALF proteome induced by dexamethasone revealed increases in the APPs alpha-2-HS-glycoprotein, alpha-1-antichymotrypsin, alpha-1-antitrypsin, and AGP in treated animals when compared to controls (Mitchell et al., 2007).

To avoid some of the limitations imposed by a 2D-GE-MALDI-TOF/MS proteomic experiment, more recent proteomic analyses of bovine milk have been accomplished through the use of LC-MS/MS (Boehmer et al., 2010; Danielsen et al., 2010; Smolenski et al., 2007). The first attempt to characterize proteins related to host defense in mastitic bovine milk did result in the identification of the APPs serum albumin, fibrinogen, and SAA, but very few biological replicates were used in the analyses, and the objectives were strictly proteome coverage, not comparisons between the healthy and diseased states (Smolenski et al., 2007). The two most recent comparative proteomic analyses of normal versus mastitic bovine milk, however, have not only identified several APPs in milk, but tracked changes in APPs over the course of infection, and quantified modulation in relative abundance of APPs during disease (Boehmer et al, 2010; Danielsen et al., 2010).

Protein	Accession Number	Species	Fluid	Method of Detection
Inter-α-trypsin inhibitor heavy chain-4	P79263	Swine	Plasma	2D-GE-MALDI-TOF/MS
Haptoglobin	Q8SPS7	Swine	Plasma	2D-GE-MALDI-TOF/MS
α-2-HS-glycoprotein	P29700	Swine	Plasma	2D-GE-MALDI-TOF/MS
Serum albumin	P08835	Swine	Plasma	2D-GE-MALDI-TOF/MS
Apolipoprotein-A1	P18648	Swine	Plasma	2D-GE-MALDI-TOF/MS
Serum Amyloid A	P35541	Bovine	Milk	LC-MS/MS
Haptoglobin	Q2TBU0	Bovine	Milk	LC-MS/MS
α-1-acid glycoprotein	Q3SZR3	Bovine	Milk	LC-MS/MS, 2D-GE MALDI-TOF/MS
		Bovine	BALF[1]	2D-GE MALDI-TOF/MS
Serum albumin	P02769	Bovine	Milk	LC-MS/MS, 2D-GE MALDI-TOF/MS
Serotransferrin	Q29443	Bovine	Milk	LC-MS/MS, 2D-GE MALDI-TOF/MS
α-2-HS-glycoprotein	P12763	Bovine	Milk	LC-MS/MS, 2D-GE MALDI-TOF/MS
		Bovine	BALF[1]	LC-MS/MS
α-2 Macroglobulin	Q7SIH1	Bovine	Milk	LC-MS/MS
Inter-α-trypsin inhibitor heavy chain-4	Q3T052	Bovine	Milk	LC-MS/MS
Apolipoprotein-A1	P15497	Bovine	Milk	LC-MS/MS, 2D-GE MALDI-TOF/MS
α-1- Antitrypsin	P34955	Bovine	Milk	2D-GE MALDI-TOF/MS
		Bovine	BALF[1]	2D-GE MALDI-TOF/MS
α-1- Antichymotrypsin	Q28921	Bovine	BALF[1]	LC-MS/MS
Fibrinogen	P02672	Bovine	Milk	LC-MS/MS, 2D-GE MALDI-TOF/MS

BALF[1] = Bronchoalveolar lavage fluid (Mitchell et al., 2008; 2007)

Table 2. Acute phase proteins identified disease in food animals using proteomic strategies

4.1 Quantification of acute phase proteins in bovine milk using proteomics

Relative and absolute quantification of changes in the abundance of potential biomarkers identified in biological matrices using proteomic strategies is a topic that has garnered significant attention in recent years (Simpson et al., 2009; Mueller et al., 2008; Fenselau, 2007; Roe and Griffin, 2006). Several strategies exist for the quantification of individual proteins in complex mixtures using proteomics; however, quantification methods can be assigned to one of two broad categories: a labeling approach that requires the incorporation of labels into proteins or peptides prior to MS analysis, or the use of a label-free method such as ion intensities or spectral counts (Simpson et al., 2009). The modulation of the APPs HPT and SAA during mastitis have been evaluated in bovine milk using both a labeled (Danielsen et al., 2010) and a label-free approach (Boehmer et al., 2010). Despite different experimental approaches in the *in vivo* challenge portion of the studies, both proteomic analyses of mastitic bovine milk detected changes in the concentration of SAA and HPT in within hours after challenge. Following infection with LPS, nearly 3-fold changes were detected in both SAA and HPT in bovine milk as early as 7 h after induction of disease (Danielsen et al., 2010). Unlike previous ELISA analyses that were limited to the evaluation of only targeted APP, changes were likewise detected in the APPs serum albumin, alpha-2-macroglobulin, alpha-2-HS-glycoprotein, and serotransferrin in bovine milk during clinical mastitis using the incorporation of isotopic labels and proteomic identification strategies (Danielsen et al., 2010).

In the proteomic analyses of a longitudinal set of bovine milk samples collected over the course of clinical mastitis following intra-mammary infusion with Gram-negative *E. coli*, modulation in the APPs serum albumin, SAA, HPT, alpha-2-HS-glycoprotein, AGP, inter-alpha trypsin inhibitor heavy chain-4 (ITIH4), serotransferrin, apolipoprotein- A1, and the α-, β-, and γ-chains of fibrinogen, (Figure 1) were evaluated using spectral counts. The theory behind spectral counting, or the number of MS/MS spectra that contribute to the identification of a given protein, is that the abundant proteins, when proteolytically digested, will yield numerous copies of the same peptide (Zybailov et al., 2005; Liu et al., 2004). Furthermore, the probability that abundant peptides will trigger multiple MS/MS events is higher than the likelihood of repeatedly sampling a peptide from a lower abundance protein. In previous investigations into the accuracy and linearity of spectral counts, the spectral counts for peptides from proteins spiked into yeast samples at known concentrations exhibited linearity over two orders of magnitude, and were highly correlated to relative protein abundance (Liu et al., 2004).

Spectral counts were used to evaluate the expression of the APPs HPT and SAA in bovine milk over the course of clinical mastitis, and trends revealed by spectral counts were compared to quantification of the APPs using commercially available ELISAs (Figure 2). Though the comparison indicated slight advantages in the sensitivity of the ELISA to detect the presence of APPs in milk at earlier time points than MS, overall trends were similar. Furthermore, the fact that peptides from relatively low abundance acute phase proteins were detected in an extremely biologically complex matrix using LC-MS/MS supported the use of spectral counts to track changes in proteins for which no antibody or ELISA currently exists.

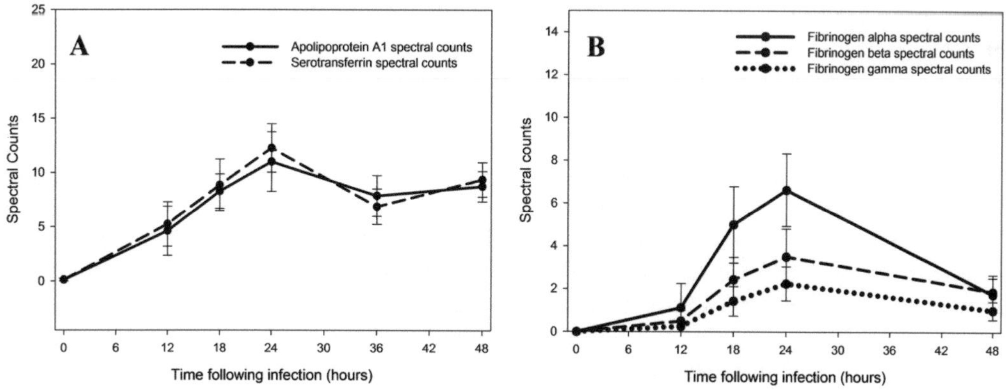

Fig. 1. Boehmer et al., 2010. Temporal expression patterns of proteins involved in the acute phase response following experimental induction of mastitis in bovine milk determined using total spectral counts (mean spectral counts ± standard error) for (A) apolipoprotein-A1 and serontransferrin, and (B) the three chains of the blood coagulation protein fibrinogen.

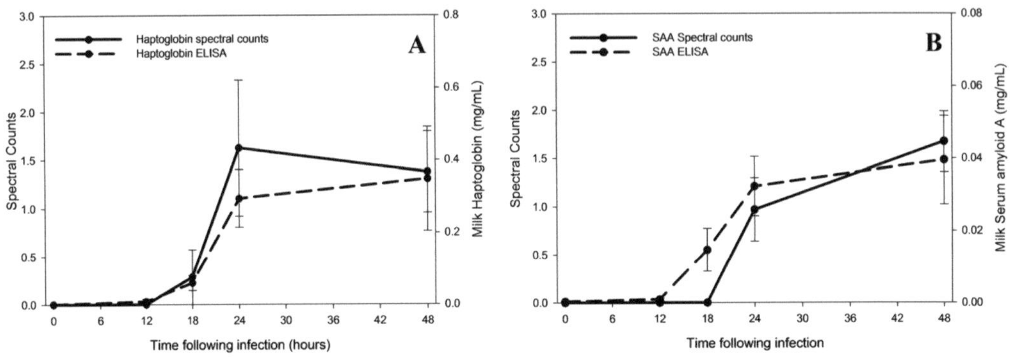

Fig. 2. Boehmer et al., 2010. Comparison of temporal expression patterns of low abundance acute phase proteins determined using ELISA and total spectral counts (mean spectral counts ± standard error) for (A) milk Haptoglobin and (B) milk serum amyloid A. Though sensitivity levels differ, the correspondence of the overall patterns exhibited by the LC-MS/MS data and the ELISA data indicates that spectral counts can be used as a screening tool to profile changes in biologically relevant proteins without a reliance on antibodies.

The added advantage of using proteomics to characterize APP expression during disease was the identification and characterization of the APP ITIH4, a potentially novel biomarker of coliform mastitis. Prior reports of ITIH4 in cattle were limited to isolation of the APP from the serum of heifers with experimentally induced summer mastitis (Pineiro et al., 2004). The association of ITIH4 with innate immunity has, however, been studied in models of acute inflammation in swine (Gonzalez-Ramon et al., 2000), and ITIH4 was recently reported to be a novel marker of acute ischemic stroke in humans (Kashyap et al., 2009). Previous research and similarity to a human homolog led to the classification of ITIH4 as a plasma kallikrein-sensitive glycoprotein, but the exact role and function of ITIH4 in the bovine mammary gland during inflammation associated with coliform mastitis is not yet clear (Nishimura et al., 1995).

As with any analytical method, drawbacks exist regarding the use of proteomic strategies to characterize proteins involved in the acute phase response during disease in livestock species. However, given the fact that the majority of previous reports of APP expression during mastitis and other food animal diseases have used data derived from ELISAs, and that there are only a limited number of commercially available antibodies for livestock species, proteomic strategies afford clear advantages over traditional methods for the detection and characterization of APP during animal disease. Additionally, proteomic strategies offer the opportunity to evaluate the post-translational modification of APP during disease, which could lead to the establishment of specific relationship between the modification of APP and select animal diseases.

5. Detection of the modification of acute phase proteins using proteomics

Modification of the glycosylation patterns of APPs has been implicated in a number of inflammatory diseases in humans and food animals (Gruys et al., 2005). Because post-translational modifications often dictate the biological activity of certain proteins, the characterization of glycosylation patterns of APPs during disease may advance current knowledge of the mechanisms involved in food animal disease, and aid in the development of new therapeutics. Glycosylation is the most diverse PTM involved in the modulation of protein function (Ohtsubo et al., 2006). Glycosylation is a site specific enzymatic process which covalently binds sugar moieties to proteins in two ways, either through linkage of polysaccharides to the amide nitrogen of asparagine side chains, or to the oxygen atoms of serine, threonin, or tyrosine, which forms N-linked or O-linked glycans, respectively. N-linked glycosylation modulates protein folding and stability through a variety of mechanisms, whereas O-linked glycosylation plays important roles in protein localization, trafficking, and solubility (Spiro 2002).

5.1 Post-translational modification of acute phase proteins during human disease

The majority of published reports detailing the proteomic analysis of the PTM of APPs have focused on the glycosylation pattern of serum proteins associated with human inflammatory diseases (Higai, et al., 2003; Brinkman-van der Linden et al., 1996; Turner et al., 1992), and different forms of cancer (Mazhar et al., 2006; Saldova,et al., 2007; Latif et al., 2002). Modification of the biantennary structures and the α1, 3 fucosylated N-glycan structures of alpha-1-acid-glycoprotein (AGP) have been reported in patients with acute inflammation (Turner et al., 1992), and chronic conditions such as rheumatoid arthritis and diabetes mellitus (Higai, et al., 2003). A remarkable feature of AGP is the microheterogeneity of its sugar moieties and the modification of these sugars during disease. AGP has five N-linked complex type glycans which may be present as bi-, tri-, and tetra-antenary structures (Gornik et al., 2008). Studies have indicated significant enhancement of bi-antennary complex glycans and alpha-1-3fucosylated bi-, tri-, and tetra-antennary glycans, as well as decreases in tri-antennary glycans of AGP, in patients with inflammatory diseases. However, the modifications of AGP in patients with diabetes were not disease-specific (Higai, et al., 2003).

Different forms of human cancer have likewise been associated with alterations in the glycosylation patterns of APPs. The most well characterized N-glycosylation changes in APPs have been studied in AGP. Modulation of glycan branching, which is the number of N-acetylglucosamine (GlcNAc) residues attached to the chitobiose core, and the levels of Sialyl Lewis X (SLex) structures has been reported (Van Dijk et al., 1994; Chandrasekaran et al., 1984,; Katnik et al., 1988). Lung cancer patients were reported to exhibit significant alterations in N-linked glycosylation in total blood serum (Arnold, et al., 2011). In contrast, decreases were observed in core-fucosylated biantennary glycans, with some being detectable as early as Stage I lung cancer. In the same study, the N-linked glycan profile of HPT revealed similar modifications to those detected in the total serum glycome (Arnold, et al., 2011). Specific HPT isoforms have also been evaluated in serum from patients with small cell lung cancer (Shah et al., 2010). The human form of HPT was reported to have only one type of beta subunit, but two different isoforms of its alpha subunit (Shah et al., 2010). Higher circulatory levels of alpha HPT were reported in patients with small cell lung cancer when compared to healthy control subjects. Additionally, a beta chain variant of HPT was discovered that appears to be differentially expressed only in small cell lung cancer patient serum (Shah et al., 2010). Changes in the glycosylation patterns of APPs have also been reported for ovarian cancer (Saldova et al., 2007). Reported findings indicated that the changes in glycosylation patterns of APPs associated with ovarian cancer involved doubling the amount of core fucosylated, galactosyl biantennary glycans and sialyl Lewis X.

5.2 Post-translational modification of acute phase proteins during animal disease

In veterinary research, differential expression and increased abundance of fucosylated peptides have been reported for lymphoma and transitional cell carcinoma (TCC) in dogs (Wilson et al., 2008). The progression of canine lymphoma was monitored during the course of disease, and it was discovered that the same fucosylated peptides that increased during the pre-chemotherapy period were reduced post-chemotherapy treatments. Additionally, the same peptides increased in abundance upon recurrence of the lymphoma. Furthermore, the comparison of all fucosylated peptides detected in lymphoma and TCC, revealed only two common peptides for the two different forms of cancer. The results of the study indicated the power of glycoproteomics in discriminating between fucosylation of specific glycopeptides in two different types of cancer in dogs (Wilson et al., 2008).

Modulation in the glycosylation of the APP HPT in serum from dogs with several diseases including anaemia, inflammation, lymphoma, and chronic progressive hepatitis has also been reported (Anderssen et al., 2001). Following pretreatment of serum with a fucose-specific lectin, abnormal microeterogeiety in the glycosylation pattern of HPT was detected using iso-electric focusing (IEF) and immunoblotting. The major modification of HPT was increased fucosylation, and was predominantly observed in dogs with anaemia, but also to a lesser extent in dogs with inflammation and lymphoma. Conversely, dogs with liver disease exhibited reduction of sialic acid residues in HPT (Andersson et al, 2001).

Similar to the PTM of HPT, glycosylation of AGP is also altered during animal diseases. During inflammation, increases in plasma concentrations of AGP, as well as many structural modifications including the glycoslyation pattern and the degree of branching and fucosylation of AGP have been reported (Ceceliani et al., 2007). The structure of the glycoprotein AGP has been analyzed in several species including cows, sheep and rats, with the results indicating that the glycosylation pattern of AGP was quite variable (Nakano et al., 2004). Using MALDI-TOF MS, it was determined that in sheep the mono- and disialodiantennary carbohydrate chains of AGP were elevated, while the abundance of tri- and tetra-sialo triantennary carbohydrate chains were decreased. Some novel carbohydrate chains containing both N-acetylneuraminic acid and N-glycolylneuraminic acid were observed in bovine AGP. No triantennary carbohydrate chains were detected in bovine AGP, however, elevated abundance of diantennary carbohydrate chains with tri- or tetra-sialyl residues were observed. In rats, a complex mixture of disialo carbohydrate chains of N, O-acetylneuraminic acids were detected on AGP (Nakano et al., 2004). The glycosylation pattern of AGP in cats was investigated in animals with feline immunodeficiency virus and feline leukemia virus. Increased sialylation of AGP was observed in cats with lymphoma; however, decreased sialylation of AGP was detected in animals with feline infectious peritonitis (Pocacqua et al., 2005; Ceciliani et al., 2004).

Due to complexity and the fact that low abundant N-glycosylated proteins or peptides exist in complex mixtures among a large excess of nonglycosylated counterparts, complete analysis of these markers in a clinical laboratory is still not feasible. In the research laboratory setting, enrichment methods including lectin-affinity chromatography or chemical linkage of the carbohydrate to surfaces are used to isolate glycosylated proteins from complex mixtures (Abbott, et al., 2010; Ito et al., 2009). However, peptide enrichment combined with proteomic strategies such as LC-MSMS is the latest technology for large-scale analysis of glycosylated proteins. In particular the use of fragmentation strategies including CID and ETD has shown to dramatically improve detection and characterization of the post-translational modification of glycoproteins (Alley et al., 2009 and Zielinska et al,

2010). All data available to date indicate that in both human and veterinary medical research, identification of APPs and characterization of the alteration in glycosylation patterns could provide valuable clinical information for use as specific biomarkers of many divergent diseases.

6. Conclusion

While results of comparative proteomic analyses conducted on biological samples collected from food animals during naturally-occurring and experimentally-induced disease have revealed promising candidate acute phase protein biomarkers and identified PTMs that are potentially disease specific, inherent roadblocks still exist that have precluded the validation of APPs as biomarkers of food animal disease. Caveats to proteomic strategies include the complexity of biological matrices, both before and during disease, the intense dynamic range of proteins present in most biological fluids, the lack of a universal analyses platform (i.e. the use of different instrument systems), as well as the intrinsic variability apparent across biological replicates during *in vivo* challenge models. Nonetheless, the data generated on APPs during recent comparative proteomic analyses of biological fluids collected from food animals is more comprehensive than information compiled from previous research, due in large part to the fact that LC-MS/MS methodologies allow for peptide identification and subsequent protein discovery without a reliance on antibody availability. Likewise, innovations in MS ion fragmentation strategies, including the use of ETD to elucidate modified amino acid residues, have advanced current capabilities to characterize post-translational modifications using MS, and show promise as a means to determine the specificity of APP as biomarkers of disease. Some attempts have been made to conduct comparative proteomic analyses of disease specific PTMs of APPs and glycopeptides for veterinary applications, but the specificity of APP modifications as biomarkers of disease is still an emerging area of research. Further development of sample preparation strategies designed to isolate glycoproteins and glycopeptides, coupled with advances in the capabilities of both LC and MS instrumentation to separate, detect, and characterize the post-translational modifications of APPs will undoubtedly broaden current knowledge of the role of APPs in inflammation, and aid in the establishment of APPs as specific biomarkers of disease.

7. References

Abbott, K.L.; & Pierce, J.M. (2010). Lectin-based glycoproteomic techniques for the enrichment and identification of potential biomarkers. *Methods Enzymology*, Vol.480, pp.461-476.

Alley, W.R.; Mechref, Y.; & Novotny, M.V. (2009). Characterization of glycopeptides by combining collision-induced dissociation and electron-transfer dissociation mass spectrometry data. *Rapid Communication of Mass Spectrometry*, Vol 23, pp.161-170.

Amory, J.R.; Mackenzie, A.M.; Eckersall, P.D.; Stear, M.J.; & Pearce G.P. (2007). Influence of rearing conditions and respiratory disease on haptoglobin levels in the pig at slaughter. *Research in Veterinary Science*, Vol 83, No.3, pp.428-35.

Andersson, M.; & Sevelius, E. (2001). Abnormal microheterogeneity of haptoglobin in serum from dogs with various diseases. *Veterinary Record,* Vol 48, pp.14-17.

Arnold, J.N.; Saldova, R.; Galligan, M.C.; Murphy, T.B.; Mimura-Kimura, Y.; Telford, J.E.; Godwin, A.K.; & Rudd, P.M. (2011). Novel Glycan Biomarkers for the Detection of Lung Cancer. *Journal of Proteome Research,* Article ASAP, Jan 7.

Bannerman, D.D.; Paape, M.J.; Lee, J.W.; Zhao, X.; Hope, J.C.; & Rainard, P. (2004). Escherichia coli and Staphylococcus aureus elicit differential innate immune responses following intramammary infection. *Clinical and Diagnostic Laboratory Immunology,* Vol 11, No.3, pp.463-72.

Bannerman, D.D.; Paape, M.J.; Hare, W.R.; & Sohn, E.J. (2003). Increased levels of LPS-binding protein in bovine blood and milk following bacterial lipopolysaccharide challenge. *Journal of Dairy Science,* Vol 86, pp.3128-3137.

Bell, L.N.; Lee, L.; Saxena, R.; Bemis, K.G,, Wang, M.; Theodorakis, J.L.; Vuppalanchi, R.; Alloosh, M.; Sturek, M.; & Chalasani, N. (2010). Serum proteomic analysis of diet-induced steatohepatitis and metabolic syndrome in the Ossabaw miniature swine. *American Journal of Physiology Gastrointestinal Liver Physiology,* Vol 298, pp.G746–G754.

Bendixen, E.; Danielsen, M.; Hollung, K.; Gianazza, E.; & Miller, I. (2011). Farm animal proteomics- A review. *Journal of Proteomics,* Vol 74, pp.282-293.

Boehmer, J.L.; DeGrasse, J.A.; McFarland, M.A.; Tall, E.A.; Shefcheck, K.J.; Ward, J.L.; & Bannerman, D.D. (2010). The proteomics advantage: label-free quantification of proteins expressed in bovine milk during experimentally induced coliform mastitis. *Veterinary Immunology and Immunopathology,* Vol 138, No.4, pp.252-266.

Brinkman-van der Linden, E.C., van Ommen, E.C.; &Van Dijk, W. (1996). Glycosylation of alpha 1-acid glycoprotein in septic shock: changes in degree of branching and in expression of sialyl Lewis(x) groups. *Glycoconjugate Journal,* Vol 13, pp.27–31.

Ceceliani, F.; & Pocacqua, V. (2007). The acute phase protein 1-Acid Glycoprotein: A model for altered glycosylation during diseases. *Current Protein and Peptide Science,* Vol 8, pp.91-108.

Ceciliani, F.; Pocacqua, V.; Provasi, E.; Comunian, C.; Bertolini, A.; Bronzo, V.; Moroni, P.; & Sartorelli, P. (2005). Identification of the bovine alpha1-acid glycoprotein in colostrum and milk. *Veterinary Research,* Vol 36, pp.735-746.

Ceciliani, F.; Grossi, C.; Giordano, A.; Pocacqua, V.; Paltrinieri, S. (2004). Decreased sialylation of the acute phase protein a1-acid glycoprotein in feline infectious peritonitis (FIP). *Veterinary Immunology and Immunopathology,* Vol 99, pp.229–236.

Chan, J.P.; Chang, C.C.; Hsu, W.L.; Liu, W.B.; & Chen, T.H. (2010). Association of increased serum acute-phase protein concentrations with reproductive performance in dairy cows with postpartum metritis. *Veterinary Clinical Pathology,* Vol 39, No.1, pp.72-78.

Chandrasekaran, E.V.; Davila, M.; Nixon, D.; & Mendicino, J. (1984). Structures of the oligosaccharide chains of two forms of crl-acid glycoprotein from liver metastasis of lung colon and breast tumours. *Cancer Research,* Vol 44, pp.1557-1567.

Colantonio, D.A.; & Chan, D.W. (2005). The clinical application of proteomics. *Clinica.Chimica.Acata,* Vol 357, pp.151-158.

Danielsen, M.; Codrea, M.C.; Ingvartsen, K.L.; Friggens, N.C.; Bendixen, E.; & Røntved, C.M. (2010). Quantitative milk proteomics--host responses to lipopolysaccharide-mediated inflammation of bovine mammary gland. *Proteomics,* Vol 10, No.12, pp.2240-2249.

Danielsen, M.; Hornshoj, H.; Siggers, R.H.; Jensen, B.B.; van Kessel, A.G.; & Bendixen, E. (2007). Effects of bacterial colonization on the porcine intestinal proteome. *Journal of Proteome Research,* Vol 6, pp.2596–2604.

Danielsen M., Thymann T., Jensen B.B., Jensen O.N., Sangild P.T., & Bendixen E. (2006). Proteome profiles of mucosal immunoglobulin uptake in inflamed porcine gut. *Proteomics,* Vol 6, pp.6588–6596.

Eckersall, P.D; & Bell, R. (2010). Acute phase proteins: Biomarkers of infection and inflammation in veterinary medicine. *The Veterinary Journal,* Vol 185, pp.23-27.

Eckersall, P.D.; Lawson, F.P.; Bence, L.; Waterston, M.M.; Lang, T.L.; Donachie, W.; & Fontaine, M.C. (2007). Acute phase protein response in an experimental model of ovine caseous lymphadenitis. *BioMed Central Veterinary Research,* Vol 19, No.3, pp.35-40.

Eckersall, P.D.; Young, F.J.; Nolan, A.M.; Knight, C.H.; McComb, C.; Waterston, M.M.; Hogarth, C.J.; Scott, E.M.; & Fitzpatrick, J.L. (2006). Acute phase proteins in bovine milk in an experimental model of Staphylococcus aureus subclinical mastitis. *Journal of Dairy Science,* Vol 89, No.5, pp.1488-1501.

Eckersall, P.D.; Young, F.J.; McComb, C.; Hogarth, C.J.; Safi, S.; Weber, A.; McDonald, T.; Nolan, A.M.; &Fitzpatrick, J.L. (2001). Acute phase proteins in serum and milk from dairy cows with clinical mastitis. *Veterinary Record,* Vol 148, pp.35-41.

Eckersall, P.D.; Saini, P.K.; & McComb, C. (1996). The acute phase response of acid soluble glycoprotein, α_1-acid glycoprotein, ceruloplasmin, haptoglobin, and C-reactive protein, in the pig. *Veterinary Immunology and Immunopathology,* Vol 51, pp. 377-385.

Fenselau, C. (2007). A review of quantitative methods for proteomic studies. *Journal of Chromatography B.,* Vol 855, pp.14-20.

Ferguson, L.P.; & Smith, R.D. (2003). Proteome analysis by mass spectrometry. *Annual Review of Biophysics and Biomolecular Structure,* Vol 32, pp.399-424.

González, F.H.D.; tecles, F.; Martínez-Subiela, S.; Tvarijonaviciute, A.; Soler, L.; & Cerón, J.J. (2008). Acute phase protein response in goats. *Journal of Veterinary Diagnostic Investigation,* Vol 20, pp. 580-584.

Gonzalez-Ramon, N.; Hoebe, K.; Alava, M.A.; van Leengoed, L.; Pineiro, M.; Carmona, S.; Iturralde, M.; Lampreave, F.; & Pineiro, A. (2000). Pig MAP/ITIH4 and haptoglobin are interleukin-6-dependent acute-phase plasma proteins in porcine primary cultured hepatocytes. *European Journal of Biochemistry,* Vol 267, No.6, pp.1878-1885.

Gornik, O.&Lauc, G. (2008). Glycosylation of serum proteins in inflammatory disease. *Disease Markers,* Vol 25, pp.267-278.

Griffin, T.J.; Gygi, S.P.; Ideker, T.; Rist, B.; Eng, J.; Hood, L.; &Aebersold, R. (2002). Complementary profiling of gene expression at the transcriptome and proteome levels in Saccharomyces cerevisiae. *Molecular and Cellular Proteomics,* Vol 1, pp.323-333.

Grönlund, U.; Hultén, C.; Eckersall, P.D.; Hogarth, C.; Persson Waller, K. (2003). Haptoglobin and serum amyloid A in milk and serum during acute and chronic experimentally induced Staphylococcus aureus mastitis. *Journal of Dairy Research,* Vol 70, No.4, pp.379-386.

Grönlund, U.; Hallén, C.; Sandgren C.; & Persson Waller, K. (2005). Haptoglobin and serum amyloid A in milk from dairy cows with chronic sub-clinical mastitis. *Veterinary Research,* Vol 36, No.2, pp.191-198.

Gruys, E.; Toussaint, M.J.M.; Niewold, T.A.; & Kooplmans, S.J. (2005). Review: Acute phase reaction and acute phase proteins. *Journal of Zhejiang University-SCIENCE B.*, Vol 6, pp.1045–1056.

Gygi, S.P.; Rist, B.; Gerber, S.A.; Turecek, F.; Gelb, M.H.; & Aebersold, R. (1999). Quantitative analysis of complex protein mixtures using isotope-coded affinity tags. *Nature Biotechnology*, Vol 17, pp.994-999.

Heegaard, P.M.; Godson, D.L.; Toussaint, M.J.M.; Tjørnehøj, K.; Larsen, L.E.; Viuff, B.; & Rønsholt, L. (2000). The acute phase response of haptoglobin and serum amyloid A (SAA) in cattle undergoing experimental infection with bovine respiratory syncytial virus. *Veterinary Immunology and Immunopathology*, Vol 77, pp. 151-159.

Heegaard, P.M.; Klausen, J.; Nielsen, J.P.; González-Ramon, N.; Pineiro, M.; Lampreave, F.; & Alava, M.A. (1998). The porcine acute phase response to infection with Actinobaccilus pleuropneumonia. Haptoglobin, C-reactive protein, major acute phase protein and serum amyloid A protein are sensitive indicators of infection. *Comparative Biochemistry and Physiology B- Biochemistry & Molecular Biology*, Vol 119, No. 2, pp. 365-373.

Higai, K.; Azuma, Y.; Aoki, Y, & Matsumoto, K. (2003). Altered glycosylation of alpha1-acid glycoprotein in patients with inflammation and diabetes mellitus. *Clinical Chimica Acta*, Vol 329, pp.117–125.

Hirvonen J, Eklund K, Teppo AM, Huszenicza G, Kulcsar M, Saloniemi H, Pyörälä S. (1999). Acute phase response in dairy cows with experimentally induced Escherichia coli mastitis. *Acta Veterinaria Scandinavica*, Vol 40, No.1, pp.35-46.

Hiss, S.; Mueller, U.; Neu-Zahren, A.; & Sauerwein, H. (2007). Haptoglobin and lactate dehydrogenase measurements in milk for the identification of subclinically diseased udder quarters. *Veterinarni Medicina*, Vol 52, No.6, pp.245-252.

Hiss, S.; Mielenz, M.; Bruckmaier, M.; &Sauerwein, H. (2004). Haptoglobin concentrations in blood and milk after endotoxin challenge and quantification of mammary Hp mRNA expression. *Journal of Dairy Science*, Vol 87, pp.3778-3784.

Hogarth, C.J.; Fitzpatrick, J.L.; Nolan, A.M.; Young, F.J.; Pitt, A.; & Eckersall, P.D. (2004). Differential protein composition of bovine whey: A comparison of whey from healthy animals and from those with clinical mastitis. *Proteomics*, Vol 4, No.7, pp.2094-2100.

Horadogoda, N.U; Knox, K.M.G.; Gibbs, H.A.; Reid, S.W.J.; Horadagoda, A.; Edwards, S.E.R.; & Eckersall, P.D. (1999). Acute phase proteins in cattle: discrimination between acute and chronic inflammation. *The Veterinary Record*, Vol 144, pp.437-441.

Horadagoda, A.; Eckersall, P.D.; Hodgson, J.C.; Gibbs, H.A.; & Moon, G.M. (1994). Immediate responses in serum TNF alpha and acute phase protein concentrations to infection with Pasteurella haemolytica A1 in calves. *Research in Veterinary Science*, Vol 57, No.1, pp.129-132.

Hultén, C.; Johansson, E.; Fossum, C.; & Wallgren, P. (2003). Interleukin 6, serum amyloid A and haptoglobin as markers of treatment efficacy in pigs experimentally infected with *Actinobacillus pleuropneumoniae*. *Veterinary Microbiology*, Vol 95, pp. 75-89.

Ideker, T.; Thorsson, V.; Ranish, J.A.; Christmas, R.; Buhler, J.; Eng, J.K.; Bumgarner, R.; Goodlett, D.R.; Aebersold, R.; & Hood, L. (2001). Integrated genomic and proteomic analyses of a systematically perturbed metabolic network. *Science,* Vol 255, pp.929-934.

Ito,S.; Hayama, K.; & Hirabayashi, J. (2009). Enrichment Strategies for Glycopeptides. *Methods in Molecular Biology,* Vol 534, pp.1-10.

Jacobsen, S.; Niewold, T.A.; Kornalijnslijper, E.; Toussaint, M.J.; & Gruys, E. (2005). Kinetics of local and systemic isoforms of serum amyloid A in bovine mastitic milk. *Veterinary Immunology and Immunopathology,* Vol 104, pp.21-31.

Jensen, O.N.; Wilm, M.; Shevchenko, A.; & Mann, M. (1999). Sample preparation methods for mass spectrometry peptide mapping directly from 2-DE gels. *Methods in Molecular Biology,* Vol 112, pp.513-530.

Karas, M.; & Krüger, R. (2003). Ion formation in MALDI: the cluster ionization method. *Chemical Reviews,* Vol 103, pp.427-440.

Kashyap, R.S.; Nayak, A.R.; Deshpande, P.S.; Kabra, D.; Purohit, H.J.; Taori, G.M.; & Daginawala, H.F. (2009). Inter-α-trypsin inhibitor heavy chain 4 is a novel marker of acute ischemic stroke. *Clinical Chimica Acta,* Vol 402, pp.160-163.

Katnik, I.; Gerber, J.; Dobryszycka, W. (1988). Microheterogeneity of olt-acid glycoprotein in the sera of patients with cancer or inflammatory states of the ovaries. *Archivum Immunologiae et Therapiae Experimentalis,* Vol 136, pp.1-6.

Kaufmann, R.; Kirsch, D.& Spengler, B. (1994). Sequencing of peptides in a time-of-flight MS: Evaluation of post source decay following matrix-assisted laser desorption ionization (MALDI). *International Journal of Mass Spectrometry and Ion Processes,* Vol 131, pp.355–385.

Larsen, M.A.; Weber, A.; Weber, A.T.; & McDonald, T.L. (2006). Differential expression and secretion of bovine serum amyloid A3 (SAA3) by mammary epithelial cells stimulated with prolactin or lipopolysaccharide. *Veterinary Immunology and Immunopathology,* Vol 107, pp.255-264.

Latif Z.; McMillan D.C.; Wallace A.M.; Sattar N.; Mir K.; Jones G.; & Underwood M.A. (2002). The relationship of circulating insulin-like growth factor 1, its binding protein-3, prostate specific antigen and C reactive protein with disease stage in prostate cancer. *British Journal of Urology International,* Vol 89, pp.396-399.

Liu, H.; Sadygov, R.G.; & Yates, J.R.III. (2004). A model for random sampling and estimation of relative protein abundance in shotgun proteomics. *Analytical Chemistry,* Vol 76, No.14, pp.4193–4201.

Mann, M.; Hendrickson, R.C.; & Pandey, A. (2001). Analysis of proteins and proteomes by mass spectrometry. *Annual Review of Biochemistry,* Vol 70, pp.437-473.

Mazhar, D.; & Ngan, S. (2006). C-reactive protein and colorectal cancer. *Quarterly Journal of Medicine,* Vol 99, pp.555-559.

Miller, I.; Wait, R.; Sipos, W.; & Gemeiner, M.A. (2009). Proteomic reference map for pig serum proteins as a prerequisite for diagnostic applications. *Research in Veterinary Science,* Vol 86, pp.362–367.

Mitchell, G.B.; Clark, M.E.; & Caswell, J.L. (2007). Alterations in the bovine bronchoalveolar lavageproteome induced by dexamethasone. *Veterinary Immunology and Immunopathology,* Vol 118, pp.283–293.

Mitchell, G.B.; Clark, M.E.; Siwicky, M.; & Caswell, J.L. (2008). Stress alters the cellular and proteomic compartments of bovine bronchoalveolar lavage fluid. *Veterinary Immunology and Immunopathology,* Vol 125, pp.111–125.

Mueller, L.N.; Brusniak, M-Y.; Mani, D.R.; & Aebersold, R. (2008). An assessment of software solutions for the analysis of mass spectrometry based quantitative proteomics data. *Journal of Proteome Research,* Vol 7, No.1, pp.51-61.

Murata, H.; Shimada, N.; & Yoshioka, M. (2004). Current research on acute phase proteins in veterinary diagnostics: an overview. *The Veterinary Journal,* Vol 168, pp.28-40.

Nakano, M.; Kakehil, N.; Tsai, M-H.; & Lee, Y.C. (2004). Detailed structural features of glycan chains derived from alpha1-acid glycoproteins of several different animals: the presence of hypersialylated, O-acetylated sialic acids but not disialyl residues. *Glycobiology,* Vol 14, pp.431-441.

Nazifi, S.; tabande, M.R.; Hosseinian, S.A.; Ansari-Lari, M.; & Safari, H. (2011). Evaluation of sialic acid and acute phase proteins (haptoglobin and serum amyloid A) in healthy and avian infection bronchitis virus-infected chicks. *Comparative Clinical Pathology,* Vol 20, pp. 69-73.

Nishimura, T. (2003). Expression of potential lymphocytes trafficking mediator molecules in the mammary gland. *Veterinary Research,* Vol 34, pp.3-10.

Ohtsubo, K.& Marth,J.D. (2006). Glycosylation in cellular mechanisms of health and disease. *Cell1,* Vol 26, pp.855–867.

Orro, T.; Pohjanvirta, T.; Rikula, U.; Huovilainen, A.; Alasuutari, S.; Sihvonen, L.; Pelkonen, S.; & Soveri, T. (2011). Acute phase protein changes in calves during an outbreak of respiratory disease by bovine respiratory syncytial virus. *Comparative Immunology, Microbiology and Infectious Diseases,* Vol 24, pp. 23-29.

Petersen, H.H.; Nielsen, J.P.; & Heegaard, P.M.H. (2004). Application of acute phase protein measurements in veterinary clinical chemistry. *Veterinary Research,* Vol 35, pp.163-187.

Pineiro, M.; Andres, M.; Iturralde, M.; Carmona, S.; Hirvonen, J.; Pyorala, S.; Heegard, P.M.H.; Tjornehoj, K.; Lampreave, F.; Pineiro, A.; & Alava, M.A. (2004). ITIH4 (Inter-alpha-trypsin inhibitor heavy chain 4) is a new acute-phase potein isolated from cattle during experimental infection. *Infection and Immunity,* Vol 72, No.7, pp.3777-3782.

Pocacqua, V.; Provasi, E.Paltrinieri,S.Gelain, E.; Comunian, C.; & Ceciliani, F. (2005). Glycan moiety modifications of feline a1-acid glycoprotein in retrovirus (FIV, FeLV) affected cats. *Veterinary Immunology and Immunopathology,* Vol 107, pp.17–26.

Rahman, M.M.; Miranda-Ribera, A.; Lecchi, C.; Bronzo, V.; Sartorelli, P.; Franciosi, F.; & Ceciliani, F. (2008). Alpha-1-acid glycoprotein is contained in bovine neutrophil granules and released after activation. *Veterinary Immunology and Immunopathology,* Vol 125, pp.71-81.

Roe, M.R.; &Griffin, T.J. (2006). Gel-free mass spectrometry-based high throughput proteomics: tools for studying biological response of proteins and proteomes. *Proteomics,* Vol 6, pp.4678-4687.

Safi, S.; Khoshvaghti, A.; Jafarzadeh, S.R.; Bolourchi, M.; & Nowrouzian, I. (2009). Acute phase proteins in the diagnosis of bovine subclinical mastitis. *Veterinary Clinical Pathology,* Vol 38, No.4, pp.471-476.

Saldova R.; Royle L.; Radcliffe C.M.; Abd Hamid U.M.; Evans R.; Arnold J.N.; Banks R.E.; Hutson R.; Harvey D.J.Antrobus R.; Petrescu S.M.; Dwek R.A.; & Rudd P.M. (2007). Ovarian cancer is associated with changes in glycosylation in both acute-phase proteins and IgG. *Glycobiology,* Vol 17, pp.1344-1356.

Simpson, K.; Whetton, A.D.; & Dive, C. (2009). Quantitative mass spectrometry-based techniques for clinical use: biomarker identification and quantification. *Journal of Chromatography B.,* Vol 877, No.13, pp.1240-1249.

Smolenski, G.; Haines, S.; Y.-S.Kwan, F.; Bond, J.; Farr, V.; Davis, S.R.; Stelwagen, K.; & Wheeler, T.T. (2007). Characterization of host defense proteins in milk using a proteomic approach. *Journal of Proteome Research,* Vol 6, No.1, pp.207-215.

Sorensen, N.S.; Tegtmeier, C.; Andresen, L.O.; Pineiro, M.; Toussaint, M.J.M.; Campbell, F.M.; Lampreave, F.; & Heegaard, P.M.H. (2006). The porcine acute phase response to acute clinical and subclinical infection with Streptococcus suis. *Veterinary Immunology and Immunopathology,* Vol 113, pp. 157-168.

Spiro, R.G. (2002). Protein glycosylation: nature, distribution, enzymatic formation, and disease implications of glycopeptide bonds. *Glycobiology,* Vol 12, pp.43R-56R.

Suojala, L.; Orro, T.; Järvinen, H.; Saatsi, J.; & Pyörälä, S. (2008). Acute phase response in two consecutive experimentally induced E.coli intramammary infection in dairy cows. *Acta Veterinaria Scandinavica,* Vol 50, No.1, pp.18- 27.

Syka, J.E.; Coon J.J.; Schroeder, M.J.; Shabanowitz, J.; & Hunt, D.F. (2004). Peptide and protein sequence analysis by electron transfer dissociation mass spectrometry. *Proceedings of the National Academy of Science,* Vol 101, pp.9528–9533.

Talamo, F.; D'Ambrosio, C.; Arena, S.; Del Vecchio, P.; Ledda, L.; Zehender, G.; Ferrara, L.; & Scaloni A. (2003). Proteins from bovine tissues and biological fluids: defining a reference electrophoresis map for liver, kidney, muscle, plasma and red blood cells. *Proteomics,* Vol 3, pp.440–460.

Tian, Q.; Stephaniants, S.B.; Mao, M.; Weng, L.; Feetham, M.C.; Doyle, M.J.; Yi, E.C.; Dai, H.; Thorsson, V.; Eng, J.; Goodlett, D.; Berger, J.P.; Gunter, B.; Linseley, P.S.; Stoughton, R.B.; Aebersold, R.; Collins, S.J.; Hanlon, W.A.; & Hood, L.E. (2004). Integrated genomic and proteomic analyses of gene expression in mammalian cells. *Molecular Cell Proteomics,* Vol 3, pp. 960-969.

Thongboonkerd, V.; Chiangjong, W.; Mares, J.; Moravec, J.; Tuma, Z.; Karvunidis, T.; Sinchaikul, S.; Chen, S.T.; Opatrný, K.; & Matejovic, M. (2009). Altered plasma proteome during an early phase of peritonitis-induced sepsis. *Clinical Science,* Vol 116, pp.721–730.

Turner, G.A. (1992). N-glycosylation of serum proteins in disease and its investigation using lectings. *Clinical Chimica Acta,* Vol 208, pp.149-171.

Van den Bergh, G.; & Arckens, L. (2005). Recent advances in 2D electrophoresis: an array of possibilities. *Expert Review of Proteomics,* Vol 2, pp.243-252.

Van Dijk, W.; Turner, G.A.; & Mackiewicz, A. (1994). Changes in glycosylation of acute-phase proteins in health and disease: occurrence, regulation and function. *Glycosylation & Disease,* Vol 1, pp.5-14.

Thongboonkerd, V.; Chiangjong, W.; Mares, J.; Moravec, J.; Tuma, Z.; Karvunidis, T.; Sinchaikul, S.; Chen, S.T.; Opatrný, K.; & Matejovic, M. (2002). Strategies for proteomics with incompletely characterized genomes: The proteome of Bos taurus serum. *Electrophoresis,* Vol 23, No.19, pp.3418–3427.

Wang, D.; Hincapie, M.; Rejtar, T.; & Karger, B.L. (2011). Ultrasensitive characterization of site-specific glycosylation of affinity-purified haptoglobin from lung cancer patient plasma using 10 μm i.d.porous layer open tubular liquid chromatography-linear ion trap collision-induced dissociation/electron transfer dissociation mass spectrometry. *Analytical Chemistry,* Vol 83, No.6, pp.2029-2037.

Wang X, Ou D, Yin J, Wu G, & Wang J. (2009). Proteomic analysis reveals altered expression of proteins related to glutathione metabolism and apoptosis in the small intestine of zinc oxide-supplemented piglets. *Amino Acids,* Vol 37, pp.209–218.

Washburn, M.P.; Wolters, D.; & Yates, J. (2001). Large-scale analysis of the yeast proteome by multidimensional protein identification technology. *Nature Biotechnology,* Vol 19, pp.242-247.

Wilm, M.; & Mann, M. (1996). Analytical properties of the nanoelectrospray ion source. *Analytical Chemistry,* Vol 68, pp.1-8.

Wilson, C.R.; Regnier, F.E.; Knapp, D.W.; Raskin, R.E.; Andrews.D.A.; & Hooser, S.B. (2008). Glycoproteomic profiling of serum peptides in canine lymphoma and transitional cell carcinoma. *Veterinary and Comparative Oncology,* Vol 6, No.3, pp.171-181.

Yang, Y.X.; Zhao, X.X.; & Zhang, Y. (2009). Proteomic analysis of mammary tissues from healthy cows and clinical mastitic cows for identification of disease-related proteins. *Veterinary Research Communications,* Vol 33, pp.295–303.

Zielinska, D.; Gnad, F.; Wisniewski, J.; & Mann, M. (2010). Precision Mapping of an In Vivo N-Glycoproteome Reveals Rigid Topological and Sequence Constraints. *Cell,* Vol 141, pp.897-907.

10

Acute Phase Proteins in Dairy Cows and Sows During the Peripartурient Period

Gabriel Kováč, Csilla Tóthová,
Oskar Nagy and Herbert Seidel
University of Veterinary Medicine and Pharmacy in Košice
Slovak Republic

1. Introduction

Acute phase proteins have been used as biomarkers of diseases for decades in human medicine, but have been relatively under-utilised in the veterinary medicine. Over recent years, significant progress has been made in studies on acute phase response in farm animal medicine, including the detection, measurement and application of acute phase proteins as biomarkers of diseases in both cattle and pigs. Acute phase proteins are blood proteins primarily synthesized by hepatocytes as part of the acute phase response. The acute phase response is a complex systemic early-defense system activated by impaired homeostasis, trauma, tissue injury, infection, inflammation, stress or neoplasia (Cray et al., 2009). This response leads to a range of metabolic activities and alterations in a wide variety of biochemical processes. One of the most important metabolic changes during the acute phase response is the strongly increased or decreased production and secretion of some plasma proteins from the liver, the acute phase proteins (Murata et al., 2004). Although non-specific, the acute phase response serves as a core of the innate immune reactions involving physical and molecular barriers and responses with the goal to prevent infection, clear potential pathogens, and contribute to the resolution and healing processes (Petersen et al., 2004).

Much of the recent attention on the assessment of acute phase proteins in farm animals has resulted not only from the advances described above, but also because they have been recognized as valuable markers of diseases. As indicators of inflammation, the assays of acute phase proteins provide valuable additional information to more traditional haematological and biochemical investigations (Skinner et al., 1991; Eckersall, 2000). Application of acute phase protein analyses in disease investigations also in farm animals has shown that it has a major diagnostic contribution to make in the evaluation of various inflammatory, as well as non-inflammatory diseases (Gruys et al., 2005). In the clinical field, acute phase proteins may serve as non-specific indicators of health status and surveillance of animals at the herd level. In the last decade, emphasis has been laid also on the application of blood test for acute phase reactants to monitor animals suffering from specified classes of diseases. However, the behavior of acute phase proteins in some disease, as well as physiological conditions, e.g. during the reproduction cycle of cows and sows, particularly around the parturition, still remain to be uncovered. Moreover, the pathophysiology of the changes in the concentrations of acute phase proteins in relation to some metabolic and biochemical reactions, as well as the relationships between immune functions and metabolic adaptations during some disease and physiological conditions are less well documented. These conditions involve e.g. changes in the concentrations of acute phase proteins in relation to altered metabolism, especially energetic metabolism in dairy cows around the parturition.

2. Acute phase proteins in farm animals

Animals undergoing external or internal challenge to their state of health manifest a vigorous response including activation of both the innate and acquired immune systems. The natural immunity is phylogenetic older, and is characterized by uniform nature to any intruder, and by immediate response (Janeway et al., 2001). The mechanisms of natural immunity defend an organism since the very first second of a danger. The defence mechanisms of innate immunity are numerous; the acute phase response belongs to those of the most important (Murata et al., 2004). It is designed to hold the infection in check until the adaptive, highly specialized immune response is initiated, which is followed by repairing processes terminating the episode of inflammation bringing the organism back to its physiological state (Baumann & Gauldie, 1994).

The varied reactions of the host to disturbances in its homeostasis caused by infection, tissue injury, trauma or surgery, neoplastic growth or immunological disorders are collectively known as the acute phase response, and encompass a wide range of pathophysiological responses (Johnson, 1997; Gruys et al., 1999) (Fig. 1). At the site of invasion by microorganisms and at the place of tissue injury, a number of responses of the tissue itself are initiated (Koj, 1996; Cray et al., 2009). Pro-inflammatory cytokines are released, subsequently, to activation of the immune and the vascular systems (Bellomo, 1992; Gruys et al., 2005). Another systemic response to injury is an increase or decrease in the production of a number of plasma proteins produced by the liver, which are known as acute phase proteins (Whicher & Westacott, 1992). These biomarkers are highly sensitive indicators of inflammation, but there are major differences among species in their acute phase response (Pyörälä, 2000). As described by Eckersall & Bell (2010), haptoglobin and serum amyloid A are the diagnostically most valuable acute phase proteins in cattle. In the pig, C-reactive protein, haptoglobin, and α_1-acid glycoprotein were identified as the major acute phase proteins (Du Clos, 2004).

Acute phase proteins might be applied as non-specific markers of clinical infections, and for prognostic purposes (Lauritzen et al., 2003). Measurement of acute phase proteins can detect or confirm the presence of infection or pathological lesion, but a major role for these analytes could be in the monitoring of the health status of animals in the production. Acute phase proteins can detect the presence of sub-clinical diseases, which are the cause of reduced growth rate and lost production (Eckersall, 2000). In the pig production system, health status is usually accepted that individuals are infectious agents-free. However, the pigs might be frequently infected leading to poor health despite high health declarations that may cause suboptimal growth and decreased welfare (Toussaint et al., 2000). Acute phase protein testing offers a tool for assessing health estimation based on the extent of inflammation and tissue damage (Petersen et al., 2004).

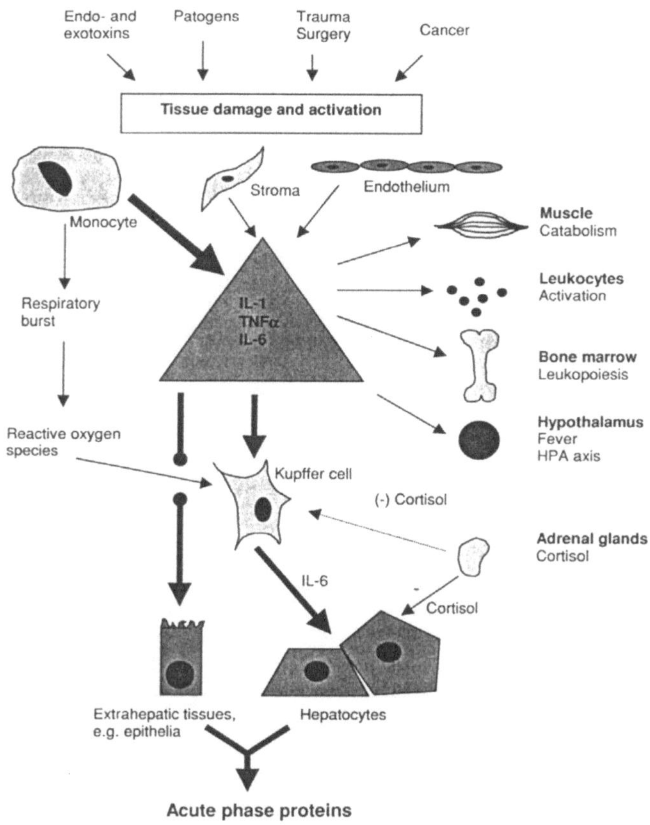

Fig. 1. The acute phase response (Jacobsen, 2003)

3. Acute phase proteins and the period after parturition in dairy cows

The period after parturition is the most critical period in dairy cows regarding health status and production. Factors such as pregnancy, parturition, blood calcium concentrations, initiation of lactation and feed intake all affect the ability of the cow's immune system to efficiently combat infections. The periparturient period is the time where complex physiological changes occur simultaneously, having a significant effect on the animal's health (Cai et al., 1994; Lippolis, 2008). Parturition, changes in homeostasis, metabolic and physiological challenges occuring in this stressful period, as well as other external and internal harmful stimuli may contribute to the activation of host immune system and inflammatory responses, including the initiation of the production of acute phase proteins.

Acute phase proteins have various activities by which contribute to germs destruction, to reduce tissue damage and help its regeneration (Pyörälä, 2000). Major bovine acute phase proteins, haptoglobin and serum amyloid A, play an important role also in the reproductive processes, they intensify the phagocytosis process against the pathogens introduced into the uterus, and help by the reconstruction of the endometrium (Regassa & Noakes, 1999; Krakowski & Zdzisińska, 2007).

Moreover, the transition of pregnancy to lactation, with the concomitant negative energy balance during early lactation, requires substantial adaptation of the cow, including metabolic and physiological adaptations, and is accompanied by changes in whole metabolism (Hachenberg et al., 2007; Leroy et al., 2008). It has been described in human medicine that physiological reactions around parturition, as well as metabolic changes are known to trigger several key events that can initiate and promote uncontrolled systemic inflammation (Gatzka et al., 2002; Sordillo et al., 2009). Yaqoob & Calder (2007) reported that in humans, altered lipid metabolism, increased circulating concentrations of non-esterified fatty acids and oxidative stress are factors that significantly contribute to both systemic inflammation and development of inflammatory-dependent diseases. Dairy cows undergo similar metabolic adaptations and changes in homeostasis after parturition. However, the pathophysiology of the aforementioned metabolic events and changes in immune functions are less clear.

4. Acute phase proteins in relation to the reproduction cycle of sows

Reproductive state and parity are important factors influencing most of the biochemical parameters of sows (Reese et al., 1984). In general, the time around parturition is the most challenging period of the reproduction cycle. Nutritional and metabolic stress around parturition is an increasingly important phenomenon because during this period the physiological balance of the animal is challenged. These phenomena and underlying mechanisms can be reflected in several endocrinological, immunological and biochemical parameters. Moreover, animals may react to disturbances in their homeostasis not only with systemic reactions, but also with increased production of acute phase proteins (Marnell et al., 2005).

In sows, there are very scarce data about the changes in the concentrations of acute phase proteins in connection to the reproduction cycle. It has been described in humans that the concentrations of most of the acute phase proteins do not change during pregnancy, but increase at parturition (Berkova et al., 2001). It is important to realize that physiologically, acute phase proteins may react at parturition also in animals (Alsemgeest et al., 1993). The time around parturition and its metabolic challenges constitute a potentially stressful period, if stress is defined as the impact of external and internal stimuli that challenge homeostasis (Moberg, 2000). Animals react to disturbances in their homeostasis with a set of physiological changes and systemic reactions like fever, alterations of appetite, and decreases in serum concentrations of iron and zinc. The most striking phenomenon, however, is the changing concentration in a number of serum proteins, particularly acute phase proteins (Petersen et al., 2004).

The stress due to prefarrowing dislocation and farrowing might activate subclinically present chronic urogenital infections, resulting in postparturient diseases of sows (Glock & Bilkei, 2005). Urinary tract infection, postparturient swine urogenital diseases, chronic endometritis, and mastitis-metritis-agalactia syndrome are the most important diseases affecting the sows in the early postparturient period (Thornton et al., 1998; Waller et al., 2002). These important disorders of the sows may cause increased values of acute phase proteins and may contribute to lower number of piglets in litter, inadequate lactation, even to sow mortality (Mirko & Bilkei, 2004). However, the influence of reproduction stage, predominantly parturition on the concentrations of acute phase proteins in sows is less well documented.

Therefore, here we propose a two-phases study. The first objective was the assessment of concentrations of some selected acute phase proteins and variables of energetic metabolism in dairy cows after parturition, as well as at the evaluation of the relationships between the activated acute phase response, characterized by higher concentrations of acute phase proteins, and between altered energetic metabolism shortly after calving. The second objective of this study was to evaluate the concentrations of selected acute phase proteins - haptoglobin and C-reactive protein in blood serum of sows during different stages of reproduction cycle, including the period before and after farrowing, as well as after weaning.

5. Material and methods

5.1 Relationships between acute phase proteins and altered energetic metabolism in dairy cows after calving

5.1.1 Animals and clinical examination

The evaluation of the relationships between the concentrations of acute phase proteins and some variables of energetic metabolism shortly after parturition was performed in 195 dairy cows of a Slovak spotted breed and its crossbreeds on a farm of high yielding dairy cows. The monitored cows were in a period of 1 - 2 weeks after parturition. The animals were housed loosely, and fed twice a day individual feeding rations according to the phase of lactation with free access to water. Before sample collection, the cows were examined clinically using standard clinical examination procedures (Jackson & Cockcroft, 2002). The evaluated cows showed no health disorders during the observation.

5.1.2 Laboratory analyses

The laboratory analyses of evaluated parameters were performed in blood samples. Blood for the investigations was taken by direct puncture of *v. jugularis*. Blood samples were collected into plastic serum tubes with clot activator and gel without anticoagulant. The separated serum was stored at -20 °C until analyzed. Blood serum was analyzed for selected acute phase proteins - haptoglobin (Hp, mg/ml) and serum amyloid A (SAA, µg/ml), and variables of energetic metabolism - glucose (Glu, mmol/l), total cholesterol (TCH, mmol/l), total lipids (TL, g/l), triglycerides (TG, mmol/l), non-esterified fatty acids (NEFA, mmol/l), and β-hydroxybutyrate (BHB, mmol/l).

Haptoglobin was assessed using commercial colorimetric kits (Tridelta Development, Maynooth, Ireland) in microplates, based on Hp-haemoglobin binding and preservation of the peroxidase activity of the bound haemoglobin at low pH. Serum amyloid A was analyzed by method of sandwich enzyme linked immunosorbent assay using commercial ELISA kits (Tridelta Development, Maynooth, Ireland). The reading of absorbancies and the consecutive calculation of final concentrations of both acute phase proteins were performed on automatic microplate reader Opsys MR (Dynex Technologies, Chantilly, USA). The concentrations of Glu, TCH, TG, and BHB were determined using commercial diagnostic kits (Randox) on automatic biochemical analyser ALIZE (Lisabio, Pouilly en Auxois, France). Total lipids were analyzed using commercial diagnostic kits (Ecomed, Zilina, Slovak Republic) by spectrophotometric method. The concentrations of NEFA were assessed according to Curtius (1974) by spectrophotometric method.

5.1.3 Study groups

The obtained results from evaluated cows were divided into two groups according to the measured concentrations of NEFA: Group A (n = 108) - cows with serum concentrations of NEFA below 0.35 mmol/l; Group B (n = 87) - cows with serum concentrations of NEFA above 0.35 mmol/l.

5.1.4 Statistical analyses

Statistical analyses of experimental results were performed by assessment of average values (x) and standard deviations (SD) in each group of cows. The significance of the differences in the obtained results (P) of corresponding variables between monitored groups of animals was evaluated by Mann-Whitney nonparametric test. The relationships between the concentrations of evaluated variables in the monitored cows were calculated by linear regression and Spearman (R) correlations coefficient, including significance of the correlation. Statistical analyses were done in the programme GraphPad Prism V5.02 (GraphPad Software Inc, San Diego, USA).

5.2 The concentrations of selected acute phase proteins during the reproduction cycle of sows

5.2.1 Animals and sample collection

The evaluation of the influence of different stages of the reproduction cycle on the concentrations of selected acute phase proteins included 24 sows, which were crossbreeds of large white and landrace after 1–5 farrowings. The animals were fed complete feedstuff according to corresponding stages of reproduction cycle twice a day, and they had free access to drinking water. Before each sample collection, the animals were clinically examined by standard clinical examination procedures (Jackson & Cockcroft, 2002).

The monitored sows were divided into 4 groups according to different stages of reproduction cycle at the beginning of the evaluation: Group I (n = 6) - sows 4 weeks before farrowing, Group II (n = 6) - sows 1 week before farrowing, Group III (n = 6) - sows 1 week after farrowing, Group IV (n = 6) - sows 1 week after weaning.

Blood for the investigations was collected by direct puncture of *v. cava cranialis* into plastic serum tubes with clot activator and gel without anticoagulant. Blood samples were taken in each group of sows four times at intervals of two weeks (Table 1).

Groups of sows	**Sample collections**			
	1st	**2nd**	**3rd**	**4th**
I	4 weeks *a.p.*	2 weeks *a.p.*	1–2 days *p.p.*	2 weeks *p.p.*
II	1 week *a.p.*	1 week *p.p.*	3 weeks *p.p.*	1 week *p.* wean.
III	1 week *p.p.*	3 weeks *p.p.*	1 week *p.*wean.	3 weeks *p.*wean.
IV	1 week *p.*wean.	3 weeks *p.*wean.	5 weeks *p.*wean.	7 weeks *p.*wean.

a.p. - ante partum, p.p. - post partum, p. wean. - post weaning

Table 1. Time-table of blood sample collections within the evaluated groups of sows

In the first part of the study, we evaluated the dynamics of changes in the concentrations of measured acute phase proteins during the reproduction cycle in the mentioned groups of sows. In the second part of the study, we summarised the individual values of acute phase proteins from these groups of sows according to four selected periods of reproduction cycle - 4 weeks *ante partum*, 1 week *ante partum*, 1 week *post partum* and 1 week *post* weaning.

5.2.2 Laboratory analyses

Venous blood samples were centrifuged at 3.000 g for 30 minutes. Serum was separated and stored at -18 °C until laboratory analyses could be performed. Blood serum was analyzed for selected acute phase proteins - haptoglobin (Hp, mg/ml), and C-reactive protein (CRP, ng/ml).

Haptoglobin was assessed using commercial colorimetric kits (Tridelta Development, Maynooth, Ireland) in microplates. Blood serum samples were initially diluted 1:5. C-reactive protein was analyzed by method of sandwich enzyme linked immunosorbent assay using commercial ELISA kits (Tridelta Development, Maynooth, Ireland). Serum samples for the determination of CRP were diluted 1:500 prior to assay. The optical densities were read on the automatic microplate reader Opsys MR (Dynex Technologies, Chantilly, USA) at 630 nm for Hp, and at 450 nm using 630 nm as reference for CRP.

5.2.3 Statistical analyses

Statistical evaluation of the obtained results was performed by assessment of means (x) and standard deviations (SD) in each monitored group of sows according to the sample collection. The significance of the differences in measured values (P) of the investigated variables in relation to the corresponding monitored periods of reproduction was evaluated by one way analysis of variance (ANOVA). The significance of differences in measured values between the sample collections in the groups was evaluated by Student's paired test (the 1st part of the study), and the significance of differences in the obtained concentrations between selected periods of reproduction cycle was evaluated by Student's unpaired test (the 2nd part of the study).

6. Results

6.1 Relationships between acute phase proteins and altered energetic metabolism in dairy cows after calving

The results of the concentrations of selected acute phase proteins, and variables of energetic metabolism characterised by average values (x) and standard deviations (SD), as well as the evaluation of the significance of differences in the obtained results (P) between two groups of cows are given in Table 2, and on Fig. 2 and 3. The analyses of relationships between monitored variables in cows are summarised in Table 3 and are shown on Fig. 4 - 7.

Soluble factors	**Group of cows**		**P**
	A (n = 108)	**B** (n = 87)	
Hp (mg/ml)	0.067 ± 0.113	0.607 ± 0.610	< 0.001
SAA (μg/ml)	30.77 ± 20.95	93.94 ± 43.64	< 0.001
Glu (mmol/l)	4.19 ± 0.57	3.95 ± 0.44	< 0.001
TCH (mmol/l)	3.25 ± 1.11	3.05 ± 1.12	n. s.
TL (g/l)	3.48 ± 1.44	3.43 ± 1.31	n. s.
TG (mmol/l)	0.14 ± 0.11	0.12 ± 0.09	n. s.
NEFA (mmol/l)	0.21 ± 0.09	0.65 ± 0.25	< 0.001
BHB (mmol/l)	0.46 ± 0.26	0.65 ± 0.35	< 0.001

Group A - cows with serum concentrations of NEFA below 0.35 mmol/l; Group B - cows with serum concentrations of NEFA above 0.35 mmol/l

P - significance of the differences in the obtained results between the groups of cows, n. s. - non significant

Table 2. Comparison of the concentrations of Hp, SAA and selected variables of energetic metabolism in two groups of dairy cows (x ± SD)

In cows with serum concentrations of NEFA above 0.35 mmol/l we found significantly higher mean value of haptoglobin than in cows with NEFA concentrations below 0.35 mmol/l ($P < 0.001$, Table 2). It is shown on Fig. 2 that while in cows with serum NEFA concentrations below 0.35 mmol/l (Group A) the median Hp concentration was 0.029 mg/ml and the individual values ranged from 0.001 to 0.697 mg/ml, in cows with NEFA values above 0.35 mmol/l (Group B) we recorded higher median Hp concentration (0.470 mg/ml), as well as markedly wider range of individual values with minimum concentration of 0.006 mg/ml and maximum value of 2.540 mg/ml. By more detailed analysis of individual Hp concentrations we found that while in Group A 50 % of measured values ranged from 0.010 mg/ml to 0.067 mg/ml, in Group B this range was from 0.162 mg/ml to 0.834 mg/ml.

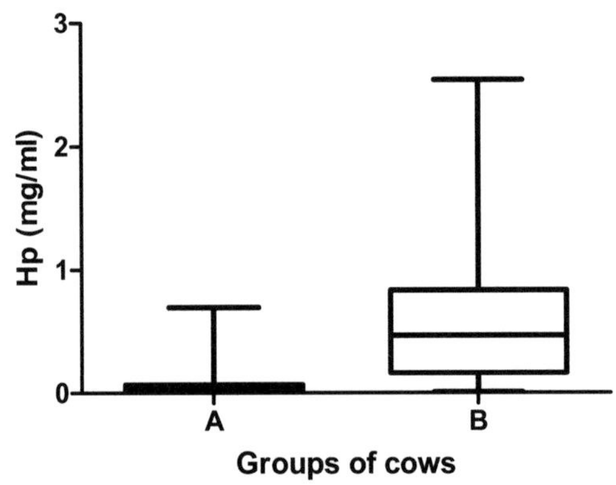

Fig. 2. The concentrations of Hp in serum from cows with NEFA concentrations below 0.35 mmol/l (Group A) and above 0.35 mmol/l (Group B). The plots show the median (line within box), 25th and 75th percentiles (box)), minimum and maximum values (whiskers)

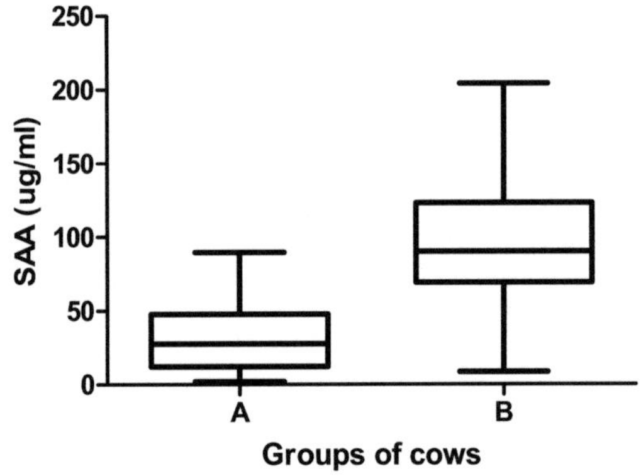

Fig. 3. The concentrations of SAA in serum from cows with NEFA concentrations below 0.35 mmol/l (Group A) and above 0.35 mmol/l (Group B). The plots show the median (line within box), 25th and 75th percentiles (box), minimum and maximum values (whiskers)

In cows with concentrations of NEFA above 0.35 mmol/l, significantly higher mean serum concentration was found also for SAA ($P < 0.001$). The median SAA concentration in cows from Group A was 27.70 μg/ml, and the individual values ranged from 1.95 μg/ml to 89.78 μg/ml (Fig. 3). The median SAA concentration in cows from Group B was higher (90.30 μg/ml), and the measured concentrations showed wider range of individual values (from 8.38 μg/ml to 204.00 μg/ml).

Trend of significantly higher values in cows with NEFA concentrations above 0.35 mmol/l was found also in the serum concentrations of BHB ($P < 0.001$). On the other hand, cows with higher values of NEFA showed significantly lower mean concentration of glucose ($P < 0.001$). In mean concentrations of total cholesterol, total lipids, and triglycerides we observed no significant differences between two groups of cows.

By the assessment of correlations we recorded a significant positive correlation between the concentrations of both measured acute phase proteins – Hp and SAA, and the values of NEFA ($R = 0.716$, $P < 0.001$; $R = 0.710$, $P < 0.001$, respectively), as well as the values of BHB ($R = 0.291$, $P < 0.001$; $R = 0.300$, $P < 0.001$, respectively) (Figs. 4 - 7).

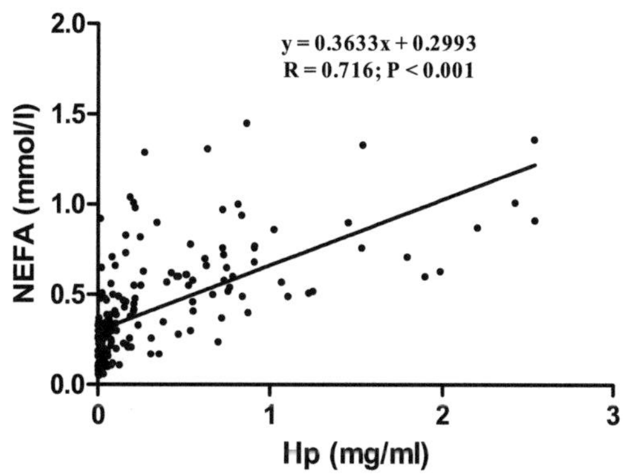

Fig. 4. Correlation and regression analysis between Hp and NEFA concentrations

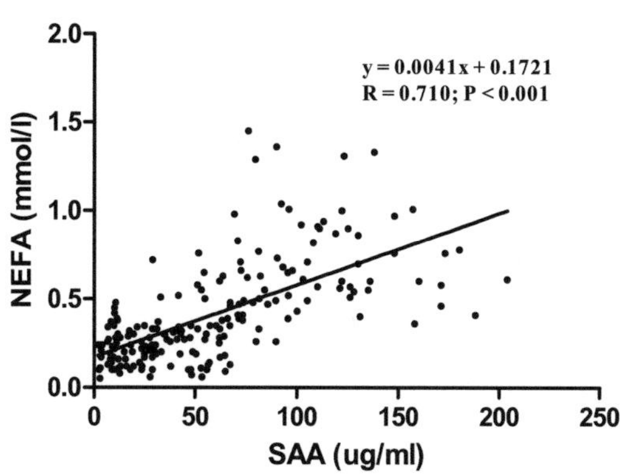

Fig. 5. Correlation and regression analysis between SAA and NEFA concentrations

Significant negative correlations was found between the concentrations of both acute phase proteins and the values of glucose (R = -0.247, P < 0.001; R = -0.249, P < 0.001, respectively), as well as the concentrations of total cholesterol (R = -0.181, P < 0.05; R = -0.241, P < 0.001, respectively). Moreover, the concentrations of Hp in cows shortly after parturition significantly positively correlated with the values of SAA (R = 0.647, P < 0.001). Significant correlations we observed also between some variables of energetic metabolism, which are listed in Table 3.

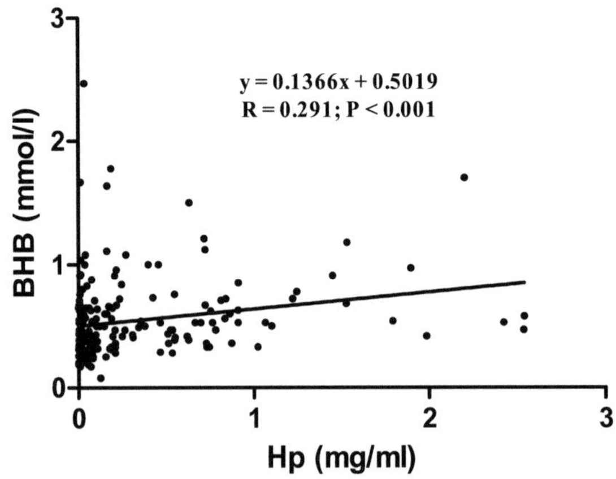

Fig. 6. Correlation and regression analysis between Hp and BHB concentrations

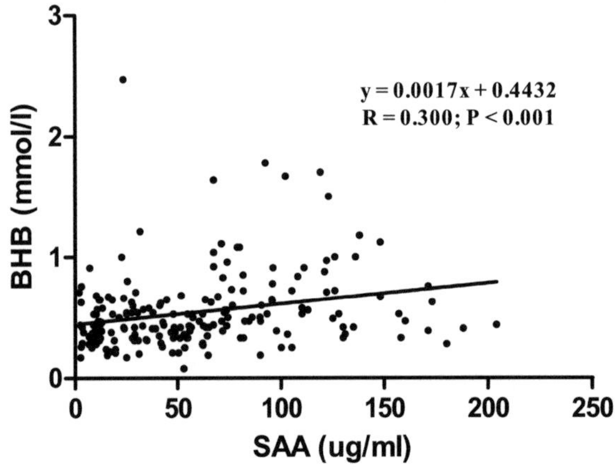

Fig. 7. Correlation and regression analysis between SAA and BHB concentrations

	Hp	SAA	Glu	TCH	TL	TG	NEFA	BHB
Hp	-	0.647^{c}	-0.247^{c}	-0.181^{a}	-0.137	-0.069	0.716^{c}	0.291^{c}
SAA	0.647^{c}	-	-0.249^{c}	-0.214^{c}	-0.041	-0.024	0.710^{c}	0.300^{c}
Glu	-0.247^{c}	-0.249^{c}	-	0.179^{a}	0.043	0.195^{b}	-0.27^{c}	-0.175^{a}
TCH	-0.181^{a}	-0.214^{b}	0.179^{a}	-	0.663^{c}	0.197^{b}	-0.125	-0.331^{c}
TL	-0.137	-0.041	0.043	0.663^{c}	-	0.205^{b}	-0.049	-0.196^{b}
TG	-0.069	-0.024	0.195^{b}	0.197^{b}	0.205^{b}	-	-0.093	-0.100
NEFA	0.716^{c}	0.710^{c}	-0.277^{c}	-0.125	-0.049	-0.093	-	0.320^{c}
BHB	0.291^{c}	0.300^{c}	-0.175^{a}	-0.331^{c}	-0.196^{b}	-0.100	0.320^{c}	-

a, b, c indexes show statistical significance of correlations: a – $P < 0.05$; b – $P < 0.01$; c – $P < 0.001$

Table 3. The correlations between selected acute phase proteins and variables of energetic metabolism

6.2 The concentrations of selected acute phase proteins during the reproduction cycle of sows

The results of the determination of selected acute phase proteins during the reproduction cycle of sows, characterized by average values (x), standard deviations (SD), and the statistical evaluation of the obtained results (P) are summarised in Tables 4 and 5.

In the Group I, by the evaluation of the serum concentrations of Hp we recorded in sows 2 weeks *ante partum* (2nd sample collection) markedly higher mean value compared with the 1st sampling (Table 4), However, the values differed not significantly. By other sample collections (*post partum*), there was a continuous decrease in its concentrations. In CRP concentrations, we found in sows by the 3rd and 4th sample collections nonsignificantly higher values compared with the 1st and 2nd samplings (Table 5). The highest average concentration of CRP was recorded in sows after farrowing (3rd sampling). The changes in average concentrations of Hp and CRP during the monitored period in this group of sows were not significant. All animals from this group were clinically healthy throughout the whole monitored period.

Groups of sows	Sample collection				ANOVA P
	1st	2nd	3rd	4th	
I	1.27 ± 0.45	2.30 ± 1.83	1.63 ± 0.40	1.57 ± 0.44	n. s.
II	1.76 ± 0.21^{a}	1.79 ± 0.44	1.63 ± 0.45	1.16 ± 0.16^{a}	n. s
III	$2.96 \pm 1.06^{a,b,B}$	$1.91 \pm 0.65^{a,A}$	1.27 ± 0.40^{b}	$1.20 \pm 0.59^{A,B}$	< 0.01
IV	$2.10 \pm 0.68^{a,b}$	1.44 ± 0.94	1.00 ± 0.71^{b}	0.99 ± 0.86^{a}	n. s.

The same indexes in lines mean statistical significance of differences in measured values between the groups of sows: a, A – $P < 0.05$; b, B – $P < 0.01$

P – significance of the differences in the obtained results, n. s. – non significant

Table 4. The changes in the concentrations of Hp (mg/ml) in blood serum of sows during different stages of reproduction cycle (x ± SD)

In the Group II, the analyses of the serum Hp concentrations showed no significant changes in its values from the period of 1 week before farrowing until 3 weeks after farrowing.

Significantly lower mean Hp concentrations compared with the 1st sampling was found 5 weeks after farrowing (4th sampling, $P < 0.05$). In the concentrations of CRP we found a nonsignificant increase of values by the 2nd and 3rd sample collection with consecutive more marked, but statistically not significant decrease of its average concentration bellow the level of initial values by the 4th sampling. The changes in the obtained results of Hp and CRP concentrations in this group of sows throughout the whole monitored period were not significant. All animals from this group were clinically healthy during the monitored period, and didn't exhibit changes in reproductive system after farrowing.

In the Group III, we recorded a trend to decrease Hp concentrations from the 1st (1 week *p.p.*) till the 4th sample collection (7 weeks *p.p.*). The mean value of Hp by the 1st sampling was significantly higher compared with its average concentrations recorded by the 3rd ($P < 0.05$) and 4th samplings ($P < 0.01$). The average Hp concentration in sows 3 weeks after farrowing (2nd sampling) was also significantly higher compared with the mean value obtained in animals by the 4th sampling ($P < 0.05$). Similarly, decreasing trend of values was found also in the concentrations of CRP. The average concentration of CRP in sows by the 1st sample collection was significantly higher compared with the mean value found by the 3rd sampling ($P < 0.05$). The changes in the concentrations of Hp and CRP in this group of sows during the monitored period were significant ($P < 0.01$ and $P < 0.05$). Almost in all of the animals from this group, clinical signs of mastitis-metritis-agalactia syndrome (MMA) were found by the 1st collection of specimens (1 week *p.p.*), characterized by a decreased food intake, discharge from vagina, erythema, and firmness of mammary gland. By the 2nd, 3rd and 4th sample collections, we did not record in these animals clinically evident changes in the reproductive system.

Group of the sows	Sample collection				ANOVA P
	1st	2nd	3rd	4th	
I.	16.27 ± 9.38	15.97 ± 12.35	27.19 ± 21.96	20.85 ± 10.16	n. s.
II.	23.97 ± 11.84	31.92 ± 37.20	49.98 ± 39.04	9.83 ± 7.36	n. s.
III.	64.92 ± 60.10[a]	14.47 ± 14.82	7.78 ± 8.76[a]	4.10 ± 3.39	< 0.05
IV.	23.59 ± 17.67[a]	52.44 ± 48.27[A]	8.25 ± 7.68[a]	6.93 ± 12.91[A]	< 0.05

The same indexes in lines mean statistical significance of differences in measured values between the groups of sows: a, A – $P < 0.05$

P – significance of the differences in the obtained results, n. s. – non significant

Table 5. The changes in the concentrations of CRP (ng/ml) in blood serum of sows during different stages of reproduction cycle (x ± SD)

In the Group IV, different changes in the concentrations of evaluated acute phase proteins were found. The analyses of serum Hp concentrations showed a trend of decreasing values. The concentrations of Hp by the 1st sample collection (1 week *post* weaning) were significantly higher compared with the values obtained by the 3rd and 4th samplings (5 and 7 weeks *post* weaning, $P < 0.05$). In the concentrations of C-reactive protein, after a non-significant increase of average value by the 2nd sampling, we recorded repeated decrease of its values by the 3rd and 4th samplings. While the changes in the concentrations of Hp in this group of sows during the whole monitored period were not significant, the values of CRP showed significant changes throughout the monitored period (P < 0.05). By the 1st sample collection, we found in one animal from this group inflammatory changes on the carpal joint, the others were clinically healthy. The clinical examination of the evaluated animals by next samplings did not reveal any disorders of general health state.

Variable	Sample collections				ANOVA P
	4 weeks *a.p.*	1 week *a.p.*	1 week *p.p.*	1 week *p.*wean.	
Hp	1.27 ± 0.45[b]	2.09 ± 1.40	2.17 ± 0.93[a,b]	1.55 ± 0.64[a]	n.s.
CRP	16.27 ± 9.38[a]	19.17 ± 12.19	42.52 ± 44.34[a,A]	14.22 ± 14.05[A]	< 0.05

The same indexes in lines mean statistical significance of differences in measured values between the groups of sows: a, A – P < 0.05; b – P < 0.01

P – significance of the differences in the obtained results, n. s. – non significant; a.p. – ante partum; p.p. – post partum;, p. wean. – post weaning

Table 6. The average concentrations of Hp and CRP in blood serum of sows in selected periods of reproduction cycle (x ± SD)

A more detailed analysis of the individual concentrations of measured acute phase proteins from the evaluated groups of sows according to selected stages of reproduction cycle is summarised in Table 6. The highest average concentration of Hp (2.17 mg/ml) we found in sows 1 week after the farrowing. This value was significantly higher compared with average concentrations recorded in sows 4 weeks before parturition and 1 week after the weaning (P < 0.01 and P < 0.05, respectively). By the evaluation of the concentrations of CRP we found a similar trend of significantly increasing values with the highest mean value in sows 1 week *post partum*. While the differences in the concentrations of haptoglobin between the sows in different stages of reproduction cycle were not significant, in the values of C-reactive protein we found significant differences (P < 0.05).

7. Discussion

7.1 Relationships between acute phase proteins and altered energetic metabolism in dairy cows after calving

The immune system is significantly affected during pregnancy. There are significant interactions between the immune system and cells and tissues of the reproductive system that are critical for the maintenance of pregnancy, but are responsible for immune suppression that is associated with increased risk of diseases (Kehrli et al., 1990; Lippolis, 2008). Parturition with following metabolic challenges constitutes a potentially stressful event for the dairy cow. One of the ways how an animal can manifest its stress state is by activating its acute phase response, mainly by an increased production of acute phase proteins by the liver. According to Alsemgeest et al. (1993), the physiological processes taking place around the time of parturition are mainly responsible for higher concentrations of acute phase proteins in blood serum. Regassa & Noakes (1999) and Rottmann (2006) reported that higher values of acute phase proteins could be related to the tissue damage occuring due to the increased myometrial activity during expulsion of the calf, involution of the uterus, as well as degeneration and regeneration of the endometrium. Young et al. (1995) found that higher concentrations of these proteins, determined in the last phase of pregnancy and after calving may be connected with the changing hormone profile (the influence of estrogens and progesterone). According to Alsemgeest et al. (1996), increased acute phase protein concentrations in cattle may be due to the increased concentrations of cortisol as part of the response to stress.

However, even if this response conserved it exhibit varations from one animal to another, some of them respond markedly, other have moderate or minor responses. Therefore, the differences between two groups of evaluated dairy cows, observed in our study in the concentrations of both measured acute phase proteins, may be due to numerous differences in the inflammatory responses to various external or internal stimuli. Pyörälä (2000) reported also that the production of acute phase proteins vary not only among different animal species, but also within them. Higher values of standard deviations obtained in both groups of cows reflect the different reactivity of acute phase proteins. The wider range of individual values of Hp, as well as SAA, suggests also the differences in the variability of animals reacting to both injury and impaired homeostasis.

Moreover, homeostais of all the energy substrates and the whole metabolism is altered during the time around parturition. Hardardottir et al. (1994) reported also that the acute phase response initiated by processes occuring around parturition is associated with numerous changes in lipid and glucose metabolism, such as decreased cholesterol, accelerated lipolysis, and increased NEFA concentrations in plasma. Investigations in human medicine showed that altered lipid metabolism, increased concentrations of non-esterified fatty acids in blood serum, and oxidative stress may markedly influence the systemic inflammatory response, and the development of inflammatory-based diseases (Sordillo et al., 2009). Our study showed highly positive correlation between the concentrations of Hp and SAA, as well as between both measured acute phase proteins and the concentrations of NEFA in dairy cows after calving. Kushibiki et al. (2002) stated that administration of tumor necrosis factor α to dairy cattle, promotes the production of acute phase proteins and is associated with decreased appetite and cachexia, and increased release of NEFA from adipose tissue into the plasma. Therefore, higher concentrations of non-esterified fatty acids in serum could be related to the activation of the immune system. Ametaj (2005) and Ametaj et al. (2005) reported that higher concentrations of haptoglobin and serum amyloid A after parturition correlate positively with total lipids in the liver, and proposed that fatty liver found in cows could be a response to non-specific inflammation associated to parturition.

The periparturient period is characterized by a sudden increase in energy requirements imposed by the onset of lactation and by a decrease in voluntary dry matter intake which results in negative energy balance (Leroy et al., 2008). A significant adaptation to the negative energy balance during the transition period is the mobilization of fat from body stores and the release of non-esterified fatty acids into the blood stream, which constitute important sources of energy in this period. Animals may react to these disturbances in their homeostasis and changes in metabolism with a set of physiological changes, including changes in the concentration of some plasma proteins, especially acute phase proteins. However, according to Bernabucci et al. (2005) and Sordillo et al. (2009), increased circulating NEFA concentrations are directly associated with increased systemic inflammatory conditions, and large amounts of adipose stores during time of energy deficiency are linked with adverse health effects on the transition cow. Other authors demonstrated also a clear relationship among nutrition, inflammation and disease susceptibility, and that elevated NEFA concentrations are positive risk factors for many inflammatory periparturient diseases in dairy cows (Goff, 2006; Calder, 2008; Wood et al., 2009).

Highly significant positive correlation was found also between Hp, SAA and β-hydroxybutyrate, as well as between NEFA and BHB. These relationships may be explained by metabolic changes after parturition, since fat-derived substances are important sources of energy, because the majority of available glucose is redirected to the mammary gland for lactose synthesis (Herdt, 2000). However, further studies are needed to explain the aforementioned relationships with the immune response, characterized by changes in the concentrations of acute phase proteins in dairy cows after calving, and with the altered energetic metabolism.

Our study showed also a network of energetic metabolism factors, reflecting mutiple overlapping metabolic reactions, and physiological adaptations of the cow in the period after calving. Seifi et al. (2007) reported that after calving there is a positive correlation between NEFA and TG, as well as between NEFA and BHB. While between glucose and the other energetic profile factors no correlation was established.

7.2 The concentrations of selected acute phase proteins during the reproduction cycle of sows

Reproductive state and gravidity are important factors influencing most of the biochemical parameters of sows, including acute phase proteins (Lampreave et al., 1994; Verheyen et al., 2007). At present, physiological reference values for haptoglobin and C-reactive protein in pigs are not definitely established. However, it appeared that the time of sampling (before or after farrowing) has an important influence on most of the acute phase proteins.

Many researchers reported that concentrations of acute phase proteins undergo significant changes associated to parturition (Alsemgeest et al., 1993; Ametaj, 2005). In horses and cows the highest concentrations of major acute phase proteins were observed at day 1 *post partum* (Gymnich et al., 2003). Data from sows during parturition are lacking. Our results suggest that in sows there are also important changes in the concentrations of acute phase proteins associated to the reproduction cycle. In sows, at the week 1 after farrowing, significantly higher average concentrations of Hp, as well as CRP were found, as compared with samples analyzed before and later after parturition. Kostro et al. (2003) reported similar findings. According to Verheyen et al. (2007), serum Hp concentrations showed a significant increase one week after farrowing over 2.09 g/l. On the other hand, the aforementioned authors reported that, similarly to our results, the concentrations of Hp on the 94th and 108th day of gestation are roughly uniform (1.36 and 1.54 g/l). The increased Hp concentration *post partum* could be explained by physiological events during the *puerperium*. Moreover, higher values of Hp and CRP, recorded after parturition, may be consequences of increased cortisol production in adrenal cortex, as part of the response of the organism to stress (Uchida et al., 1993; Burger et al., 1998). According to Busch et al. (2003), Hp concentrations in young sows increase 2–8 weeks before farrowing, and the elevations are higher than in older sows. Verheyen et al. (2007) reported also that parity one sows showed higher Hp concentrations. This finding is in contrast whit the results presented by Petersen *et al.* (2002), who reported an increase in concentrations of acute phase proteins with age.

The reproductive tract of sows is susceptible to infection after farrowing because of the periparturient increase in the number of both nonpathogenic microflora and facultative pathogens in the caudal vagina and urinary bladder (Bilkei et al., 1994). Elevated concentrations of Hp and CRP in sows may reflect the inflammation in the reproductive tract and mammary gland. Mirko & Bilkei (2004) evaluated sows without postparturient complications of normal process of *puerperium* and sows suffering from MMA syndrome after parturition. In both groups they recorded an increase of the concentrations of Hp and α_1-acid glycoprotein in postparturient period. The concentrations of the aforementioned acute phase proteins on the 1st and 5th day after parturition were higher in sows suffering from MMA syndrome compared with sows without clinical signs of reproductive disorders. Friendship & Bilkei (2005) stated that in sows with MMA syndrome and other urogenital diseases the Hp concentrations were higher on the 1st and 5th day of lactation. Therefore, monitoring the concentrations of these indicators during the first days after parturition may be used to diagnose early stages of the MMA syndrome and to start suitable therapy (Gymnich et al., 2003).

In general, the acute phase response is considered to be useful tool in prevention of microbial growth, and may help in recovery of the organism. In addition, an active cell immune response in sow, indirectly negatively influence growth rate in preweaning piglets, probably due to decreased milk production (Bilkei, 1995; Segales et al., 2004).

8. Conclusion

Our present results indicate strong relationships between acute phase proteins and some variables of energetic metabolism in cows shortly after parturition. In this critical period, we recorded significant correlations between evaluated acute phase proteins and non-esterified fatty acids, as well as β-hydroxybutyrate. Understanding how all these factors interact with the immune system will help in developing disease control and management strategies that will aid in maintaining good health in dairy cattle, resulting in greater production.

The aforementioned results suggest that acute phase proteins, haptoglobin and serum amyloid A, may be potential candidates for monitoring the around parturition time. However, future possibilities for acute phase reactants depend on basic new molecular mechanims involving known proteins, as well as new discoveries such as organ-specific components, and new technological possibilities for rapid immunological or chemical multi-analyses.

The aforementioned results suggest that the reproductive state influences the production of acute phase proteins, and indicates that around parturition in sows there are important changes in the concentrations of diagnostically useful acute phase proteins. In the monitored period we recorded significant changes in the values of haptoglobin and C-reactive protein with their highest concentrations shortly after parturition. However, the interpretation of these metabolites should always be performed together with a thorough anamnesis and clinical evaluation of individual animals.

The advantages and uses of acute phase protein assays are well supported in the human medicine. Unfortunately, because of the practical limitations of current technology, clinical application of acute phase protein analyses in veterinary medicine is not widespread. Continuing challenges include the need for automated assays and standardization of tests across laboratories. However, many potential uses are possible for acute phase protein measurements to assess the health state, poor hygiene and welfare in pig production processes. In addition, acute phase proteins seem to be a promising marker of health status by reflecting a broad spectrum of ongoing clinically declared, as well as asymptomatic diseases. Exceptionally sensitive, but non-specific markers of diverse inflammatory etiologies, acute phase proteins are excellent candidates to monitor both animal health, and animal wellbeing.

9. Acknowledgment

This work was supported by VEGA Scientific Grant No 1/0614/09 from the Ministry of Education, and by Slovak Research and Development Agency under contract No. APVV-0475-10.

10. References

Alsemgeest, S.P.M., Taverne, M.A.M., Boosman, R., van der Weyden, B. & Gruys, E. (1993). Peripartum acute-phase protein serum amyloid-A concentration in plasma of cows and fetuses, *American Journal of Veterinary Research*, Vol.54, pp. 164-167

Alsemgeest, S.P.M., vant Clooster, G.A.E., van Miert, A.S.J.P.A.M., Huslkamp-Koch, C.K. & Gruys, E. (1996). Primary bovine hepatocytes in the study of cytokine induced acute-phase protein secretion *in vitro*, *Veterinary Immunology and Immunopathology*, Vol.53, pp. 179-184

Ametaj, B. (2005). A new understanding of the causes of fatty liver in dairy cows, *Advances in Dairy Technology*, Vol.17, pp. 97-112

Ametaj, B.N., Bradford, B.J., Bobe, G., Nafikov, R.A., Lu, Y., Young, J.W. & Beitz, D.C. (2005). Strong relationships between mediators of the acute phase response and fatty liver in dairy cows, *Canadian Journal of Animal Sciences*, Vol.85, pp. 165-175

Baumann, H. & Gauldie, J. (1994). The acute phase response, *Immunology Today*, Vol.15, pp. 74-80

Bellomo, R. (1992). The cytokine network in the critically ill, *Anaesthesia and Intensive Care*, Vol.20, pp. 288-302

Berkova, N., Lemay, A., Dresser, D.W., Fontaine, J.Y., Kerizit, J. & Goupil, S. (2001). Haptoglobin is present in human endometrium and shows elevated levels in the decidua during pregnancy, *Molecular Human Reproduction*, Vol.7, pp. 747-754

Bernabucci, U., Ronchi, B., Lacetera, N. & Nardone, A. (2005). Influence of body condition score on relationships between metabolic status and oxidative stress in periparturient dairy cows, *Journal of Dairy Science*, Vol.88, pp. 2017-2026

Bilkei, G. (1995). Herd health strategy for improving the reproductive performance of pigs, *Proceedings of the 8th „In-between" Symposium of the International Society for Animal Hygiene, Hungarian Veterinary Journal*, Vol.10, pp. 766-768

Bilkei, G., Bölcskei, A. & Goos, T. (1994). Bericht über den peripartalen Krankheitskomplex der Muttersau in der industriellen Schweinezucht. 1ste Mitteilung: Peripartaler Verlauf der Bakteriurie der Sauen mit vaginal-vulvalem Ausfluss in einem modernen Schweinezuchtbetrieb, *Berliner und Münchener Tierärztliche Wochenschrift*, Vol.107, pp. 327-330

Burger, W., Ewald, C. & Fennert, E.M. (1998). Increase in C-reactive protein in the serum of piglets (pCRP) following ACTH or corticosteroid admimistration, *Journal of Veterinary Medicine Series B*, Vol.45, pp. 1-6

Busch, M.E., Baekbo, P. & Wachmann, H. (2003). Haptoglobin levels in sows and associations with clinical signs of disease around farrowing, *Proceedings of the Fourth European Colloquium on Acute Phase Proteins*, p. 33, Segovia, Spain

Cai, T.Q., Weston, P.G., Lund, L.A., Brodie, B., McKenna, D.J. & Wagner, W.C. (1994). Association between neutrophil functions and periparturient disorders in cows, *American Journal of Veterinary Research*, Vol.55, pp. 934-943

Calder, P.C. (2008). The relationship between the fatty acid composition of immune cells and their function, *Prostaglandins Leukotrienes and Essential Fatty Acids*, Vol.79, pp. 101-108

Cray, C., Zaias, J. & Altman, N.H. (2009). Acute phase response in animals : a review, *Comparative Medicine*, Vol.59, No.6, pp. 517-526

Du Clos, T.W. (2004). C-reactive protein. An activator of innate imunity and a modulator of adaptive imunity, *Immunolological Research*, Vol.30, pp. 261-277

Eckersall, P.D. (2000). Recent advances and future prospects for the use of acute phase proteins as markers of disease in animals, *Revue de Médicine Véterinarie*, Vol.151, No.7, pp. 577-584

Eckersall, P.D. & Bell, R. (2010). Acute phase proteins : Biomarkers of infection and inflammation in veterinary medicine, *The Veterinary Journal*, Vol.185, pp. 23-27

Friendship, P.Z.E. & Bilkei, G. (2005). Acute phase proteins and serum cortisol levels in sows affected with mastitis, metritis, agalactia (MMA) and swine urogenital disease (SUGD), *The Pig Journal*, Vol.55, pp. 9-18

Gatzka, C., Bremerich, D., Kaufmann, M. & Ahr, A. (2002). Isolated decrease in haptoglobin during pregnancy: diagnosis by chance or pathological? *Zentralblatt für Gynakologie*, Vol.124, pp. 120-122

Glock, X.T.P. & Bilkei, G. (2005). The effect of postparturient urogenital diseases on the lifetime reproductive performance of sows, *Canadian Veterinary Journal*, Vol.46, pp. 1103-1107

Goff, J.P. (2006). Major advances in our understanding of nutritional influences on bovine health, *Journal of Dairy Science*, Vol.89, pp. 1292-1301

Gruys, E., Touissant, M.J.M., Landman, W.J.M., Tivapasi, M., Chamanza, R. & van Veen, L. (1999). Infection, inflammation and stress inhibit growth. Mechanism and non-specific assessment of the processes by acute phase proteins, In: *Production diseases in farm animals*, T. Wensing (Ed.), 72-87, Wageningen Press, The Netherlands

Gruys, E., Toussaint, M.J.M., Niewold, T.A. & Koopmans, S.J. (2005). Acute phase reaction and acute phase proteins, *Journal of Zhejiang University Science*, Vol.6B, No.11, pp. 1045-1056, ISSN 1009-3095

Gymnich, S., Hiss, S., Sauerwein, H. & Petersen, B. (2003). Haptoglobin in sows at parturition, *Proceedings of the Fourth European Colloquium on Acute Phase Proteins*, p. 136, Segovia, Spain

Hachanberg, S., Weinkauf, C., Hiss, S. & Sauerwein, H. (2007). Evaluation of classification modes potentially suitable to identify metabolic stress in healthy dairy cows during the peripartal period, *Journal of Animal Sciences*, Vol.85, pp. 1923-1932

Hardardottir, I., Grunfeld, C. & Feingold, K.R. (1994). Effects of endotoxin and cytokines on lipid metabolism, *Current Opinion in Lipidology*, Vol.5, pp. 207-215

Herdt, T.H. (2000). Ruminants adaptation to negative energy balance. Influences on the etiology of ketosis and fatty liver, *Veterinary Clinics of North America: Food Animal Practice*, Vol.16, pp. 215-230

Jackson, P.G.G. & Cockcroft, P.D. (2002). *Clinical examination of farm animals*. Blackwell Science Ltd., Blackwell Publishing Company, ISBN 0-632-05706-8, Oxford, United Kingdom

Jacobsen, S. (2003). The bovine acute phase response to endotoxin and Gram-negative bacteria, Ph.D. thesis, 162 pp., Samfundslitteratur Grafik, Frederiksberg, Denmark

Janeway, C.A., Travers, P., Walport, M. & Schlomschik, M.J. (2001). *Immunobiology*, 5th ed., Taylor & Francis, London, United Kingdom

Johnson, R.W. (1997). Inhibition of growth by pro-inflammatory cytokines; an integrated view, *Journal of Animal Science*, Vol.75, pp. 1244-1255

Kehrli, M.E.Jr., Goff, J.P., Harp, J.A., Thurston, J.R. & Norcross, N.L. (1990). Effects of preventing periparturient hypocalcemia in cows by parathyroid hormone administration on hematology, immunoglobulin, and shedding of *Staphylococcus aureus* in milk, *Journal of Dairy Science*, Vol.73, pp. 2103-2111

Koj, A. (1996). Initiation of acute phase response and synthesis of cytokines, *Biochemical and Biophysical Acta*, Vol.1317, pp. 84-94

Kostro, K., Wawron, W., Szczubial, M., Luft-Deptula, D. & Glinski, Z. (2003). C-reactive protein in monitoring and evaluation of effects of therapy of the MMA syndrome of sows, *Polish Journal of Veterinary Science*, Vol.6, pp. 235-238

Krakowski, L. & Zdzisińska, B. (2007). Selected cytokines and acute phase proteins in heifers during the ovarian cycle course and in different pregnancy periods, *Bulletin of the Veterinary Institue Pulawy*, Vol.51, pp. 31-36

Kushibiki, S., Hodate, K., Shingu, H., Hayashi, T., Touno, E., Shimoda, M. & Yokomizo, Y. (2002). Alterations in lipid metabolism induced by recombinant bovine tumor necrosis factor-alpha administration in dairy heifers, *Journal of Animal Sciences*, Vol.80, pp. 2151-2157

Lampreave, F., Gonzalez-Ramon, N., Martinez-Ayensa, S., Hernandez, M.-A., Lorenzo, H.-K., Garcia-Gil, A. & Pineiro, A. (1994). Characterisation of the acute phase serum protein response in pigs, *Electrophoresis*, Vol.15, pp. 672-676

Lauritzen, B., Lykkesfeldt, J., Skaanild, M.T., Angen, Ø., Nielsen, J.P. & Friis, C. (2003). Putative biomarkers for evaluating antibiotic treatment of *Actinobacillus pleuropneumoniae* infection in pigs, *Research in Veterinary Science*, Vol.74, pp. 271-277

Leroy, J.I., Vanholder, T., Van Knegsel, A.T., Garcia-Ispierto, I. & Bols, P.E. (2008). Nutrient prioritization in dairy cows early postpartum: mismatch between metabolism and fertility. *Reproduction in Domestic Animals*, Vol.43, pp. 96-103

Lippolis, J.D. (2008). Immunological signaling networks: integrating the body's immune response, *Journal of Animal Sciences*, Vol.86, pp. E53-E63

Marnell, L., Mold, C. & Du Clos, T.W. (2005). C-reactive protein: Ligands, receptors and role in inflammation, *Clinical Immunology*, Vol.117, pp. 104-111

Mirko, C.P. & Bilkei, G. (2004). Acute phase proteins, serum cortisol and preweaning litter performance in sows suffering from periparturient disease, *Acta Veterinaria Beograd*, Vol.54, pp. 153-161

Moberg, G.P. (2000). Biological response to stress: Implications for animal welfare, In: *The Biology of Animal Sress*, G.P. Moberg & J.A. Mench (Eds.), 1-21, CABI Publishing, New York, USA

Murata, H., Shimada, N. & Yoshioka, M. (2004). Current research on acute phase proteins in veterinary diagnosis : an overview, *The Veterinary Journal*, Vol.168, pp. 28-40

Petersen, H.H., Ersbøll, A.K., Jensen, C.S. & Nielsen, J.P. (2002). Serum haptoglobin concentration in Danish slaughter pigs in different health status, *Preventive Veterinary Medicine*, Vol.54, pp. 325-335

Petersen, H.H., Nielsen, J.P. & Heegaard, P.M.H. (2004). Application of acute phase protein measurements in veterinary clinical chemistry, *Veterinary Research*, Vol.35, pp. 136-187

Pyörälä, S. (2000). *Hirvonen's thesis on acute phase response in dairy cattle*, University of Helsinki, ISBN 951-45-9104-6, Helsinki, Finnland

Reese, D.E., Peo, E.R., Lewis, A.J. & Hogg, A. (1984). Serum chemical values of gestating and lactating swine: reference values, *American Journal of Veterinary Research*, Vol.45, pp. 978-980

Regassa, F. & Noakes, D.E. (1999). Acute phase protein response of ewes and the release of PGFM in relation to uterine involution and the presence of intrauterine bacteria.,*Veterinary Record*, Vol.144, pp. 502-506

Rottmann, S. (2006). *Einfluss von nichtsteroidalen Antiphlogistika (NSAID) auf hämatologische und klinisch-chemische Parameter bei Rindern mit Dystokie,* Inaugural-Dissertation, Veterinärmedizinische Fakultät der Universität Leipzig, Leipzig, Germany

Segales, J., Pineiro, C., Lampreave, F., Nofrarias, M., Mateu, E., Calsamiglia, M., Andres, J., Morales, M., Pineiro, M. & Domingo, M. (2004). Haptoglobin and pig-major acute protein are increased in pigs with postweaning multisystemic wasting syndrome (PMWS), *Veterinary Research,* Vol.35, pp. 275-282

Seifi, H.A., Gorji-Dooz, M., Mohri, M., Dalir-Naghaden, B. & Farzaneh, N. (2007). Variations of energy-related biochemical metabolites during transition period in dairy cows, *Comparative Clinical Pathology,* Vol.16, pp. 253-258

Skinner, J.G., Brown, R.A.L. & Roberts, L. (1991). Bovine haptoglobin response in clinically defined field conditions, *Veterinary Record,* Vol.128, pp. 147–149

Sordillo, L.M., Contreras, G.A. & Aitken, S.L. (2009). Metabolic factors affecting the inflammatory response of periparturient dairy cows, *Animal Health Research Revue,* Vol.10, pp. 53-63.

Thornton, E.J., Wilson, R.J. & Connaughton, I. (1998). Effect of subclinical urogenital infection on reproductive performance in the sow, *Proceedings of the 15th International Pig Veterinary Society Congress,* p.236, Birmingham, England

Toussaint, M.J.M., Eckersall, P.D., Alava, M., Madec, F., Meleon, R.H. & Gruys, E. (2000). Acute phase protein assays as tool in assessment of health in pigs, *Revue de Medicine Veterine,* Vol.151, pp. 780

Uchida, E., Katoh, N. & Takahashi, K. (1993). Appearance of haptoglobin in serum from cows at parturition, *Journal of Veterinary Medical Science,* Vol.55, pp. 893-894

Yaqoob, P. & Calder, P.C. (2007). Fatty acids and immune functions: new insights into mechanisms, *British Journal of Nutrition,* Vol.98, pp. S41-S45

Young, C.R., Eckersall, P.D., Saini, P.K. & Stanker, L. (1995). Validation of immunoassays for bovine haptoglobin, *Veterinary Immunology and Immunopathology,* Vol.49, pp. 1-13

Verheyen, A.J.M., Maes, D.G.D., Mateusen, B., Deprez, P., Janssens, G.P.J., de Lange, L. & Counotte, G. (2007). Serum biochemical reference values for gestating and lactating sows, *The Veterinary Journal,* Vol.174, pp. 92-98

Waller, C.M., Bilkei, G. & Cameron, R.D.A. (2002). Effect of periparturient disease and/or reproductive failure accompained by excessive vulval discharge and weaning to mating interval on sow reproductive performance, *Australian Veterinary Journal,* Vol.80, pp. 545-549

Whicher, J.T. & Westacott, C.I. (1992). The acute phase response, In: *Biochemistry of inflammation,* J.T. Whicher & S.W. Evans, (Eds.), 243-271, Kluwer Academic, London, United Kingdom

Wood, I.G., Scott, H.A., Garg, M.I. & Gibson, P.G. (2009). Innate immune mechanisms linking non-esterified fatty acids and respiratory disease, *Progress in Lipid Research,* Vol.48, pp. 27-43

11

Acute Phase Proteins as Markers of Diseases in Farm Animals

Csilla Tóthová, Oskar Nagy,
Herbert Seidel and Gabriel Kováč
University of Veterinary Medicine and Pharmacy in Košice
Slovak Republic

1. Introduction

Acute phase proteins have been studied widely in human medicine, especially as biomarkers of diseases, inflammatory processes and various infections, to diagnose and monitor the success of diseases, as well as to follow-up the treatment in clinical praxis (Hilliquin, 1995; Deans & Wigmore, 2005; Endre & Westhuyzen, 2008). However, the possible influence of inflammatory conditions on the concentrations of acute phase proteins, and the use of these indicators in the monitoring of animal health and detection of diseases in veterinary medicine, especially in farm animal medicine is less well documented. Therefore, an increased focus on the application of acute phase proteins in veterinary clinical practice has recently been developed. Recently studies show their functions, and influences on the organism (Murata et al., 2004; Petersen et al., 2004).

The acute phase response is in animal species, by which the organism respond to impaired homeostasis, caused by tissue injury or inflammation, leading to a range of metabolic activities and biochemical processes (Whicher & Westacott, 1992 ; Baumann & Gauldie, 1994). One of the most important metabolic changes during the acute phase response is the strongly plasma-increased or decreased liver production and secretion of the acute phase proteins. These biomarkers are non-specific but highly sensitive exhibiting strong differences in their production between different animal species (Eckersall & Bell, 2010).

For this reason, the objective of this article is provide an integrated overview about the diagnostic value of acute phase proteins levels in farm animals along with some clinical aspects of veterinary practices.

2. The acute phase response

All vertebrates demonstrate an early and non-specific complex of reactions to injury known as the acute phase response. The acute phase response is a cascade of host responses, which is induced by any process that leads to tissue damage e.g. bacterial and viral infection, parasite infestation, trauma, surgery, ischemic necrosis, burns, neoplastic growth (Baumann & Gauldie, 1994; Suffredini et al., 1999). The acute phase response is characterized by numerous local and systemic changes and involves a variety of cell types and organs (Koj, 1996; Gabay & Kushner, 1999). The reactions of the acute phase response are part of the non-specific immune system and thus the first line of defense against invading pathogens. It is designed to hold the infection in check until the adaptive, highly specialized immune response is initiated (Fearon & Locksley, 1996).

Blood monocytes and tissue macrophages are central to initiating the acute phase response. After being activated by "alarm molecules" e.g. arachidonic acid metabolites and modified host proteins recognized as foreign, released from injured cells and tissues, monocytes and macrophages produce a vast number of inflammatory mediators, among which the cytokines play very important roles (Bellomo, 1992). The local, paracrine effects and the distant, endocrine effects of cytokines propagate the continuation of the acute phase response by stimulating various other cell types to the secondary release of cytokines responsible for the start of the systemic inflammatory response (Janeway et al., 2001; Cray et al., 2009).

During the acute phase response, the metabolic effort is directed at removal of the inflammatory stimulus, promotion of healing and repair processes and restoration of the homeostasis (Murata et al., 2004). However, the acute phase response is not uniformly beneficial. For example, iron sequestration and catabolism may result from prolonged cytokine production and cause anemia and impaired growth and weight loss (Jennings & Elia, 1996). Furthermore, when pro-inflammatory cytokines are produced in excessive amounts – as may occur during sepsis – shock and even death may ensue. The acute phase response thus needs to be tightly controlled.

2.1 Stimulation of the acute phase response

The acute phase response is stimulated by the release of pro-inflammatory cytokines such as interleukin-1 beta (IL1-β), interleukin-6 (IL-6) and tumor necrosis factor α (TNF-α) from macrophages and monocytes at the site of inflammatory lesions or infection (Heinrich et al., 1990). Cytokines are soluble proteins, which act at picomolar to nanomolar concentrations to regulate host inflammatory functions (Nathan & Sporn, 1991). Cytokines exert their effects mainly over shorter distances, but they may also affect cells far from their site of synthesis (Hagiwara et al., 2001). They have a short half-life span, their continue synthesis is a requisite for sustained elevated concentrations of cytokines. In addition, active inhibition through anti-inflammatory mediators such as IL-4, IL-10 and IL-13 is involved in termination of the acute phase response (Koj, 1996). The disease outcome depends on the balance between pro- and anti-inflammatory activities (Adrie & Pinsky, 2000). If their effects are not properly modulated or if they are synthesized in excessive amounts, the pro-inflammatory cytokines are potent enough to cause tissue injury, organ failure and death (Taniguchi et al., 1999).

2.2 Acute phase response and homeostasis

Cytokines activate receptors on different target cells leading to systemic inflammatory reactions, including hormonal, metabolic or biochemical reactions, and resulting in a number of changes clinically characterized by fever, anorexia, weight loss or slow-wave sleep (Gruys et al., 2005). These symptoms reflect multiple changes in the homeostatic control of the diseased animals, such as increased production of adrenocorticotrophic hormone and glucocorticoids, activation of the complement cascade and blood coagulation system, decreased serum concentrations of calcium, zinc, iron, vitamin A and α-tocopherol, and changes in the concentrations of some plasma proteins (Pyörälä, 2000). One of the most important metabolic changes is the strongly increased synthesis of a group of plasma proteins, namely acute phase proteins, by the liver (Raynes, 1994).

3. Acute phase proteins

Acute phase proteins are phylogenetically old and may be found not only in mammals, but also in other vertebrates such as birds, marsupials, and fish. In general, acute phase proteins are a group of blood proteins that change in concentrations in animals subjected to external or internal challenges, such as infection, inflammation, trauma or stress (Murata et al., 2004).

By definition, the serum concentrations of acute phase proteins increase (positive acute phase proteins) or decrease (negative acute phase proteins) with at least 25 % during the acute phase response (Ceron et al., 2005; Eckersall & Bell, 2010). Moreover, there are large differences in the responsibility of various acute phase proteins, some of them respond markedly to inflammatory stimuli, another have moderate or minor responses (Petersen et al., 2004). Major acute phase proteins have low concentrations in the serum of healthy animals, but with their concentrations increase over 100- or 1000-fold on stimulation, reaching a peak 24 - 48 hours after the insult and fall rapidly during recovery (Niewold et al., 2003). Moderate acute phase proteins are present in the blood of healthy animals, but after stimulation their concentrations increase 5 - 10 fold, reaching a peak concentration 2 - 3 days after stimulation and decrease more slowly than major acute phase proteins (Eckersall, 2006). Minor acute phase proteins show a gradual increase of 50 - 100 % of normal values.

The functions of the acute phase proteins are varied and combined to defend the host against pathological damage and assist in the homeostasis restoration. A number of acute phase proteins are likely to participate directly in the protection of the host. Some of the acute phase proteins (α_1-antitrypsin, α_2-macroglobulin) have anti-protease activity designed to inhibit proteases released by phagocytes or pathogens to minimize damage to normal tissues (Pyörälä, 2000). Another acute phase proteins (haptoglobin, serum amyloid A, C-reactive protein) have scavenging activities and bind metabolites released from cellular degradation so they can re-enter host metabolic processes rather than be utilized by pathogen (Wagener et al., 2001). Other acute phase proteins (α_1-acid glycoprotein) are characterized by anti-bacterial activity and by the ability to influence the course of the immune response (Eckersall, 2006a).

3.1 Acute phase proteins in cattle

Despite the uniform nature of the acute phase response, there are numerous differences in the acute phase characteristics between different animal species (Pyörälä, 2000). C-reactive protein is a good example of this phenomenon: in healthy humans it is practically negligible, but has a high relative increase during infections, whereas in healthy cattle it is present, but does not increase markedly during the acute phase response (Steel & Whitehead, 1994). Acute phase proteins have typically their representatives in different species (Table 1). In cattle, haptoglobin and serum amyloid A were identified as major acute phase proteins.

Animal species	Major APPs	Moderate APPs
Cat	SAA	AGP, Hp
Dog	CRP, SAA	Hp, AGP
Horse	SAA	Hp
Cattle	Hp, SAA	AGP
Pig	CRP, MAP, SAA	Hp

Table 1. Acute phase proteins in different animal species (Eckersall, 2007)

3.1.1 Haptoglobin

Haptoglobin (Hp) is a glycoprotein composed of 2 α and 2 β subunits. The α subunit has a molecular weight of 16 - 23 kDa and the β subunit 35 - 40 kDa. The subunits combine in the form of a β-α-α-β tetramer chain. Human Hp has 3 subtypes known to be genetic polymorphism (Hp 1-1, Hp 1-2, Hp 2-2). In animals, Hp tetramers have noticeable species differences. Haptoglobin in carnivores and omnivores is thought to be similar to human Hp 1-1, while bovine Hp has closer similarities to Hp 2-2 (Morimatsu et al., 1991). In circulation, Hp is highly polymerized having a molecular weight of approximately 1000 - 2000 kDa, and exists also as polymer associated with albumin (Godson et al., 1996).

The primary function of Hp is to bind free hemoglobin in the blood. The affinity of Hp for hemoglobin is one of the major protein transporters (Bowman, 1992). By removing from the circulation any free hemoglobin, which has inherent peroxidase activity, Hp prevents oxidative damage of tissues (Yang et al., 2003). The Hp-hemoglobin binding also reduces the availability of the heme residue from bacterial growth and therefore Hp has an indirect anti-bacterial activity (Murata et al., 2004).

Many studies have indicated the significance of Hp as a clinically useful parameter for measuring the occurrence and severity of inflammatory responses in cattle with mastitis, pneumonia, enteritis, peritonitis, endocarditis, abscesses, endometritis and other natural or experimental infectious situations (Ohtsuka et al., 2001; Eckersall, 2006). Haptoglobin is used to monitor the treatment efficacy of antibiotics in cows with toxic puerperal metritis (Smith et al., 1998). Hp is also used to determine the effect of anti-inflammatory drugs following the castration of bull calves, the relative effects of bacterial contamination and involution of the uterus in dairy cows after calving, the effects of treatment in transport-stressed feedlot cattle, the effects of tail docking or surgical castration, and the changes in the blood profile of neonatal calves (Carter et al., 2002).

Haptoglobin is also induced in cows with fatty liver syndrome, by starvation, and in calves following stress associated with road transport (Katoh et al., 2002).

3.1.2 Serum amyloid A

Serum amyloid A (SAA) is a small hydrophobic protein (9 - 14 kDa), which is found in serum associated with high density lipoprotein. In humans, four separate isoforms have been identified (Jensen & Whitehead, 1998). Of these, SAA1 and SAA2 respond to an acute phase reaction with increased production from the liver. In contrast, SAA4 is a constitutive protein that is produced normally at low concentrations and is not affected by the acute phase response. The SAA3 isoform is expressed in non-hepatic tissues during the acute phase response with increases found in lung, adipose tissue, ovarian granulosa, as well as in the mammary gland (Weber et al., 2006). The mammary isoform (M-SAA3) has also been detected in bovine colostrum (McDonald et al., 2001).

Serum amyloid A is the precursor of amyloid A and is therefore implicated in the pathogenesis of amyloidosis (Uhlar & Whitehead, 1999). Among the functions ascribed to SAA have been reverse transport of cholesterol from tissue to hepatocytes, inhibition of phagocyte oxidative burst and platelet activation (Petersen et al., 2004). Recently, a direct antibacterial action of SAA was identified, in which SAA was found to bind to Gram-negative bacteria leading to opsonisation of the target pathogen (Hari-Dass et al., 2005). The M-SAA3 isoform found in colostrum stimulates the production of mucin from intestinal cells assisting the initiation of secretions from the neonatal intestine and helping to prevent bacterial colonization (Mack et al., 2003).

Serum amyloid A is a valuable acute phase protein in diagnosing cattle with inflammation. Increased milk SAA concentrations can be detected in cows with mastitis (Eckersall et al., 2001). Moreover, SAA in conjunction with haptoglobin may be useful markers of milk quality. Elevated serum SAA concentrations are also found in cows at parturition or in cattle subjected to physical stress, suggesting that the acute phase response is also activated under conditions unrelated to inflammation (Alsemggest et al., 1993). In cattle, it was raised also by experimental infection with *Mannheimia haemolytica* and with bovine respiratory syncytial virus (Heegaard et al., 2000). The mammary isoform M-SAA3 is secreted in milk from the mammary gland of dairy cows with mastitis, which suggests a potential role of this biomarker for this condition (Jacobsen et al., 2005).

3.1.3 Fibrinogen

Fibrinogen (Fbg), a precursor of fibrin, is also an acute phase protein, which has been used for many years to evaluate inflammatory and traumatic diseases in cattle, and is characterized by markedly increased synthesis in response to infection (Hirvonen & Pyörälä, 1998). Fibrinogen is involved in homeostasis, providing a substrate for fibrin formation, and in tissue repair, providing a matrix for the migration of inflammatory-related cells (Thomas, 2000).

Fibrinogen is used in cattle and sheep as a reliable indicator of the presence of inflammation, bacterial infection or surgical trauma (Cheryk et al., 1998). It increases in various inflammatory conditions of cattle, such as peritonitis, endocarditis, pericarditis, pneumonia, and nephritis, or *E. coli* infection in calves (Jafarzadeh et al., 2004). However, plasma Fbg concentrations can also remain unchanged or decrease during acute inflammatory conditions of cattle. This may reflect consumption of the protein at the inflamed area which transiently can exceed the production (Welles et al., 1993).

3.1.4 Albumin

Serum albumin is the major negative acute phase protein. During the acute phase response the demand for amino acids for synthesis of the positive acute phase proteins is markedly increased, which necessitates reprioritization of the hepatic protein synthesis: albumin synthesis is down-regulated and amino acids are shunted into synthesis of positive acute phase proteins (Aldred & Schreiber, 1993). It has been reported that during the acute phase response 30 to 40 % of the hepatic protein synthesizing capacity is used for production of positive acute phase proteins, and the production of other proteins thus need to be diminished (Mackiewicz, 1997).

3.2 Acute phase proteins in small ruminants

The acute phase proteins in small ruminants have not been studied in as much detail as in cattle, but it appears that the acute phase response is similar. Experimental studies showed that caseous lymphadenitis in sheep can cause a marked increase of Hp and SAA concentrations, which is accompanied by lower and more lasting increase of the concentrations of α_1-acid glycoprotein (Eckersall, 2007). Haptoglobin has proven useful as prognostic indicator of dystocia in sheep, and can be used to investigate the relationship between uterine involution and the presence of intrauterine bacteria in ewes (Scott et al., 1992). A recent study reports that vaccination of lambs causes an acute phase response that reaches a peak within 24-48 hours, and could have a role to play in the assessment of vaccine efficacy (Dowling et al., 2004).

3.3 Acute phase proteins in pigs

In pigs, C-reactive protein, haptoglobin, α_1-acid glycoprotein, and pig specific major acute phase protein were identified as the diagnostically most important acute phase proteins.

3.3.1 C-reactive protein

In pigs, as in dogs and humans, C-reactive protein (CRP) is the prototypical acute phase protein with major diagnostic value. Tillet and Francis (1930) discovered CRP over 70 years ago in the blood of pacients with *Streptococcus pneumoniae* infection, as a substance that precipitated the C-polysaccharide of the cell wall of the pneumococcus and they called it C-reactive substance, which was later changed to C-reactive protein (Du Clos, 2004). C-reactive protein plays important roles in the protection against infection, clearence of damaged tissues, and regulation of the inflammatory response (Mold et al., 2002). Structurally, CRP is a cyclic pentamer which binds with a variety of pathogenic bacteria or intracellular antigens of damaged cells, thus recognizing foreign molecules and altered self (Murata et al., 2004).

In pigs, CRP is considered to be one of the best markers for the identification of inflammatory lesions. It can be used as a parameter for monitoring a pig's general state of health, including for stress assessment (Burger et al., 1998). Serum CRP concentrations increased following aseptic inflammation and during the experimental infection with *Actinobacillus pleuropneumoniae* (Lampreave et al., 1994). Porcine CRP has also been found to rise in experimental models of *Mycoplasma hyorhinis*, *Toxoplasma gondii*, *Streptococcus suis* and porcine reproductive and respiratory syndrome virus infection (Eckersall, 2006).

3.3.2 Alpha$_1$-acid glycoprotein

The precise function of α_1-acid glycoprotein (AGP) is not yet clear, but it does bind to a number of metabolites such as heparin, histamine and serotonin, steroids and catecholamines (Israili and Dayton, 2001). It is also known to bind to pharmacological compounds which may have therapeutic implications as the amount bound can affect the metabolically active fraction of the drug. Increased AGP due to an acute phase response thus may reduce the concentration of free drugs, thus affecting their pharmacokinetics.

3.3.3 Pig specific major acute phase protein

Specifically in pigs, a specific acute phase protein (pig MAP) of unknown function has been reported as a sensitive indicator of infection. Increased levels in pig MAP have been shown during infections with *Actinobacillus pleuropneumoniae*, in post weaning multisystemic wasting disorder as well as following animal transportation (Segales et al., 2004).

4. The usefulness of the evaluation of acute phase proteins in the veterinary clinical practice

The measurement of the concentrations of acute phase proteins can detect or confirm the presence of infection or pathological lesion, but a major role for these analytes in farm animal medicine could be in the monitoring of the health status of animals in production. Acute phase proteins can detect the presence of sub-clinical disease which is the cause of reduced growth rate and losses in the production (Petersen et al., 2004). Use of an acute phase index, by combining the results of both positive and negative acute phase proteins has been suggested as a means to increase the sensitivity of detection of sub-clinical disease (Toussaint et al., 2000). In the clinical field, acute phase proteins may serve as indicators of prognosis and effect of treatment. The magnitude and duration of the acute phase response reflect the severity of the infection and underlying tissue damage (Heegaard et al., 2000).
Acute phase proteins have been extensively investigated in various inflammatory and non-inflammatory conditions. However, there are many more areas of enquiry which can be pursued to deepen our knowledge about the acute phase response and also to develop novel applications for the acute phase proteins, e.g. in various physiological conditions (after birth), during some less frequently studied diseases of young (diarrhoea, omphalophlebitis) and adult cattle (laminitis, mastitis), as well as not only in acute infections, but also in chronic inflammatory conditions.

5. Material and methods

5.1 Animals used in the study, clinical examination, sample collection, and the evaluated parameters

5.1.1 Acute phase proteins in relation to the growth and development of calves

The evaluation of the dynamics of age-dependent changes in the concentrations of selected acute phase proteins during the first 6 months of life was performed in seven clinically healthy calves (three males, four females) on a farm near to the University of Veterinary Medicine and Pharmacy in Kosice. The calves were of a low-land black spotted breed and its crossbreeds. The observation of the calves started at the age of 1 month and body weight of 45 - 51 kg. The animals were kept loosely in individual pens and fed ordinary whole milk 2 times a day. The transition to a solid diet lasted until the age of 2.5 month. During this period, the calves were fed gradually decreasing amounts of milk, and increasing amounts of meadow hay, and concentrates (transitional feeding period). At the age of 3 months, they were moved to a stable and housed loosely in larger groups of animals, and fed hay and grain with free access to water. Before each sample collection, the calves were examined clinically using standard clinical examination procedures (Jackson & Cockcroft, 2002). The evaluated calves showed no health disorders during the whole time of observation.
The analyses of evaluated parameters were performed in blood samples. Blood samples were taken monthly by jugular venipuncture during the first 6 months of life. The first collection was established at the age of 1 month. Blood samples were collected into plastic tubes with gel and clot activator. Serum was stored at -20 °C until analysis of haptoglobin (Hp, mg/ml) and serum amyloid A (SAA, μg/ml). Moreover, blood samples were collected also into tubes with sodium citrate, and the separated plasma was used for the analysis of the concentrations of fibrinogen (Fbg, g/l) immediately after the separation without storage.

5.1.2 Acute phase proteins in calves suffering from various inflammatory diseases

Sixty-nine sick calves with clinical signs of various inflammatory diseases such as respiratory diseases, diarrhoea or omphalophlebitis were used in this study. The calves were of a Slovak spotted breed, low-land black spotted breed, or their crossbreeds at the age from 2 weeks to 6 months. The evaluated calves were sent to the Clinic for Ruminants of the University of Veterinary Medicine and Pharmacy in Kosice (Slovak Republic) by privat veterinarian from three different conventional dairy farms. On the clinic, the animals were housed individually, fed twice a day with free access to water.

After the arrival to the clinic, all calves were thoroughly clinically examined using standard clinical examination procedures, oriented to the examination of general health state (body temperature, food intake, behaviour), and than specially to the respiratory system, gastrointestinal tract and umbilicus, including the recording of the clinical signs of the diseases (Jackson & Cockcroft, 2002). The evaluation of acute phase proteins was performed in 4 groups of calves grouped on the basis of the clinical examination: Group A - calves with clinical signs of respiratory diseases (n = 46); Group B - calves with diarrhoea (n = 10); Group C - calves with omphalophlebitis (n = 5); Group D - calves with multisystemic diseases (n = 8). This group of calves consisted of animals with more than one affected organ (respiratory system, digestive tract, navel, joints). To compare the evaluated variables between sick and healthy animals, twenty-eight clinically healthy calves (Group H) of the same age and breed, in good general health without any obvious disease were used as a group of controls.

Blood samples were taken from both healthy and sick animals once after initial clinical examination, when the clinical signs of the disease in sick animals were apparent. Blood samples were collected by direct puncture of *v. jugularis*, subseqeuntly haptoglobin (Hp, mg/ml), serum amyloid A (SAA, µg/ml), and fibrinogen (Fbg, g/l) were assessed.

5.1.3 The influence of chronic respiratory diseases on the concentrations of acute phase proteins in calves

The influence of chronic respiratory diseases on the concentrations of selected acute phase proteins was investigated in twenty-seven sick calves of a low-land black spotted breed and its crossbreeds at the age of 3 - 6 months, which were clinical cases suffering from chronic respiratory diseases of various degree, and were hospitalized on the Clinic for Ruminants of the University of Veterinary Medicine in Kosice (Slovak Republic). The animals were submitted to the clinic by privat veterinarian from three dairy farms localized in the district of the university. The feeding regime of the animals on these farms was similar. On the clinic, the animals were kept in individual pens, fed twice a day with free access to water. The body weight of the calves was 85 - 140 kg.

In this study, calves with clinical signs manifested for more than 2 weeks despite antimicrobial, antiinflammatory, and supportive therapy done by private veterinarians of the farm were analyzed. The duration of the disease in animals was estimated from the history of the disease process. Diagnosis was done by clinical examination and in some cases by ultrasound as well as endoscope examination by the same veterinarian. Clinical examination was oriented predominantly to the examination of general health state (body temperature, food intake, behaviour), and the respiratory system by visual inspection (breathing rate, nasal discharges, type of breathing, dyspnoe, coughing) and auscultation (increased or decreased loudness of the breathing sounds, abnormal sounds). The calves did not show pathological lesions on other organ systems. On the clinic we performed further therapy of sick calves by antibiotics (marbofloxacine, amoxicillin, tetracycline, benzylpenicillin, streptomycine), antiinflammaatory drugs (flunixin-meglumine), supportive remedies (vitamins), and infusions.

Blood samples for the investigations were taken from calves once during the study period, after the clinical examination and including the animals into the study. Blood samples were collected by direct puncture of *v. jugularis*. subseqeuntly Hp and SAA, were assessed.

Calves were divided into two groups according to their health state during the treatment: Group A (n = 16) - calves with observable response to treatment and improvement of general health state (normal body temperature, improved appetite, intermittent coughing, less marked abnormal breathing sounds, but not in a comparable general condition as healthy calves); Group B (n = 11) - calves with no response to treatment, which despite long lasting antibiotic, anti-inflammatory, and supportive therapy during the treatment died, or because of poor prognosis (as a consequence of persistent disturbance of general health state and marked changes on the respiratory system) were euthanised. The control group consist in fifteen clinically healthy calves of the same age, nutrition and breed.

5.1.4 Acute phase proteins in the laboratory diagnosis of mastitis in dairy cows

To assess the relationship between clinical and sub-clinical mastitis and concentrations of milk amyloid A in milk samples, and selected acute phase proteins in blood serum 41 dairy cows (of a low-land black spotted breed and its crossbreeds with various clinical findings on the mammary gland) were studied. These cows were in the 3rd - 4th lactation, but not in the period shortly after parturition. Clinical examination of the mammary gland was performed by visual inspection and palpation, using standard physical methods of examination. Clinical mastitis was diagnosed by the presence of observable signs of inflammation in the infected quarter such as swelling, heat, pain or redness, and by the presence of clots and flakes in the milk, or by its abnormal color or consistency. To detect sub-clinical mastitis the Californian Mastitis Test (CMT) was performed. According to the results of the clinical examination of the udder and to the results of CMT the animals were divided into 4 groups: Group I - cows without clinical changes on the mammary gland and with negative CMT (n = 7), Group II - cows without clinical changes on the mammary gland and with weakly positive CMT (n = 12), Group III - cows without clinical changes on the mammary gland and with strongly positive CMT (n = 13), Group IV - cows with clinical changes on the mammary gland and changes in milk appearance (n = 9).

Milk samples were collected into plastic tubes by hand-stripping. Blood samples were collected by direct puncture of *v. jugularis*. Milk samples were used to assess concentrations of milk amyloid A (M-SAA, ng/ml) and Hp and SAA were assessed in blood samples.

5.1.5 Acute phase proteins in heifers affected by hoof diseases

Selected acute phase proteins were assessed in 35 heifers of a low-land black spotted breed and its crossbreeds, with various clinical findings on hoofs. These animals were hospitalized on the Clinic for Ruminants of the University of Veterinary Medicine and Pharmacy in Kosice (Slovak Republic). The animals were submitted to the clinic by private veterinarian from a private farmer. On the clinic, the heifers were housed individually, fed twice a day and had *ad libitum* access to water.

All heifers were clinically examined using standard clinical examination procedures, oriented to the examination of general health state (body temperature, food intake, behaviour, gait, and movement). Hoof disorders were diagnosed by orthopedic inspection performed according to the method described by Jackson & Cockcroft (2002). In the evaluated heifers pododermatitis, laminitis, sole ulcer, and digital dermatitis were the most often diagnosed diseases, and they did not show pathological lesions on other organ systems. Another 23 clinically healthy animals of the same age and breed, in good general health without any obvious disease, including lameness, as evaluated by routine clinical inspection were used as controls to compare the evaluated variables between sick and healthy animals.

Blood samples were collected by direct puncture of *v. jugularis* into plastic tubes with gel and clot activator for serum (analysis of haptoglobin and serum amyloid A), and into special tubes with sodium citrate for plasma (analysis of fibrinogen).

5.2 APP analyses

5.2.1 Haptoglobin

Haptoglobin was assessed using commercial colorimetric kits (Tridelta Development, Ireland) in microplates, based on Hp-haemoglobin binding and preservation of the peroxidase activity of the bound haemoglobin at low pH. The optical densities were read on automatic microplate reader Opsys MR (Dynex Technologies, USA) at an optical density of 630 nm.

5.2.2 Serum amyloid A

Serum amyloid A was analysed by a commercial ELISA kit (Tridelta Development, Ireland). The optical densities were read on automatic microplate reader Opsys MR (Dynex Technologies, USA) at 450 nm using 630 nm as reference.

5.2.3 Milk amyloid A

The concentrations of M-SAA were analyzed according to the method described in the section 5.2.2, modified by the manufacturer for the determination of amyloid A in milk samples.

5.2.4 Fibrinogen

The determination of fibrinogen was performed on the semi-automatic 4-channel coagulometer Behnk CL-4 (Behnk Elektronik GmbH & Co., Germany) using commercial diagnostic kits (Diagon Kft, Hungary), based on the principle of electromagnetic detection of fibrin formation.

5.2.5 Californian Mastitis Test

The Californian Mastitis Test was performed using equal volumes of milk and alkyl-aryl-sulphonate by the same person in each cow.

5.3 Statistical analyses

Statistical analyses were done in the programme GraphPad Prism V5.02 (GraphPad Software Inc.) by assessment of arithmetic means (x) and standard deviations (SD) for each

evaluated parameter and each group of animals, calculated using descriptive statistical procedures.
The significance of the influence of age (P) on the evaluated variables during the whole monitored period was analyzed by the non-parametric Friedman's rank sum test. The significance of the differences in values between the sample collections was evaluated by the Dunn`s Multiple Comparisons Test.
The analysis of the significance of differences in measured values between calves with various inflammatory diseases was performed by Kruskal-Wallis nonparametric ANOVA test and Dunn's Multiple Comparisons Test. The aforementioned statistical methods were used also by the evaluation of the differences between cows with various clinical findings on the mammary gland.
The assessment of the significance of differences in measured values of the evaluated variables between healthy animals and calves affected by chronic respiratory diseases was peformed by Mann-Whitney non-parametric test. Similar statistical methods were used for the analyses of differences between healthy animals and heifers with hoof diseases.

6. Results

6.1 Acute phase proteins in relation to the growth and development of calves

Concentrations of acute phase proteins during the first six months of calves life were monitored. The results showed significant changes in haptoglobin, serum amyloid A, as well as fibrinogen concentrations (P < 0.05, P < 0.05, and P < 0.01, respectively). The serum concentrations of Hp during the first three months of life and in the 5th month of age were roughly uniform. More marked changes in the mean Hp concentrations were recorded in the 4-month-old calves (increase) and in the 6-month-old ones (decrease).
Serum concentrations of SAA in calves gradually and significantly decrease (P < 0.05). The mean concentrations of SAA in the first three months of life were more than two-fold higher than those in older animals. The highest mean concentration of Fbg (3.14 g/l) in blood plasma of calves was recorded in the 2nd month of age. In the 3rd month of age a repeated decrease of the values measured with the lowest mean Fbg concentrations (2.17 g/l) was observed in the 6-month-old calves.

Variable		Age of the calves (months)						*P*
		1	2	3	4	5	6	
Hp (mg/ml)	x	0.068^{A}	0.064	0.056	0.213	0.062	0.021^{A}	< 0.05
	± SD	0.021	0.026	0.024	0.344	0.081	0.018	
SAA (µg/ml)	x	59.12^{a}	53.37	39.71	21.20	10.51^{a}	19.86	< 0.05
	± SD	35.61	21.43	26.65	19.97	10.36	27.42	
Fbg (g/l)	x	2.31	3.14^{a}	2.55	2.87	2.82^{b}	$2.17^{a,b}$	< 0.01
	± SD	0.76	0.75	0.32	0.57	0.40	0.20	

The same superscripts in rows mean statistical significance of differences in concentrations between the columns: a, b – P < 0.05, A – P < 0.01
P – significance of the differences

Table 2. Age-related changes in the concentrations of evaluated APPs in clinically healthy calves from the 1st till 6th month of age

6.2 Acute phase proteins in calves suffering from various inflammatory diseases

Hp exhibited significant differences between clinically healthy calves and calves suffering from various inflammatory diseases (P < 0.001, Table 3). The highest mean value among the sick animals was found in calves with clinical signs of respiratory diseases (Group A). The Hp concentrations obtained in calves with respiratory signs were significantly higher than the values recorded in clinically healthy animals (Group H, P < 0.001). Higher mean concentration we found also in calves with multisystemic diseases (Group D), but the obtained results were not significantly different compared with values recorded in clinically healthy animals. The mean concentrations found in calves with diarrhoea (Group B) and in calves with omphalophlebitis (Group C) were roughly uniform and lower than in the above mentioned animals from the Group A and D.

Significant differences between the evaluated groups of calves were found also for SAA (P < 0.001, Table 3), with concentrations in samples from calves with clinical signs of respiratory diseases (Group A) being significantly higher than in clinically healthy calves (Group A, P < 0.001). Markedly higher mean concentration of SAA compared with healthy animals was found also in calves with omphalophlebitis (Group C), with the maximum individual concentration of 106.00 μg/ml. The SAA concentrations recorded in calves with signs of diarrhoea (Group B) and in calves affected by multisystemic diseases (Group D) were the lowest among the evaluated groups of calves, and were nearly similar.

Variables		Groups of calves					K-W
		H	A	B	C	D	*P*
Hp (mg/ml)	x	0.04[a]	0.73[a]	0.10	0.13	0.43	< 0.001
	SD	0.03	0.78	0.16	0.16	0.78	
SAA (μg/ml)	x	29.78[a]	93.38[a]	51.47	74.94	42.02	< 0.001
	SD	24.62	50.96	25.05	26.16	28.21	
Fbg (g/l)	x	2.31[a]	3.86[a]	2.84	2.81	3.16	< 0.001
	SD	0.41	1.55	0.77	0.51	1.22	

The same superscripts in rows mean statistical significance of differences in measured concentrations between the groups of calves: a – P < 0.001
K-W – Kruskal-Wallis analysis; P – significance of the analysis
Groups of calves: H – clinically healthy calves, A – calves with clinical signs of respiratory diseases, B – diarrhoeic calves, C – calves with omphalophlebitis, D – calves with multisystemic diseases

Table 3. Comparison of the concentrations of Hp, SAA and Fbg between clinically healthy calves and calves affected by various inflammatory diseases

Similarly, the concentrations of Fbg in blood plasma differed significantly between the evaluated groups of calves (P < 0.001). Significantly higher concentrations of Fbg compared with clinically healthy calves we observed in calves suffering from respiratory diseases (Group A, P < 0.001). Trend of higher Fbg concentrations was observed also in calves affected by multisystemic diseases (Group D) with the maximum individual concentration of 5.04 g/l in this group of calves. Higher values of Fbg were found also in calves suffering from diarrhoea (Group B), as well as in calves with navel inflammation (Group C). However, the differences between these groups of animals and the healthy ones were not significant.

6.3 The influence of chronic respiratory diseases on the concentrations of acute phase proteins in calves

The average Hp concentration was significantly higher (P < 0.001) in calves suffering from chronic respiratory diseases as compared with healthy animals (Table 4). Moreover, the analyses of results in sick animals showed significantly higher serum concentration of Hp in died, or euthanised calves (Group B; P < 0.05) as compared with those in improved health state (Group A, Table 5).

Variables	Group of calves		P
	Healthy (n = 15)	**Sick** (n = 27)	
Hp (mg/ml)	0.05 ± 0.06	1.11 ± 0.80	< 0.001
SAA (ʃg/ml)	28.02 ± 20.60	63.19 ± 39.42	< 0.01

P - significance of the differences in measured values between healthy and sick animals, n. s. - non significant

Table 4. Concentrations of Hp, and SAA in healthy animals and calves suffering from chronic respiratory diseases (x ± SD)

SAA levels (P < 0.01) in sick calves were significantly higher than in healthy individuals. The mean value of this variable in calves with poor prognosis (Group B) was about two-fold higher (P < 0.01) compared with the mean in the Group A (Table 5).

Variables	Group of sick calves		P
	A (n = 16)	**B** (n = 11)	
Hp (mg/ml)	0.81 ± 0.60	1.56 ± 0.86	< 0.05
SAA (µg/ml)	44.70 ± 30.78	90.07 ± 35.73	< 0.01

Groups of calves: A - group of calves with improved general health state; B - group of died or euthanised calves

P - significance of the differences in measured values between two groups of sick calves, n. s. - non significant

Table 5. Comparison of concentrations of Hp, and SAA between two groups of sick calves (x ± SD)

6.4 Acute phase proteins in the laboratory diagnosis of mastitis in dairy cows

M-SAA concentrations in milk samples differed significantly between the groups (P < 0.001), with concentrations in samples from cows with clinical mastitis (group IV) being significantly higher than in samples from groups I and II (P < 0.001 and P < 0.05, respectively, Table 6). The concentrations of M-SAA in milk samples increased with increasing CMT score.

The serum concentrations of Hp showed also tendency of gradual significant increase with increasing CMT score and clinical changes on the mammary gland (P < 0.05, Table 6). The highest mean Hp concentration we found in cows with clinically manifested signs of mastitis. Similarly, SAA concentrations differed significantly between the evaluated groups of cows (P < 0.05), with the highest mean concentration in animals with clinical signs of mastitis. However, the differences in the obtained results of Hp and SAA concentrations between the evaluated groups of cows were less significant (P < 0.05) compared with M-

SAA concentrations. The mean SAA concentrations found in cows from group I and group II were roughly uniform.

Variable		Groups of cows				K-W P
		I. (n=7)	**II.** (n=12)	**III.** (n=13)	**IV.** (n=9)	
M-SAA ng/ml	x	325.7[A,B]	1433.1[a]	3910.4[A]	6073.8[B,a]	< 0.001
	± SD	173.8	949.2	2145.8	4414.0	
Hp mg/ml	x	0.046	0.122	0.299	0.329	< 0.05
	± SD	0.053	0.263	0.314	0.339	
SAA µg/ml	x	29.7	27.6[a]	48.2	71.5[a]	< 0.05
	± SD	27.6	28.0	42.5	31.5	

The same superscripts in rows mean statistical significance of differences in measured concentrations between the groups of cows: a – P < 0.05; A, B – P < 0.001
K-W – Kruskal-Wallis analysis; P – significance of the analysis
Groups of cows: I – cows without clinical findings on the mammary gland and with negative CMT, II – cows without clinical findings on the mammary gland and with weakly positive CMT, III – cows without clinical findings on the mammary gland and with strongly positive CMT, IV – cows with clinical changes and changes in the milk appearance

Table 6. The concentrations of M-SAA, Hp, and SAA in dairy cows with various findings on the mammary gland

6.5 Acute phase proteins in heifers affected by hoof diseases

The data referring to the concentrations of evaluated acute phase proteins in healthy animals and heifers with hoof diseases are presented in Table 7. In affected animals, the concentrations of Hp, SAA, as well as Fbg were significantly higher than in healthy animals (P < 0.05, P < 0.001, and P < 0.001, respectively).

Variables	Groups of animals		P
	Healthy (n = 23)	**Sick** (n = 35)	
Hp (mg/ml)	0.094 ± 0.086	0.450 ± 0.601	< 0.05
SAA (µg/ml)	12.70 ± 16.80	113.90 ± 55.66	< 0.001
Fbg (g/l)	2.19 ± 0.37	2.95 ± 0.65	< 0.001

P – significance of the differences in measured values between healthy and sick animals, n. s. – non significant

Table 7. Comparison of the concentrations of evaluated acute phase proteins in healthy animals and heifers with hoof diseases (x ± SD)

7. Discussion

7.1 Acute phase proteins in relation to the growth and development of calves

A high number of biochemical parameters in calves have been investigated earlier by several authors, stating that growth and development of the organism is accompanied by dynamic changes in the values of various haematological parameters (Hugi & Blum, 1997; Knowles et al., 2000). The evaluation of metabolic disorders in calves is helpful for interpreting results of biochemical parameters regarding physiological processes. These processes include development, nutrition, functional immaturity of various organs, unstableness of the homeostasis, and immunological reactions. However, there are only scarce data about the possible influence of age on the concentrations of other parameters, including APP.

After birth, newborns and young animals go through a period of rapid growth and development, and adapt their life outside the uterus. This transition from foetal to neonatal life and then from newborn to young animal necessitates major physiological adjustments (Bittrich et al., 2004). Young calves must adapt to various environmental factors, including nutrition which changes from a primarily carbohydrate-based energy supply during the foetal period to a high fat and relatively low carbohydrate nutritional energy supply in colostrum and milk, and then from milk to solid diet (Odle, 1997). The exposure to the new environment and foreign antigens requires the establishment of appropriate defence responses. The neonate is immunocompetent, but the adaptive immune system is immature (Morein et al., 2002). Non-specific defence mechanisms, including the reactions of the acute phase response may thus be important for the adaptation to complicated physiological processes during growth and development of calves. Therefore, the concentrations of acute phase proteins were expected to be also influenced by the age of evaluated animals. The concentrations measured in young calves thus may differ from the values in adult cattle.

The results presented here indicate that there are significant changes in the concentrations of the evaluated acute phase proteins in calves. The most pronounced changes were observed in the concentrations of SAA. The highest mean of SAA concentration was observed at the age of 1 month followed by a gradual decrease up to 5th month of life. Orro et al. (2008) reported higher mean serum concentrations of SAA shortly after birth, being the highest at the age of 7 days (112.0 mg/l), decreasing after 10 days of age. According to the aforementioned authors, possible factors contributing to the higher serum SAA concentrations in newborn and young calves include neonatal synthesis of acute phase proteins in the liver due to the birth trauma or intake of colostral inducers such as cytokines. Studies performed by Hagiwara et al. (2001) have shown that colostrum contains high amounts of pro-inflammatory cytokines, which are the main inducers of the APP production by the liver. These inflammatory mediators present in colostrum may stimulate the hepatic production of acute phase proteins. On the other hand, the higher serum concentrations of SAA in newborn and young calves could also be caused by direct transfer of this protein from the colostrum to the calf, similarly to immunoglobulins, as colostrum of healthy cows contains mammary-associated amyloid A (McDonald et al., 2001). These age-dependent changes of SAA concentrations in young calves may reflect physiological adaptation mechanisms to the new environment, that are not necessarily a sign of a disease. The higher values of standard deviations obtained in calves reflect the different reactivity of acute phase proteins to various external or internal stimuli. The wider range of individual values of measured acute phase proteins, predominantly SAA, also suggests the differences in the variability of animals reacting to impaired homeostasis. Pyörälä (2000) reported a significant variation between the different APP profiles and that the production of these proteins varies not only among different animal species, but also within them.

There are only few studies available about the serum concentrations of Hp in newborn and young calves, and the data are contradictory. The results obtained in calves showed less pronounced changes in the Hp concentrations during the first three months of life than those observed in the serum SAA concentrations. The concentrations of Hp in the blood serum of calves in the first three months after birth were roughly uniform, and the values were comparable with the concentrations measured in healthy adult cattle. Similar findings were reported by Hyvönen et al. (2006). Orro et al. (2008) stated also that serum Hp concentrations after birth were more stable compared with serum amyloid A. Slightly higher mean Hp concentration was observed by above-mentioned authors at the age of 3 days, and then (after a small decrease) the serum concentrations of Hp remained relatively stabile. On the other hand, Knowles et al. (2000) reported considerable fluctuation and high Hp concentrations during the first two weeks of life. According to Dobryszycka (1997) lower concentrations of Hp shortly after birth may be related to the increased consumption of Hp due to haemolysis of foetal red cells and the functional immaturity of the neonatal liver to compensate for this. A more pronounced increase in serum Hp concentrations was observed in calves aged of 4 months with repeated decrease of values approximately to the initial concentrations. These higher Hp concentrations can be explained by sub-clinical infections, other stressors (e.g. displacement of calves from individual pens to stable, larger groups of animals), or possible effect of exposure to changing environmental factors.

Studies performed by Knowles et al. (2000) showed that mean Fbg concentrations in calves increased during the first 2 weeks after birth, although the rise was relatively small, and the concentrations did not exceed the general reference limit used for healthy cattle. Very similar transient and relatively small increases in Fbg concentrations during the first 2 weeks of life in calves have been reported by Gentry et al. (1994). Our results showed a transient increase in the plasma concentrations of fibrinogen at the age of 2 months, which was followed by a repeated decrease of mean Fbg concentrations, and the obtained values were similar to those usually measured in healthy adult cattle. Higher concentrations of Fbg in calves, obtained in our study at the age of 2 months, may be related to the exposure of calves to changing nutritional and rearing factors and may be associated with the normal process of growth.

7.2 Acute phase proteins in calves suffering from various inflammatory diseases

In this study results suggest that among the evaluated diseases of calves, respiratory diseases induce the most marked acute phase response as measured by significantly higher concentrations of haptoglobin, serum amyloid A, as well as fibrinogen compared with clinically healthy animals. Higher concentrations of Hp, SAA and Fbg in blood samples observed in this study agree with previous findings which reported that the concentrations of these proteins rise in cattle with repiratory diseases (Godson et al., 1996; Wittum et al., 1996). Carter et al. (2002) indicated also the usefulness of APP as important diagnostic factors in calves with respiratory infections, and suggested them as valuable markers for differentiating animals with respiratory signs from healthy ones.

In the presented study, significantly higher concentrations of the evaluated acute phase proteins in calves with clinical signs of respiratory diseases were found for Hp, SAA, as well as fibrinogen, although there was a considerable variation between the aforementioned inflammatory proteins in the ability to react to an acute phase response causing event. The most marked differences between healthy calves and calves suffering from respiratory diseases we found in the concentrations of haptoglobin. While the mean serum Hp concentration in calves affected by respiratory diseases was more than eighteen fold higher than the average concentration recorded in the group of clinically healthy animals, the average concentration of SAA in calves with respiratory signs was about three fold higher compared with healthy calves. The findings correspond to the data presented by Angen et al. (2009), who obtained higher concentrations of Hp, as well as SAA in calves affected by harmful agents in the respiratory tract compared with healthy animals, but the serum SAA concentrations in diseased calves were much closer to those of the healthy calves than what was found for haptoglobin. Therefore, the aforementioned authors concluded that Hp is a more sensitive indicator of diseases in the investigated herds. Similarly, Carter et al. (2002) suggested that even if SAA is more sensitive and rapidly reacting biomarker, haptoglobin might be preferable in the field, its bigger and more prolonged response is giving rise to its usefulness to detecting disease.

The usefulness of the measurement of plasma Fbg concentrations in cattle has been demonstrated mostly by the diagnosis of traumatic conditions, monitoring of postoperative complications, e.g. peritonitis, as well as by the differentiation of traumatic reticuloperitonitis from other gastrointestinal disorders (Jafarzadeh et al., 2004). The results presented show that the determination of the concentrations of Fbg may be useful also in the monitoring of respiratory diseases, as in calves with clinical signs of respiratory diseases we found significantly higher concentrations of Fbg than in clinically healthy calves. However, the differences in the concentrations of Fbg between healthy calves and calves with respiratory signs were in means less marked than the differences observed in the concentrations of Hp and SAA. On the other hand, marked increase in plasma Fbg concentrations was found in calves after infection with *Dictyocaulus viviparus*, *Mannheimia haemolytica* or bovine viral diarrhoea virus (Gänheim et al., 2003). Therefore, in this area of research, further investigations are needed to deepen our knowledge about the synthesis of fibrinogen in calves suffering from respiratory diseases.

Although the evaluated calves with clinical signs of respiratory disorders were found to have higher concentrations of measured acute phase proteins compared with healthy calves, in sick animals we observed a markedly wider range of individual values of Hp, SAA, as well as Fbg. The higher values of standard deviations recorded in our study may reflect the different reactivity of various acute phase proteins to impaired homeostasis. Similarly, considerable individual variations in acute phase response to respiratory tract infections were reported by Wittum et al. (1996). Lomborg et al. (2008) reported also that animals can vary in their acute phase response to the same exposure. Different disease severity (i.e. more severe diseases are accompanied by higher concentrations of acute phase proteins) might be another reason for higher values of standard deviations of measured acute phase proteins (Young et al., 1996).

The influence of other disease conditions on the concentrations of acute phase proteins in calves is less well documented, and there are only scarce data reporting some results in this area of interest. Experimental *Salmonella* infection in young calves has been shown to cause an increase in the production of haptoglobin (Deignan et al., 2000). However, the Hp values following *Salmonella* infection, obtained by the aforementioned authors, did not reach the concentrations seen in other disease conditions in cattle. In our study, presented results showed in calves with clinical signs of diarrhoea a slightly higher mean SAA concentration compared with clinically healthy calves. However, in Hp and Fbg concentrations we found no marked differences between healthy and diarrhoeic calves. Thus, these findings indicate that the disturbances in the homeostasis, inflammatory reactions of the organism, and tissue damage caused by diarrhoea did not evoke sufficient inflammatory response giving a more marked systemic increase in the concentrations of measured acute phase proteins. Similarly, according to Muller-Doblies et al. (2004), Hp requires a stronger stimulation to induce an increase in serum concentrations.

Seeing that the inflammation of the navel, the tissue damage and other pathologic lesions in the associated structures may cause inflammatory reactions, we expected that omphalophlebitis in calves may affect the concentrations of major acute phase proteins. However, to the best of our knowledge, there are no published reports describing the influence of omphalophlebitis on the concentrations of acute phase proteins. In our study, the presented results showed in calves with clinical signs of omphalophlebitis, similarly to the calves with diarrhoea, more markedly higher mean concentration of SAA than in clinically healthy calves, but in the concentrations of Hp and Fbg we did not find marked differences between these two groups of calves. These findings might be a consequence of a different initiation of the production of various acute phase proteins, seeing that SAA is a more sensitive acute phase protein than Hp in cattle, with rapid increase in serum concentrations after the inflammatory stimulus (Werling et al., 1996). An opposite trend with more markedly higher mean concentrations of Hp and Fbg was observed in calves affected by multisystemic diseases, while the mean SAA concentration obtained in this group was only slightly higher compared with clinically healthy calves. Similar findings were reported by Gänheim et al. (2007), who found higher concentrations of Hp and Fbg in calves with diarrhoea at the same time as respiratory symptoms compared to those that had signs of only respiratory diseases or diarrhoea. Because of only scarce data available about the changes in the concentrations of acute phase proteins in calves affected by diarrhoea, omphalophlebitis, as well as multisystemic diseases, further investigations in larger animal groups are needed to yield satisfactory results.

7.3 The influence of chronic respiratory diseases on the concentrations of acute phase proteins in calves

Most of the investigations about the synthesis of acute phase proteins in respiratory diseases have been focused on the immediate or acute phase response to the infection (Wittum et al., 1996; Carter et al., 2002). However, only a few reports on the acute phase protein production in chronic inflammatory conditions have been published, and the data are not uniform. Horadagoda et al. (1999) found that the concentrations of Hp, SAA, and α_1- acid glycoprotein were higher in cases of acute compared with chronic inflammation. In contrast, Alsemgeest et al. (1994) indicated that serum Hp concentrations and Hp:SAA ratios were elevated in cases of chronic rather than acute inflammation. Our results indicate that in chronic inflammatory processess, especially chronic diseases of the respiratory tract, increased serum concentrations of Hp and SAA are generally observed. However, the response to chronic inflammation varies from one protein to another. Similarly, in general, Horadagoda et al. (1999) observed differences in the inducibility of SAA and haptoglobin by chronic disorders. Our results suggest that Hp is more typical indicator for chronic conditions than SAA, as in calves suffering from chronic respiratory diseases we found more than twentyfold higher mean Hp concentration compared with healthy animals, whereas average concentration of SAA in sick calves were significantly higher, but compared with Hp only about twofold higher than in healthy calves. Alsemgeest et al. (1994) found that Hp did not increase in very acute inflammatory conditions such as peracute pneumonia. They found the largest Hp concentrations in animals with serious, often chronic inflammatory diseases, at which bovine SAA was a more sensitive indicator of acute disease than haptoglobin. This may be consequence of a different initiation of the production of various APPs, as Hp is characterised by a later increase in serum concentration after stimulus remaining elevated for longer period. On the other hand, SAA is rapidly reacting acute phase protein characterised by a dramatic increase in serum concentration after the inflammatory stimulus and a relatively rapid normalisation (Petersen et al., 2004).

The aforementioned results indicate that serum concentrations of acute phase proteins, particularly Hp, may reflect the severity of the disease and may be useful as a prognostic indicator, as in calves, which during the treatment died or were euthanised, we found significantly higher mean concentrations of measured acute phase proteins, compared with those with good response to treatment and improved general health state. Eckersall et al. (2007) concluded that investigation of a range of acute phase proteins could provide additional diagnostic information on the progress of the disease, and could be sensitive marker of respiratory infections in calves. Similar findings for haptoglobin are reported by Godson et al. (1996). On the other hand, Berry et al. (2004) questioned the efficacy of SAA as a diagnostic tool because it may be elevated under stressful situations. Heegaard et al. (2000) found that the magnitude and duration of serum Hp concentration correlated well with the severity of experimental respiratory infection, whereas serum SAA concentrations increased more rapidly following infection. Carter et al. (2002) and Gånheim et al. (2007) concluded that measurement of blood Hp concentrations is a better way to predict morbidity in calves than SAA. However, our results obtained in serum concentrations of Hp and SAA in calves affected by chronic respiratory diseases indicate that both indices may be useful in the determination of the severity and prognosis of the disease. The aforementioned results suggest that Hp concentrations in the range of 1 - 3 mg/ml, and SAA concentrations around 100 μg/ml predict severe course of the disease with poor prognosis. Similar findings in calves are reported by Heegaard et al. (2000). Skinner et al. (1991) found that haptoglobin concentrations of more than 0.2 mg/ml indicated mild infection, values above 0.4 mg/ml diagnosed severe infection, while extended pathological conditions were typically associated with Hp concentrations in the range of 1 - 2 mg/ml. These results closely correlate with our observations in sick calves.

7.4 Acute phase proteins in the laboratory diagnosis of mastitis in dairy cows

The results of our study indicate that inflammatory diseases of the mammary gland lead to an increase in the concentrations of M-SAA. Raised levels of Hp and SAA have previously been shown in milk from cows with clinical mastitis as a result of the leakage of these proteins from the blood to the milk (Hirvonen et al., 1999; Eckersall et al., 2001). On the other hand, M-SAA is synthesized directly in the mammary epithelia of the udder in response to infection (Jacobsen et al., 2005). Therefore, M-SAA is believed to be a more sensitive indicator of mastitis; it accumulates in milk only during mammary inflammation. Petersen et al. (2005) reported that M-SAA concentrations, similarly to our results, were higher in quarters with mastitis compared to healthy quarters. On the other hand, Nazifi et al. (2008) presented markedly higher mean M-SAA concentrations for clinically healthy cows and for cows with sub-clinical mastitis (6.96 and 54.53 mg/ml, respectively). These contradictory data indicate that further studies are necessary to deepen our knowledge about the behavior of M-SAA in such conditions.

Mastitis can be caused by different microbial agents, mostly bacteria. Some bacteria invading a cow's mammary gland absorb milk nutrients, and some of them can produce endotoxins that destroy mammary tissue (Haltia et al., 2006). If these toxins escape the gland and spread throughout the cow's body, they may activate systemic inflammatory reactions. Moreover, other inflammatory mediators, e.g. cytokines released in response to infection and injury may activate systemic inflammatory reactions, including the induction of the synthesis of acute phase proteins by the liver (Baumann & Gauldie, 1994). The results of our study showed that the concentrations of Hp and SAA were higher in serum from cows with clinical mastitis, and increased with increasing CMT score. The increases observed in the concentrations of these proteins in serum of cows with mastitis are in line with several previous studies (Hirvonen et al., 1999; Eckersall et al., 2001). It appears that localized severe inflammation of the udder is sufficiently intense to induce a measurable systemic acute phase response. The concentrations of measured acute phase proteins had a tendency to be higher in the serum from the cows with local signs of mastitis and also in cows without clinical changes on the mammary gland, but with positive CMT. However, the finding that the differences in Hp and SAA concentrations observed between the groups of cows were less significant than the differences in M-SAA concentrations means that the measuring of serum concentrations of some acute phase proteins would be less useful to the evaluation of the severity of mastitis than the measuring of the concentrations of M-SAA directly in milk samples.

7.5 Acute phase proteins in heifers affected by hoof diseases

Presented results indicate that hoof diseases in cattle, accompanied by various local changes, lameness, as well as systemic reactions may induce increased production of some acute phase proteins. Smith et al. (2009) reported that sole ulcers, white line disease, and lameness in cows may cause not only decreased milk production and reproduction problems, but may have also a marked impact on the synthesis of acute phase proteins as a result of a generalized acute phase response. On the other hand, in the study of Laven et al. (2004), no increased concentrations of acute phase proteins were found in cattle with hoof haemorrhages.

In the presented study, significantly higher concentrations of the measured acute phase proteins in heifers affected by hoof disorders were found for Hp, SAA, as well as Fbg. However, marked differences between the aforementioned inflammatory proteins were observed in the ability to react to an acute phase response causing event. The most marked differences between healthy and sick animals we recorded in the concentrations of serum amyloid A. The mean SAA concentration in heifers with hoof diseases was about nine fold higher than the average concentration recorded in the group of clinically healthy animals. On the other hand, the average serum concentration of Hp in heifers with clinical signs of hoof diseases and lameness was about fivefold higher compared with healthy ones. These findings correspond partially to the data presented by Kujala et al. (2010). The aforementioned authors showed higher mean concentration of SAA in lame cows due to sole ulcer and white line disease than in healthy animals. However, in Hp concentrations they found no significant differences between healthy and lame cows. Therefore, the authors suggested that SAA is a better indicator for claw disorders than haptoglobin. Werling et al. (1996) reported also that SAA is a more sensitive acute phase protein than Hp in cattle with rapid increase in serum concentrations after the inflammatory stimulus.

According to Muller-Doblies et al. (2004), Hp requires a stronger stimulation to induce an increase in serum concentrations. On the other hand, Smith et al. (2009) described, similarly to our results, elevated serum Hp concentrations in lame cows with claw disorders.
The influence of hoof diseases and lameness on the plasma Fbg concentrations in cattle is less well documented. The usefulness of the measurement of the Fbg concentrations in cattle has been demonstrated by other, predominantly gastrointestinal disorders (Jafarzadeh et al., 2004). The presented study suggest that the determination of the concentrations of fibrinogen may be also useful by the diagnosis of other diseases, as we found higher plasma Fbg concentrations in heifers affected by hoof disorders compared with clinically healthy animals. However, the differences in the concentrations of Fbg between the two groups of animals were less marked than the differences observed in the concentrations of Hp and SAA. Increased concentrations of Fbg have been recently described but only in 14 lame cows with clinical signs of claw diseases (Jawor et al., 2008). Therefore, in this area of research, further investigations are needed to deepen our knowledge about the synthesis of some acute phase proteins in cattle with hoof diseases and lameness.

8. Conclusion

In the study presented results indicate that most of the evaluated acute phase proteins were pronouncedly related to the age of clinically healthy calves. Therefore, these data suggest that the age of evaluated animals should be taken into consideration during the diagnostic procedure, and by the interpretation of measured values of acute phase proteins when using these proteins as disease markers. Our data support the usefulness of APP assessments to monitor animals with respiratory diseases, and indicate their use as sensitive markers to identify calves with various inflammatory diseases.
Our findings also indicate that not only acute diseases of the respiratory tract, but also chronic cases are characterized by an increased production of some acute phase proteins. Moreover, diseases with severe clinical signs and poor prognosis (death or euthanasia) are associated with markedly higher Hp and SAA concentrations. Therefore, the aforementioned data suggest that the measurement of some acute phase proteins may serve as prognostic indicator in respiratory diseases.
Generated data also suggest the usefulness of milk amyloid A for diagnosis of bovine sub-clinical mastitis, as well as in the determination of the severity of mastitis. Moreover, presented results indicate that hoof diseases and lameness in heifers may be also associated with a systemic acute phase response characterized by elevated concentrations of some APP, suggesting that their assessment as a part of the laboratory diagnosis would be a valuable supplementation to the proper clinical diagnosis and determination of other blood laboratory parameters regarding to a better evaluation of the systemic status.
Although at present, the routine use of APP to monitor the herd health state, as well as healthy individual has not been a current veterinary diagnosis, presented data suggest their usefulness also in the veterinary medicine. The aforementioned findings may deepen our knowledge about the production of these proteins in a variety of physiological conditions, as well as during some inflammatory disease conditions in farm animals.

9. Acknowledgment

This work was supported by VEGA Scientific Grant No 1/0614/09 from the Ministry of Education, and by Slovak Research and Development Agency under contract No. APVV-0475-10.

10. References

Adrie, C. & Pinsky, M.R. (2000). The inflammatory balance in human sepsis, *Intensive Care Medicine*, Vol.26, pp. 364-375

Aldred, A.R. & Schreiber, G. (1993). The negative acute phase protein, In: *Acute phase proteins. Molecular biology, biochemistry, and clinical applications,* A. Mackiewicz, I. Kushner & H. Baumann, (Eds.), 21-37, CRC Press, Boca Raton, Florida, USA

Alsemgeest, S.P.M., Taverne, M.A.M., Boosman, R., van der Weyden, B.C. & Gruys, E. (1993). Peripartum acute-phase protein SAA concentration in plasma of cows and fetuses, *American Journal of Veterinary Research*, Vol.54, pp. 164-167

Alsemgeest, S.P.M., Kalsbeek, H.C., Wensing, T.H., Koeman, J.P., van Ederen, A.M. & Gruys, E. (1994). Bovine serum amyloid A (SAA) and haptoglobin (Hp) plasma concentrations in the diagnosis of inflammatory diseases, *Veterinary Quarterly*, Vol.16, pp. 21–24

Angen, Ø., Thomsen, J., Larsen, L.E., Larsen, J., Kokotovic, B., Heegaard, P.M.H. & Enemark, J.M.D. (2009). Respiratory disease in calves: Microbiological investigations on trans-tracheally aspirated bronchoalveolar fluid and acute phase protein response, *Veterinary Microbiology*, Vol.137, pp. 165-171

Baumann, H. & Gauldie, J. (1994). The acute phase response, *Immunology Today*, Vol.15, pp. 74-80

Bellomo, R. (1992). The cytokine network in the critically ill, *Anaesthesia and Intensive Care*, Vol.20, pp. 288-302

Berry, B.A., Confer, A.W., Krehbiel, C.R., Gill, D.R., Smith, R.A. & Montelongo, M. (2004). Effects of dietary energy and starch concentrations for newly received feedlot calves: II. Acute-phase protein response, *Journal of Animal Science*, Vol.82, pp. 845–850

Bittrich, S., Philipona, C., Hammon, H.M., Romé, V., Guilloteau, P., Blum, J.W. (2004). Preterm as compared with full-term neonatal calves are characterized by morphological and functional immaturity of the small intestine, *Journal of Dairy Science*, Vol.87, pp. 1786-1795

Bowman, B.H. (1992). *Hepatic plasma proteins*, Academic Press, New York, USA

Burger, W., Ewald, C. & Fennert, E.M. (1998). Increase in C-reactive protein in the serum of piglets (pCRP) following ACTH or corticosteroid admimistration, *Journal of Veterinary Medicine Series B*, Vol.45, pp. 1-6

Carter, J.N., Meredith, G.L., Montelongo, M., Gill, D.R., Krehbiel, C.R., Payton, M.E. & Confer, A.W. (2002). Relationship of vitamin E supplementation and antimicrobial treatment with acute-phase protein responses in cattle affected by naturally acquired respiratory tract disease, *American Journal of Veterinary Research*, Vol.63, pp. 1111-1117

Ceron, J.J., Eckersall, P.D. & Martinez-Subiela, S. (2005). Acute phase proteins in dogs and cats : current knowledge and future perspectives, *Veterinary Clinical Pathology*, Vol.34, pp. 85-99

Cheryk, L.A., Hooper-McGrevy, K.E. & Gentry, P.A. (1998). Alterations in bovine platelet function and acute phase proteins induced by *Pasterella haemolytica* A1, *Canadian Journal of Veterinary Research*, Vol.62, pp. 1-8

Cray, C., Zaias, J. & Altman, N.H. (2009). Acute phase response in animals : a review, *Comparative Medicine*, Vol.59, No.6, pp. 517-526

Deans, C. & Wigmore, S.J. (2005). Systemic inflammation, cachexia, and prognosis in patients with cancer, *Current Opinion in Clinical Nutrition Metabolic Care,* Vol.8, pp. 265-269

Deignan, T., Alwan, A., Kelly, J., McNair, J., Warrens, T. & O'Farrelli, C. (2000) Serum haptoglobin: an objective indicator of experimentally-induced *Salmonella* infection in calves, *Research in Veterinary Science*, Vol.69, pp. 153-158

Dobryszycka, W. (1997). Biological functions of haptoglobin, new pieces to an old puzzle, *European Journal of Clinical Chemistry and Clinical Biochemistry*, Vol. 35, pp. 647-654

Dowling, A., Hodgson, J.C., Dagleish, M.P., Eckersall, P.D. & Sales, J. (2004). Pathophysiological and immune cell responses in calves prior to and following lung challenge with formalin killed *Pasteurella multocide* biotype A3 and protection studies involving subsequent homologous live challenge, *Veterinary Immunology and Immunopathology*, Vol.100, pp. 197-207

Du Clos, T.W. (2004). C-reactive protein. An activator of innate imunity and a modulator of adaptive imunity, *Immunolological Research*, Vol.30, pp. 261-277

Eckersall, P.D., Young, F.J., McComb, C., Hogarth, C.J., Safi, S., Weber, A., McDonald, T., Nolan, A.M. & Fitzpatrick, J.L. (2001). Acute phase proteins in serum and milk from dairy cows with clinical mastitis, *Veterinary Record*, Vol.148, pp. 35-41

Eckersall, P.D. (2006). Measurement of acute phase proteins as biomarkers of disease in production animals, *Proceedings of the 57th Annual Meeting of the American College of Veterinary Pathologists and the 41st Annual Meeting of the American Society for Veterinary Clinical Pathology*, Tucson, Arizona, USA, December 2-6, 2006, Available from www.ivis.org

Eckersall, P.D. (2006a). Acute phase proteins: form, function and analysis, *Proceedings of the 57th Annual Meeting of the American College of Veterinary Pathologists and the 41st Annual Meeting of the American Society for Veterinary Clinical Pathology*, Tucson, Arizona, USA, December 2-6, 2006, Available from www.ivis.org

Eckersall, P.D. (2007). Acute phase proteins as monitoring tools in farm animals, In: *Production Diseases in Farm Animals*, M. Fürll (Ed.), *Proceedings of the 13th International Conference on Production Diseases*, pp. 374-380, Leipzig, Germany

Eckersall, P.D. & Bell, R. (2010). Acute phase proteins : Biomarkers of infection and inflammation in veterinary medicine, *The Veterinary Journal*, Vol.185, pp. 23-27

Endre, Z.H. & Westhuyzen, J. (2008). Early detection of acute kidney injury : emerging new biomarkers, *Nephrology (Carlton)*, Vol.13, pp. 91-98

Fearon, D.T. & Locksley, R.M. (1996). The instructive role of innate imunity in the acquired immune response, *Science*, Vol.272, pp. 50-54

Gabay, C. & Kushner, I. (1999). Acute-phase proteins and other systemic responses to inflammation, *New England Journal of Medicine*, Vol.340, pp. 448-454

Gänheim, C., Hultén, C., Carlsson, U., Kindahl, H., Niskanen, R. & Pesson Waller, K. (2003). The acute phase response in calves experimentally infected with bovine viral dirrhoea virus and/or *Mannheimia haemolytica, Veterinary Medicine B*, Vol.50, pp. 1-8

Gänheim, C., Alenius, S. & Persson Waller, K. (2007). Acute phase proteins as indicators of calf herd health, *The Veterinary Journal*, Vol.173, pp. 645-651

Gentry, P.A., Ross, M.L. & Hayatgheybi, H. (1994). Competency of blood coagulation in the newborn calf, *Research in Veterinary Science*, Vol.57, pp. 336-342

Godson, D.L., Campos, M., Attah-Poku, S.K., Redmond, M.J., Cordeiro, D.M., Sethi, M.S., Harland, R.J. & Babiuk, L.A. (1996). Serum haptoglobin as an indicator of the acute phase response in bovine respiratory disease, *Veterinary Immunology and Immunopathology*, Vol.51, pp. 277-302

Gruys, E., Toussaint, M.J.M., Niewold, T.A. & Koopmans, S.J. (2005). Acute phase reaction and acute phase proteins, *Journal of Zhejiang University Science*, Vol.6B, No.11, pp. 1045-1056, ISSN 1009-3095

Hagiwara, K., Yamanaka, H., Hisaeda, K., Taharaguchi, S., Kirisawa, R. & Iwai, H. (2001). Concentration of IL-6 in serum and whey from healthy and mastitic cows, *Veterinary Research Communication*, Vol.25, pp. 99-108

Haltia, L., Honkanen-Buzaiski, T., Spiridonova, I., Olkonen, A. & Myllys, V. (2006). A study of bovine mastitis, milking procedures and management practices on 25 Estonian dairy herds, *Acta Veterinaria Scandinavica*, Vol.48, pp. 22

Hari-Dass, R., Shah, C., Meyer, D.J. & Raynes, J.G. (2005). Serum amyloid A protein binds to outer membrane protein A of Gram-negative bacteria, *Journal of Biological Chemistry*, Vol.280, pp. 18562-18567

Heegaard, P.M.H., Godson, D.L., Toussaint, M.J.M., Tjornehoj, K., Larsen, L.E., Viuff, B. & Ronsholt, L. (2000). The acute phase response of haptoglobin and serum amyloid A (SAA) in cattle undergoing experimental infection with bovine respiratory syncytial virus, *Veterinary Immunology and Immunopathology*, Vol.77, pp. 151-159

Heinrich, P.C., Castell, J.C. & Andus, T. (1990). Interleukin-6 and the acute phase response, *Biochemical Journal*, Vol.265, pp. 621-636

Hilliquin, P. (1995). Biological amrkers in inflammatory rheumatic diseases, *Cellular and Molecular Biology (Noisy-Le-Grand)*, Vol.41, pp. 993-1006

Hirvonen, J. & Pyörälä, S. (1998). Acute phase response in dairy cows with surgically-treated abdominal disorders, *The Veterinary Journal*, Vol.155, pp. 53-61

Hirvonen, J., Eklund, K., Teppo, A.M., Huszenicza, G., Kulcsar, M., Saloniemi, H. & Pyörälä, S. (1999). Acute phase response in dairy cows with experimentally induced *Escherichia coli* mastitis, *Acta Veterinaria Scandinavica*, Vol.40, pp. 35-46

Horadagoda, N.U., Knox, K.M., Gibbs, H.A., Reid, S.W., Horadagoda, A., Edwards, S.E. & Eckersall, P.D. (1999). Acute phase proteins in cattle: Discrimination between acute and chronic inflammation, *Veterinary Record*, Vol.144, pp. 437–441

Hugi, D. & Blum, J.W. (1997). Changes of blood metabolites and hormones in breeding calves associated with weaning, *Journal of Veterinary Medicine*, Vol.44, pp. 99-108

Hyvönen, P., Suojala, L., Orro, T., Haaranen, J., Simola, O., Røntved, C. & Pyörälä, S. (2006). Transgenic cows that produce recombinant human lactoferrin in milk are not protected from experimental *Escherichia coli* intramammary infection, *Infection and Immunity*, Vol.74, pp. 6206-6212

Israili, Z.H. & Dayton, P.G. (2001). Human Alpha-1-Glycoprotein and its interactions with drugs, *Drug Metabolites Revue*, Vol.33, pp. 161-235

Jackson, P.G.G. & Cockcroft, P.D. (2002). *Clinical examination of farm animals*. Blackwell Science Ltd., Blackwell Publishing Company, ISBN 0-632-05706-8, Oxford, United Kingdom

Jacobsen, S., Niewold, T.A., Kornalijnslijper, E., Toussaint, M.J.M. & Gruys, E. (2005). Kinetics of local and systemic isoforms of serum amyloid A in bovine mastitic milk, *Veterinary Immunology and Immunopathology*, Vol.104, pp. 21-31

Jafarzadeh, S.R., Nowrouzian, I., Khaki, Z., Ghamsari, S.M. & Adibhashemi, F. (2004). The sensitivities and specificities of total plasma protein and plasma fibrinogen for the diagnosis of traumatic reticuloperitonitis in cattle, *Preventive Veterinary Medicine*, Vol.65, pp. 1-7

Janeway, C.A., Travers, P., Walport, M. & Schlomschik, M.J. (2001). *Immunobiology*, 5th ed., Taylor & Francis, London, United Kingdom

Jawor, P., Steiner, S., Stefaniak, T., Baumgartner, W. & Rzasa, A. (2008). Determination of selected acute phase proteins during the treatment of limb diseases in dairy cows, *Veterinary Medicine - Czech*, Vol.53, pp. 173-183

Jennings, G. & Elia, M. (1996). Changes in protein distribution in normal and protein-deficient rats during an acute-phase „injury" response, *British Journal of Nutrition*, Vol.76, pp. 123-132

Jensen, L.E. & Whitehead, A.S. (1998). Regulation of serum amyloid A protein expression during the acute phase response, *Biochemical Journal*, Vol.334, pp. 489-503

Katoh, N., Oikawa, S., Oohashi, T., Takahashi, H. & Itoh, F. (2002). Decreases of apolipoprotein B-100 and A-1 concentrations and induction of haptoglobin and serum amyloid A in nonfed calves, *Journal of Veterinary Medical Science*, Vol.64, pp. 51-55

Knowles, T.G., Edwards, J.E., Bazeley, K.J., Brown, S.N., Butterworth, A. & Warriss, P.D. (2000). Changes in the blood biochemical and haematological profile in neonatal calves with age, *Veterinary Record*, Vol.18, pp. 593-598

Koj, A. (1996). Initiation of acute phase response and synthesis of cytokines, *Biochemical and Biophysical Acta*, Vol.1317, pp. 84-94

Kujala, M., Orro, T. & Soveri, T. (2010). Serum acute phase proteins as a marker of inflammation in dairy cattle with hoof diseases, *Veterinary Record*, Vol.166, pp. 240-241

Laven, R.A., Livesey, C.T. & May, S.A. (2004). Relationship between acute phase proteins and hoof horn haemorrhages in postpartum first-lactation heifers. *Veterinary Record*, Vol.154, pp. 135-138

Lampreave, F., Gonzalez-Ramon, N., Martinez-Ayensa, S., Hernandez, M.-A., Lorenzo, H.-K., Garcia-Gil, A. & Pineiro, A. (1994). Characterisation of the acute phase serum protein response in pigs, *Electrophoresis*, Vol.15, pp. 672-676

Lomborg, S.R., Nielsen, L.R., Heegaard, P.M.H. & Jacobsen, S. (2008). Acute phase proteins in cattle after exposure to complex stress, *Veterinary Research Communications*, Vol.32, pp. 575-582

Mack, D.R., McDonald, T.L., Larson, M.A., Wei, S. & Weber, A. (2003). The conserved TFLK motif of mammary-associated serum amyloid A is responsible for up-regulation of intestinal MUC3 mucin expression *in vitro*, *Pediatric Research*, Vol.53, pp. 137-142

Mackiewicz, A. (1997). Acute phase proteins and transformed cells, *International Review of Cytology*, Vol.170, pp. 225-300

McDonald, T.L., Larson, M.A., Mack, D.R. & Weber, A. (2001). Elevated extrahepatic expression and secretion of mammary-associated serum amyloid A 3 (M-SSA3) into colostrum, *Veterinary Immunology and Immunopathology*, Vol.83, pp. 203-211

Mold, C., Rodriguez, W., Rodic-Polic, B. & Du Clos, T.W. (2002). C-reactive protein mediates protection from lipopolysaccharide through interactions with Fc-gammaR, *Journal of Immunology*, Vol.169, pp. 7019-7025

Morein, B., Abusugra, I., Blomquist, G. (2002). Immunity in neonates, *Veterinary Immunology and Immunopathology*, Vol.87, pp. 207-213

Morimatsu, M., Syuto, B., Shimada, N., Fujinaga, T., Yamamoto, S., Saito, M. & Naiki, M. (1991). Isolation and characterisation of bovine haptoglobin from acute phase sera, *Journal of Biological Chemistry*, Vol.266, pp. 11833-11837

Muller-Doblies., D., Arquint, A., Schaller, P., Heegaard, P.M.H., Hilbe, M., Albini, S., Abril, C., Tobler, K., Ehrensperger, F., Peterhans, E., Ackermann, M. & Metzler, A. (2004). Innate immune responses of calves during transient infection with a noncytopathic strain of bovine viral diarrhoea virus, *Clinical and Diagnostic Laboratory Immunology*, Vol.11, pp. 302-312

Murata, H., Shimada, N. & Yoshioka, M. (2004). Current research on acute phase proteins in veterinary diagnosis : an overview, *The Veterinary Journal*, Vol.168, pp. 28-40

Nathan, C. & Sporn, M. (1991). Cytokines in context, *Journal of Cell Biology*, Vol.113, pp. 981-986

Nazifi, S., Khoshvaghti, A. & Gheisari, H.R. (2008). Evaluation of serum and milk amyloid A in some inflammatory diseases of cattle, Iranian *Journal of Veterinary Research*, Vol.9, pp. 222-226

Niewold, T.A., Toussaint, M.J.M. & Gruys, E. (2003). Monitoring health by acute phase proteins, *Proceedings of the Fourth European Colloquium on Acute Phase Proteins*, pp. 57-67, Segovia, Spain

Odle, J. (1997). New insights into the utilization of medium-chain triglycerides by the neonate: observation from a piglet model, *Journal of Nutrition*, Vol.127, pp. 1061-1067

Ohtsuka, H., Kudo, K., Mori, K., Nagai, F., Hatsugaya, A., Tajima, M., Tamura, K., Hoshi, F., Koiwa, M. & Kawamura, S. (2001). Acute phase response in naturally occuring coliform mastitis, *Journal of Veterinary Medical Science*, Vol.63, pp. 675-678

Orro, T., Jacobsen, S., LePage, J-P., Niewold, T., Alasuutari, S. & Soveri, T. (2008). Temporal changes in serum concentrations of acute phase proteins in newborn dairy calves, *The Veterinary Journal*, Vol.176, pp. 182-187

Petersen, H.H., Nielsen, J.P. & Heegaard, P.M.H. (2004). Application of acute phase protein measurements in veterinary clinical chemistry, *Veterinary Research*, Vol.35, pp. 136-187

Petersen, H.H., Gardner, I.A., Rossitto, P., Larsen, H.D. & Heegaard, P.M.H. (2005). Accuracy of milk amyloid A (MAA) concentration and somatic cell count for diagnosing bovine mastitis, *Proceedings of the 5th International Colloquium on Animal Acute Phase Proteins*, pp. 43-44, Dublin, Ireland, March 14-15, 2005

Pyörälä, S. (2000). *Hirvonen's thesis on acute phase response in dairy cattle*, University of Helsinki, ISBN 951-45-9104-6, Helsinki, Finnland

Raynes, J.G. (1994). The acute phase response, *Biochemical Society Transactions*, Vol.22, pp. 69-74

Scott, P.R., Murray, L.D. & Penny, C.D. (1992). A preliminary studie of serum haptoglobin concentrtaion as a prognostic indicator of ovine dystocia cases, *British Veterinary Journal*, Vol.148, pp. 351-355

Segales, J., Pineiro, C., Lampreave, F., Nofrarias, M., Mateu, E., Calsamiglia, M., Andres, J., Morales, M., Pineiro, M. & Domingo, M. (2004). Haptoglobin and pig-major acute protein are increased in pigs with postweaning multisystemic wasting syndrome (PMWS), *Veterinary Research*, Vol.35, pp. 275-282

Skinner, J.G., Brown, R.A.L. & Roberts, L. (1991). Bovine haptoglobin response in clinically defined field conditions, *Veterinary Record*, Vol.128, pp. 147–149

Smith, B.I., Donovan, G.A., Risco, C.A., Young, C.R. & Stanker, L.H. (1998). Serum haptoglobin concentrations in Holstein dairy cattle with toxic puerperal metritis, *Veterinary Record*, Vol.142, pp. 83-865

Smith, B.I., Kauffold, J. & Sherman, L. (2009). Serum haptoglobin concentrations in dairy cattle with lameness due to claw disorders, *The Veterinary Journal*, doi: 10.1016/j.tvjl.2009.08.012

Steel, D.M. & Whitehead, A.S. (1994). The major acute phase reactants: C-reactive protein, serum amyloid P component and serum amyloid A protein, *Immunology Today*, Vol.15, pp. 81-88

Suffredini, A.F., Fantuzzi, G., Badolato, R., Oppenheim, J.J. & O`Grady, N. (1999). New insights into the biology of the acute phase response, *Journal of Clinical Immunology*, Vol.19, pp. 203-214

Taniguchi, T., Koido, Y., Aiboshi, J., Yamashita, T., Suzaki, S. & Kurokawa, A. (1999). Changes in the ratio of interleukin-6 to interleukin-10 predicts a poor outcome in patients with systemic inflammatory response syndrome, *Critical Care Medicine*, Vol.27, pp. 1262-1264

Thomas, J.S. (2000). Overview of plasma proteins, In: *Schalm's Veterinary Hematology*, B.F. Feldman, J.G. Zinkl, & N.C. Jain, (Eds.), 891-898, Lippincott Williams, Wilkins, Philadelphia, USA

Tillet, W.S. & Francis, T. (1930). Serological reactions in pneumonia with a nonprotein fraction from pneumococcus, *Journal of experimental Medicine*, Vol. 52, pp. 561-571

Toussaint, M.J.M., Eckersall, P.D., Alava, M., Madec, F., Meleon, R.H. & Gruys, E. (2000). Acute phase protein assays as tool in assessment of health in pigs, *Revue de Medicine Veterine*, Vol.151, pp. 780

Uhlar, C.M. & Whitehead, A.S. (1999). Serum amyloid A, the major vertebrate acute-phase reactant, *European Journal of Biochemistry*, Vol.265, pp. 501-523

Wagener, F.A., Eggernt, A., Boerman, O.C., Oyen, W.J., Verhofstad, A., Abraham,N.G., Adema, G., van Kooyk, Y., de Witte, T. & Figdor, C.G. (2001). Heme is a potent inducer of inflammation in mice and is countected by heme oxygenase, *Blood*, Vol.98, pp. 1802-1811

Weber, A., Weber, A.T., McDonald, T.L. & Larson, M.A. (2006). *Staphylococcus aureus* lipotechoic acid induces differential expression of bovine serum amyloid A3 (SAA3) by mammary epithelial cells: Implications of early diagnosis of mastitis, *Veterinary Immunology and Immunopathology*, Vol.109, pp. 79-83

Welles, E.G., Williams, M.A., Tyler, J.W. & Lin, H.C. (1993). Hemostasis in cows with endotoxin-induced mastitis, *American Journal of Veterinary Research,* Vol.54, pp. 1230-1234

Werling, D., Sutter, F., Arnold, M., Kun, G., Tooten, P.C., Gruys, E., Kreuzer, M. & Langhans, W. (1996). Characterisation of the acute phase response of heifers to a prolonged low dose infusion of lipopolysaccharide, *Research in Veterinary Science,* Vol.61, pp. 252-257

Whicher, J.T. & Westacott, C.I. (1992). The acute phase response, In: *Biochemistry of inflammation,* J.T. Whicher & S.W. Evans, (Eds.), 243-271, Kluwer Academic, London, United Kingdom

Wittum, T.E., Young, C.R., Stanker, L.H., Friffin, D.D., Perino, L.J. & Littledike, E.T. (1996). Haptoglobin response to clinical respiratory tract disease in feedlot cattle, *American Journal of Veterinary Research,* Vol.57, pp. 646-649

Yang, F.M., Haile, D.J., Berger, F.G., Herbert, D.C., Van Beveren, E. & Ghio, A.J. (2003). Haptoglobin reduces lung injury associated with exposure to blood, *American Journal of Physiology and Lung Cell Molecular Physiology,* Vol.284, pp. L402-L409

Young, C.R., Wittum, T.E., Stanker, L.H., Perio, L.J., Griffin, D.D. & Littledike, T. (1996). Serum haptoglobin concentrations in a population of feedlot cattle, *American Journal of Veterinary Research,* Vol.57, pp. 138-141

12

Acute Phase Proteins as Biomarkers in Animal Health and Welfare

Jaime Gómez-Laguna[1], Francisco J. Salguero[2], Francisco J. Pallarés[3], Irene M. Rodríguez-Gómez[4], Inmaculada Barranco[4] and Librado Carrasco[4]

[1]CICAP, Agri-food Research Centre, Pozoblanco, Córdoba
[2]Veterinary Laboratories Agency, New Haw, Addlestone, Surrey
[3]Department of Anatomy and Comparative Pathology, Faculty of Veterinary Medicine, Murcia University, Murcia
[4]Department of Anatomy and Comparative Pathology, Faculty of Veterinary Medicine, Córdoba University, Córdoba
[1,3,4]Spain
[2]United Kingdom

1. Introduction

The acute phase proteins (APPs) are reactants synthesized during an acute phase response (APR) against several stimuli like infection, inflammation, stress, trauma or tissue damage (Petersen et al., 2004; Cerón et al., 2005). The main role of the APR is to restore the normal homeostasis of the organism after any of the stimuli mentioned above. In this sense, the APR is considered as part of the innate immune system triggering off functions just as leukocytosis, fever, chelation of serum zinc and iron, or opsonization (Cerón et al., 2005). During the APR organic concentrations of APPs may change, and measuring APPs levels is being used widely nowadays both in human and in veterinary medicine. The concentration of APPs may increase or decrease after an appropriate stimulus being classified as positive, moderate or negative APPs depending on the enhancement of its concentration. Thus, a positive APP may show up to 100-1000-fold increase in its serum concentration in 1-2 days; a moderate APP displays a 5 to 10-fold increase in 2-3 days; and a minor APP increase between 50% and 100%. Negative APPs are those which decrease after a specific stimulus (Petersen et al., 2004; Cray et al., 2009; Eckersall & Bell, 2010).
Serum samples are the most common sample used to measure the levels of APPs in both companion and farm animals. Recently, other specimens such as saliva or meat juice has been successfully used as samples for APPs measurements in dog (Parra et al., 2005) and pig (Gutiérrez et al., 2008; 2009). Saliva presents the advantage of being a non-invasive, easier and less stressful sampling method for the animals and meat juice represent a suitable alternative to serum or blood samples and simplifies the process of sampling collection at slaughter.

In this sense, the extrahepatic synthesis of APPs is one of the recent subjects of study in the field of the APR. The synthesis of APPs is regulated by both endogenous glucocorticoids and the production of proinflammatory cytokines, mainly interleukin-1 (IL-1), IL-6 and tumor necrosis factor-alpha (TNF-α), which activate specific cells to synthesize APPs. The liver is the main target for the production of APPs, specially the hepatocytes; however, several extrahepatic sites have been reported. An extrahepatic synthesis of haptoglobin (Hp) has been reported in airway epithelial cells and immigrated leucocytes (Hiss et al., 2008) and extrahepatic production of C-reactive protein (CRP) has been observed in vascular smooth muscle cells (Kuji et al., 2007), pulmonary fibroblast and endothelial cells in the lung (Päiväniemi et al., 2009). In our group an extrahepatic expression of both Hp (Gutiérrez et al., 2011) and CRP (unpublished data) has been observed in epithelial cells from the respiratory tract, in the parotid salivary gland and in diaphragmatic myofibers from sick pigs (Fig. 1).

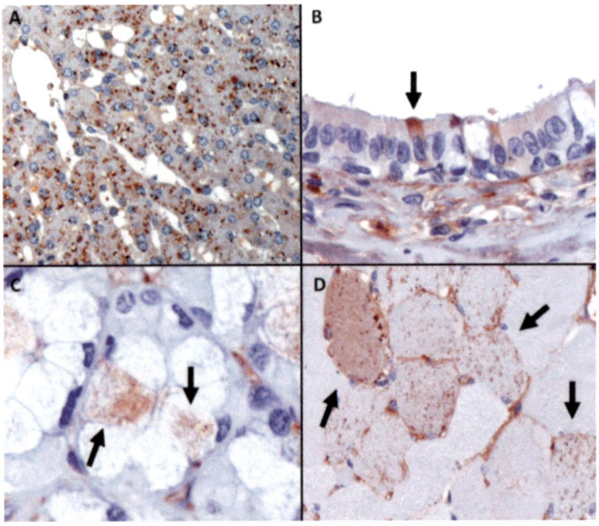

Fig. 1. Immunohistochemical haptoglobin expression in hepatocytes (1A), airway epithelial cells (1B, arrow), epithelial glandular cells (1C, arrows), and diaphragmatic myofibers (1C, arrows).

Before describing the role of APPs in veterinary medicine, it should be useful to remind some of the functions of the main APPs. The main biological function of Hp consists on prevention of iron loss by the formation of haemoglobin-iron complexes (Ceciliani et al., 2002; Petersen et al., 2004). Therefore, Hp develops a bacteriostatic effect reducing the level of available iron for the microorganisms (Petersen et al., 2004). The expression of Hp has also been related to the secretion of anti-inflammatory cytokines, particularly IL-10, through the interaction with CD163, a haemoglobin scavenger receptor that is solely present in cells of monocyte/macrophage lineage (Moestrup & Moller, 2004; Philippidis et al., 2004). However, the exact mechanism used by Hp as modulator of the immune response is not clear, acting as suppressor of lymphocyte proliferation in bovine (Murata & Miyamoto, 1993), and as supporter of B and T lymphocytes proliferation and differentiation in Hp-deficient C57BL/6J mice (Huntoon et al., 2008).

Serum amyloid A (SAA) shows more than 100-fold increase after any injury, which triggers off the APR (Petersen et al., 2004). SAA carries out several functions related with the inflammatory response, just as cholesterol removal from the local site of inflammation and transport to hepatocytes; chemotaxis of monocytes, polymorphonuclear leukocytes and T cells; inhibitory effect on fever, oxidative burst, platelet activation and in vitro immune response (Ceciliani et al., 2002; Petersen et al., 2004). Secondary amyloidosis is triggered by a conformational change of SAA into an insoluble peptide, AA, which takes place when there is a marked high expression of SAA (Ceciliani et al., 2002).

CRP was first discovered in the serum of patients which suffered a pneumococcal infection, as a substance which reacted with C polysaccharide (Petersen et al., 2004). In the acute phase response, CRP increases often more moderately than Hp or SAA, showing between 1 to 10 times increase (Petersen et al., 2004). Although some authors consider CRP as a useful tool to differentiate between a bacterial or a viral infection, other authors could not detect such differences because of the individual variability (Petersen et al., 2004). CRP participates in the innate immune response removing bacteria and damaged cells by complement activation and opsonisation, activating monocyte/macrophage to inflammatory cytokines production, and preventing neutrophils migration (Ceciliani et al., 2002; Petersen et al., 2004). Since CRP is a component of the innate response, it may be considered as an early bioindicator of health status in swine herds (Stevenson et al., 2006).

This chapter will deal with the role of APPs in domestic animal species, as well as their role in animal welfare, in disease and in the evaluation of prophylactic and therapeutic strategies.

2. Useful acute phase proteins in domestic animal species

As mentioned above, APPs are classified as positive, moderate, minor or negative depending on either the enhancement or the decrease in their serum concentration during the APR (Petersen et al., 2004; Cray et al., 2009; Eckersall & Bell, 2010). The synthesis and role of APPs may differ depending on the animal species. In this sense, whereas an APP may act as a positive APP in one species, it may not suffer any change in other species, such as CRP in swine and in cattle, respectively (Table 1).

Species	Major APP	Moderate APP	Minor APP	Negative APP
Dog	CRP, SAA	AGP, Hp, Cp, Fb	-	Albumin, Tf
Cat	AGP, SAA	Hp	-	Albumin, Tf
Horse	SAA	Hp, Fb	-	Albumin
Swine	Pig-MAP, Hp, SAA	AGP, CRP	Fb	Albumin, Apo A-I
Cattle	Hp, SAA	AGP, MAP	Fb	Albumin
Sheep	Hp, SAA	AGP	Fb, Cp	Albumin
Goat	Hp, SAA	Fb, ASG	Cp	Albumin

CRP: C-reactive protein; SAA: serum amyloid A; AGP: α_1-acid glycoprotein; Hp: haptoglobin; Cp: ceruloplasmin; Fb: fibrinogen; Tf: transferrin; Pig-MAP: pig major acute phase protein; Apo A-I: apoliprotein A-I; MAP: major acute phase protein; ASG: acid soluble glycoprotein.

Table 1. Expression of APPs in different species according to their degree of importance.

It is well established that albumin participates as a negative APP in most of the animal species. On the other hand, Hp and fibrinogen (Fb) are considered as positive APPs, although the enhancement shown by the former may be up to ten times higher than the one observed by the latter. CRP is a really useful biomarker in human for monitoring the course of different clinical processes, and its measure is also of interest in swine and dog. Nonetheless, the serum concentration of CRP does not suffer big changes in the APR in bovine or in cat. Therefore, the selection of the appropriate APP for each species is of key importance.

2.1 APPs of significance in small animals

The APR is mounted in a similar way both in dogs and cats; however they show few differences with respect to the behaviour of some APPs. Whereas Hp, SAA, and α_1-acid glycoprotein (AGP) are considered as positive APPs in both species, CRP acts as a positive APP in dogs but usually shows no changes in cats (Petersen et al., 2004; Cerón et al., 2005; Eckersall and Bell, 2010). In addition, Fb is a positive APP in dogs, but no information is available in cats (Petersen et al., 2004; Cerón et al., 2005). Finally, albumin participates as a negative APP in all mammalian species (Mackiewicz, 1997).

2.1.1 Canine APPs

In the dog the main APPs to consider are CRP and SAA, as positive APPs; AGP, Hp and ceruloplasmin (Cp), as moderate APPs; and albumin and transferrin, as negative APP (Petersen et al., 2004; Cerón et al., 2005) (Table 1). No age- or sex-related differences have been observed in the concentration of CRP for dogs (Yamamoto et al., 1994), however, adult dogs respond to inflammation with a higher enhancement in the concentration of both CRP and AGP than young animals do (Hayashi et al., 2001).

The concentration of APPs has been reported to rise after several bacterial, viral or parasitic infections, in autoimmune disorders and in neoplasia (just as lymphoma) (Table 2). In this sense, the magnitude of the increase of different APPs has been reported as a valuable tool to monitor parvoviral (Kocaturk et al., 2010) and *Erlichia canis* (Rikihisa et al., 1994) infections. Moreover, a correlation has been observed between the levels of APPs and the remission of the autoimmune hemolytic anemia (Mitchell et al., 2009). Some studies have been focused on the role of APPs in the monitoring of mammary tumors in the bitch but the results are contradictory. In these reports, the changes observed in the concentration of APPs have been related mainly to the inflammation associated to the tumor (Planellas et al., 2009; Tecles et al., 2009).

In the same way, it is interesting to take into account that the measure of APPs may not be of help in several processes. Nakamura et al. (2008) performed a study to determine the role of CRP in different diseases, concluding that the measure of CRP was not useful in neurological and endocrine processes.

2.1.2 Feline APPs

The APR has not been thoroughly studied in cats. However some relevant data are available in the literature. AGP and SAA act as positive APPs in the APR in cats, whereas Hp participates as a moderate APP and albumin and transferring as negative APPs (Petersen et al., 2004; Cerón et al., 2005; Paltrinieri, 2008) (Table 1). No age-related differences have been observed in the concentration of APPs in cats (Campbell et al., 2004).

Although scarce studies have been carried out to determine the role of APPs in feline species, there are several studies available concerning the role of APPs in feline infectious peritonitis (FIP) (Table 3). Thus, a persistent increase in the concentration of AGP, SAA and Hp has been reported in cats suffering from FIP (Giordano et al., 2004; Paltrinieri et al.,

	Disorder	Acute Phase Protein	Reference
Inflammation	Acute pancreatitis	CRP	Nakamura et al., 2008
	Pyometra	CRP, Hp, SAA	Dabrowski et al., 2009
	Polyarthritis	CRP	Tvarijonaviciute et al., 2011
	Inflammatory bowel disease	CRP	Jergens at al., 2003
	Rhinitis	CRP, Hp	Sheahan et al., 2010
	Surgery	CRP , Hp, Cp	Serin & Ulutas, 2010
Bacteria	*Bordetella bronchiseptica*	CRP	Yamamoto et al., 1994
	Escherichia coli	CRP, SAA, Hp	Dabrowski et al., 2009
	Staphylococcus aureus	CRP, SAA, Hp	Dabrowski et al., 2009
	Leptospira interrogans	CRP, Hp	Mastrorilli et al., 2007
Viruses	Parvovirus	CRP, SAA, AGP	Yule et al., 1997 Kocaturk et al., 2010
Parasites	Babesiosis	CRP, SAA, AGP	Lobetti et al., 2000; Matjako et al., 2007
	Erlichia canis	CRP, AGP	Rikihisa et al., 1994
	Leishmania infantum	CRP, Hp, Cp	Martínez-Subiela et al., 2002
	Trypanosomiasis	CRP, Hp	Ndung'u et al., 1991
	Granulocytic anaplasmosis	CRP	Pantchev, 2010
Neoplasia	Round cell tumor (lymphoma) Carcinoma Sarcoma	CRP, AGP	Ogilvie et al., 1993 Mischke et al., 2007 Nakamura et al., 2008 Yuki et al., 2011
Endocrine	Cushing's syndrome	Hp, Fb	Caldin et al., 2009
Autoimmune	Autoimmune hemolytic anemia	CRP	Caspi et al., 1987
	Rheumatoid arthritis	Cp	Tecles et al., 2005

CRP: C-reactive protein; Hp: haptoglobin; SAA: serum amyloid A; CP: ceruloplasmin; AGP: α_1-acid glycoprotein.

Table 2. Main canine disorders and specific APPs that play a significant role in each disease (modified from Cerón et al., 2005).

2007b). Moreover, AGP has been shown to be useful in monitoring the early interferon (IFN) treatment of parvoviral infected cats (Paltrinieri et al., 2007a). SAA has been reported as a useful tool in the diagnosis, monitoring and treatment of feline pancreatitis (Tamamoto et al., 2009). An enhancement in the concentration of AGP and Hp has been observed in anemic cats suffering from pyothorax, abscesses or fat necrosis (Ottenjann et al., 2006). Some studies have been focused on the expression of APPs in cats with neoplasia, however, whereas some authors describe no changes in APPs concentration in cats with lymphoma (Correa et al., 2001) others show a significant increase of AGP or SAA in cats bearing carcinomas, sarcomas or round cell tumors (Selting et al., 2000; Tamamoto et al., 2008).

Disorder		Acute Phase Protein	Reference
Inflammation	Pancreatitis	SAA	Tamamoto et al., 2008, 2009
	Reactive amyloidosis	AGP, SAA, Hp	Kajikawa et al., 1999
	Renal failure, FLUTD[1]	SAA	Sasaki et al., 2003
	Abscesses, pyothorax, fat necrosis	AGP, Hp	Ottenjann et al., 1996
	Lipopolysaccharide	AGP, SAA, Hp	Kajikawa et al., 1999
	Injury, liver disorders	SAA	Sasaki et al., 2003
	Surgery	AGP, SAA, Hp	Kajikawa et al., 1999
Bacteria	*Chlamydophila psittaci*	AGP	Terwee et al., 1998
Viruses	Feline infectious peritonitis	AGP, SAA, Hp	Duthie et al., 1997 Giordano et al., 2004 Paltrinieri et al., 2007b
	Feline immunodeficiency	AGP, Hp	Duthie et al., 1997
	Parvovirosis	AGP	Paltrinieri et al., 2007a
	Feline calicivirus	AGP	Terwee et al., 1997
Neoplasia	Lymphoma Malignant mesothelioma Carcinoma Sarcoma	SAA, AGP	Selting et al., 2000 Sasaki et al., 2003 Tamamoto et al., 2008
Endocrine	Hyperthyroidism Diabetes mellitus	SAA	Sasaki et al., 2003 Tamamoto et al., 2008
Autoimmune	Autoimmune hemolytic anemia	SAA	Paltrinieri, 2007
	Polycystic disease Familial amyloidosis		Tamamoto et al., 2008

[1] FLUTD: Feline Low Urinary Tract Disease; SAA: serum amyloid A; AGP: α_1-acid glycoprotein; Hp: haptoglobin.

Table 3. Main APPs related with the diagnosis of feline disorders.

2.2 APPs of significance in large animals

In large animals, besides all the research carry out concerning the role of APPs in inflammatory and infectious disease, there is an intense ongoing investigation on the APR triggered off by the stress related to several conditions, such as transport, feeding or housing conditions. These studies are valuable in order to determine the animal welfare status of the herds in order to both improve the production and obtain products of higher quality.

2.2.1 Equine APPs

As in cats, there are just few studies concerning the role of APPs in horses. SAA is the main APP in equines participating in the APR as a major APP, whereas both Hp and Fb acts as moderate APPs. Similar to other mammalian species, albumin is considered as a negative APP (Cray et al., 2009; Eckersall & Bell, 2010) (Table 1). Attention must be paid to the age were the concentration of APPs is going to be measured. Thus, in the first week of life of the foal there is a physiological enhancement in the level of SAA, as well as in the mare just after foaling (Nunokawa et al., 1993; Paltrinieri et al., 1998). In addition, an increase of SAA is observed after vaccination (Andersen et al., 2011).

	Disorder	Acute Phase Protein	Reference
Inflammation	Surgery	SAA, Fb	Jacobsen et al., 2009
	Colic	SAA	Vandenplas et al., 2005
	Non-infectious arthritis	SAA, Hp, Fb	Hultén et al., 2002
	Infectious arthritis	SAA	Jacobsen et al., 2006a; 2006b
	Laminitis	Hp	Petersen et al., 2004
	Equine dysautonomia	Hp, Cp	Milne et al., 1991
Bacteria	*Escherichia coli* (endometritis)	SAA, Fb	Mette et al., 2010
	Streptococcus zooepidemicus (bronchopneumonia)	SAA	Hobo et al., 2007
	Septicemia	SAA	Paltrinieri et al., 2008
Viruses	Equine Influenza	SAA	Hultén et al., 1999
Stress	Training	Fb, Hp	Fazio et al., 2010
Others	Early embrionary death	SAA, Hp	Krakowski et al., 2011
	Vaccination	SAA, Fb	Andersen et al., 2011

AGP: α_1-acid glycoprotein; SAA: serum amyloid A; Hp: haptoglobin.

Table 4. Equine disorders and specific APPs for their diagnosis and monitoring.

Changes in the concentration of SAA have been reported in horses in several conditions, just as non-septic arthritis, laminitis, colic, or influenza infection. Other conditions which may lead to an increase in the level of this and/or another APPs in horses are shown in Table 4.

However, there are several conditions in which the use of APPs is not completely justified. In foals it is controversial if the measure of SAA may be a useful tool for the diagnosis of bronchopneumonia associated to *Rhodococcus equi* (Hultén & Demmers, 2002; Cohen et al., 2005). In addition, other plasmatic proteins, such as the plasma iron, have been reported to better reflect acute inflammation than do APPs (Borges et al., 2007). On the other hand, the levels of APPs are not affected by selenium dose or source (Calamari et al., 2010).

2.2.2 Bovine APPs

In bovines it is important to take into consideration that some APPs, just as CRP, are not useful tools to measure the APR. The major APPs in cattle are Hp and SAA, acting both AGP and major acute phase protein (MAP) as moderate APPs and Fb as a minor APP. Albumin participates in the APR as a negative responder (Petersen et al., 2004; Eckersall & Bell, 2010) (Table 1).

There are several factors that may imply variations in the expression of APPs. In this sense, the breed of the animals has to be considered before carrying out an analysis since, for example, the Holsteins show a prolonged production of the AGP, which is only slightly elevated in the Sahiwals (Glass & Jensen, 2007). In another study, differences with respect to the level of Cp in both calves and cows were observed between Angus and Romosinuano breeds in response to weaning and transportation (Qiu et al., 2007). Another factor to consider is the age of the animals, being increased the levels of the APPs at calving and reaching baseline values during the first 3 weeks of life (Orro et al., 2008).

Disorder		Acute Phase Protein	Reference
Inflammation	Lameness	Hp, SAA	Kujala et al., 2010; Smith et al., 2010
	Postpartum	Hp, SAA	Gabler et al., 2010; Humbledt et al., 2006
			Tóthová et al., 2010
	Chronic respiratory disease	Hp, SAA	Huzzey et al., 2009; Chan et al., 2010
	Metritis	Hp, SAA	Carroll et al., 2009
			Tabrizi et al., 2008
	LPS	Hp, SAA	Safi et al., 2008; Tabrizi et al., 2008
	Clinical mastitis	Fb, Cp	
	Subclinical mastitis	MAA, MHp, Fb	Nazifi et al., 2009a
	Traumatic reticuloperitonitis	SAA, Hp	
Bacteria	*Escherichia coli* (mastitis)	SAA, Hp, LBP*	Suojala et al., 2008
	Staphylococcus aureus (subclinial mastitis)	SAA, HP*	Eckersall et al., 2006
	Mannheimia haemolytica	SAA, Hp, Fb	Gånheim et al., 2003
	Pasteurella multocida	SAA, Hp, AGP	Dowling et al., 2004
Viruses	Bovine viral diarrhea virus	SAA, Hp, Fb	Gånheim et al., 2003
	BRSV[1]	SAA, Hp	Heegard et al., 2000
	Foot and mouth disease virus	Hp	Höfner et al., 1994
Parasites	*Trypanosoma congolense*	SAA	Meade et al., 2009
	Theileria annulata	SAA, Hp, Cp, Fb	Nazifi et al., 2009b
Stress	Weaning	Hp, Fb	Lynch et al., 2010
	Housing	Hp	Lynch et al., 2010
	Feeding (ruminal acidosis)	SAA, Hp, LBP	Khafipour et al., 2009
	Transport	SAA, Hp	Lomborg et al., 2008
Other	Fatty liver (F.l.)	Hp	Katoh & Nakagawa, 1999
	F.l. + abomasal displacement	Hp, SAA	Guzelbektes et al., 2010

[1]BRSV: bovine respiratory syncytial virus; *All the three APPs increased both in milk and serum. Hp: haptoglobin; SAA: serum amyloid A; Cp: ceruloplasmin; Fb: fibrinogen; MAA: milk A amyloid; MHp: milk haptoglobin; LBP: lipopolysaccharide-binding protein; AGP: α_1-acid glycoprotein.

Table 5. Main APPs reported in different disorders in cattle useful for their diagnosis and/or monitoring.

Several studies are available concerning the role of APPs in different disorders affecting bovine species (Table 5). Many of them are focused on the APR in mastitis, being interesting the higher concentration of Hp and LBP response triggered off in mastitis caused by gram negative bacteria than in those caused by gram positive bacteria (Wen et al., 2010). Some of these studies determine the differences between the concentration of APPs in serum and in

milk. As it could be expected in cases of mastitis, the concentration of APPs is much higher in milk than in serum (Tabrizi et al., 2008; Safi et al., 2009).
Other studies are also focused on the changes experimented by APPs against different stressors or metabolic conditions, such as hepatic lipidosis (fatty liver) (Table 5).

2.2.3 APPs in small ruminants

The APR in small ruminants is poorly described. The different APPs may play a similar role both in sheep and goat but some differences have been reported. Hp and SAA are considered as major APPs and Cp as a minor APP in both ovine and caprine APRs. Nonetheless, Fb participates as a minor APP in sheep but as a moderate APP in goat. AGP and acid soluble glycoprotein (ASG) are also moderate APPs of the ovine and caprine APRs, respectively (Table 1). In both species the concentration of albumin diminishes after an appropriate stimulus (González et al., 2008; Cray et al., 2009).
Most of the studies performed on sheep are focused on the role of APPs after several inflammatory stimuli, being carried out few studies concerning specific bacterial, viral or parasitic infections (Table 6). Some studies are focused on the expression of APPs against lentiviral infections, being observed a local expression of SAA (Sack & Zink, 1992) but no serum enhancement of Hp or Fb concentrations (de la Concha et al., 2000).
Few studies have been focused on the changes of APPs in milk secretions of sheep. Whereas SAA levels in milk may be useful for the diagnosis on subclinical mastitis in individual ewes further studies are needed to determine its usefulness from bulk milk (Winter et al., 2006). Interestingly, opposite to bovine, the changes in the concentration of SAA in ewes with mastitis experimentally induced by *Staphylococcus epidermidis* are observed earlier in serum than in milk (Winter et al., 2003).
In goats the studies are rather limited than in sheep. The measure of APPs has been shown to not imply any advantage against the traditional markers observed for the diagnosis of pregnancy toxemia (González et al., 2011). Moreover, an increase of several APPs has been observed in the Alpine ibex with sarcoptic mange (Rahmann et al., 2010), which probably would act in the same way in domestic goats.

2.2.4 Porcine APPs

In swine there is an extensive literature available concerning the usefulness of APPs as a tool for monitoring both the health status of a herd as well as its welfare conditions. In pigs there are three major APPs, namely Hp, SAA and pig-major acute phase protein (Pig-MAP), whereas CRP and AGP are considered as moderate APPs and Fb as a minor APP (Petersen et al., 2004; Cray et al., 2009). Gender differences have been reported in swine exposed to stressors, being observed significantly higher concentrations of CRP and Hp in females than in males, although males tend to have higher Pig-MAP concentrations (Piñeiro M et al., 2007).
As it has just been said, APPs have been tested in pigs after exposure to stress (Salamano et al., 2008) and after natural (Chen et al., 2003; Parra et al., 2006) or experimental infections (Francisco et al., 1996; Asai et al., 1999; Magnusson et al., 1999; Knura-Deszczk et al., 2002; Van Gucht et al., 2005; Stevenson et al., 2006). Increased levels of different APPs have been reported in porcine viral and bacterial infections. The most significant of them are summarized in Table 7. As occurred in other species, inflammation or bacterial diseases trend to trigger off a more marked APR with a higher increase in the concentration of APPs

	Disorders in ovine	Acute Phase Protein	Reference
Inflammation	Peptidoglycan-polysaccharide	Hp, SAA	Dow et al ., 2010
	Uterine involution	Hp	Regassa & Noakes, 1999
	Pneumonia	Hp, Cp, Fb	Pfeffer & Rogers, 1989
	Chronic pneumonia	SAA	Kingston et al., 1982
	Subclinical mastitis	SAA	Winter et al., 2006
	Intrathoratic yeast inyection	Hp, Cp, Fb	Pfeffer et al., 1993
	Surgery	Hp, Cp, Fb	Pfeffer & Rogers, 1989
	Castration	Hp	Paull et al., 2009
Bacteria	*Corynebacterium pseudotuberculosis*	Hp, SAA, AGP	Pépin et al., 1991; Eckersall et al., 2007
	Mannheimia haemolytica	Hp, SAA, CRP, Cp	Ulutas & Ozpinar, 2006
	Staphylococcus epidermidis (mastitis)	SAA	Winter et al., 2003
Viruses	Lentivirus	SAA	Sack & Zink, 1992
Parasites	Myasis	SAA, Hp, Fb	Colditz et al., 2001; O'meara et al., 1995
Stress	Feeding	SAA	Eckersall et al., 2008
Other	Mulesing	Hp, SAA, Fb	Lepherd et al., 2011
	Carprofen + mulesing	Hp	Colditz et al., 2009
	NSAIDs + mulesing	Hp	Paull et al., 2008
	Vaccination	Hp, SAA	Eckersall et al., 2008
	Disorders in goats	**Acute Phase Protein**	**Reference**
Inflammation	Pregnancy toxemia	Hp	González et al., 2011
	Turpentine oil	Hp, SAA, ASG, Fb	González et al., 2008
Viruses	Lentivirus	SAA	Sack & Zink, 1992
Parasites	*Sarcoptes scabiei*	SAA, AGP, Hp, Cp	Rahmann et al., 2010
	Trichuris spp. + *Trichostrongylidae* spp. + *Fasciola* spp.	SAA, Hp	Ulutaş et al., 2008

Hp: haptoglobin; SAA: serum amyloid A; Cp: ceruloplasmin; Fb: fibrinogen; AGP: α_1-acid glycoprotein; CRP: C-reactive protein; ASG: acid soluble glycoprotein.

Table 6. Main APPs reported in different disorders in small ruminants.

than viral infections, however, the infection with specific porcine viruses such as porcine circovirus type 2 induces an enhancement in APPs comparable to the one observed in inflammation or *Mycoplasma hyopneumoniae* infection (Parra et al., 2006).

Recently, an interesting paper regarding the role of APPs in the diagnosis of infectious diseases in pigs has been published. In this paper the authors demonstrate specific combinations of APPs which may help to the diagnosis of porcine infectious diseases better than the analysis of individual APPs (Heegard et al., 2011).

	Disorder	Acute Phase Protein	Reference
Inflammation	Lipopolysaccharide		Dritz et al., 1996
	Surgery	CRP, Hp	Hernandez-Richter et al., 2001
Bacteria	*Actinobacillus pleuropneumoniae*	SAA, CRP	Skovgaard et al., 2009
	Mycoplasma hyopneumoniae	Pig-MAP, Hp, CRP	Parra et al., 2006
	Streptococcus suis	SAA, CRP	Sorensen et al., 2009
	Bordetella bornchiseptica +		Francisco et al., 1996
	Pasteurella multocida type D	Hp	Magnusson et al., 1999
	Mycoplasma hyorhinis	Hp	Jacobson et al., 2004
	Brachyspira hyodysenteriae	SAA, Hp	
Viruses	PRRS[1]	Pig-MAP, Hp	Gómez-Laguna et al., 2010a
	PCV2[2]	Pig-MAP, Hp	Grau-Roma et al., 2009
	Influenza	Hp, CRP	Barbé et al., 2011
	Aujeszky	Hp	Parra et al., 2006
Parasites	*Toxoplasma gondii*	Hp	Jungersen et al., 1999
Stress	Transportation	Pig-MAP, Hp	Piñeiro et al., 2007
	Housing	Hp, CRP	Salamano et al., 2008
	Slaughter	SAA, CRP, Pig-MAP, Hp	Piñeiro M et al., 2007
Others	Gestation	Fb	Sorrels et al., 2007

[1]PRRS: porcine reproductive and respiratory síndrome; [2]PCV2: porcine circovirus type 2; CRP: C-reactive protein; Hp: haptoglobin; SAA: serum amyloid A; Pig-MAP: pig-major acute phase protein; Fb: fibrinogen.

Table 7. Main conditions and APPs increased in the early response in pigs.

Although several studies are being conducted to determine the welfare status of several potential stressors in pigs, just as transportation, housing conditions, feeding or slaughter, a lack of an evident APR is reported in some investigations (Johnson et al., 2008; Weber et al., 2008). In the Table 7 appear some conditions which may evoke an increase in APPs.

3. Acute phase proteins as biomarkers of animal welfare

Stress is considered to be the most important factor to control on animal welfare. Hans Selye was the first author to introduce the concept of stress in 1936, as the non-specific response of the body to external challenges such as pathogens or a harsh physical environment (Selye, 1998). Nowadays in the animal production systems some aspects related to the housing and feeding system, changes in diet and transportation are considered as causes of stress, which compromise the welfare of animals (Broom & Johnson, 1993). Also, stress causes a risk in the animal homeostasis which results in an inflammatory response leading to immunosupression. This immunosupression favors the appearance of diseases such as shipping fever of feedlot cattle and Glasser's disease in pigs. Additionally, poor welfare may conduct to losses in performance and meat quality. Recently, the population has a significant and increasing concern for animal welfare where consumers prefer to pay higher prices for those products whose quality is guaranteed.

Animal welfare can be measured by different parameters such us mortality in the herd, presence of injuries, behavioral assessment, plasma glucocorticoid concentrations and heart rate (Broom & Johnson, 1993). Nonetheless, a high number of measured factors should be done to establish a reliable evaluation (Grandin, 1997). Different studies have shown that APPs are a useful tool in the assessment of animal welfare (Eckersall, 2000; Murata et al., 2004). With the measure of APPs, a rapid diagnosis can be made before the behavioral signs appear, as a result an effective treatment can be performed in order to solve losses in performance.

Firstly, it is definitely important to know the baseline APPs concentrations in healthy animals just to establish the reference ranges for the proteins. Different studies (Heegaard et al., 1998; Petersen et al., 2002; Campbell et al., 2005; Carpintero et al., 2005; Martín et al., 2005; Clapperton et al., 2007; Piñeiro et al., 2007, 2009) have determined the baseline ranges of APPs in pigs, these results were summarized by Diack et al. (2011).

There is no agreement if the age of the animal can modify the baseline levels of APPs. Thus, Piñeiro C et al. (personal communication) pointed to not changes in APPs values, whereas Alsemgeest et al. (1993, 1995) and Orro et al. (2008) showed significant differences depending on the age in calves. Also, there were significant differences between genetic lines for CRP, Pig-MAP and transthyretin in pigs, the same finding was reported by Frank et al. (2005), Shutterland et al. (2006), and Clapperton et al. (2005, 2007). These results highlight that APPs concentrations should be adjusted for factors such as age, sex, genetic line or individual herds, being needed the determination of a reference range which allow a reliable use of APPs measurement. Even, it has been reported that the same stressor can cause differences among animals (Von Borell, 1995).

Recently, some authors have shown that it is more significant to study the correlation between two APPs than the changes of the level of only one APP following a stressful situation. In this sense, significant correlations have been found between Hp and CRP (Diack et al., 2011), between Hp and Pig-MAP (Clapperton et al., 2007; Diack et al., 2011) and between CRP and Pig-MAP (Diack et al., 2011) in pigs.

3.1 APPs and welfare in small animals

Dogs and cats also experience changes in their homeostasis due to stressors (Eckersall, 2000). Although it has not been reported any article about the behaviour of APPs in dogs and cats, cortisol levels have been reported to increase when dogs are introduced to novel kennels (Rooney et al., 2007) and where cats are maintained in non-enrichment shelter (McCobb et al., 2005). Knowing that APPs are sensitive biomarkers of welfare, it may be possible that an increase in APP concentration occurs after these conditions.

As a conclusion, not only transportation but also the stress of adapting to new environment comprising feeding, housing and different stock densities may cause an enhancement in APP concentration levels. Thus, the measure of APPs results in a useful parameter in order to assess animal's welfare, particularly in farm animals where the analysis of APPs could help to assess if the new automation machines are according to welfare conditions or in contrast are a cause of stress in animals and taking into account that a decrease in the APPs levels can express an adaptation to the stressful situation.

3.2 APPs and welfare in large animals

3.2.1 Bovine APPs of importance in stress and welfare

The majority of studies concerning to APPs performed in this species suffer from baseline ranges which allowed to compare the experimental results with the healthy situation.

Indeed, the absence of some control animals in the experiments carried out in matter of transportation and mixing animals, does not allow having a clear understanding of the APP behaviour. However, it is important to highlight that SAA suggests being the better APP to determine changes in weaning, feeding and housing systems in cattle.
Conner et al. (1988) described the increase of APPs in response to stress stimuli in calves. Table 8 summarized the studies performed in different possible stressful situations in this species.

Conditions	Acute Phase Proteins	Reference
3 hours transport after weaning	↑ SAA, Fb, Cp	Arthington et al., 2003
Road and sea transport	NC Hp, Fb	Earley & Murray, 2010
Mixing animals	NC Fb, Cp, AGP	Arthington et al., 2003
Dietary differences on diet	NC Hp, Fb, SAA	Berry et al., 2004
Different housing and feeding systems	↑ SAA NC Hp	Saco et al., 2008
Housing (different number of heifers per concentrate feeding place)	↑ Hp	González et al., 2008
Housing (different types of floor)	↑ SAA NC Hp	Alsemgeest et al., 1995
Parturition	↑ SAA, Hp, AGP, LPS	Orro et al., 2008

↑ : increased expression; NC: no change in expression; SAA: serum amyloid A; Fb: fibrinogen; Cp: ceruloplasmin; Hp: haptoglobin; AGP: α_1-acid glycoprotein; LPS: lipopolysaccharide.

Table 8. APPs levels depend on the studied stressor.

Regarding transportation, Arthington et al. (2003) showed changes in APPs levels, these changes were transient and not significantly altered. Also, the absence of a weaning control does not allow establishing a solid conclusion.
In cattle, it has been reported that competition for food can result in poor welfare and production losses (Miller & Wood-Gush, 1991). The results showed that the energy level of the diet does not induce changes in APP concentrations. The genetics background has also proven to be important in cows, where SAA levels showed an increase in semi-feral cows in comparison with feed type selected breed.
SAA was the main protein enhanced depending on the housing system, this major APP in cattle may be a better biomarker of the health status.
The results found in bibliography about parturition are controversial. Nonetheless, concentrations of APPs were higher in those calves which needed the use of forceful extraction, so we conclude that parturition increases the levels of APPs.

3.2.2 APPs of importance in small ruminants stress and welfare

The number of studies about welfare and APPs in this species of animals is scarce. In ewes, it has been reported that sheep which were transported for 30 and 48 hours, exhibit greater total plasma protein concentrations than those transported for 12 hours. Hp and albumin were considered within the total plasma protein levels (Fisher et al., 2010). More studies should be performed in this topic in order to assess the use of APPs as biomarkers of welfare in sheep and goats.

3.2.3 Porcine APPs of importance in stress and welfare

Pigs belong to the species in which more studies have been carried out regarding animal welfare. In fact, there is a tight European Union Legislation which regulates the conditions of raising animals to assess the well-being.

Condition	Acute Phase Proteins	Reference
Average time transport (24h) + poor transport conditions	↑ Pig-MAP, Hp	Saco et al., 2003 Piñeiro M et al., 2007
Long time transport (48h) + great transport conditions	↑ Pig-MAP	Saco et al., 2003 Piñeiro M et al., 2007
Short time transport (6-12h) + commercial conditions	↑ Pig-MAP, Hp, CRP, SAA ↓ Apo A-I	Saco et al., 2003 Piñeiro M et al., 2007
Long time transport + management and new accommodation	↑ Pig-MAP, Hp, CRP	Salamano et al., 2008
Changes in pattern of food	↑ Pig-MAP, Hp, CRP (males) ↓ Apo A-I (males)	Piñeiro C et al., 2007
Organic versus conventional food	NC Hp	Millet et al., 2005
Housing (gestation crates)	NC Hp, Fb, AGP	Sorrels et al., 2007
Group versus cages	NC Pig-MAP	Rodríguez-Gómez et al., (unpublished data)
Organic versus conventional housing	↑ Hp	Millet et al., 2005
Different stock densities housing	↑ Pig-MAP NC Hp, CRP, Apo A-I	Marco-Ramell et al., 2011

↑: increased expression; ↓: decrease expression; NC: no change in expression; Pig-Map: pig-major acute phase protein; Hp: haptoglobin; CRP: C-reactive protein; SAA: serum amyloid A; Apo A-I: apoliprotein A-I; Fb: fibrinogen; AGP: α_1-acid glycoprotein.

Table 9. APPs changes depend on the stressful condition studied.

Different studies have shown that shipment of animals can result in an APP response related to the stress of transportation. Stress in transportation can affect meat quality and as a result, the value of the commercial product (Warris, 1998, 2003). Table 9 summarizes the different studies performed according to the stressful condition studied. In general, APP levels are extremely sensitive to shipment in pigs. Although all major APPs experience changes in their levels, the variation in Pig-MAP and Hp concentrations were constant in the different situations. Apoliprotein A-I (Apo A-I), as a negative APP, was a good biomarker too (Saco et al., 2003; Piñeiro M et al., 2007). APP levels not only were increased after the trip but also as a result of the adaptation to the unfamiliar accommodation, handling procedures and mixing of the animals (Salamano et al., 2008).

The appearance of gastric ulcer is related to stress conditions such as poor management and changes in feeding. This damage leads to huge economical losses in porcine industry. In one study, feeding changes were transient and only in males, possibly due to a higher manifestation of behavior, where the fight, dominance and competition for the food between males are more evident than in females (Piñeiro C et al., 2007). Also, the implementation of organic food did not show any advantage with respect to conventional food (Millet et al., 2005).

Other controversial topic which is in constant study is the type of gestation crates used during gestation in pigs. It is well-known that stress related to gestation can result in weird behaviour to the offspring and disturbances in the immune response leading to higher susceptibility to diseases (Eicher & Burton, 2005). In the majority of the studies performed, no changes were found in APP levels. Only Hp and Pig-MAP proteins altered their concentrations as a result of changes in housing or stock densities housing, respectively. It should be expected that changes between organic versus conventional housing are more patent due to the intention to reproduce natural conditions. However, these results should be interpreted carefully due to some important stressors were not taken into account.

In summary, Pig-MAP and Hp should be considered the best biomarkers of welfare in pig production due to that their analysis can reflect a stressful situation.

4. Disease and acute phase proteins

The discovery of new biomarkers which allow the clinical monitoring of different diseases is nowadays encouraged in order to improve the treatment and therapeutics in each phase of the disease. Therefore, the use of APPs in diagnosis and their application in monitoring of treatments is considered as one of the most interesting applications of these proteins. In this sense, APPs have been widely used in human medicine as biomarkers of inflammation, infection or trauma; however, their use in veterinary medicine is more recent. Thus, a significant progress has been made in the detection, measurement and application of APPs as biomarkers in both companion and farm animals over recent years.

The monitoring of two or more APPs is highly valuable in different diseases as each APP may display a different kinetic after the infection or trauma in the animal (Eckersall, 2000). This information may be of interest to evaluate the progress of the disease and may help in the prognosis of the animal or herd health.

4.1 Disease and APPs in small animals

4.1.1 Disease and APPs in dogs

CRP, SAA, Hp and/or AGP are the main APPs in dogs which may show changes after different infectious diseases, inflammation or other disorders, just as neoplasia (Table 2). For example, an increase of CRP has been observed in parvovirus infection, and in this disease the magnitude of the increase in APPs could be a useful indicator of the prognosis, being CRP a potent predictor of mortality due to this process (Kocaturk et al., 2010).

High levels of CRP have been related to the onset of sepsis in several disease models in dogs. Thus, the marked increased of CRP reported in dogs infected by canine parvovirus type 2 were due to the appearance of sepsis in these animals (Kocaturk et al., 2010). In fact, the levels reported in this study were similar to those observed previously in dogs with septic processes (Caldin et al., 2009), and deal with the knowledge that usually bacterial infections elicit a much higher APR than viral infections do (Gruys et al., 2005). However, in the previous study (Kocaturk et al., 2010) the use of CRP was evaluated as diagnostic tool for differentiation of survivors versus non survivors displaying a high sensitivity (91%) but a low specificity (61%). For these reasons, the role of CRP as useful marker of sepsis in dogs although indicative of a septic disease remains still controversial.

Serum levels of SAA have been used in the monitoring of responses to treatments as hyperadrenocorticism treatment (Arteaga et al., 2010) or possible complications in postoperative periods as after surgery because of pyometra (Dabrowski et al., 2009). Due to the particular sensitivity of Hp to effects of corticoid in the dog, elevated concentrations of Hp are found after corticosteroids treatments or in cases of hyperadrenocorticism so this protein could be used as a method of screening for canine hyperadrenocorticism but not in monitoring of inflammation because of steroid treatments could interfere with results interpretation (Arteaga et al., 2010; Eckersall & Bell 2010).

In dogs with a fracture or subjected to percutaneous gastrostomy, serum CRP and AGP levels correlated with the condition of the dogs and may be useful in routine testing for inflammation, in preclinical studies and in veterinary clinical biochemistry (Hayashi et al., 2001).

Changes in CRP and Hp have been reported in dogs with lymphatic neoplasia (Mischke et al., 2007). Dogs with mammary neoplasia have high CRP, SAA and Hp levels but the increased concentrations of APPs could be stimulated by different factors, such as metastasis, large size of the primary mass and ulceration or secondary inflammation of the neoplasm (Planellas et al., 2009; Tecles et al., 2009). Serum levels of these APPs are of use in the diagnosis and management of steroid responsive meningitis-arteritis (SRMA), particularly in relation to identifying relapse (Lowrie et al., 2009). Dog with gastric mucosa injury present elevated serum CRP, SAA and Hp levels and may be potentially useful together with gastroscopy in the diagnosis and monitoring of gastric injury (Bayramli & Ulutas, 2008).

4.1.2 Disease and APPs in felines

Feline serum SAA, AGP and/or Hp levels increase in infectious diseases, such as feline infectious peritonitis (FIP), and others inflammatory conditions (Table 3). The serum concentration of SAA may be also a useful marker for evaluating response to treatment and disease exacerbation in feline pancreatitis (Tamamoto et al., 2009).

Elevated concentrations of AGP have been also found in serum of cats with lymphoma although did not provide useful information regarding response or survival of affected animals (Correa et al., 2001).

Increased levels of Hp have been seen in cats affected by FIP (Giordano et al., 2004). In cats experimentally inoculated with feline infectious peritonitis virus Hp levels increased very early and then slight decreased, but two weeks after experimental induction of the disease increased concentrations were found again (Stodddart et al 1988). Besides Hp, increased levels of AGP have also been reported in cats suffering from FIP, as it has been mentioned above. AGP may trigger several functions related with the regulation of the immune response. In this sense, the sialic acid content has been associated to the defensive functions proposed for AGP, favoring the competition of AGP for cell surface receptors, blocking the binding and the invasion of infectious agents (Ceciliani et al., 2004). Interestingly, it has been postulated that the enhancement in AGP concentrations observed in FIP may play a significant role in the immunopathogenesis of the disease. As stated before, AGP and its glycosylation pattern are associated with resistance or susceptibility to some viral diseases (Rabehi et al 1995). Furthermore, a hyposialylitation of feline AGP has been reported in cats with FIP (Ceciliani et al 2004). Following these results, Paltrinieri et al. (2007c) hypothesized that cats with endemic FCoV infection respond to increased viral burden by increasing the production of AGP and only cats with hyposialylated AGP have persistently increased AGP levels and develop FIP.

4.2 Disease and APPs in large animals

4.2.1 Disease and APPs in equines

The measurement of APPs has potential use in the study of inflammatory disorders in equine medicine (Crisman et al., 2008). Increased serum concentrations of SAA have been found in horses affected by arthritis and a local synthesis of this protein has also been reported in the inflamed joint (Jacobsen et al., 2006a). Synovial fluid SAA concentration seems to be a good marker of infectious arthritis and present advantages as ease and speed of measurement and the fact that concentrations in synovial fluid were not influenced by repeated arthrocentesis in healthy horses (Jacobsen et al., 2006b). High levels of SAA in serum and an increased expression in endometrium have been reported in mares with experimentally induced endometritis (Mette et al., 2010). The serum concentration of SAA has demonstrated its utility for identification of the clinical condition of horses with bacterial pneumonia (Hobo et al., 2007). Horses with enteritis or colitis and conditions characterized by chronic inflammation (e.g. abdominal abscesses, peritonitis, or rectal tears) had SAA concentrations significantly greater than those for horses with other conditions so evaluation of SAA concentrations may be of use in identifying horses with colic attributable to diseases that have inflammation as a primary component of pathogenesis (Vandenplas et al., 2005).

In foals, increased concentrations of SAA have been found in septicaemic animals (Paltrinieri et al., 2008) and has been observed that foals with a strong suspicion of sepsis have significantly higher concentrations of SAA than compromised foals with non-infectious inflammatory disease (Duggan, 2008). The measurement of SAA could be a useful tool in the early diagnosis of neonatal septicaemia (Paltrinieri et al., 2008).

Surgical trauma produces an acute phase response and elective and non-elective surgery induces an increase in the serum levels of SAA (Pollock et al., 2005). The concentration of SAA have shown to reflect the intensity of the surgical trauma and may be useful for comparing surgical trauma associated with novel versus well-established surgical techniques (Jacobsen et al., 2009).

Elevated serum Hp levels have been reported in processes such as experimental aseptic arthritis, experimental local aseptic inflammation, experimentally induced noninfectious laminitis, grass sickness (equine dysautonomia) or castration (Petersen et al., 2004) (Table 4).

4.2.2 Disease and APPs in cattle

In ruminants, the acute phase response is different from other species since Hp is considered as a major APP (Eckersall & Bell 2010). Hp serum levels have been found increased in several inflammatory diseases such as endometritis, pneumonia, enteritis, peritonitis, mastitis and endocarditis (Murata et al., 2004; Petersen et al., 2004) (Table 5). In the case of metritis Hp values may assist in the early detection of the disease, providing increased opportunities for early treatment and prevention (Huzzey et al., 2009). Lameness due to claw disorders can be associated with a systemic acute phase response and elevated serum Hp in dairy cattle and the values of this protein can be used for monitoring the effectiveness of different treatments (Smith et al., 2010). In lame cows as a result of hoof disease increased concentrations of serum SAA were found while Hp values did not increased significantly what could mean that a greater stimulation associated with inflammation is needed for serum haptoglobin to increase (Kujala et al., 2010).

The serum values of SAA seem to be more sensitive marker for acute inflammation than Hp values (Horadagoda et al., 1999). In calves with chronic respiratory diseases elevated concentrations of Hp and SAA were found, and were significantly higher in dead or euthanized calves compared with calves in improved health status during therapy, so their evaluation could be useful in the determination of prognosis of the respiratory disease (Tóthová et al., 2010). In the case of viral pneumonias, the concentration of both proteins are elevated but the magnitude and duration of the Hp response was found to correlate well with the severity of clinical signs (fever) and with the extent of lung consolidation while SAA responded most rapidly to infection, so this last protein seems to be a more sensitive marker for viral pneumonia (Heegaard et al., 2000). In experimental infection with *Mannheimia haemolytica*, SAA was found to be more rapidly induced than Hp (Horadagoda et al.,1994), but in field cases, Hp produce a bigger and more prolonged response giving rise to its higher sensitivity in detecting disease (Angen et al., 2009).

The serum concentrations of Hp and SAA are increased in cases of mastitis (Gerardi et al., 2009; Petersen et al., 2004; Safi et al., 2009). In animals suffering from this disorder, the levels of these proteins have been also measured in milk. Hp levels in milk in cows affected by clinical mastitis were higher in cows with moderate to severe versus mild systemic disease (Wenz et al., 2010). In a study carried out by Safi et al. (2009) in Holstein cows from 7 different dairy farms the levels of Hp and amyloid A were measured in milk (AAM) and serum in order to evaluate the use and compare the accuracy of both APPs in these specimens for the diagnosis of subclinical mastitis based on bacterial culture results and with comparison with the California mastitis test (CMT) and somatic cell counts (SCC). The results of the study showed that the bacteria most found in the cases of subclinical mastitis were *Streptococcus agalactiae* and *Staphylococcus aureus* and the most accurate test for the diagnosis was AAM followed by CMT, SCC, HP in milk, SAA in serum and Hp in serum. Therefore test on milk generally were more accurate than test in serum in the diagnosis of subclinical mastitis. In another study carried out by Gerardi et al. (2009) about the use of SAA and AAM for the diagnosis of subclinical mastitis, the levels of AAM measured with a milk ELISA kit were significantly different between cows with subclinical and clinical mastitis and resulted to be a better tool for distinguishing subclinical from clinical mastitis than AAM measured with a serum ELISA kit. The results of this study also showed that the measurement of AAM could allow the identification of subclinical mastitis in equal or higher measure than SCC so the control of AAM and SAA on dairy farms could reduce both the laboratory costs and the time required for milk analysis.

Serum levels of Hp and SAA have been measured in cows with left displaced abomasum, right displaced abomasum or abomasal volvulus and the values were most strongly associated with liver fat percentage than with the alteration in abomasums so an increase in SAA or Hp may indicate the presence of hepatic lipidosis in cattle with abomasal displacement (Guzelbektes et al., 2010)

AGP is considered as moderate APP in cow. Elevated serum levels of this protein have been reported in cows with respiratory disease (Nikunen et al., 2007). In experimental infections with *Pasteurella multocida* increases in the concentrations of AGP have been found to be more gradual and to remain elevated for longer than those observed for SAA or Hp (Dowling et al., 2002). Elevated serum levels of AGP have been also reported in animals with mastitis (Eckersall et al., 2001).

CRP serum levels have shown their utility as a marker or tool for evaluating the health status of a herd and could also be considered as useful criteria to assess the stress levels as well as in early surveillance of disease conditions in a dairy herd (Lee et al., 2003).

Another utility of APPs could be the assessment of animal health and welfare as an aid to meat inspections (Eckersall & Bell, 2010). Hp and SAA serum concentrations al slaughter have been found increased in cows with infectious and metabolic diseases compared to animal with minor lesions and animal with acute lesions compared with healthy animals (Hirvonen et al., 1997; Tourlomousis et al., 2004).

4.2.3 Disease and APPs in small ruminants

In goats, Hp and SAA can be considered as major APPs, while ASG and Fb can be considered as moderate (Table 1). Increase in Hp, SAA, ASG, and Fb serum concentrations have been found after inducing an inflammatory response by subcutaneous injection of turpentine oil (González et al., 2008). Elevated serum levels of Hp have been reported in experimentally induced pregnancy toxemia in goats (González et al., 2011) (Table 6).

In sheep, serum Hp seems to be useful as a marker for the presence of bacterial infection (Skinner & Roberts, 1994). Serum Hp, SAA and AGP were increased in an experimental model of caseous lymphadenitis, suggesting the results that AGP could have a role as a marker for chronic conditions in sheep (Eckersall et al., 2007). Increased serum CRP, Hp, Cp and Fb levels have been reported in animals infected with *M. haemolytica* (Ulutas & Ozpinar, 2006) (Table 6).

4.2.4 Disease and APPs in swine

Increased serum levels of APPs have been reported in pigs experimentally and naturally infected with different virus and bacteria. Hp, CRP, SAA and Pig-MAP increased serum levels have been recently reported in pigs experimentally infected with porcine reproductive and respiratory syndrome virus (PRRSV) by our research group (Gómez-Laguna et al., 2010b). In this study we found an increase at 10 days post inoculation (dpi) in the serum levels of Hp and Pig-MAP. The serum levels of CRP and SAA showed a delayed increase at 17 dpi, being this last APP which reached the highest increase. The increase in the serum concentrations of Hp coincided with the highest titer of viraemia and a light enhancement in the levels of IL-6 and TNF-α, and might be related with and increased expression of IL-10. CRP participates in the complement activation and opsonization, and induces cytokine production by macrophages, whereas SAA is chemotactic for monocytes, T cells and polymorphonuclear, so the delayed increased expression found in both APPs may contribute to the establishment of an impaired non-efficient host-immune response. The result of our study suggested a modulation of the immune response by the enhanced expression of Hp, and the poor or/and delayed expression of TNF-α, CRP and SAA making feasible a prolonged viraemia and an inefficient PRRSV clearance. Another study carried out by our research group showed that the values of Hp and CRP in saliva and meat juice showed a similar kinetic than in serum in PRRSV-infected animals, so these samples could serve as complementary or alternative biomarkers in this disease (Gómez-Laguna et al., 2010a). The serum levels of these proteins are also increased in swine influenza virus (SIV) experimentally infected animals (Barbé et al., 2011). In pigs experimentally infected with classical swine fever and African swine fever viruses the serum concentrations of Hp, CRP and SAA were increased, being the levels of this last protein what more increase presented in the animals infected by both viruses (Sánchez-Cordón et al., 2007).

In animals naturally infected by PRRSV serum levels of Hp, CRP and SAA were found increased but not Pig-MAP concentrations. This APPs did not present any change when compared with Specific Pathogen Free (SPF) pigs taken as controls. In animals affected with Aujeszky's disease virus (ADV) only Hp showed increased levels, whereas pigs with porcine circovirus type 2 (PCV2) showed marked modifications in all APPs tested. The increases in the concentrations of APPs were higher in animals with clinical signs and concurrent bacterial processes (Parra et al., 2006). In a study in farms with animals clinically affected by Postweaning Multisystemic Wasting Syndrome (PMWS) caused by PCV2, the serum levels of Hp and Pig-MAP correlate with PCV2 viremia and the clinical course of the disease, concluding that Pig-MAP, in the conditions of this study, was better indicator of the PMWS status than Hp (Grau-Roma et al., 2009). In another study in farms affected by PMWS the increase in the viral load did not induce any SAA response (Wallgren et al., 2009).

In pigs experimentally infected by *Streptococcus suis* showed increased serum concentrations of Hp, CRP, SAA and Pig-MAP (Sorensen et al., 2006). In an experimental infection with *Actinobacillus pleuropneumoniae* increased serum levels of CRP and SAA were found but extrahepatic expression of these two proteins and of Hp and Pig-MAP was also detected in peripheral lymphoid tissues by PCR (Skovgaard et al., 2009). Extrahepatic presence of Hp has been also detected in lung by immunohistochemistry (Hiss et al., 2008). In field cases of enzootic pneumonia (EP) caused by *Mycoplasma hyopneumoniae* elevated serum levels of Hp, CRP, SAA and Pig-MAP have been reported (Parra et al., 2006) (Table 7).

In slaughter-aged pigs, the serum levels of Pig-MAP resulted to be more sensitive marker than Hp to differentiate animals suffering of pleuritis and cranio-ventral pulmonary consolidations (Saco et al., 2010). In a study carried out at slaughter by our research group serum levels of Hp and CRP in apparently healthy pigs were significantly higher in animals with lesions than those without lesions. In this same study was found that the extent and severity of lung lesions were related to serum levels of Hp (Pallarés et al., 2008). In another study the findings indicative of lesions compatible with enzootic pneumonia were associated with increased serum Hp at slaughter (Amory et al., 2004). In pigs with carcass condemnations due to abscesses increased serum APPs have been also reported (Heinonen et al., 2010). The use of APPs in finishing pigs just before sacrifice could provide information to the veterinary inspector about the possible appearance of lesions in these pigs and could serve as a tool to the meat industry to differentiate pigs with different health status that probably will match with different quality of carcasses (Pallarés et al., 2008).

5. Conclusion: APP in the evaluation of prophylaxis and therapeutic strategies

APPs may act as biomarkers of inflammation allowing us to study the progression of the inflammatory response which is evoked during the acute phase of several diseases. The application of different therapeutic agents should diminish the intensity and the length of the inflammation and, therefore, the APR. Monitoring diseases and their treatments by means of APPs, may allow us to determine the efficiency and efficacy of a specific treatment. In this sense, Arteaga et al. (2010) monitored the response of canine hyperadrenocorticism to trilostane, and concluded that whereas only Hp (together with cholesterol and alkaline phosphatase) give some information about the control of the disease, no information was obtained from SAA or CRP, despite the former also decreased after the treatment. On the other hand, CRP represents an interesting parameter to measure in other processes, just as in canine lymphoma, where a significant decrease in CRP values was associated to remission after treatment with specific cytotoxic drugs (Nielsen et al., 2007). Specific APPs have been reported as value tools in monitoring both infectious diseases, just as CRP and Cp (but not SAA or Hp) in leishmaniasis (Martínez-Subiela et al., 2003) or CRP (but not Hp) in trypanosomiasis (N'dungu et al., 1991), and inflammatory processes, just as SAA in feline acute pancreatitis (associated with remission and recurrence) (Tamamoto et al., 2009) or Hp in bovine respiratory disease (Carter et al., 2002). In other conditions, just as canine hemolytic anemia, the changes in APPs were not useful to monitor the success of specific treatments (Griebsch et al., 2009; Mitchell et al., 2009).

On the other side, some prophylactic strategies are carried out in order to prevent the disease. One of the most common prophylactic strategies is the use of vaccines, which may prepare the organism to fight against a specific pathogen. Some vaccines are made with peptidic fragments from the microorganism or with the whole microorganism inactivated by different methods. Thus, vaccines may develop also an APR which may have an adverse effect and limit the efficacy and safety of these prophylactic strategies (Gruys et al., 2005). For these reasons, APPs may be used to determine the usefulness of vaccines as prophylactic agents, determining the magnitude of the inflammatory response evoked by their use. Moreover, aminoacids are required for the production of APPs, specifically phenylalanine, tryptophan and tyrosine may be detected in high percentage in some positive APPs. Therefore, vaccination may limit in some cases the recovery of the diseased animal acting opposite to the anabolism of the muscle (Gruys et al., 2005).

The inflammatory and the acute phase responses have been measured in cattle vaccinated with different clostridial vaccine candidates, being observed a higher expression of Hp and a decrease in feed consumption when a multiple clostridial- instead of a mono-clostridial vaccine was used, which points to the potential negative effects of multiple clostridial-vaccinations (Stokka et al., 1994). Moreover, the utility of Hp values have been shown in the follow-up of the trimming and antibiotic treatment against several claw disorders (Smith et al., 2000).

In pigs, monitoring the APPs has been widely used to determine the usefulness of specific vaccines against both bacteria and viruses. A panel of APPs (Pig-MAP, Hp, CRP and Apo A-I) has been used in order to monitor pigs challenge against both the bacteria *Hameophilus parasuis* and commercial and non-commercial bacterins finding a lower expression of APPs in vaccinated animals together with a shorter course of the disease and higher survival rates (Martín de la Fuente et al., 2010). Apo A-I and Pig-Map has been shown to be useful tools to monitor vaccination against Aujeszky's disease, showing the vaccinated animals none or only mild clinical signs, a less pronounced APR and recovered earlier to normal values (Carpintero et al., 2007). Nonetheless, further studies are required in order to assess the predictive value of APPs in vaccine testing.

Although a wide range of studies have been carried out to determine the role of APPs in several conditions just as stress, inflammation, infection or vaccination there is still necessity for establishing reference values which allow interpreting the results from the different studies and disorders. Some of this information may be available for some species of domestic animal; however, there is no still a global consensus to accept specific ranges for each APP in each species, as well as, validation of specific analytical techniques which enable the interlaboratory comparison of results.

6. Acknowledgements

This work was supported financially by the Spanish Ministry of Education and Science, project number AGL2009-12438/GAN.

7. References

Alsemgeest, S.P.; Lambooy, I.E., Wierenga, H.K., Dieleman, S.J., Meerkerk, B., van Edern A.M., Niewold, T.A. (1995). Influence of physical stress on the plasma concentration of erum amyloid-A (SAA) and haptoglobin (Hp) in calves. *The Veterinary Quarterly* Vol. 17, No. 1, pp. 9-12, ISSN 0165-2176

Alsemgeest, S.P.M., Taverne, M.A.M., Boosman, R., van der Weyden, G.C., Gruys, E., 1993. Peripartum acute-phase protein serum amyloid-A concentration in plasma of cows and fetuses. *American Journal of Veterinary Research* Vol. 54, pp. 164-167, ISSN 0891-6640

Alsemgeest, S.P.M.; Jonker, F.H., Taverne, M.A.M., Kalsbeek, H.C., Wensing, Th., Gruys, E., 1995. Serum amyloid-A (SAA) and haptoglobin (HP) plasma concentrations in newborn calves. *Theriogenology* Vol. 43, pp. 381-387, ISSN 0093-691X

Amory, J.R.; Mackenzie, A.M.,. Eckersall, P.D., Stear, M.J. & Pearce, G.P. (2007). Influence of rearing conditions and respiratory disease on haptoglobin levels in the pig at slaughter. *Research in Veterinary Science* Vol. 83, No. 3, (December 2007), pp. 428-435, ISSN 0034-5288

Andersen, S.A.; Petersen, H.H., Ersbøll, A.K., Falk-Rønne, J. & Jacobsen, S. (2011). Vaccination elicits a prominent acute phase response in horses. *The Veterinary Journal*, doi:10.1016/j.tvjl.2011.01.019, ISSN 1090-0233

Angen, O.; Thomsen, J., Larsen, L.E., Larsen, J., Kokotovic, B., Heegaard, P.M. & Enemark, J.M. (2009). Respiratory disease in calves: microbiological investigations on trans-tracheally aspirated bronchoalveolar fluid and acute phase protein response. *Veterinary Microbiology* Vol. 137, No. 1-2, (May 2009), pp. 165-171, ISSN 0378-1135

Arteaga, A., Dhand, N.K., McCann, T., Knottenbelt, C.M., Tebb, A.J., Evans, H., Eckersall, P.D. & Ramsey IK. (2010). Monitoring the response of canine hyperadrenocorticism to trilostane treatment by assessment of acute phase protein concentrations. *Journal of Small Animal Practice* Vol. 51, No. 4, (April), pp. 204-209, ISSN 1748-5827

Arthington, J.D., Eicher, S.D., Kunkle, W.E., Marin, F.G. (2003). Effect of transportation and commingling on the acute-phase protein response, growth, and feed intake of newly waned beef calves. *Journal of Animal Science* Vol. 81, No. 5, (May 2003), pp.1120-1125, ISSN 0021-8812

Asai, T.; Mori, M., Okada, M., Uruno, K., Yazawa, S. & Shibata, I. (1999). Elevated serum haptoglobin in pigs infected with porcine reproductive and respiratory syndrome virus. *Veterinary Immunology and Immunopathology* Vol. 70, No 1-2, pp. 143-148, ISSN 0165-2427

Barbé, F.; Atanasova, K. & Van Reeth, K. (2011). Cytokines and acute phase proteins associated with acute swine influenza infection in pigs. *The Veterinary Journal*, Vol. 187, No. 1, (January 2011), pp. 48-53, ISSN 1090-0233

Bayramli, G. & Ulutas, B. (2008). Acute phase protein response in dogs with experimentally induced gastric mucosal injury. *Veterinary Clinical Pathology*, Vol. 37, No. 3, (September 2008), pp. 312-316, ISSN 0275-6382

Berry, B.A., Confer, A.W., Krehbiel, C.R., Gill, D.R., Smith, R.A., Montelongo, M., (2004). Effects of dietary energy and starch concentrations for newly received feedlot calves: II. Acute-phase protein response. *Journal of Animal Science*, Vol. 82, No. 3 (March 2004), pp. 845-850, ISSN 0021-8812

Borges, A.S.; Divers, T.J., Stokol, T. & Mohammed, O.H. (2007). Serum iron and plasma fibrinogen concentrations as indicators of systemic inflammatory diseases in horses. *Journal of Veterinary Internal Medicine* Vol. 21, No 3, (May-June 2007), pp. 489-494, ISSN 0891-6640

Broom, D.M. & Johnson, K.G. (1993). Stress and Animal Welfare. In: *Animal Behaviour Series*. Chapman and Hall, ISBN 0813816599, London

Calamari, L.; Abeni, F. & Bertin, G. (2010). Metabolic and hematological profiles in mature horses supplemented with different selenium sources and doses. *Journal of Animal Science* Vol. 88, No. 2, (February 2010), pp. 650-659, ISSN 1523-3163

Caldin, M.; Tasca, S., Carli, E., Bianchini, S., Furlanello, T., Martinez-Subiela, S. & Cerón, J.J. (2009). Serum acute phase protein concentrations in dogs with hyperadrenocorticism with and without concurrent inflammatory conditions. *Veterinary Clinical Pathology* Vol. 38, No. 1, (March 2009), pp. 63-68, ISSN 0275-6382

Campbell, D.J., Rawlings, J.M., Koelsch, S., Wallace, J., Strain, J.J. & Hannigan, B.M. (2004). Age-related differences in parameters of feline immune status. *Veterinary Immunology and Immunopathology* Vol. 100, No. 1-2, (July 2004), pp. 73-80, ISSN 0165-2427

Campbell, F.M., Waterston, M., Andresen, L.O., Sorensen, N.S., Heegaard, P.M., Eckersall, P.D. (2005). The negative acute phase response of serum transthyretin following *Streptococcus suis* infection in the pig. *Veterinary Research* Vol. 36, No. 4, (July-August 2005), pp. 657-664, ISSN 0928-4249

Carpintero, R., Piñeiro, M., Andrés, M., Iturralde, M., Alava, M.A., Heegaard, P., Jobert, J.L., Madec, F., Lampreave, F. (2005). The concentration of apolipoprotein A-I decreases during experimentally induced acute processes in pigs. *Infection and Immunity* Vol. 73, No. 5, (May 2005), pp. 3184-3187, ISSN 1098-5522

Carpintero, R.; Alonso, C., Piñeiro, M., Iturralde, M., Andrés, M., Le Potier, M.F., Madec, F., Alava, M.A., Piñeiro, A. & Lampreave, F. (2007). Pig major acute-phase protein and apolipoprotein A-I responses correlate with the clinical course of experimentally induced African Swine Fever and Aujeszky's disease. *Veterinary Research* Vol. 38, No. 5, (September-October 2007), pp. 741-753, ISSN 0891-6640

Carter, J.N.; Meredith, G.L., Montelongo, M., Gill, D.R., Krehbiel, C.R., Payton, M.E. & Confer, A.W. (2002). Relationship of vitamin E supplementation and antimicrobial treatment with acute-phase protein responses in cattle affected by naturally acquired respiratory tract disease. *American Journal of Veterinary Research* Vol. 63, No. 8, (August 2002), pp. 1111-1117, ISSN 0891-6640

Caspi, D.; Snel, F.W., Batt, R.M., Bennett, D., Rutteman, G.R., Hartman, E.G., Baltz, M.L., Gruys, E. & Pepys, M.B. (1987). C-reactive protein in dogs. *American Journal of Veterinary Research* Vol. 48, No. 6, (June 1987), pp. 919-921, ISSN 0891-6640

Ceciliani, F.; Giordano, A. & Spagnolo, V. (2002). The systemic reaction during inflammation: the acute-phase proteins. *Protein and peptide letters* Vol.9, No.3, (June 2002), pp.211-223, ISSN: 0929-8665

Ceciliani, F.; Grossi, C., Giordano, A., Pocacqua, V. & Paltrinieri, S. (2004). Decreased sialylation of the acute phase protein alpha1-acid glycoprotein in feline infectious peritonitis (FIP). *Veterinary Immunology and Immunopathology* Vol. 99, No. 3-4, (June 2004), pp. 229-236, ISSN 0165-2427

Cerón, J.J.; Eckersall, P.D. & Martínez-Subiela, S. (2005). Acute phase proteins in dogs and cats: current knowledge and future perspectives. *Veterinary Clinical Pathology*, Vol. 34, No. 2, (June 2005), pp. 85-99, ISSN 0275-6382

Chan, J.P., Chang, C.C., Hsu, W.L., Liu, W.B. & Chen, T.H. (2010). Association of increased serum acute-phase protein concentrations with reproductive performance in dairy cows with postpartum metritis. *Veterinary Clinical Pathology* Vol. 39, No. 1, (March 2010), pp. 72-78, ISSN 0275-6382

Chen, H.H., Lin, J.H., Fung, H.P., Ho, L.L., Yang, P.C., Lee, W.C., Lee, Y.P. & Chu, R.M. (2003). Serum acute phase proteins and swine health status. *Canadian Journal of Veterinary Research* Vol. 67, No. 4, (October 2003), pp. 283-290, ISSN 0830-9000

Clapperton, M., Bishop, S.C., Glass, E.J. (2005). Innate immune traits differ between Meishan and Large White pigs. *Veterinary Immunology and Immunopathology*, Vol. 104, No. 3-4, (April 2005), pp. 131-144, ISSN 0165-2427

Clapperton, M., Bishop, S.C., Piñeiro, M., Campbell, F.M., Glass, E.J. (2007). The association between plasma levels of acute phase proteins, hatoglobin, alpha-1 acid glycoprotein (AGP), Pig-MAP, transthyretin and serum amyloid A (SAA) in Large White and Meishan pigs. *Veterinary Immunology and Immunopathology*, Vol. 119, No. 3-4, (October 2007), pp. 303-309, ISSN 0165-2427

Cohen, N.D.; Chaffin, M.K., Vandenplas, M.L., Edwards, R.F., Nevill, M., Moore, J.N. & Martens, R.J. (2005). Study of serum amyloid A concentrations as a means of achieving early diagnosis of *Rhodococcus equi* pneumonia. *Equine Veterinary Journal* Vol. 37, No. 3, (May 2005), pp.212-216, ISSN 2042-3306

Colditz, I.G.; Lloyd, J.B., Paull, D.R., Lee, C., Giraudo, A., Pizzato, C. & Fisher, A.D. (2009). Effect of the non-steroidal anti-inflammatory drug, carprofen, on weaned sheep following non-surgical mulesing by intradermal injection of cetrimide. *Australian Veterinary Journal* Vol. 87, No. 1, (January-February 2009), pp. 19-26, ISSN 1751-0831

Colditz, I.G.; Walkden-Brown, S.W., Daly, B.L. & Crook, B.J. (2005). Some physiological responses associated with reduced wool growth during blowfly strike in Merino sheep. *Australian Veterinary Journal* Vol. 83, No. 11, (November 2005), pp. 695-699, ISSN 1751-0831

Conner, J.G., Eckersall, P.D., Wiseman, T.C., Aitchison, T.C., Douglas, T.A. (1988). Bovine acute phase response following turpentine injection. *Research in Veterinary Science*, Vol. 44, No. 1, (January 1988), pp. 82-88, ISSN 1540-2681

Correa, S.S.; Mauldin, G.N.; Mauldin, G.E. & Mooney, S.C. (2001). Serum alpha 1-acid glycoprotein concentration in cats with lymphoma. *Journal of the American Animal Hospital Association*, Vol. 37, No. 2, (March 2001), pp. 153-158, ISSN 0587-2871

Crisman, M.V.; Scarratt, W.K. & Zimmerman, K.L. (2008). Blood proteins and inflammation in the horse. *Veterinary Clinics of North America: Equine Practice*, Vol. 24, No. 2, (August 2008), pp. 285-297, ISSN 0749-0739

Dabrowski, R.; Kostro, K.; Lisiecka, U.; Szczubiał, M. & Krakowski, L. (2009). Usefulness of C-reactive protein, serum amyloid A component, and haptoglobin determinations in bitches with pyometra for monitoring early post-ovariohysterectomy complications. *Theriogenology*, Vol. 72, No. 4, (September 2009), pp. 471-476, ISSN 0093-691X

de la Concha-Bermejillo, A.; Singh, B., Whitney, M.S. & Bazer, F.W. (2000). Acute-phase proteins and hematologic values in ovine lentivirus-infected lambs treated with recombinant ovine IFN-tau. *Journal of Interferon & Cytokine Research* Vol. 20, No. 1, (January 2000), pp. 41-53, ISSN 1557-7465

Diack, A.B., Gladney C.D., Mellencamp, M.A., Stear M.J., Eckersall, P.D. (2011). Characterisation of plasma acute phase protein concentrations in a high health boar herd. *Veterinary Immunology and Immunopathology*, Vol. 139, No. 2-4 (February 2011), pp. 107-112, ISSN 0165-2427

Dow, T.L.; Rogers-Nieman, G., Holásková, I., Elsasser, T.H. & Dailey, R.A. (2010). Tumor necrosis factor-alpha and acute-phase proteins in early pregnant ewes after challenge with peptidoglycan-polysaccharide. *Domestic Animal Endocrinology* Vol. 39, No. 2, (August 2010), pp. 147-154, ISSN 0739-7240

Dowling, A.; Hodgson, J.C.; Schock, A.; Donachie, W.; Eckersall, P.D. & Mckendrick, I.J. (2002). Experimental induction of pneumonic pasteurellosis in calves by intratracheal infection with *Pasteurella multocida* biotype A:3. *Research in Veterinary Science*, Vol. 73, No. 1, (August 2002), pp. 37-44, ISSN 0034-5288

Duggan, V. (2008). Serum amyloid A in the neonatal foal: the significance of peri-parturient events. *The Veterinary Journal*, Vol. 176, No.3, (June 2008), pp. 267-269, ISSN 1090-0233

Duthie, S.; Eckersall, P.D.; Addie, D.P.; Lawrence C.E. & Jarret, O. (1997). Value of α1-acid glycoprotein in the diagnosis of feline infectious peritonitis. *Veterinary Record*, Vol. 141, No. 12, (September 1997), pp. 299-303, ISSN 2042-7670

Earley, B., and Murray, M. (2010). The effect of road and sea transport on inflammatory, adrenocoritcal, metabolic and behavioural responses of weanling heifers. *BMC Veterinary Research* Vol. 6, No.1, (July 2010), pp. 36, ISSN 1746-6148

Eckersall, P.D. & Bell, R. (2010). Acute phase proteins: biomarkers of infection and inflammation in veterinary medicine. *The Veterinary Journal*, Vol. 185, No. 1, (July 2010), pp. 23-27, ISSN 1090-0233

Eckersall, P.D. (2000). Acute phase proteins as markers of infection and inflammation: monitoring animal health, animal welfare and food safety. *Irish Veterinary Journal, Vol.* 53, No. 6, (June 2000), pp. 307–311, ISSN 0368-0762

Eckersall, P.D. (2000). Recent advances and future prospects for the use of acute phase proteins as markers of disease in animals. *Revue de Médicine Vétérinaire* Vol. 151, pp. 577-584, ISSN 0035-1555

Eckersall, P.D.; Lawson, F.P., Bence, L., Waterston, M.M., Lang, T.L., Donachie, W. & Fontaine, M.C. (2007). Acute phase protein response in an experimental model of ovine caseous lymphadenitis. *BMC Veterinary Research,* Vol. 3, No. 35, (December 2007), doi:10.1186/1746-6148-3-35, ISSN 1746-6148

Eckersall, P.D.; Lawson, F.P., Kyle, C.E., Waterston, M., Bence, L., Stear, M.J. & Rhind, S.M. (2008). Maternal undernutrition and the ovine acute phase response to vaccination. *BMC Veterinary Research* Vol. 15, No. 4, (January 2008), pp. 1, ISSN 1746-6148

Eckersall, P.D.; Young, F.J., Nolan, A.M., Knight, C.H., McComb, C., Waterston, M.M., Hogarth, C.J., Scott, E.M. & Fitzpatrick, J.L. (2006). Acute phase proteins in bovine milk in an experimental model of *Staphylococcus aureus* subclinical mastitis. *Journal of Dairy Science* Vol. 89, No. 5, (May 2006), pp. 1488-1501, ISSN 0022-0302

Eckersall, P.D.; Young, F.J.; McComb, C.; Hogarth, C.J.; Safi, S.; Weber, A.; McDonald, T.; Nolan, A.M. & Fitzpatrick, J.L. (2001). Acute phase proteins in serum and milk from dairy cows with clinical mastitis. *Veterinary Record,* Vol. 148, No. 2, (January 2001), pp. 35-41, ISSN 2042-7670

Eicher, S.D. & Burton, J.L. (2005). Immune system: stress effects, In. *Encyclopedia of Animal Science.* Pond and Bell, pp. 541-547, ed. Marcel Dekker, ISBN 0-8247-4796-8, New York, NY

Fazio, F.; Assenza, A., Tosto, F., Casella, S., Piccione, G. & Caola, G. (2010). Modifications of some acute phase proteins and the white blood cell count in thoroughbreds during training. *Veterinary Record* Vol. 167, No. 10, (September 2010), pp. 370-373, ISSN 0042-4900

Fisher, A.D., Niemeyer, D.O., Lea, J.M., Lee, C., Paull, D.R., Reed, M.T., Ferguson, D.M. (2010). The effects of 12, 30 or, 48 hours or road transport on the physiological and behavioural responses of sheep. *Journal of Animal Science* Vol. 88, No. 6, (June 2010), pp. 2144-2152, ISSN 1525-3163

Francisco, C.J.; Shryock, T.R., Bane, D.P. & Unverzagt, L. (1996). Serum haptoglobin concentration in growing swine after intranasal challenge with *Bordetella bronchiseptica* and toxigenic *Pasteurella multocida* type D. *Canadian Journal of Veterinary Research* Vol. 20, N0. 3, (July 1996), pp. 222-227, ISSN 0830-9000

Frank, J-W., Mellencamp, M.A., Carroll, J.A., Boys, R.D., Allee, G.L., (2005). Acute feed intake and acute-phase responses following a lipopolysaccharide challenge in pigs from two dam lines. *Veterinary Immunology Immunopathology* Vol. 107, No. 3-4, (September 2005), pp.179-187, ISSN 0165-2427

Gabler, C., Fischer, C., Drillich, M., Einspanier, R. & Heuwieser, W. (2010). Time-dependent mRNA expression of selected pro-inflammatory factors in the endometrium of primiparous cows postpartum. *Reproduction Biology and Endocrinology* Vol. 22, No.8, (December 2010), pp. 152, ISSN 1477-7827

Gånheim, C.; Hultén, C., Carlsson, U., Kindahl, H., Niskanen, R. & Waller, K.P. (2003). The acute phase response in calves experimentally infected with bovine viral diarrhoea virus and/or *Mannheimia haemolytica. Journal of Veterinary Medicine B, Infectious Diseases and Veterinary Public Health* Vol. 50, No. 4, (May 2003), pp. 183-190, ISSN 0931-1793.

Gerardi, G.; Bernardini, D., Azzurra Elia, C., Ferrari, V., Iob, L. & Segato, S. (2009). Use of serum amyloid A and milk amyloid A in the diagnosis of subclinical mastitis in dairy cows. *Journal of Dairy Research*, Vol. 76, No. 4, (November 2009), pp. 411-417, ISSN 0022-0299G

Giordano, A.; Spagnolo, V., Colombo, A. & Paltrinieri, S. (2004). Changes in some acute phase protein and immunoglobulin concentrations in cats affected by feline infectious peritonitis or exposed to feline coronavirus infection. *The Veterinary Journal*, Vol. 167, No. 1, (July 2010), pp. 38-44, ISSN 1090-0233

Glass E.J. & Jensen, K. (2007). Resistance and susceptibility to a protozoan parasite of cattle--gene expression differences in macrophages from different breeds of cattle. *Veterinary Immunology and Immunopathology* Vol. 120, No. 1-2, (November 2007), pp. 20-30, ISSN 0165-2427

Gómez-Laguna, J.; Gutiérrez, A.; Pallarés, F.J.; Salguero, F.J.; Cerón, J.J. & Carrasco, L. (2010a). Haptoglobin and C-reactive protein as biomarkers in the serum, saliva and meat juice of pigs experimentally infected with porcine reproductive and respiratory syndrome virus. *The Veterinary Journal*, Vol. 185, No. 1, (July 2010), pp. 83-87, ISSN 1090-0233

Gómez-Laguna, J.; Salguero, F.J.; Pallarés, F.J.; Fernández de Marco, M.; Barranco, I.; Cerón, J.J.; Martínez-Subiela, S.; Van Reeth, K. & Carrasco, L. (2010b). Acute phase response in porcine reproductive and respiratory syndrome virus infection. *Comparative Immunology, Microbiology and Infectious Diseases*, Vol. 33, No. 6, (December 2010), pp. e51-e58, ISSN 0970-9320

González, F.H.; Hernández, F.; Madrid, J., Martínez-Subiela, S., Tvarijonaviciute, A., Cerón, J.J. & Tecles, F. (2011). Acute phase proteins in experimentally induced pregnancy toxemia in goats. *Journal of Veterinary Diagnostic Investigation*, Vol. 23, No. 1, (January 2011), pp. 57-62, ISSN 1040-6387

González, F.H.; Tecles, F., Martínez-Subiela, S., Tvarijonaviciute, A., Soler, L. & Cerón, J.J. (2008). Acute phase protein response in goats. *Journal of Veterinary Diagnostic Investigation*, Vol. 20, No. 5, (September 2008), pp. 580-584, ISSN 1040 6387

González, L.A., Ferret, A., Manteca, X., Ruíz de la Torre, J.L., Calsamiglia, S., Devant, M., Bach, A. (2008). Performance, behavior, and welfare of Friesian heifers housed in pens with two, four, and eight individuals per concentrate feeding place. *Journal of Animal Science* Vol. 86, No. 6, (June 2008), pp. 1446-1458, ISSN 0021-8812

Grandin, T. (1997). Assessment of stress during handling and transport. *Journal of Animal Science* Vol. 75, No. 1, (January 1997), pp. 249-257, ISSN 0021-8812

Grau-Roma, L.; Heegaard, P.M.; Hjulsager, C.K.; Sibila, M.; Kristensen, C.S.; Allepuz, A.; Piñeiro, M.; Larsen, L.E.; Segalés, J. & Fraile, L. (2009). Pig-major acute phase protein and haptoglobin serum concentrations correlate with PCV2 viremia and the clinical course of postweaning multisystemic wasting syndrome. *Veterinary Microbiology* Vol. 138, No. 1-2, (July 2009), pp. 53-61, ISSN 0378-1135

Griebsch, C.; Arndt, G., Raila, J., Schweigert, F.J. & Kohn, B. (2009). C-reactive protein concentration in dogs with primary immune-mediated hemolytic anemia. *Veterinary Clinical Pathology* Vol. 38, No. 4, (December 2009), pp. 421-425, ISSN 0275-6382

Gruys, E.; Toussaint, M.J., Upragarin, N., Van, E.A., Adewuyi, A.A., Candiani, D., Nguyen, T.K. &, Sabeckiene, J. (2005). Acute phase reactants, challenge in the near future of animal production and veterinary medicine. *Journal of Zhejiang University SCIENCE B* Vol. 6, No. 10, (October 2005), pp. 941-947, ISSN 1673-1581

Gutiérrez, A.M.; Martínez-Subiela, S.; Eckersall, P.D. & Cerón, J.J. (2009). C-reactive protein quantification in porcine saliva: a minimally invasive test for pig health monitoring. *The Veterinary Journal*, Vol. 181, No. 3, (September 2009), pp. 261-265, ISSN 1090-0233

Gutiérrez, A.M.; Martínez-Subiela, S.; Montes, A.; Parra, M.D. & Cerón, J.J. (2008). C-reactive protein measurements in meat juice of pigs. *Veterinary Immunology and Immunopathology*, Vol. 122, No. 3-4, (April 2008), pp. 250-255, ISSN 0165-2427

Gutiérrez, A.M.; Yelamos, J., Pallarés, F.J., Gómez-Laguna, J. & Cerón, J.J. (2011) Monoclonal antibody development and its use for local identification of porcine haptoglobin in salivary gland and diaphragmatic muscle tissues. *Histology and Histopathology (in press)*, ISSN 1699-5848

Guzelbektes, H.; Sen, I., Ok, M., Constable, P.D., Boydak, M. & Coskun, A. (2010). Serum amyloid A and haptoglobin concentrations and liver fat percentage in lactating dairy cows with abomasal displacement. *Journal of Veterinary Internal Medicine*, Vol. 24, No. 1, (January-February 2010), pp. 223-219, ISSN 0891-6640

Hayashi, S.; Jinbo, T., Iguchi, K., Shimizu, M., Shimada, T., Nomura, M., Ishida, Y. & Yamamoto, S. (2001). A comparison of the concentrations of C-reactive protein and alpha1-acid glycoprotein in the serum of young and adult dogs with acute inflammation. *Veterinary Research Communications*, Vol. 25, No. 2, (February 2001), pp. 117-126, ISSN 0165-7380

Heegaard, P.M., Klausen, J., Nielsen, J.P., González-Ramón, N., Piñeiro, M., Lampreave, F., Alava, M.A. (1998). The porcine acute phase response to infection with Actinobacillus pleuropneumoniae. Haptoglobin, C-reactive protein, major acute phase protein and serum amyloid A protein are sensitive indicators of infection. *Comparative Biochemistry and Physiology B* Vol. 119, No. 2, (February 1998), pp. 365-373, ISSN 0305-0491

Heegaard, P.M.; Godson, D.L., Toussaint, M.J., Tjørnehøj, K., Larsen, L.E., Viuff, B. & Rønsholt, L. (2000). The acute phase response of haptoglobin and serum amyloid A (SAA) in cattle undergoing experimental infection with bovine respiratory syncytial virus. *Veterinary Immunology and Immunopathology* Vol. 77, No. 1-2, (November 2000), pp. 151-159, ISSN 0165-2427

Heegaard, P.M.; Stockmarr, A., Piñeiro, M., Carpintero, R., Lampreave, F., Campbell, F.M., Eckersall, P.D., Toussaint, M.J., Gruys, E. & Sorensen, N.S. (2011). Optimal combinations of acute phase proteins for detecting infectious disease in pigs. *Veterinary Research* Vol. 42, No. 1, (March 2011), pp.50, ISSN 0165-7380

Heinonen, M.; Orro, T., Kokkonen, T., Munsterhjelm, C., Peltoniemi, O. & Valros, A. Tail biting induces a strong acute phase response and tail-end inflammation in finishing pigs. *The Veterinary Journal*, Vol. 184, No. 3, (June 2010), pp. 303-307, ISSN 1090-0233

Hernandez-Richter, T.M.; Wichmann, M.W.; Schrödl, W., Angele, M.K., Heinritzi, K. & Schildberg, F.W. (2001). The acute phase response following implantation of triclosan-bonded vascular prostheses. *Clinical and Experimental Medicine* Vol. 1, No. 1, (March 2001), pp. 35-41, ISSN 1940-5901

Hirvonen, J.; Hietakorpi, S. & Saloniemi, H. (1997). Acute phase response in emergency slaughtered dairy cows. *Meat Science,* Vol. 46, No. 3; (July 1997), pp. 249-257, ISSN 0309-1740

Hiss, S.; Willbrenning, G.S., Suntz, M., Reinacher, M. & Sauerwein, H. (2008). Immunohistochemical localization of haptoglobin in porcine lungs. *Anatomia Histologia Embryologia,* Vol. 37, No. 3, (June 2008), pp. 166-169, ISSN 1439-0264

Hobo, S.; Niwa, H., & Anzai, T. (2007). Evaluation of serum amyloid A and surfactant protein D in sera for identification of the clinical condition of horses with bacterial pneumonia. *Journal of Veterinary Medical Science,* Vol. 69, No. 8; (August 2007), pp. 827-830, ISSN 0916-7250

Höfner, M.C.; Fosbery, M.W., Eckersall, P.D. & Donaldson, A.I. (1994). Haptoglobin response of cattle infected with foot-and-mouth disease virus. *Research in Veterinary Science* Vol. 57, No. 1, (July 1994), pp.125-128, ISSN 0034-5288

Horadagoda, A.; Eckersall, P.D., Hodgson, J.C., Gibbs, H.A. & Moon, G.M. (1994). Immediate responses in serum TNF alpha and acute phase protein concentrations to infection with *Pasteurella haemolytica* A1 in calves. *Research in Veterinary Science,* Vol. 57, No. 1, (July 1994), pp. 129-132, ISSN 0034-5288

Horadagoda, N.U.; Knox, K.M.; Gibbs, H.A.; Reid, S.W.; Horadagoda, A.; Edwards, S.E. & Eckersall, P.D., (1999). Acute phase proteins in cattle: discrimination between acute and chronic inflammation. *Veterinary Record,* Vol. 144, No. 16, (April 1999), pp. 437-441, ISSN 2042-7670

Hultén, C. & Demmers, S. (2002). Serum amyloid A (SAA) as an aid in the management of infectious disease in the foal: comparison with total leucocyte count, neutrophil count and fibrinogen. *Equine Veterinary Journal* Vol. 34, No. 7, (November 2002), pp. 693-698, ISSN 2042-3306

Hultén, C.; Grönlund, U., Hirvonen, J., Tulamo, R.M., Suominen, M.M., Marhaug, G. & Forsberg, M. (2002). Dynamics in serum of the inflammatory markers serum amyloid A (SAA), haptoglobin, fibrinogen and alpha2-globulins during induced noninfectious arthritis in the horse. *Equine Veterinary Journal* Vol. 34, No. 7, (November 2002), pp. 699-704, ISSN 2042-3306

Hultén, C.; Sandgren, B., Skiöldebrand, E., Klingeborn, B., Marhaug, G. & Forsberg, M. (1999). The acute phase protein serum amyloid A (SAA) as an inflammatory marker in equine influenza virus infection. *Acta Veterinaria Scandinavica* Vol. 40, No. 4, pp. 323-333, ISSN 0044-605X

Humblet, M.F.; Guyot, H., Boudry, B., Mbayahi, F., Hanzen, C., Rollin, F. & Godeau, J.M. Relationship between haptoglobin, serum amyloid A, and clinical status in a survey of dairy herds during a 6-month period. *Veterinary Clinical Pathology* Vol. 35, No. 2, (June 2006), pp. 188-193, ISSN 0275-6382

Huntoon, K.M.; Wang, Y., Eppolito, C.A., Barbour, K.W., Berger, F.G., Shrikant, P.A. & Baumann, H. (2008). The acute phase protein haptoglobin regulates host immunity. *Journal of leukocyte biology* Vol. 84, No. 1, pp. 170-181.

Huzzey, J.M.; Duffield, T.F., LeBlanc, S.J., Veira, D.M., Weary, D.M. & von Keyserlingk, M.A. (2009). Short communication: Haptoglobin as an early indicator of metritis. *Journal of Dairy Science,* Vol. 92, No. 2, (February 2009), pp. 621-625, ISSN 0022-0302

Jacobsen, S.; Halling-Thomsen, M. & Nanni, S. (2006b). Concentrations of serum amyloid A in serum and synovial fluid from healthy horses and horses with joint disease.

American Journal of Veterinary Research, Vol. 67, No. 10, (October 2006), pp. 1738-1742, ISSN 0891-6640

Jacobsen, S.; Nielsen, J.V.; Kjelgaard-Hansen, M.; Toelboell, T.; Fjeldborg, J.; Halling-Thomsen, M.; Martinussen, T. & Thoefner, M.B. (2009). Acute phase response to surgery of varying intensity in horses: a preliminary study. *Veterinary Surgery*, Vol. 38, No. 6 (August 2009), pp. 762-769, ISSN 0161-3499

Jacobsen, S.; Niewold, T.A.; Halling-Thomsen, M.; Nanni, S.; Olsen, E.; Lindegaard, C. & Andersen, P.H. (2006a). Serum amyloid A isoforms in serum and synovial fluid in horses with lipopolysaccharide-induced arthritis. *Veterinary Immunology and Immunopathology*, Vol. 110, No. 3-4 (April 2006), pp. 325-330, ISSN 0165-2427

Jacobson, M.; Fellström, C., Lindberg, R., Wallgren, P. & Jensen-Waern, M. (2004). Experimental swine dysentery: comparison between infection models. *Journal of Medical Microbiology* Vol. 53, No. Pt 4, (April 2004), pp. 273-280, ISSN 1473-5644

Jergens, A.E.; Schreiner, C.A.; Frank, D.E.; Niyo, Y.; Ahrens, F.E.; Eckersall, P.D.; Benson, T.J. & Evans, R. (2003). A scoring index for disease activity in canine inflammatory bowel disease. *Journal of Veterinary Internal Medicine*, Vol. 17, No. 3, (May 2003), pp. 291-297, ISSN 0891-6640

Johnson, A.K.; Mitloehner, F.M., Morrow, J.L. & McGlone, J.J. (2008). Effects of shaded versus unshaded wallows on behaviour, performance, and physiology of the outdoor lactating sow. *Journal of Animal Science* Vol. 86, No. 12, (December 2008), pp. 3628-3634, ISSN 1523-3163

Jungersen, G.; Jensen, L., Riber, U., Heegaard, P.M., Petersen, E., Poulsen, J.S., Bille-Hansen, V. & Lind, P. (1999). Pathogenicity of selected *Toxoplasma gondii* isolates in young pigs. *International Journal of Parasitology* Vol. 29, No. 8, (August 1999), pp. 1307-1319, ISSN 0020-7519

Kajikawa, T.; Furuta, A., Onishi, T., Tajima, T. & Sugii, S. (1999). Changes in concentrations of serum amyloid A protein, alpha 1-acid glycoprotein, haptoglobin, and C-reactive protein in feline sera due to induced inflammation and surgery. *Veterinary Immunology and Immunopathology* Vol. 68, No. 1, (March 1999), pp. 91-98, ISSN 0165-2427

Katoh, N. & Nakagawa, H. (1999). Detection of haptoglobin in the high-density lipoprotein and the very high-density lipoprotein fractions from sera of calves with experimental pneumonia and cows with naturally occurring fatty liver. *Journal of Veterinary Medical Science* Vol. 61, No. 2, (February 1999), pp. 119-124, ISSN 0916-7250

Khafipour, E.; Krause, D.O. & Plaizier, J.C. (2009). A grain-based subacute ruminal acidosis challenge causes translocation of lipopolysaccharide and triggers inflammation. *Journal of Dairy Science* Vol. 92, No. 3, (March 2009), pp. 1060-1070, ISSN 0022-0302

Kingston, R.S.; Shih, M.S. & Snyder, S.P. (1982). Secondary amyloidosis in Dall's sheep. *Journal of Wildlife Disease* Vol. 18, No. 3, (July 1982), pp. 381-383, ISSN 0090-3558

Knura-Deszczk, S.; Lipperheide, C., Petersen, B., Jobert, J.L., Berthelot-Hérault, F., Kobisch, M. & Madec, F. (2002). Plasma haptoglobin concentration in swine after challenge with *Streptococcus suis*. *Journal of Veterinary Medicine. B, Infectious Diseases and Veterinary Public Health* Vol. 49, No. 5, (June 2002), pp. 240-244. , ISSN 0931-1793.

Kocaturk, M.; Martínez, S.; Eralp, O.; Tvarijonaviciute, A.; Cerón, J. & Yilmaz, Z. (2010). Prognostic value of serum acute-phase proteins in dogs with parvoviral enteritis.

Journal of Small Animal Practice, Vol. 51, No. 9, (September 2010), pp. 478-483, ISSN 1748-5827

Krakowski, L.; Krawczyk, C., Kostro, K., Stefaniak, T., Novotny, F. & Obara, J. (2011). Serum Levels of Acute Phase Proteins: SAA, Hp and Progesterone (P4) in Mares with Early Embryonic Death. *Reproduction in Domestic Animals*. 2011 Jan 17. doi: 10.1111/j.1439-0531.2010.01715.x, ISSN 0936-6768

Kujala, M.; Orro, T. & Soveri, T. (2010). Serum acute phase proteins as a marker of inflammation in dairy cattle with hoof diseases. *Veterinary Record*, Vol. 166, No. 8, (February 2010), pp. 240-241, ISSN 2042-7670

Kuji, T.; Masaki, T., Li, L., Cheung & A.K. (2007). Expression of C-reactive protein in myointimal hyperplasia in a porcine arteriovenous graft model. Nephrology Dialisys Transplantation Vol. 22, No. 9, (September 2007), pp. 2469-2475, ISSN 1460-2385

Lee, W.C.; Hsiao, H.C.; Wu, Y.L.; Lin, J.H.; Lee, Y.P.; Fung, H.P.; Chen, H.H.; Chen, Y.H. & Chu, R.M. (2003). Serum C-reactive protein in dairy herds. *Canadian Journal of Veterinary Research*, Vol. 67, No. 2, (May 2003), pp. 102-107, ISSN 0830-9000

Lepherd, M.L.; Canfield, P.J., Hunt, G.B., Thomson, P.C. & Bosward, K.L. (2011). Assessment of the short-term systemic effect of an acute phase response to mulesing and other options for controlling breech flystrike in Merino lambs. *Australian Veterinary Journal* Vol. 89, No. 1-2, (January 2011), pp. 19-26, ISSN 1751-0831

Lobetti, R.G.; Möhr, A.J., Dippenaar, T. & Myburgh, E. (2000). A preliminary study on the serum protein response in canine babesiosis. *Journal of the South African Veterinary Association*, Vol. 71, No. 1, (March 2000), pp. 38-42, ISSN 0038-2809

Lomborg, S.R.; Nielsen, L.R., Heegaard, P.M. & Jacobsen, S. (2008). Acute phase proteins in cattle after exposure to complex stress. *Veterinary Research Communications*, Vol. 32, No. 7, (October 2008), pp. 575-582, ISSN 0165-7380

Lowrie, M.; Penderis, J., McLaughlin, M., Eckersall, P.D. & Anderson, T.J. (2009). Steroid responsive meningitis-arteritis: a prospective study of potential disease markers, prednisolone treatment, and long-term outcome in 20 dogs (2006-2008). *Journal of Veterinary Internal Medicine*, Vol. 23, No. 4, (July-August 2009), pp. 862-870, ISSN 0891-6640

Lynch, E.M.; Earley, B., McGee, M. & Doyle, S. (2010). Characterisation of physiological and immunological responses in beef cows to abrupt weaning and subsequent housing. *BMC Veterinary Research* Vol. 20, No. 6, (July 2010), pp. 37, ISSN 1746-6148

Mackiewicz, A. (1997). Acute phase proteins and transformed cells. *International Review of Cytology* Vol. 170, (1997), pp. 225–300, ISSN 0074-7696

Magnusson, U.; Wilkie, B., Artursson, K. & Mallard, B. (1999). Interferon-alpha and haptoglobin in pigs selectively bred for high and low immune response and infected with *Mycoplasma hyorhinis*. *Veterinary Immunology and Immunopathology* Vol. 68, No.2-4, (May 1999), pp. 131-137, ISSN 0165-2427

Marco-Ramell, A.; Pato, R., Peña, R., Saco, Y., Manteca, X., Ruiz de la Torre, J.L. & Bassols A. (2011). Identification of serum stress biomarkers in pigs housed at different stocking densities. *The Veterinary Journal*, doi:10.1016/j.tvjl.2011.01.003, (February 2011), ISSN 1090-0233

Martín de la Fuente, A.J.; Carpintero, R., Rodríguez Ferri, E.F., Alava, M.A., Lampreave, F. & Gutiérrez Martín, C.B. (2010). Acute-phase protein response in pigs experimentally infected with *Haemophilus parasuis. Comparative Immunology, Microbiology & Infectious Disease* Vol. 33, No. 6, (December 2010), pp. 455-465, ISSN 0970-9320

Martín, M., Tesouro, M.A., Gonz Am, N., Pi, A., Lampreave, F. (2005). Major plasma proteins in pig serum during postnatal development. Reproduction, Fertility, and Development Vol. 17, No. 4 (2005), pp. 439-445, ISSN 1031-3613

Martínez-Subiela, S.; Bernal, L.J., Cerón, J.J. (2003). Serum concentrations of acute-phase proteins in dogs with leishmaniosis during short-term treatment. *American Journal of Veterinary Research* Vol. 64, No. 8, (August 2003), pp. 1021-1026, ISSN 0891-6640

Martínez-Subiela, S.; Tecles, F., Eckersall, P.D. & Cerón, J.J. (2002). Serum concentrations of acute phase proteins in dogs with leishmaniasis. *Veterinary Record,* Vol. 150, No. 8, (February 2002), pp. 241-244, ISSN 2042-7670

Mastrorilli, C.; Dondi, F., Agnoli, C., Turba, M.E., Vezzali, E. & Gentilini, F. (2007). Clinicopathologic features and outcome predictors of *Leptospira interrogans* Australis serogroup infection in dogs: a retrospective study of 20 cases (2001-2004). *Journal of Veterinary Internal Medicine* Vol. 21, No. 1, (January-February 2007), pp. 3-10, ISSN 0891-6640

Matijatko, V.; Mrljak, V., Kis, I., Kucer, N., Forsek, J., Zivicnjak, T., Romi, Z., Simec, Z. & Ceron, J.J. (2007). Evidence of an acute phase response in dogs naturally infected with *Babesia canis. Veterinary Parasitology,* Vol. 144, No. 3-4, (March 2007), pp. 242-250, ISSN 0304-4017

McCobb, E.C., Patronek, G.J., Marder, A., Dinnage, J.D., Stone, M.S. (2005). Assessment of stress levels among cats in four animal shelters. *Journal of the American Veterinary Medical Association* Vol. 226, No. 4, (February 2005), pp. 548-555, ISSN 0003-1488

Meade, K.G., O'Gorman, G.M., Hill, E.W., Narciandi, F., Agaba, M., Kemps S.J., O'Farrellys C., MacHughs D.E (2009). Divergent antimicrobial peptide (AMP) and acute phase protein (APP) responses to *Trypanosoma congolense* infection in trypanotolerant and trypanosusceptible cattle. Mol Immunol. 2009 Dec;47(2-3):196-204.

Mette, C.; Dooleweerdt B.C., Stine, J., Miki B. A., Roenn P.M. & Henrik LJ. (2010). Evaluation of the systemic acute phase response and endometrial gene expression of serum amyloid A and pro- and anti-inflammatory cytokines in mares with experimentally induced endometritis. *Veterinary Immunology and Immunopathology,* Vol. 138, No. 1-2 (November 2010), pp. 95-105, ISSN 0165-2427

Miller, K. & Wood-Gush, D.G.M. (1991). Some effects of housing on the social behavior of dairy cows. *Animal Production* Vol. 53, pp. 271-278, ISSN 0003-3561

Millet, S., Cox, E., Buyse, J., Goddeeris, B.M., Janssens, G.P.J. (2005). Immunocompetence of fatteing pigs fed organic versus conventional diets in organic versus conventional housing. *The Veterinary Journal* Vol. 169, No. 2, (March 2005), pp. 293-299, ISSN 1090-0233

Milne, E.M.; Doxey, D.L., Kent, J.E. & Pemberton, A. (1991). Acute phase proteins in grass sickness (equine dysautonomia). *Research in Veterinary Science* Vol. 50, No. 3, (May 1991), pp. 273-278, ISSN 0034-5288

Mischke, R.; Waterston, M. & Eckersall, P.D. (2007). Changes in C-reactive protein and haptoglobin in dogs with lymphatic neoplasia. *The Veterinary Journal,* Vol. 174, No. 1, (July 2007), pp. 188-192, ISSN 1090-0233

Mitchell, K.D., Kruth, S.A., Wood, R.D. & Jefferson, B. (2009). Serum acute phase protein concentrations in dogs with autoimmune hemolytic anemia. *Journal of Veterinary Internal Medicine* Vol. 23, No. 3, pp. 585-591, ISSN 0891-6640

Moestrup, S.K. & Moller, H.J. (2004). CD163: a regulated hemoglobin scavenger receptor with a role in the anti-inflammatory response. *Annals of Medicine* Vol. 36, No. 5, pp. 347-354, ISSN 0785-3890

Murata, H. & Miyamoto, T. (1993). Bovine haptoglobin as a possible immunomodulator in the sera of transported calves. *The British Veterinary Journal* Vol. 149, No. 3, (May-June 1993), pp. 277-283, ISSN 0007-1935

Murata, H.; Shimada, N. & Yoshioka, M. (2004). Current research on acute phase proteins in veterinary diagnosis: an overview. *The Veterinary Journal*, Vol. 168, No. 1, (July 2004), pp. 28-40, ISSN 1090-0233

Nakamura, M.; Takahashi, M., Ohno, K., Koshino, A., Nakashima, K., Setoguchi, A., Fujino, Y. & Tsujimoto, H. (2008). C-reactive protein concentration in dogs with various diseases. *Journal of Veterinary Medical Science* Vol. 70, No. 2, (February 2008), pp. 127-131, ISSN 0916-7250

Nazifi, S.; Ansari-Lari, M., Asadi-Fardaqi, J. & Rezaei, M. (2009a). The use of receiver operating characteristic (ROC) analysis to assess the diagnostic value of serum amyloid A, haptoglobin and fibrinogen in traumatic reticuloperitonitis in cattle. *The Veterinary Journal* Vol. 182, No. 2, (November 2009), pp. 315-319, ISSN 1090-0233

Nazifi, S.; Razavi, S.M., Esmailnejad, Z. & Gheisari, H. (2009b). Study on acute phase proteins (haptoglobin, serum amyloid A, fibrinogen, and ceruloplasmin) changes and their diagnostic values in bovine tropical theileriosis. *Parasitology Research* Vol. 105, No. 1, (July 2009), pp. 41-46, ISSN 0932-0113

Ndung'u, J.M.; Eckersall, P.D. & Jennings, F.W. (1991). Elevation of the concentration of acute phase proteins in dogs infected with *Trypanosoma brucei*. *Acta Tropica* Vol. 49, No. 2, (June 1991), pp. 77-86, ISSN 0001-706X

Nielsen, L.; Toft, N., Eckersall, P.D., Mellor, D.J. & Morris, J.S. (2007). Serum C-reactive protein concentration as an indicator of remission status in dogs with multicentric lymphoma. *Journal of Veterinary Internal Medicine* Vol. 21, No. 6, (November-December 2007), pp. 1231-1236, ISSN 0891-6640

Nikunen, S.; Härtel, H., Orro, T., Neuvonen, E., Tanskanen, R., Kivelä, S.L., Sankari, S., Aho, P., Pyörälä, S., Saloniemi, H. & Soveri, T. (2007). Association of bovine respiratory disease with clinical status and acute phase proteins in calves. *Comparative Immunology, Microbiology and Infectious Diseases*, Vol. 30, No. 3, (May 2007), pp. 143-151, ISSN 0970-9320

Nunokawa, Y.; Fujinaga, T., Taira, T., Okumura, M., Yamashita, K., Tsunoda, N. & Hagio, M. (1993). Evaluation of serum amyloid A protein as an acute-phase reactive protein in horses. *Journal of Veterinary Medical Science* Vol. 55, No. 6, (December 1993), pp. 1011-1016, ISSN 0916-7250

Ogilvie, G.K.; Walters, L.M., Greeley, S.G., Henkel, S.E., Salman, M.D. (1993). Concentration of alpha 1-acid glycoprotein in dogs with malignant neoplasia. *Journal of the American Veterinary Medical Association* Vol. 203, No. 8, (October 1993), pp. 1144-1146, ISSN 0003-1488

O'Meara, T.J.; Nesa, M., Seaton, D.S. & Sandeman, R.M. (1995). A comparison of inflammatory exudates released from myiasis wounds on sheep bred for resistance or susceptibility to *Lucilia cuprina*. *Veterinary Parasitology* Vol. 56, No. 1-3, (January 1995), pp. 207-223, ISSN 0304-4017

Orro, T.; Jacobsen, S., LePage, J.P., Niewold, T., Alasuutari, S. & Soveri, T. (2008). Temporal changes in serum concentrations of acute phase proteins in newborn dairy calves. *The Veterinary Journal* Vol. 176, No. 2, (May 2008), pp. 182-187, ISSN 1090-0233

Ottenjann, M.; Weingart, C., Arndt, G. & Kohn, B. (2006). Characterization of the anemia of inflammatory disease in cats with abscesses, pyothorax, or fat necrosis. *Journal of Veterinary Internal Medicine*, Vol. 2, No. 5, (September-October 2006), pp. 1143-1150, ISSN 0891-6640

Päiväniemi, O.E.; Maasilta, P.K., Vainikka, T.L., Alho, H.S., Karhunen, P.J. & Salminen, U.S. (2009). Local C-reactive protein expression in obliterative lesions and the bronchial wall in posttransplant obliterative bronchiolitis. *Mediators of Inflammation* Vol. 2009, (May 2009), pp. 510254, ISSN 1466-1861

Pallarés, F.J.; Martínez-Subiela, S., Seva, J., Ramis, G., Fuentes, P., Bernabé, A., Muñoz, A. & Cerón, J.J. (2008). Relationship between serum acute phase protein concentrations and lesions in finishing pigs. *The Veterinary Journal*, Vol. 177, No. 3, (September 2008), pp. 369-373, ISSN 1090-0233

Paltrinieri, S. (2008). The feline acute phase reaction. *The Veterinary Journal*, Vol. 177, No. 1, (July 2008), pp. 26-35, ISSN 1090-0233

Paltrinieri, S.; Crippa, A., Comerio, T., Angioletti, A. & Roccabianca, P. (2007). Evaluation of inflammation and immunity in cats with spontaneous parvovirus infection: consequences of recombinant feline interferon-omega administration. *Veterinary Immunology and Immunopathology* Vol. 118, No. 1-2, (July 2007), pp. 68-74, ISSN 0165-2427

Paltrinieri, S.; Giordano, A., Tranquillo, V. & Guazzetti, S. (2007). Critical assessment of the diagnostic value of feline alpha1-acid glycoprotein for feline infectious peritonitis using the likelihood ratios approach. *Journal of Veterinary Diagnostic Investigation* Vol. 19, No. 3, (May 2007), pp. 266-272, ISSN 1040-6387

Paltrinieri, S.; Giordano, A., Villani, M., Manfrin, M., Panzani, S. & Veronesi, M.C. (2008). Influence of age and foaling on plasma protein electrophoresis and serum amyloid A and their possible role as markers of equine neonatal septicaemia. *The Veterinary Journal*, Vol. 176, No. 3, (June 2008), pp. 393-396, ISSN 1090-0233

Paltrinieri, S.; Metzger, C., Battilani, M., Pocacqua, V., Gelain, M.E. & Giordano, A. (2007c). Serum alpha1-acid glycoprotein (AGP) concentration in non-symptomatic cats with feline coronavirus (FCoV) infection. *Journal of Feline Medicine and Surgery*. Vol. 9, No. 4, (August 2007), pp. 271-277, ISSN 1098-612X

Pantchev, N. (2010). C-reactive protein as a marker in canine granulocitic anaplasmosis. *Veterinary Record*, Vol. 166, No. 20, (May 2010), p. 632, ISSN 2042-7670

Parra, M.D.; Fuentes, P., Tecles, F., Martínez-Subiela, S., Martínez, J.S., Muñoz, A. & Cerón, J.J. (2006). Porcine acute phase protein concentrations in different diseases in field conditions. *Journal of Veterinary Medicine B, Infectious Diseases and Veterinary Public Health*, Vol. 53, No. 10, (December 2006), pp. 488-493, ISSN 0931-1793

Parra, M.D.; Tecles, F.; Martínez-Subiela, S. & Cerón, J.J. (2005). C-reactive protein measurement in canine saliva. *Journal of Veterinary Diagnostic Investigation*, Vol. 17, No. 2, (March 2005), pp. 139-144, ISSN 1040-6387

Paull, D.R.; Lee, C., Atkinson, S.J. & Fisher, A.D. Effects of meloxicam or tolfenamic acid administration on the pain and stress responses of Merino lambs to mulesing. *Australian Veterinary Journal* Vol. 86, No. 8, (August 2008), pp. 303-311, ISSN 1751-0831

Paull, D.R.; Lee, C., Colditz, I.G. & Fisher, A.D. Effects of a topical anaesthetic formulation and systemic carprofen, given singly or in combination, on the cortisol and behavioural responses of Merino lambs to castration. *Australian Veterinary Journal* Vol. 87, No. 6, (June 2009), pp. 230-237, ISSN 1751-0831

Pépin, M.; Pardon, P., Lantier, F., Marly, J., Levieux, D. & Lamand, M. (1991). Experimental *Corynebacterium pseudotuberculosis* infection in lambs: kinetics of bacterial dissemination and inflammation. *Veterinary Microbiology* Vol. 26, No. 4, (February 1991), pp. 381-392, ISSN 0378-1135

Petersen, H.H., Ersboll, A.K., Jensen, C.S., Nielsen, J.P. (2002). Serum haptoglobin concentration in Danish slaughter pigs of different health status. *Preventive Veterinary Medicine* Vol. 54, No. 4, (August 2002), pp. 325-335, ISSN 0167-5877

Petersen, H.H.; Nielsen, J.P. & Heegaard, P.M. (2004). Application of acute phase protein measurements in veterinary clinical chemistry. *Veterinary Research*, Vol. 35, No. 2, (March-April 2004), pp. 163-187, ISSN 1746-6148

Pfeffer, A. & Rogers, K.M. Acute phase response of sheep: changes in the concentrations of ceruloplasmin, fibrinogen, haptoglobin and the major blood cell types associated with pulmonary damage. *Research in Veterinary Science* Vol. 46, No. 1, (January 1989), pp. 118-124, ISSN 0034-5288

Pfeffer, A.; Rogers, K.M., O'Keeffe, L. & Osborn, P.J. (1993). Acute phase protein response, food intake, liveweight change and lesions following intrathoracic injection of yeast in sheep. *Research in Veterinary Science* Vol. 55, No. 3, (November 1993), pp. 360-366, ISSN 0034-5288

Philippidis, P.; Mason, J.C., Evans, B.J., Nadra, I., Taylor, K.M., Haskard, D.O. & Landis, R.C. (2004). Hemoglobin scavenger receptor CD163 mediates interleukin-10 release and heme oxygenase-1 synthesis: antiinflammatory monocyte-macrophage responses in vitro, in resolving skin blisters in vivo, and after cardiopulmonary bypass surgery. *Circulation Research* Vol. 94, No. 1, pp. 119-126, ISSN 0009-7300

Piñeiro, C., Piñeiro, M., Morales, J., Andres, M., Lorenzo, E., Pozo, M.D., Alava, M.A., Lampreave, F. (2009). Pig-MAP and haptoglobin concentration reference values in swine from commercial farms. *The Veterinary Journal* Vol. 179, No. 1, (January 2009), pp. 78-84, ISSN 1090-0233

Piñeiro, C., Piñeiro, M., Morales, J., Carpintero, R., Campbell, F.M., Eckersall, P.D., Toussaint, M.J.M., Alava, M.A. & Lampreave, F. (2007). Pig acute-phase protein levels after stress induced by changes in the pattern of food administration. *Animal* Vol. 1, pp. 133-139, ISSN 1751-7311

Piñeiro, M.; Piñeiro, C., Carpintero, R., Morales, J., Campbell, F.M., Eckersall, P.D., Toussaint, M.J. & Lampreave, F. (2007). Characterisation of the pig acute phase protein response to road transport. *The Veterinary Journal*, Vol. 173, No. 3, (May 2007), pp.669-674, ISSN 1090-0233

Planellas, M.; Bassols, A., Siracusa, C., Saco, Y., Giménez, M., Pato, R. & Pastor, J. (2009). Evaluation of serum haptoglobin and C-reactive protein in dogs with mammary tumors. *Veterinary Clinical Pathology*, Vol. 38, No. 3, (September 2009), pp. 348-352, ISSN 0275-6382

Pollock, P.J.; Prendergast, M., Schumacher, J. & Bellenger, C.R. (2005). Effects of surgery on the acute phase response in clinically normal and diseased horses. *Veterinary Record*, Vol. 156, No. 17, (April 2005), pp. 538-542, ISSN 2042-7670

Qiu, X.; Arthington, J.D., Riley, D.G., Chase, C.C. Jr., Phillips, W.A., Coleman, S.W. & Olson, T.A. (2007). Genetic effects on acute phase protein response to the stresses of weaning and transportation in beef calves. *Journal of Animal Science* Vol. 85, No. 10, (October 2007), pp. 2367-2374, ISSN 1523-3163

Rabehi, L.; Ferriere, F., Saffar, L. & Gattegno, L. (1995). alpha 1-Acid glycoprotein binds human immunodeficiency virus type 1 (HIV-1) envelope glycoprotein via N-linked glycans. *Glycoconjugate Journal* Vol. 12, No. 1, (February 1995), pp. 7-16, ISSN 0282-0080

Rahman, M.M.; Lecchi, C., Fraquelli, C., Sartorelli, P. & Ceciliani, F. Acute phase protein response in Alpine ibex with sarcoptic mange. *Veterinary Parasitology* Vol. 168, No. 3-4, (March 2010), pp. 293-298, ISSN 0304-4017

Regassa, F. & Noakes, D.E. (1999). Acute phase protein response of ewes and the release of PGFM in relation to uterine involution and the presence of intrauterine bacteria. *Veterinary Record* Vol. 144, No. 18, (May 1999), pp. 502-506, ISSN 2042-7670

Rikihisa, Y.; Yamamoto, S., Kwak, I., Iqbal, Z., Kociba, G., Mott, J. & Chichanasiriwithaya, W. (1994). C-reactive protein and alpha 1-acid glycoprotein levels in dogs infected with *Ehrlichia canis*. *Journal of Clinical Microbiology* Vol. 32, No. 4, (April 1994), pp-912-917, ISSN 0095-1137

Rooney, N.J., Gaines, S.A., Bradshaw, J.W. (2007). Behavioural and glucocorticoid responses of dogs (Canis familiaris) to kennelling: Investigating mitigation of stress by prior habituation. *Physiology & Behavior* Vol. 92, No. 5, (December 2007), pp. 847-854, ISSN 0031-9384

Sack, G.H.Jr. & Zink, M.C. (1992). Serum amyloid A gene transcription in synovial cells during retroviral arthritis. *American Journal of Pathology* Vol. 141, No. 3, (September 1992), pp. 525-529, ISSN 0002-9173

Saco, Y.; Docampo, M., Fàbrega, E., Manteca, X., Diestre, A., Lampreave, F. & Bassold, A. (2003). Effect of transport stress on serum haptoglobin and Pig-MAP in pigs. *Animal Welfare* Vol. 12, No. 3, (August 2003), pp. 403-409, ISSN 0962-7286

Saco, Y.; Fina, M., Giménez, M., Pato, R., Piedrafita, J., Bassols, A. (2008). Evaluation of serum cortisol, metabolic parameters, acute phase proteins and faecal corticosterone as indicators of stress in cows. *The Veterinary Journal* Vol. 177, No. 3, (September 2008), pp. 439-441, ISSN 1090-0233

Saco, Y.; Fraile, L., Giménez, M., Alegre, A., López-Jimenez, R., Cortey, M., Segalés, J. & Bassols, A. (2010). Serum acute phase proteins as biomarkers of pleuritis and cranio-ventral pulmonary consolidation in slaughter-aged pigs. *Research in Veterinary Science*, doi:10.1016/j.rvsc.2010.08.016, ISSN 0034-5288

Safi, S.; Khoshvaghti, A., Jafarzadeh, S.R., Bolourchi, M. & Nowrouzian, I. (2009). Acute phase proteins in the diagnosis of bovine subclinical mastitis. *Veterinary Clinical Pathology*, Vol. 38, No. 4, (December 2009), pp. 471-476, ISSN 0275-6382

Salamano, G.; Mellia, E., Candiani, D., Ingravalle, F., Bruno, R., Ru, G. & Doglione, L. (2008). Changes in haptoglobin, C-reactive protein and pig-MAP during a housing period following long distance transport in swine. *The Veterinary Journal*, Vol. 177, No. 1, (July 2008), pp.110-115, ISSN 1090-0233

Sánchez-Cordón, P.J.; Cerón, J.J., Núñez, A., Martínez-Subiela, S., Pedrera, M., Romero-Trevejo, J.L., Garrido, M.R. & Gómez-Villamandos, J.C. (2007). Serum concentrations of C-reactive protein, serum amyloid A, and haptoglobin in pigs inoculated with African swine fever or classical swine fever viruses. *American Journal of Veterinary Research*, Vol. 68, No. 7, (July 2007), pp. 772-777, ISSN 0891-6640

Sasaki, K.; Ma, Z.Y., Khatlani, T.S., Okuda, M., Inokuma H. & Onishi, T. (2003). Evaluation of feline serum amyloid A (SAA) as an inflammatory marker. *Journal of Veterinary Medical Science*, Vol. 65, No. 4; (April 2003), pp. 545-548, ISSN 0916-7250

Selting, K.A.; Ogilvie, G.K., Lana, S.E., Fettman, M.J., Mitchener, K.L., Hansen, R.A., Richardson, K.L., Walton, J.A. & Scherk, M.A. (2000). Serum alhpa 1-acid glycoprotein concentrations in healthy and tumor-bearing cats. *Journal of Veterinary Internal Medicine* Vol. 14, No. 5, (September-October 2000), pp. 503-506, ISSN 0891-6640

Selye, H. (1998). A syndrome produced by diverse nocuous agents. 1936. *The Journal of Neuropsychiatry and Medical Neuroscience* Vol. 10, No. 2, (Spring 1998), pp. 230-231, ISSN 1545-7222

Serin, G. & Ulutas, P.A. (2010). Measurement of serum acute phase proteins to monitor postoperative recovery in anoestrous bitches after ovariohysterectomy. *Veterinary Record* Vol. 166, No. 1, (January 2010), pp. 20-22, ISSN 2042-7670

Sheahan, D.; Bell, R., Mellanby, R.J., Gow, A.G., Friend, E., Heller, J., Bence, L.M. & Eckersall, P.D. (2010). Acute phase protein concentrations in dogs with nasal disease. *Veterinary Record*, Vol. 167, No. 23, (December 2010), pp. 895-899, ISSN 2042-7670

Skinner, J.G. & Roberts, L. (1994). Haptoglobin as an indicator of infection in sheep. *Veterinary Record*, Vol. 134, No. 2, (January 1994), pp. 33-36, ISSN 2042-7670

Skovgaard, K.; Mortensen, S., Boye, M., Poulsen, K.T., Campbell, F.M., Eckersall, P.D. & Heegaard, P.M. (2009). Rapid and widely disseminated acute phase protein response after experimental bacterial infection of pigs. *Veterinary Research*, Vol. 40, No. 3, doi: 10.1051/vetres/2009006, (May-June 2009), ISSN 1297-9716

Smith, B.I.; Kauffold, J. & Sherman, L. (2010). Serum haptoglobin concentrations in dairy cattle with lameness due to claw disorders. *The Veterinary Journal*, Vol. 186, No. 2, (November 2010), pp.162-165, ISSN 1090-0233

Sorensen, N.S.; Tegtmeier, C., Andresen, L.O., Piñeiro, M., Toussaint, M.J., Campbell, F.M., Lampreave, F. & Heegaard, P.M. (2006). The porcine acute phase protein response to acute clinical and subclinical experimental infection with *Streptococcus suis*. *Veterinary Immunology and Immunopathology*, Vol. 113, No. 1-2, (September 2006), pp. 157-168, ISSN 0165-2427

Sorrells, A.D.; Eicher, S.D., Harris, M.J., Pajor, E.A. & Richert, B.T. (2007). Periparturient cortisol, acute phase cytokine, and acute phase protein profiles of gilts housed in groups or stalls during gestation. *Journal of Animal Science* Vol. 85, No. 7, (July 2007), pp. 1750-1757, ISSN 1523-3163

Stevenson, L.S., McCullough, K., Vincent, I., Gilpin, D.F., Summerfield, A., Nielsen, J., McNeilly, F., Adair, B.M. & Allan, G.M. (2006). Cytokine and C-reactive protein profiles induced by circovirus type 2 experimental infection in 3-week-old piglets. *Viral Immunology* Vol. 19, No. 2, (Summer 2006), pp. 189-195, ISSN 0882-8245

Stoddart, M.E.; Whicher, J.T. & Harbour, D.A. (1988). Cats inoculated with feline infectious peritonitis virus exhibit a biphasic acute phase plasma protein response. *Veterinary Record*, Vol. 123, No. 24, (December 1988), pp. 622-624, ISSN 2042-7670

Stokka, G.L.; Edwards, A.J., Spire, M.F., Brandt, R.T.Jr. & Smith, J.E. (1994). Inflammatory response to clostridial vaccines in feedlot cattle. *Journal of American Veterinary Medical Association* Vol. 204, No. 3, (February 1994), pp. 415-419, ISSN 0003-1488

Suojala, L.; Orro, T., Järvinen, H., Saatsi, J. & Pyörälä, S. (2008). Acute phase response in two consecutive experimentally induced *E. coli* intramammary infections in dairy cows. *Acta Veterinaria Scandinavica* Vol. 13, No. 50, (June 2008), pp. 18, ISSN 0044-605X

Sutherland, M.A., Niekamp, S.R., Rodríguez-Zas, S.L., Salak-Johnson, J.L. (2006). Impacts of chronic stress and social status on various physiological and performance measures in pigs of different breeds. *Journal of Animal Science* Vol. 84, No. 3, (March 2006), pp. 588-596, ISSN 0021-8812

Tabrizi, A.D.; Batavani, R.A., Rezaei, S.A. & Ahmadi, M. (2008). Fibrinogen and ceruloplasmin in plasma and milk from dairy cows with subclinical and clinical mastitis. *Pakistan Journal of Biological Sciences* Vol. 11, No. 4, (February 2008), pp. 571-576, ISSN 1028-8880

Tamamoto, T.; Ohno, K., Ohmi, A., Seki, I. & Tsujimoto, H. (2009). Time-course monitoring of serum amyloid A in a cat with pancreatitis. *Veterinary Clinical Pathology*, Vol. 38, No. 1, (March 2009), pp. 83-86, ISSN 0275-6382

Tecles, F.; Caldín, M., Zanella, A., Membiela, F., Tvrijonaviciute, A., Martínez-Subiela, S. & Cerón, J.J. (2009). Serum acute phase protein concentrations in female dogs with mamary tumors. *Journal of Veterinary Diagnostic Investigation*, Vol. 21, No. 2; (March 2009), pp. 214-219, ISSN 1040-6387

Tecles, F.; Spiranelli, E., Bonfanti, U., Cerón, J.J. & Paltrinieri, S. (2005). Preliminary studies of serum acute-phase protein concentrations in hematologic and neoplastic diseases of the dog. *Journal of Veterinary Internal Medicine* Vol. 19, No. 6, (November-December 2005), pp. 865-870, ISSN 0891-6640

TerWee, J.; Lauritzen, A.Y., Sabara, M., Dreier K.J. & Kokjohn, K. (1997). Comparison of the primary signs induced by experimental exposure to either a pneumotrophic or a 'limping' strain of feline calicivirus. *Veterinary Microbiology* Vol. 56, No. 1-2, (May 1997), pp. 33-45, ISSN 0378-1135

TerWee, J.; Sabara, M., Kokjohn, K., Sandbulte, J., Frenchick P. & Dreier, K.J. (1998). Characterization of the systemic disease and ocular signs induced by experimental infection with *Chlamydia psittaci* in cats. *Veterinary Microbiology* Vol. 59, No. 4, (January 1998), pp. 259-281, ISSN 0378-1135

Tóthová, C.; Nagy, O., Seide, H. & Kovác, G. (2010). The effect of chronic respiratory diseases on acute phase proteins and selected blood parameters of protein metabolism in calves. *Berliner und Munchener Tierarztliche Wochenschrift*, Vol. 123, No. 7-8, (July-August 2010), pp. 307-313, ISSN 0005-9366

Tourlomousis, P.; Eckersall, P. D., Waterston, M. & Buncic, S. (2004). A comparison of acute phase protein measurements and meat inspection findings in cattle. *Foodbourne Pathogens and Disease*, Vol. 1, No. 4, (Winter 2004), pp. 281-290, ISSN 1535-3141

Tvarijonaviciute, A.; Martínez-Subiela, S., Carrillo-Sánchez, J., Tecles, F., Cerón J.J. (2011). Effects of Orchidectomy in Selective Biochemical Analytes in Beagle Dogs. *Reproduction in Domestic Animals* (March 2011), doi: 10.1111/j.1439-0531.2011.01765.x, ISSN 0936-6768

Ulutaş, P.A. & Ozpinar, A. (2006). Effect of *Mannheimia* (*Pasteurella*) *haemolytica* infection on acute-phase proteins and some mineral levels in colostrum-breast milk-fed or colostrum-breast milk-deprived sheep. *Veterinary Research Communications*, Vol. 30, No. 5, (July 2006), pp. 485-495, ISSN 0165-7380

Ulutaş, P.A.; Voyvoda, H., Ulutaş, B. & Aypak, S. (2008). Haptoglobin, serum amyloid A and ceruloplasmin concentrations in goats with mixed helminth infection. *Turkiye Parazitol Derg* Vol. 32, No. 3, pp. 229-233, ISSN 1300-6320

Van Gucht, S.; Van Reeth, K., Nauwynck, H. & Pensaert, M. (2005). Porcine reproductive and respiratory syndrome virus infection increases CD14 expression and lipopolysaccharide-binding protein in the lungs of pigs. *Viral Immunology* Vol. 18, No. 1, pp. 116-126, ISSN 0882-8245

Vandenplas, M.L.; Moore, J.N., Barton, M.H., Roussel, A.J. & Cohen, N.D. (2005). Concentrations of serum amyloid A and lipopolysaccharide-binding protein in horses with colic. *American Journal of Veterinary Research*, Vol. 66, No. 9, (September 2005), pp. 1509-1516, ISSN 0891-6640

Von Borell, E., (1995). Neuroendocrine integration of stress and significance of stress for the performance of farm animals. *Applied Animal Behaviour Science* Vol. 44, pp. 219-227, ISSN 0168-1591

Wallgren, P.; Brunborg, I.M., Blomqvist, G., Bergström, G., Wikström, F., Allan, G., Fossum, C. & Jonassen, C.M. (2009). The index herd with PMWS in Sweden: presence of serum amyloid A, circovirus 2 viral load and antibody levels in healthy and PMWS-affected pigs. *Acta Veterinaria Scandinavica,* Vol. 51, No. 13, doi:10.1186/1751-0147-51-13, (March 2007), ISSN 0044-605X

Warris, P.D. (1998). Choosing appropriate space allowance for slaughter pigs transported by road: a review. *The Veterinary Record* Vol. 142, No. 17, (April 1998), pp. 449-454, ISSN 0042-4900

Warris, P.D. (2003). Optimal lairage times and conditions for slaughter pigs: a review. *The Veterinary Record* Vol. 153, No. 6, (August 2003), pp. 170-176, ISSN 2042-7670

Weber, T.E.; Ziemer, C.J. & Kerr, B.J. (2008). Effects of adding fibrous feedstuffs to the diet of young pigs on growth performance, intestinal cytokines, and circulating acute-phase proteins. *Journal of Animal Science* Vol. 86, No. 4, (April 2008), pp. 871-881, ISSN 1523-3163

Wenz, J.R.; Fox, L.K., Muller, F.J., Rinaldi, M., Zeng, R. & Bannerman, D.D. (2010). Factors associated with concentrations of select cytokine and acute phase proteins in dairy cows with naturally occurring clinical mastitis. *Journal of Dairy Science*, Vol. 93, No. 6, (June 2010), pp. 2458-2470, ISSN 0022-0302

Winter, P., Miny, M., Fuchs, K. & Baumgartner, W. (2006). The potential of measuring serum amyloid A in individual ewe milk and in farm bulk milk for monitoring udder health on sheep dairy farms. *Research in Veterinary Science* Vol. 81, No. 3, (December 2006), pp. 321-326, ISSN 0034-5288

Winter, P.; Fuchs, K., Walshe, K. & Colditz, I.G. (2003). Serum amyloid A in the serum and milk of ewes with mastitis induced experimentally with *Staphylococcus epidermidis*. *Veterinary Record* Vol. 152, No. 18, (May 2003), pp. 558-562, ISSN 2042-7670

Yamamoto, S.; Shida, T., Honda, M., Ashida, Y., Rikihisa, Y., Odakura, M., Hayashi, S., Nomura, M. & Isayama, Y. (1994). Serum C-reactive protein and immune responses in dogs inoculated with *Bordetella bronchiseptica* (phase I cells). *Veterinary Research Communications* Vol. 18, No. 5, pp. 347-357, ISSN 0165-7380

Yamamoto, S.; Shida, T., Okimura, T., Otabe, K., Honda, M., Ashida, Y., Furukawa, E., Sarikaputi, M. & Naiki, M. (1994). Determination of C-reactive protein in serum and plasma from healthy dogs and dogs with pneumonia by ELISA and slide reversed passive latex agglutination test. *The Veterinary Quarterly* Vol. 16, No. 2, (July 1994), pp. 74-77, ISSN 0165-2176

Yuki, M.; Machida, N., Sawano, T. & Itoh, H. (2011). Investigation of serum concentrations and immunohistochemical localization of α1-acid glycoprotein in tumor dogs. *Veterinary Research Communications*, Vol. 35, No. 1, (January 2011), pp. 1-11, ISSN 0165-7380

Yule, T.D.; Roth, M.B., Dreier, K., Johnson, A.F., Palmer-Densmore, M., Simmons, K. & Fanton, R. (1997). Canine parvovirus vaccine elicits protection from the inflammatory and clinical consequences of the disease. *Vaccine*, Vol. 15, No. 6-7, (April-May 1997), pp. 720-729, ISSN 0264-410X

13

Application of Acute Phase Proteins for Monitoring Inflammatory States in Cattle

Burim N. Ametaj et al.*
University of Alberta
Canada

1. Introduction

The animal body functions in a controlled internal environment, strictly regulated by a variety of homeostatic mechanisms. However, the internal milieu is disturbed by external factors that lead to imbalance of the inner homeostasis. The host is equipped with multiple tools to abolish external challenges like tissue injury and infection by activation of various defense mechanisms; however, mobilization of all these responses is associated with alterations of the homeostatic status. The multifaceted immune and metabolic responses of the host to external challenges are commonly referred to as the acute-phase response (APR) (Kushner, 1982; Koj, 1985; Baumann & Gauldie, 1994; Moshage, 1997; Mackiewicz, 1997). The aim of the APR is to eliminate the agent(s) that caused the interference and to bring the homeostasis back to normality (Figure 1). The APR is initiated in response to a variety of stimuli including acute trauma, bacterial infection, surgery, fracture, burns, tissue necrosis, presence of a chronic disease, or ongoing inflammatory processes (Kushner, 1982; Gordon & Koj, 1985; Baumann & Gauldie, 1994; Steel & Whitehead, 1994; Boosalis et al., 1996; Mackiewicz, 1997). The APR usually resolves within a few days or weeks, however sometimes it can persist when the causal agent is defiant (Boosalis et al., 1996; Mackiewicz, 1997; Koj, 1998).

The APR is regulated by numerous compounds referred to as cytokines (Mackiewicz, 1997; Koj, 1998; Martin et al., 1999). The latter are produced by macrophages, when they are activated by bacterial endotoxin, viruses, free radicals, prostaglandins, or other factors released under different inflammatory conditions. The main cytokines released by macrophages are interleukin-1 (IL-1), IL-8, tumor necrosis factor-alpha (TNF-α), and interferon-gamma (INF-γ) (Koj, 1998; Martin et al., 1999). The release of proinflammatory cytokines, at the site of tissue injury, stimulates various other cell types to produce a cascade of other cytokines, including IL-6-type cytokines, which act to stimulate the production of acute phase proteins (APP) from liver hepatocytes or other tissues (Baigrie et al., 1991; Mackiewicz, 1997). Although the production of cytokines in the liver or other local sites is complex, it is believed that IL-1 and IL-6 are the two main stimulants of APP production (Gauldie et al., 1987; Nijsten et al., 1991; Ohzato et al., 1992).

* Afshin Hosseini, John F. Odhiambo, Summera Iqbal, Sumeet Sharma, Qilan Deng, Tran H. Lam, Umar Farooq, Qendrim Zebeli and Suzanna M. Dunn
University of Alberta, Canada

Over the years three different systems of classification of APP have been developed. The first system is based on the degree of blood elevation of the APP, referred to as positive or negative APP; the second system is based on the time when APP are released during an APR; and the third system is based on the subset of cytokines responsible for stimulating gene expression of APP (Mackiewicz, 1997; Moshage, 1997). In the first system, positive APP are classified into one of three groups based upon the degree of rise in the blood concentration: type I APP, whose concentration increases by 50% (*e.g.* ceruloplasmin (Cp), complement factor C3, and factor C4); type II APP, whose concentration increases 2- to 5-fold (*e.g.* fibrinogen and haptoglobin - Hp); and type III APP, whose quantity rises more than 5-fold the normal value [*e.g.* C-reactive protein (CRP) and serum amyloid A (SAA)]

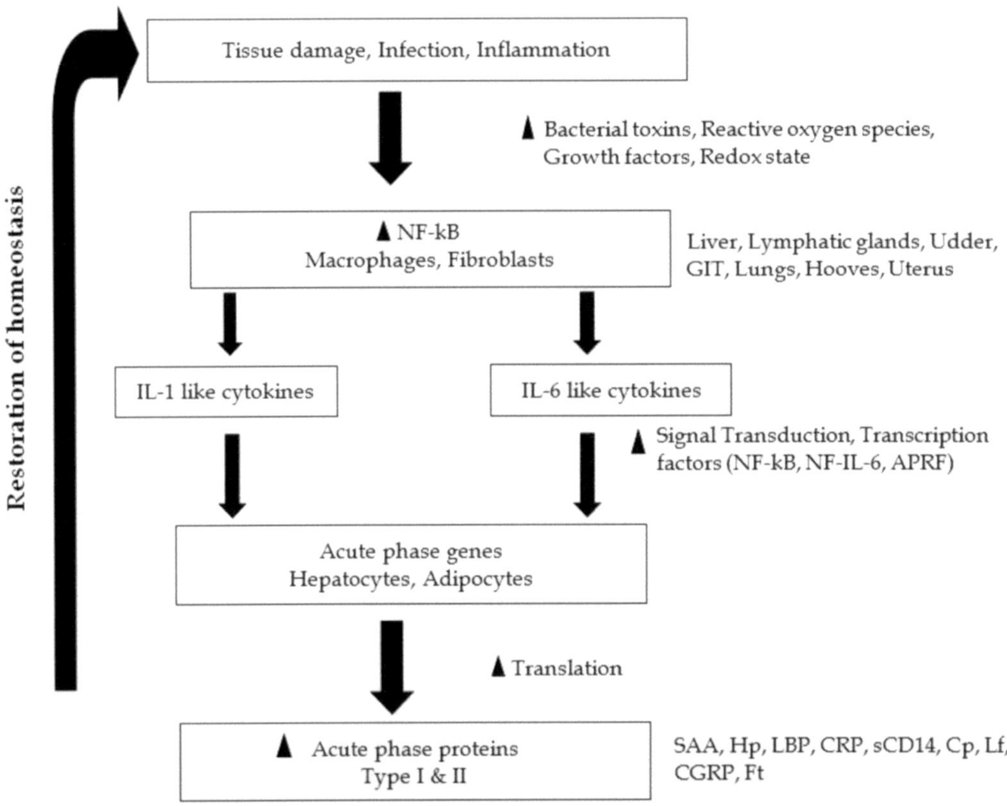

Fig. 1. Acute phase response in animals triggered by infection, tissue damage or inflammation initiates rapid activation of transcription factor NF-kB in macrophages and fibroblasts in peripheral tissues. This is followed by increased production of cytokines. Subsequent signaling cascades result in transcription of acute phase genes and ultimately, secretion of acute phase proteins that function to restore homeostasis. APRF: Acute phase protein factor; CGRP: Calcitonin gene related peptide; Cp: Ceruloplasmin; CRP: C-Reactive protein; Ft: Ferritin; Hp: Haptoglobin; IL: Interleukin; Lf: Lactoferrin; LBP: Lipopolysaccharide binding protein; SAA: Serum amyloid A; sCD14: Soluble cluster of differentiation antigen 14.

(Mackiewicz, 1997; Moshage, 1997). A few APP decrease during an APR and they are known as negative APP. The most studied negative APP include retinol binding protein (RBP), albumin, trasferrin, and transthyretin.

Based on the time when they are released APP are classified as either first- or second-phase proteins (Kushner & Mackiewicz, 1987; Mackiewicz, 1997). Examples of the first-phase APP are SAA and CRP, whose levels rise as early as 4 h after the initiation of inflammation, peak within 1-3 d, and quickly return to baseline concentrations (Mackiewicz, 1997). Examples of the second-phase APP are Hp and fibrinogen, which increase 1-3 d after the initiation of APR, peak within 7-10 d, and decrease to baseline levels within 2 or more wk (Mackiewicz, 1997; Moshage, 1997).

The third system classifies APP based on which cytokine subsets induce their gene expression (Baumann & Gauldie, 1994; Mackiewicz, 1997). Type I APP are induced by IL-1-like cytokines, including IL- 1α, IL-1β, TNF-α, and TNF-β, and synergistically by IL-6-like cytokines, while type II APP are stimulated by IL-6-like cytokines alone, including IL-6 and IL-11 (Baumann & Gauldie, 1994; Mackiewicz, 1997; Moshage, 1997). C-reactive protein, SAA, and C3 are examples of type I proteins, while type II proteins include Hp and fibrinogen.

At least forty different plasma proteins have been defined as APP. They include clotting proteins, complement factors, anti-proteases, and transport proteins (Samols, 2002). However, the number of APP commonly used in cattle research is smaller than in human research. In this chapter we will discuss only about 9 of the most studied APP in cattle.

Recent evidence also indicates that several APP are secreted extrahepatically playing important roles in immune defenses against different pathogens populating mucosal layers in the body. In the following sections we will discuss the most recent reports regarding structures, functions, tissue expression as well as various factors that affect expression and production of SAA, Hp, LBP, soluble(s)CD14, CRP, Cp, lactoferrin (Lt), calcitonin gene-related peptide (CGRP), and ferritin in cattle (i.e., dairy and beef cattle).

2. Serum amyloid A

2.1 Structure

Serum amyloid A is an APP that belongs to a family of apolipoproteins that are coded by different genes with a high degree of homology between species (Uhlar, 1994; Malle, 1993). The family of SAA proteins in mammals has a MW of 12 kDa with 104 amino acids. They are very well conserved throughout evolution and have a wide range of functions.

2.2 Functions

It is known that SAA is over expressed several orders of magnitude during infections and inflammation. Four different isoforms of SAA have been described in humans and mice (Uhlar & Whitehead, 1999) and seven different isoforms were reported in the blood of dairy cows (Takahashi, 2009). Among the known isoforms, SAA1 and SAA2 are the only ones reported to be overproduced during the APR and are known as acute phase (A)-SAA. They are mainly expressed in the liver hepatocytes. The third isoform, SAA3, is expressed extrahepatically by adipose tissue, mammary gland, intestinal epithelial cells, and macrophages and is present in the plasma at a very low level (Meek, 1992; Chiba, 2009; Eckhardt, 2010). The fourth isoform, SAA4, is constituitively expressed (de Beer, 1995) and does not respond to external stimuli. A recent investigation in cows with amyloidosis and chronic inflammation showed seven different isoforms of SAA in the serum (Takahashi,

2009). Larson (2005) reported production of SAA3 by ductal cells in the mammary gland of healthy lactating dairy cows. Moreover, Mukesh (2010) showed presence of SAA3 in the adipose tissue of dairy cows. However, the precise functions of these seven different isoforms of SAA in dairy cows are not known yet.

Serum amyloid A is transported in blood in association with lipoprotein particles, particularly high-density lipoproteins (HDL) (Eriksen, 1980; Coetzee, 1986). During an APR, SAA replaces almost 85% of the apolipoprotein-A1 (apo-A1) and becomes the main apolipoprotein on HDL (Uhlar & Whitehead, 1999; Coetzee, 1986). The reason for replacement of apo-A1 during APR is related to the fact that SAA half-life is 75-80 min compared with that of apo-A1 of 11 h (Hoffman & Benditt, 1983). It is believed that endotoxin-lipoprotein complexes are quickly removed from circulation by liver hepatocytes (Harris, 2002; Ametaj, 2010). The shorter half-life of SAA might help in expedited clearance of endotoxin-lipoprotein complexes from circulation (Harris et al., 1998).

The main known functions of SAA are to: 1) bind to lipoproteins and help in their expedited clearance from liver hepatocytes (Harris, 2002), 2) extract cholesterol from cells (van der Westhuyzen, 2007); 3) bind and activate neutrophils and macrophages (Furlaneto & Campa, 2000), 4) kill coliform bacteria (Shah, 2006). Other reported functions of SAA include suppression of lymphocyte response to antigens (Benson, 1979), inhibition of platelet aggregation (Zimlichman, 1990), and regulation of expression of tissue collagenase (Brinckerhoff, 1989). In addition, SAA has been shown to stimulate adhesion of mast cells to the extracellular matrix (Hershkoviz, 1997), migration and adhesion of T cells (Preciado-Patt, 1996), and migration, adhesion, and tissue infiltration of monocytes and neutrophils (Badolato et al., 1994). Serum amyloid A also induces mobilization of calcium (Ca) and chemotaxis in monocytes (Badolato, 1995) and enhances synthesis of eicosanoid in human monocytes (Malle, 1997).

Although early research indicated that SAA in dairy cows is increased more during acute rather than chronic inflammatory conditions (Horadagoda, 1999), recent research shows that SAA is also increased during chronic conditions (Chan, 2010). This protein is also raised following experimental infection of cattle with *Mannheimia haemolytica* and during bovine respiratory syncytial virus infections (Horadagoda, 1994; Heegaard, 2000).

2.3 Factors that affect its expression

2.3.1 Mammary gland infections

Molenaar (2009) demonstrated presence of a constituitive isoform of SAA3 in the mammary gland tissue of dairy cows. These authors reported that the expression profile of SAA3 was different in relation with stage of lactation and disease. Thus, SAA3 was high in the mammary tissue of pregnant cows, low during lactation, elevated during involution of the gland, and strongly increased during mastitis. An interesting observation of the same authors was that SAA3 was not expressed in lactational tissues of the gland (i.e., alveoli) but only in the epithelial cells lining ductal tissue of the teat. The role of SAA3 in ductal cells might be to protect the teat potential colonization of that area by bacteria during milking or suckling. Several other authors have reported elevated mammary gland SAA3 in the milk of cows and ewes with mastitis (Eckersall, 2001; Winter et al., 2003; Nielsen et al., 2004; Jacobsen et al., 2005). Moreover, experimental models of mastitis have demonstrated that SAA3 in the mammary gland is synthesized by the infected udder and is not coming from the blood (Grönlund, 2003; Eckersall, 2006). Gram-negative bacterial lipopolysaccharide (LPS) and the Gram-positive bacterial lipoteichoic acid (LTA) were shown to upregulate SAA3 in bovine mammary epithelial cells by 18.5-fold and 12.5-fold, respectively (Larson,

2006). Concentrations of SAA in the milk of normal cows were 0.5 ± 1.0 mg/mL and in cows affected by mastitis were 2.2 ± 8.6 mg/mL (Åkerstedt, 2011). Another group of investigators showed that concentrations of SAA in the serum of normal cows were 3.6-11.0 mg/mL, in those with mild mastitis 5.4-142 mg/mL, and those with moderate mastitis 5.9-141 mg/mL (Eckersall, 2001).

Molenaar (2009) tested the bacterial activity of recombinant SAA3 from the mammary gland and they reported that mammary(M)-SAA3 had antimicrobial activity against *Escherichia coli*, *Streptococcus uberis*, and *Pseudomonas aeruginosa* with the greatest activity against *E. coli*. This offers an explanation as to why the protein is expressed in the mammary gland at times where defense against bacteria is required. Another interesting report comes from Weber (2006) who showed presence of SAA3 in high concentrations in the colostrum of healthy cows. Moreover, the same authors reported that the colostral SAA3 has a unique four amino acid motif (TFLK) within the first residues that is not present in the isoforms produced in the liver (McDonald, 2001). This isoform has the ability to stimulate intestinal epithelial cells to produce a protective intestinal mucin and lower the adherence of enteropathogenic *E. coli* to these cells (Mack, 2003; Larson, 2003). This feature of SAA3 might help protect newborn calves during their first days of life from enteropathogenic bacteria.

2.3.2 Dietary factors

Recent research work conducted by our team and others has shown that feeding of high grain diets is associated with enhanced concentrations of SAA in the blood of both dairy (Emmanuel, 2008) and beef cattle (Ametaj, 2009). Dairy cows fed barley grain at 0-15% of the diet dry matter (DM) had plasma SAA concentrations between 2-12 mg/mL and those fed 30-45% of diet DM had values ranging between 19-46 mg/mL (Emmanuel, 2008). The reason for the increased SAA in the plasma of cattle fed high grain diets is suggested to be related to translocation of endotoxin into the systemic circulation which then stimulates the release of pro-inflammatory cytokines such as TNF-α, IL-1, and IL-6 by liver macrophages (Gabay & Kushner, 1999), resulting in enhanced secretion of SAA from hepatocytes (Emmanuel, 2008). Our team also showed that feeding high grain diets was associated with development of fatty liver and greater concentrations of SAA in the blood of cows diagnosed with fatty liver. We proposed a role for expedited internalization of SAA-LPS-lipoprotein complexes from liver hepatocytes in development of fatty liver (Ametaj, 2005a; 2005b). Other investigators demonstrated that plasma SAA was increased in cows affected by displaced abomasum (Guzelbektes, 2010).

In another study conducted by our team we found that concentrations of SAA in the plasma of steers, during a 12-wk period of feeding a backgrounding diet with 45% barley grain-based concentrate and 55% barley silage (DM basis), were 2.5-14 mg/mL (Ametaj, 2009). In addition, during a 15-wk period of feeding a finishing diet with 91% barley grain-based concentrate and 9% barley silage concentrations of SAA in the plasma were 8-24 mg/mL (Ametaj, 2009). Plasma SAA was greater in the group of steers fed the finishing diet compared to those fed the backgrounding diet (8.0 vs 17.0 mg/mL). Interestingly, the peak concentration of SAA in steers fed the finishing diet reached at 3 wk (21 mg/mL) after the starting of the diet (Ametaj, 2009).

2.3.3 Uterine infections

Serum amyloid A is related to infections of the uterus in postpartal dairy cows (Chan, 2010). The latter authors indicated that concentrations of SAA in the serum of cows affected by metritis reached peak values 4-7 d after calving (85 ± 23 mg/mL) compared to healthy cows (48 ± 20 mg/mL) and remained above the baseline values for 2 mo after parturition. This is the first report indicating that SAA might be produced not only during acute states of inflammation but also during chronic diseases such as metritis. Besides its role as an antibacterial compound SAA in the uterus might also activate macrophages and neutrophils to clear the tissue from bacterial infections.

2.3.4 Lameness

Lameness and hoof health is an important disease of dairy cows that affects their wellbeing and most importantly the economic efficiency of dairy farms. In a recent trial several cows were selected on the day they showed signs of lameness and if they were diagnosed with sole ulcers and/or white line abscesses. Concentrations of SAA were reported to be greater in lame dairy cows (37-60 mg/mL) than their counterparts (10-12 mg/mL) during days 0, 4, 7, and 8 of the disease (Kujala, 2010). Serum amyloid A fell on day 14, which was confirmed by healing of cows on that day. Concentration of SAA in the serum of lame cows reached values of 50 mg/mL versus lower than 10 mg/mL of the healthy cows.

2.3.5 Fatty liver and downer cow syndrome

In an investigation about the etiology and pathology of fatty liver we reported that postpartal cows affected by fatty liver had greater plasma SAA compared to the healthy ones (Ametaj et al., 2005a, 2005b). Concentration of SAA in the bloodstream of cows affected by fatty liver reached peak value of ca. 80 μg/mL (Ametaj et al., 2005a). Moreover, the average concentrations of plasma SAA in cows with fatty liver were greater than those in the control cows during days 3, 8, 12, and 27 postpartum. In the same study, we reported that after 12 d postpartum, mean plasma SAA in fatty-liver cows decreased below prepartal values, and was similar to values for control cows, ca 15 μg/mL (Ametaj et al., 2005a).

In a case study with clinical signs of downer cow syndrome we also found that plasma concentrations of SAA were between 3.3-11.5 mg/mL during day -14 and -7 before calving, respectively; they increased to 82.7 mg/mL 2 wk after calving and ranged between 11.7-27.8 mg/mL in eight normal cows. These data suggest a role of inflammation and endotoxin in the etiology and pathogenesis of the downer cow (Ametaj, 2010). Although the pathology of this disease has been a mystery for a long time, in dairy industry, the data generated from our team implicate bacterial components or proinflammatory cytokines released in response to these by-products in development of the disease. Further research would be needed to explore the role of inflammatory conditions in etiopathology of downer cows.

2.3.6 Adipose tissue

Both bovine and non-ruminant research has indicated expression of SAA3 in adipose tissue (Poitou, 2009; Mukesh, 2010). The latter authors showed that SAA3 mRNA abundance was greater in mesenteric than subcutaneous tissue of dairy cows. Expression of SAA3 has been related to gastrointestinal bacterial components such as LPS. Moreover, injection of LPS in the mammary gland or intraperitoneum was associated with enhanced SAA3 mRNA in both dairy cows and rodents (Mukesh, 2010). Data with mice support a role for SAA3 in exerting local inflammatory functions in adipose tissue from obese animals (Larson, 2006). The greater abundance of SAA3 mRNA in adipose tissue during an inflammatory challenge could play a role in lipid/steroid metabolism and/or transport (Benditt, 1989). Yang (2006) suggests that SAA has a long-term effect in stimulating basal lipolysis and that the lipolytic activity of SAA can be an autocrine feedback mechanism by which increased SAA production from enlarged adipocytes limits further triacylglycerol accumulation and increases non-esterified fatty acid (NEFA). The resulting increased release of NEFA into the circulation may contribute to insulin resistance.

2.4 Age-related changes

Alsemgeest et al. (1994) reported that SAA is present in neonatal veal calves and that serum SAA was greater in calves with different inflammatory diseases including diarrhea, pneumonia, and omphalitis. The same authors showed that concentrations of SAA in newborn calves were lower than in adult cows. Weaning and transportation was shown to affect concentrations of SAA in the serum of newly weaned beef calves (Arthington, 2003). Serum SAA were greater on d 1 and decreased steadily on d 3 and 7 (51.2, 43.8, and 28.5μg/mL, respectively) after transportation.

3. Haptoglobin

3.1 Structure

Haptoglobin (Hp) is another APP reported to be present in the blood of all mammals analyzed so far (Bowman & Kurosky 1982). The protein is synthesized mainly from liver hepatocytes as a precursor polypeptide, which after oligomerization and cleavage, is split into two types of chains, called α and β (Kurosky et al. 1980). The α-chain contains a complement control protein (CCP) domain and the β-chain contains a serine proteinase (SP) related domain. In humans, but not in other primates, the Hp gene is found in two allelic variants, Hp1 and Hp2 (Maeda et al. 1984). The shorter α-chain (α_1) forms a link to one, and the longer chain (α_2) to two other α-chains. The two alleles, therefore, give rise to three different serotypes composed of two $\alpha_1\beta$ units (in Hp1-1), two $\alpha_1\beta$ and variable numbers of $\alpha_2\beta$ units (in Hp1-2), or variable numbers of $\alpha_2\beta$ units (in Hp2-2). The sizes of the three Hp proteins are Hp1-1 ~100 kDa; Hp2-1 ~ 120-220 kDa; and Hp2-2 ~ 160-500 kDa (Carter & Worwood, 2007).

Haptoglobin of cow (*Bos taurus*) contains an α-chain, the structure of which is similar to that of the human Hp2 α-chain. Interestingly, comparison of the structure of bovine Hp and human Hp2 suggests that the bovine gene arose by a duplication of the gene segment homologous to that duplicated in human Hp2 (Wicher & Fries, 2007). In ruminants, however, multiple electrophoretic bands of Hp have been observed, which are similar to those observed after electrophoresis of human Hp2-2 (Travis & Sanders, 1972); interestingly, no other Hp phenotypes seem to exist in these animals. In addition, it has been suggested that the structure of Hp in cattle, goat, sheep, and deer is similar to that of human Hp2 (Busby & Travis, 1978).

3.2 Functions

The main reported function of Hp is to bind hemoglobin (Hb). It is known that bacteria need iron (Fe) for their growth and they have developed sophisticated means to acquire Fe from Hb, like hemolysins. Hemoglobin has four Fe atoms and one hemolysed red blood cell might release ~ 250 million Hb molecules. In addition, by binding Hb, it inhibits its oxidative activity and its passage through the glomeruli (Lim et al. 1998). Hemoglobin also is highly toxic (Alayash, 2004) and its prosthetic group, heme, is lipophilic and intercalates into cell membranes to disrupt the lipid bilayers. Iron present in heme catalyzes the generation of reactive oxygen species (ROS; Sadrzadeh et al., 1984). Moreover, Hp binds to apo A-1 to protect it from free radical-mediated damage and also to prevent HDL from forming adducts with other lipoprotein molecules (Salvatore et al., 2007). Another function of Hp is to inhibit both cyclooxygenase (COX) and lipooxygenase (LOX) activities, which provide a means to modulate responses to inflammation or infection that may be harmful to tissues (Saeed et al., 2007). Arredouani et al. (2005) showed evidence that Hp has the ability to selectively antagonize effects of LPS in vitro by suppressing monocyte production of TNF-α, IL-10, and IL-12. Haptoglobin is an established suppressor of T cell proliferation, exhibiting strong inhibition of Th2 cytokine release and weak inhibition of Th1 cytokine release (Arredouani et al., 2003).

3.3 Tissue distribution and factors that affect expression of haptoglobin

3.3.1 Tissue distribution

The expression of Hp is in abundant amounts in liver hepatocytes, which is the main source of Hp in blood (Yang et al., 1983). However, Hp has been detected in multiple tissues besides plasma such as in white and brown adipose tissue, placenta, lungs, arteries, testis, ovaries, and mammary gland tissues of dairy cows (Friedrichs et al., 1995; Kalmovarin et al., 1991; Yang et al., 1995; Hiss et al., 2004). The induction of Hp gene expression is mediated mainly by IL-6, which is the cytokine mediator for stimulation of Hp production in the liver hepatocytes of different species studied (Quaye, 2008).

3.3.2 Dietary factors

Two experiments were conducted by our team to investigate the effects of oral supplementation of the lactic acid-producing bacterium *Enterococcus faecium* EF212 alone or in combination with *Saccharomyces cerevisiae* (yeast) on mediators of the APR in feedlot steers (Emmanuel et al., 2007b). The effects of *E. faecium* alone or with yeast were evaluated. We found that feed supplementation with *E. faecium* had no effect on concentration of Hp in the plasma compared with control animals. However, feeding *E. faecium* and yeast increased plasma concentrations of Hp. Tourlomoussis et al. (2004) reported Hp concentration of 110μg/mL in the plasma of healthy beef cattle; however, cattle under different pathological conditions have average plasma Hp values of approximately 270 μg/mL. Results of *E. faecium* alone experiment, conducted by us, showed Hp concentrations of about 270 μg/mL in control group and about 225 μg/mL in experimental steers (Emmanuel et al., 2007b).

3.3.3 Mammary gland infections

Although it was believed that the liver is the main and the only source of Hp in cattle, in a recent study, Hiss et al. (2004) demonstrated that Hp also is expressed extrahepatically in mammary gland including parenchimal tissue, tissues surrounding the cisternal milk ducts, and in the teats. They also observed that milk Hp was increased 3 h after LPS challenge to one of the quarters, whereas elevation of blood Hp occurred 9 h after the challenge (Hiss et al., 2004). Concentrations of Hp in the blood and milk of cows before LPS challenge were at 32.8 and 0.9 mg/mL and increased 12 h after the LPS administration at 371.7 and 152.2 mg/mL, respectively (Hiss et al., 2004). In other studies conducted by Ohtsuka et al. (2001) and Pedersen et al. (2003) it was reported that concentrations of Hp in the milk increased in cows affected naturally from severe Gram-negative coliform mastitis and in those in which mastitis was induced experimentally with Gram-positive *Streptococcus uberis*, respectively. Eckersall et al. (2001) also showed increased concentrations of Hp in the milk of cows with naturally occurring mild and moderate mastitis. These findings suggest that milk Hp might be a good biomarker of mastitis in dairy cows. In another study conducted by Åkersted et al. (2008) milk with detectable levels of Hp showed lower total protein and casein levels and higher somatic cell counts. It is not clear whether the relationship between Hp in the milk and differences observed in the milk composition is causal or simply the result of bacterial presence.

In a recent article Wenz et al. (2010) observed that concentration of Hp in the group of cows affected by Gram-negative bacterial mastitis was approximately twice that of the group infected by Gram-positive bacteria (1,126 vs 575 mg/mL, respectively). Moreover, cows in the mid-lactation group tended to have greater concentrations of Hp in the milk compared with those in the early lactation group (470 vs 891 mg/mL, respectively). Moreover, concentration of Hp was lower in cows with clinical mastitis during the Spring (345 mg/mL) vs those with clinical mastitis in the Summer (1,362 mg/mL), or Fall (1,105 mg/mL) and tended to be lower than those in the Winter (808 mg/mL).

3.3.4 Uterine infections

Different authors have reported an association among concentrations of Hp in the blood and diseases of the reproductive tract of dairy cows. For example, Smith et al. (1998) and Sheldon et al. (2001) showed an association between elevated concentrations of Hp in the postpartum period and metritis and Huzzey et al (2009) indicated that cows with concentration of Hp of more than 1.0 g/L at 3 days in milk were 7 times more likely to develop metritis. Data from our team (unpublished) also support the fact that Hp is increased in dairy cows around calving especially in those affected by metritis. In a recent article Dubuc et al. (2010) indicated that blood Hp is a risk factor for reproductive disorders. They used a cut off concentration of Hp in blood, for cows with risk of metritis, at more than 0.8 g/L. They showed that Hp at more than 0.8 g/L, in the first 7 days of milk, is associated with more than 2 times the odds of developing metritis. In addition, the same authors found that elevated concentration of Hp is a risk factor for purulent vaginal discharges and cytological endometritis at 35 d in milk.

3.3.5 Lameness

Different investigators have reported increased concentrations of Hp in the serum of cows with claw disorders. Interestingly, most of them have suggested that all claw disorders, whether infectious or non-infectious, lead to a systemic APR (Shearer et al., 1996; Bergsten et al., 1998; Hoblet & Weiss, 2001). For example, Smith et al. (2010) showed that concentrations of Hp in the serum of healthy cows, free of lameness, were below the detection limit of <1.0 mg/dL. Lame cows, with infectious or non-infectious claw disorders, were found to have either increased serum Hp of more than 1.0 mg/dL, or found with concentrations lower than 1.0 mg/dL. Cows that tested positive for Hp had concentrations ranging between 37 and more than 100 mg/dL. Additionally, Jawor et al. (2008) demonstrated that increased concentrations of Hp in the serum are associated with lameness in cattle; however, the authors caution that there are also lame cows with undetectable Hp levels in the serum.

3.3.6 Fatty liver and downer cow syndrome

In a study conducted by us we showed that in cows fed high amounts of grain, to induce fatty liver in periparturient cows, concentrations of plasma Hp were similar to those of control cows before parturition, but after parturition plasma Hp increased markedly (ca. 200 mg/dL) and remained higher than that of control cows on days 3, 8, and 12 postpartum (Ametaj et al., 2005a). By day 14 postpartum, plasma Hp decreased to prepartal concentrations (ca. 40 mg/dL) in fatty-liver cows and remained at that level up to 36 d postpartum.

3.3.7 Age-related factors

Alsemgeest et al. (1995) showed that healthy newborn calves had no detectable amounts of Hp in the serum. On the other hand, only 25% of the newborn calves suffering from different diseases immediately after birth had detectable concentrations of Hp. It is possible that the assay for measuring Hp in the serum has affected detection of Hp during the 1990s. In 1999 Katoh & Nakagawa showed association of Hp with the high-density (HDL) and very-high density (VHDL) lipoprotein fractions but not with those of chylomicrons, VLDL, and LDL fractions in the sera of calves experimentally infected with *Pasteurella hemolytica*. Concentration of Hp in the sera of calves with pneumonia were <0.01, 194, 717, 940, 722, and 524 mg/mL on d 0, 1, 2, 3, 4, and 7 of infection with *P. hemolytica*, respectively. Orro et al. (2008) showed that Hp in the plasma of the newborn calves between 0-21 d were between 100-350 mg/mL.

4. Lipopolysaccharide-binding protein

4.1 Structure and tissue distribution

Bovine LBP is a 50-kDa polypeptide that consists of 481 amino acids (Khemlani et al., 1994). The protein is mainly synthesized by hepatocytes and is released into the bloodstream as a 60 kDa glycoprotein (Schumann et al., 1990; Khemlani et al., 1994). Its amino acid sequence reveals an 86% similarity compared to human LBP (Khemlani et al., 1994). Moreover, a recent investigation, showed that mRNA LBP is widely expressed extrahepatically, in the gastro-intestinal tract (i.e., submandibular salivary gland, rumen, reticulum, omasum and abomasum), lung, female reproductive system (i.e., ovary and uterus), thyroid gland, nervous system (i.e., brain and cerebellum), and mammary gland (i.e., parenchyma, cistern, and teat) of cattle. Moreover, research reveals that the highest expression of bovine LBP gene is observed in the reticulum (72-fold) and parotid gland (50-fold) compared with 1-fold in the liver (Rahman et al., 2010). These results show that epithelial mucosal tissues of the ruminant particularly forestomach secrete LBP and that LBP might play a significant role in mucosal immunity. It is worth mentioning that besides LBP there is another similar protein known as bactericidial permeability increasing protein (BPI) and that both LBP and BPI belong to the family of lipid transfer/LPS binding proteins (Bingle & Craven, 2004). In cattle, both genes are closely located on the chromosome 13. Interestingly, both LBP and BPI interact with bacterial endotoxin, however, the mechanism by which they deal with LPS is different. Lipopolysaccharide-binding protein causes disaggregation of LPS as part of its role in promoting LPS signaling, whereas BPI inserts itself into LPS aggregates, promotes formation of larger aggregates, and interferes with the ability of LBP to disperse large LPS aggregates (Tobias et al., 1997). Lipopolysaccharide-binding protein is considered to be proinflamatory, as it induces the LPS signaling, whereas BPI as anti-inflammatory because it removes the LPS molecules without inducing the LPS signaling (Elsbach & Weiss, 1998, Fenton & Golenbock, 1998).

4.2 Functions

The main known function of LBP is to bind and transport LPS either to immune cells or lipoprotein particles (Gallay et al., 1994). The principle mechanism by which this occurs is through the ability of LBP to dissociate LPS aggregates into LPS monomers. In this process other proteins like CD14 help LBP to transfer LPS. In fact, CD14 is found in two isoforms, as a membrane-bound (mCD14) and a free soluble molecule (sCD14). Interestingly, when blood LPS is at low concentration LBP directs it to the macrophages and when LPS is at greater concentration it directs it to lipoprotein particles, especially HDL (Gallay et al., 1994). The LBP-LPS complex interacts either with mCD14, which is expressed by monocytes, macrophages, and neutrophiles (Schumann et al., 1994) or with sCD14 that transefers LPS to HDL particles (Tobias et al., 1999). Binding of LPS to immune cells triggers the release of cytokines, which are responsible for stimulating the APR (Moshage, 1997). Toll-like receptor (TLR)-4 and MD-2 are also involved in the activation of both monocytic cells and those that do not express CD14 during binding of LPS (Chow et al., 1999). It is also known that CD14 facilitates the binding and activation of TLR4/MD-2 complex (Fitzgerald et al., 2004). Interestingly, sCD14 is also present in bovine milk. For example, milk concentration of sCD14 was shown to be increased following the LPS challenge or *Escherichia coli* infection in dairy cows (Lee et al., 2003a, b).

4.3 Factors that affect expression of LBP

4.3.1 Dietary factors

A study by our team indicated that the amount of grain in the diet affects concentration of LBP in the plasma of dairy cows (Emmanuel et al. 2008). Thus, cows fed diets containing high proportions of barley grain (45%) had greater LBP concentration (10 µg/mL) compared with control cows (5.7 µg/ mL) that were fed no barley grain. The same study reported that concentration of LBP in the plasma differed between cows fed diets containing 15% (4.6 µg/mL) and 30% (6.5 µg/mL) barley grain. Furthermore, no differences were found in plasma LBP levels between groups of cows fed 0 and 15% barley grain (i.e. 6 µg/mL). In an investigation by Khafipour et al. (2009) they showed similar results with elevated blood and milk LBP (18.2 vs 53.1 µg/mL and 3.02 vs 6.94 µg/ mL) during induced subacute ruminal acidosis (SARA). The reason for increased LBP in the blood circulation of cows fed high-grain diets has been related to translocation of endotoxin into the systemic circulation (Emmanuel et al., 2008; Khafipour et al., 2009). Research conducted in beef steers (i.e., backgrounding and feedlot cattle) has also shown that feeding high amounts of grain (i.e., barley grain) induces an inflammatory state in those animals (Ametaj et al., 2009). The same authors report that concentration of LBP in steers fed a finishing diet shows peak values of LBP within 3 wk from the initiation of the diet (23 µg/mL).

In an effort to find a solution against grain-induced inflammatory states in dairy cows we fed cows barley grain steeped in lactic acid for 48 h and found that treatment was associated with lowered concentration of LBP in the plasma (Iqbal et al. 2010). Different investigators have studied the potential application of direct-fed microbials as prophylactic tools against ruminal acidosis. In a study conducted by our team we infused *Enterococcus faecium* EF212 (*E. faecium;* 6×10^{10} cfu/d) alone or in combination with *Saccharomyces cerevisiae* (*S. cerevisiae;* 6×10^{10} cfu/d) in the diet of feedlot steers fed 87% steamed rolled barley grain and 8%

whole-crop barley silage for a period of 3 wk (Emmanuel et al., 2007b). Data showed that feeding *E. faecium* and yeast increased plasma concentrations of LBP versus controls on both day 17 and 21 of the experimental period (22 vs 10 μg/mL and 40 vs 25 μg/mL, respectively).

It is known that during early lactation the concentration of glutamine, the most abundant amino acid in the plasma and milk, is lowered in dairy cows (Meijer et al., 1993). Therefore, we conducted a blood infusion study administering daily 0 (control), 106, and 212 g/d of L-glutamin to periparturient dairy cows for 7 consecutive days starting on d 1 after calving. Data showed increased LBP concentrations by administration of L-glutamin (10.8 vs 35.6 and 50.0 μg/mL, respectively; Jafari et al., 2006).

In another investigation involving oral supplementation of feedlot cattle, fed with 86% barley grain and 9% barley silage, with four different amounts of cinnamaldehyde (0, 400, 800, and 1,600 mg/steer) we showed lowered blood concentration of LBP in relation with the amount of cinnamaldehyde in the diet (1.63, 2.36, 1.78, and 0.98 μg/mL; Yang et al., 2010).

4.3.2 Mammary gland infections

Concentrations of LBP in the serum and milk of cows with natural or induced clinical mastitis was reported to be greater than in dairy cows with healthy udders (Zeng et al., 2009). Interestingly, blood LBP increased earlier and remained longer at high levels compared with other APP such as SAA following an intramammary challenge with *Escherichia coli*, *Mycoplasma bovis*, or *Pseudomonas aeruginosa* (Bannerman et al., 2005, Kauf et al., 2007). Other investigators also have shown that intramammary challenge with LPS or *E. coli* increases both blood and milk LBP (Bannerman et al., 2004; Kauf et al., 2007). For example in a recent experiment, mastitis was induced with a dose of 1,500 cfu of *E. coli* in one quarter of six cows and inoculation was repeated in another quarter after an interval of 14 days (Suojala et al., 2008). Concentrations of LBP in both milk and blood were found to be greater in this expriment compared with those of Bannerman et al. (2004). Thus, Suojala et al. (2008) reported that the basic concentrations of serum LBP before the LPS and *E. coli* challenge were at 10.8 μg/mL after the first challenge and 10.0 μg/mL after the second one. Serum LBP started to increase rapidly in both groups of cows and peaked at 36 h after challenge, being on average 148.6 μg/mL after the first challenge and 108.9 μg/mL after the second one. Interestingly, milk LBP was associated with somatic cell counts (SCC) regardless of the infection status. Milk samples containing > 250,000 and those containing < 250,000 had blood LBP levels at 12.78 and 0.33 μg/mL, respectively.

4.3.3 Fatty liver and downer cow syndrome

As mentioned before, production of LBP is stimulated by LPS, which might affect different metabolic pathways in dairy cattle. Therefore, different metabolic disturbances might be triggered either directly by endotoxin or indirectly by the inflammatory response (i.e., cytokines) initiated by endotoxin. Previous studies have supported the hypothesis that impaired insulin sensitivity mediated by cytokines such as TNF-α activates lipolysis and decreases glucose production in cows with fatty liver (Ametaj et al., 2005a, Bradford et al., 2009).

Recent data have suggested that blood LBP might be used as a biomarker for downer cow syndrome (DCS). An observational study by Ametaj et al. (2010) showed a strong association between DCS and plasma LBP (a 10-fold increase) at 7 d before parturition. Moreover, results indicated that cows affected by DCS had lower anti-LPS IgG and greater concentrations of anti-LPS IgM. Involvement of LBP in different metabolic disturbances suggests it can be used as a valuable diagnostic biomarker in dairy cattle.

4.3.4 Age-related factors

Hoadagoda et al. (1995) and Schrödl et al. (2001) showed presence of LBP in several weeks old calves. They reported values of serum LBP ranging between 1.6 – 2.3 µg/mL. Both groups of investigators infected calves with *Mannheimia haemolytica (Pasteurella)* and observed a sharp increase (4- to 7-fold) in the serum LBP several hours (6 h) after the challenge. On the other hand they (Schrödl et al. 2001) reported that Hp was increased only 12 h after the inoculation with bacteria. Based on those results they suggested to use LBP as a biomarker of disease in calves infected by *M. haemolytica*. Furthermore, in a study conducted by Nikunen et al. (2007) calves with clinical respiratory disease (i.e., *Pasteurella multocida*) had elevated concentrations of LBP in the serum compared to noninfected healthy calves (13.5 vs 6.3 µg/mL).

5. C-reactive protein

5.1 Structure

C-reactive protein belongs to the pentraxin family of calcium-dependent ligand-binding-proteins consisting of 5 identical 23-kDa protomers arranged symmetrically around a central pore. Each protomer consists of 206 amino acids folded into 2 antiparallel β sheets. In the assembled protein, all protomers have the same orientation. Thus, each protomer has a recognition face with a phosphocholine (PCh) binding site consisting of two coordinated Ca ions adjacent to a hydrophobic pocket, and an effector face, where complement C1q binds and Fcγ receptors are presumed to bind (Shrive et al., 1996; Thompson et. al., 1999). Binding of PCh to CRP is mediated by 2 key amino acid residues: Phe-66 that provides hydrophobic linkages with methyl groups of PCh, and Glu-81 that interacts with positively charged choline nitrogen (Agrawal et al., 2002; Black et al., 2003). Asp-112 and Tyr-175 are the critical residues required for CRP binding to complement C1q (Agrawal & Volanakis, 1994; Agrawal et al., 2001).

5.2 Functions

C-reactive protein is a highly conserved plasma protein that participates in systemic responses to inflammation. It binds specifically to host molecules exposed during apoptosis or found on surfaces of pathogens. More specifically, CRP has a Ca-dependent binding specificity to PCh. The CPR synthesis increases within hours of infection or tissue injury and has thus been considered part of the APR (Black et al., 2004; Volanakis, 2001). Its ability to recognize pathogens and to mediate their elimination by recruiting the complement system proteins and phagocytic cells makes CRP an important constituent of the first line of innate host defense. Furthermore, the protein appears to play a key role in the clearance of apoptotic and necrotic host cells, thus contributing to restoration of normal structure and function of injured tissues (Volanakis, 2001). The discovery of CRP stemmed from studies of patients with *Streptococcus pneumoniea* infection where a protein was found that could precipitate the C polysaccharide of the bacterial cell wall during acute phase of the illness

(Tillet & Francis, 1930). Phosphocholine was later identified as the specific ligand for CRP in the pneumococcal C polysaccharide, part of the techoic acid of the pneumococcal cell wall (Volanakis & Kaplan, 1971).

The main biological function of CRP is particle recognition on pathogens and damaged cells of the host followed by mediation of their removal through activation of the complement cascade and phagocytosis. As mentioned previously, the main ligand of CRP is PCh, which is found on a number of bacterial species. Membrane phospholipids of eukaryotes also contain PCh but their head groups are only accessible to CRP in damaged or apoptotic state (Kaplan & Volanakis, 1974; Volanakis & Wirtz, 1979). The other well-recognized ligands of CRP are phosphoethanolamine, chromatin, histones, fibronectin, small nuclear ribonucleoproteins, laminin, and polycations (Black et al., 2004). Binding of CRP to these nuclear constituents is Ca dependent and has been observed in nuclei of necrotic cells at sites of inflammation (Gitlin et al., 1977). In addition to interacting with various ligands, CRP can activate the classical complement pathway, stimulate phagocytosis, and bind to immunoglobulin IgG receptors (FcγR). C-reactive protein bound to a multivalent ligand is recognized by C1q and can efficiently initiate the formation of a C3 convertase through the classical complement pathway (Volanakis, 2001). This cascade efficiently results in recruitment of the opsonic function of the complement system, but not its pro-inflammatory and membrane damaging effects, which requires cleavage of C5 (Volanakis, 2001). The opsonic properties of CRP have been demonstrated for both macrophages and neutrophils (Volanakis, 2001). Indeed, phagocytosis of CRP-opsonized particles by mouse monocytes and neutrophils was shown to proceed through the FcγRI (Mold et al., 2001). Enhancement of phagocytosis by CRP is also mediated indirectly by opsonic complement fragments attached to CRP ligands as a result of CRP-initiated complement activation (Edwards et al., 1982).

5.3 Factors affecting its concentration

Plasma CRP is produced mainly by hepatocytes, predominantly under transcriptional control by IL-6, although other sites of local CRP synthesis and possibly secretion have been suggested. De novo hepatic synthesis starts very rapidly after a single stimulus. The plasma half-life of CRP is about 19 h and is constant under all conditions of health and disease, so that the sole determinant of circulating CRP concentration is the synthesis rate (Vigushin et al., 1993), which thus directly reflects the intensity of the pathological process(es) stimulating production of CRP. When the stimulus for increased production completely ceases, concentrations of circulating CRP fall rapidly, at almost the rate of plasma CRP clearance. Concentrations of CRP in the serum of healthy dairy cows range between 10-30 μg/mL (Lee et al., 2003c; Morimatsu et al., 1989, 1991). However, these levels can dramatically rise following natural or experimental infections. The following factors have been reported to affect CPR levels in dairy cows.

5.3.1 Lactation

The circulating CRP was observed to increase a few days after parturition in dairy cows but it was attributed to tissue injury in the uterine epithelium (Morumatsu et al., 1991). Interestingly, serum CRP also increased gradually as milk production increased during peak lactation in dairy cows. Thus, the lactation-induced pattern of CRP might be useful in monitoring milk production and progression of mastitis in dairy cows (Morimatsu et al., 1991). In a recent article we indicated a strong relationship between rumen endotoxin and plasma CRP and suggested a potential role of CRP in milk fat depression syndrome in dairy cows (Emmanuel et al., 2008). We proposed that CRP might prevent interaction of apo-C-II with lipoprotein lipase to shift lipoprotein particles toward liver and as a result lowering transferring of lipid loads into the mammary gland (Zebeli & Ametaj, 2009).

5.3.2 Body condition score (BCS), age, and pregnancy status

An inverse relationship was found in serum CRP levels and BCS of dairy cows and subsequent regression analysis indicated that a unit increase in BCS decreased CRP level by 20.2 μg/mL (Lee et al., 2003c). On the other hand, age of the cow correlated poorly with serum CRP levels. Interestingly, concentrations of CRP in the serum increased during the first 4 mo of gestation (34.5 μg/mL) and gradually decreased to nadir levels (4.9 μg/mL) during late gestation (Lee et al., 2003c, Turk et al., 2008). Although it is not clear what is the function of CRP during gestation in cattle, human research indicates that high concentrations of CRP during pregnancy have been associated to complications during its course (Teran et al., 2001). Elevated CRP levels at first trimester may represent a risk to gestational preeclampsia (Wolf et al., 2001). On the other hand, Sacks et al. (2004) observed a very early increase of circulatory CRP at 4 wk of gestation in non-obese young pregnant women, suggesting a maternal low-grade inflammatory response during the earliest phases of ovule implantation.

5.3.3 Stress and disease

Concentration of CRP in the serum of cows is invariably affected by stress. Handling and/or sampling stress has been shown to influence serum CRP in dairy cows; however, the effect subsides within 48 h (Lee et al., 2003c). Diseases accompanied by inflammatory reactions induce greater stress and in turn elevate CRP levels in dairy cows. Lee et al. (2003c) categorized disease in dairy cows into inflammatory (for example, acute and chronic mastitis, foot rot, endometritis, and pneumonia) and non-inflammatory (for example, abortion, reproductive disorders, stillbirth, and ovarian cysts) groups. The authors reported greater concentrations of CRP in both groups of diseased cows whether classified as inflammatory or non-inflammatory, and indicated that CRP levels might be useful in monitoring herd health and disease surveillance in dairy cows. The amount of CRP (i.e., in optical density values) in the diseased cows was 3-3.5 fold greater than the healthy cows (Lee et al., 2003c).

5.3.4 Mastitis

Mastitis is an important production disease of dairy cattle commonly caused by infectious agents in the environment. The results regarding utilization of milk CRP as an indicator of mastitis have been controversial. Thus, Schrödl et al. (1995) reported as much as 10-fold increase in the concentration of CRP in the milk of cows with mastitis (1,083 ng/mL) compared to normal healthy cows (82 ng/mL). On the other hand, Hamann et al. (1997) showed that the capacity of the milk CRP to distinguish between healthy and mastitic quarters was poor, and the correlation between the concentration of the CRP in the milk and SCC was low ($r = 0.32$).

5.3.5 Age-related factors

Only a few studies have addressed blood CRP in young ruminants. Schrödl et al. (2003) showed presence of CRP in all plasma samples of calves before the first colostrum intake, and a greater concentration in the blood 1 d after colostrum application. The authors postulated that the increase of the CRP concentration (1 d postpartum) is affected by the passive transfer of CRP from colostrum to blood. The same authors showed that feeding lactulose, a prebiotic compound, further increased the levels of CRP in the plasma of calves fed colostrum.

In conclusion, CRP, like other APP, is an important constituent of the first line of innate host defense. Most evidence for these functions to date has been obtained in studies using human and murine CRP. Even though increased concentrations of bovine CRP during naturally occurring infections and a correlation with herd health status have been reported, CRP has not been fully considered as an APP in cattle.

6. Soluble cluster of differentiation 14

6.1 Structure

Soluble CD14 is a single chain protein with a molecular weight of about 50-53 kDa and spans approximately 348 amino acids in length. Structure analysis by proteolytic cleavage has shown that the molecule is made of two tightly folded domains, the main binding site for LPS (Juan et al., 1995; McGinley et al., 1995).

6.2 Functions

The bovine cluster of CD14 is an important player in host innate immunity in that it mediates host defense against Gram-negative bacterial infections and also confers immunity against viral infections (Chen et al., 1999; Haziot et al., 1996). Two forms of CD14 have been reported; a membrane bound form (mCD14) and a soluble (sCD14) form (Ulevitch & Tobias, 1995). The sCD14 helps to carry LPS in cells that lack mCD14 (e.g., endothelial and epithelial cells). The mCD14 is attached to the surface of myeloid cells (monocyte/macrophages) via glycosyl-phosphatidyinositol tail (Haziot et al., 1998). Moreover, CD14 is required for the recognition of other bacterial products including peptidoglycan, lipoteichoic acid (LTA), and lipoarabinomannan (Gupta et al., 1996; Pugin et al., 1994; Savedra et al., 1996). The CD14 gene in cattle was initially cloned and sequenced by Ikeda et al. (1997) and recently by the bovine genome project. In this review we will focus on sCD14 as an APP.

The serum sCD14 is believed to originate from enzymatic cleavage of its membrane homologue mCD14 through the action of specific phospholipases or proteases (Bazil et al., 1989, Sohn et al., 2007). It was first described by Maliszewski et al. (1985) as a culture-supernatant blocking factor, soluble My 23, an antigen from human myeloid cells that was able to block staining of monocytes by anti-CD14 monoclonal antibodies. Together with LBP, sCD14 plays a crucial role in enabling cellular responses to Gram-negative bacterial LPS by shuttling LPS between LPS micelles to HDL (Kitchens & Thompson, 2005; Wurfel et al., 1995).

Soluble CD14 facilitates transfer of LPS to lipoproteins, preventing over stimulation during the inflammatory responses (Maliszewski, 1991; Schutt et al., 1992). Transfer of LPS to HDL occurs either by the direct action of LBP or by a two-step reaction in which LPS is first transferred to sCD14 and subsequently to HDL. However, the two-step pathway of LPS transfer to HDL is strongly favored over direct transfer (Wurfel et al., 1995). Interestingly, movement of LPS from LPS-sCD14 complexes to HDL neutralizes the capacity of LPS to stimulate neutrophils.

Soluble CD14 also functions as a soluble receptor for bacterial LPS to cells that do not express CD14 such as epithelial and endothelial cells and thereby activates TLR-4 and the release of cytokines (Frey et al., 1992; Kitchens & Thompson, 2005). Toll-like receptor 4 mediates cellular responses to microbial LPS and acts as a co-receptor with mCD14 for LPS (Sohn et al., 2007).

Soluble CD14 also has pro-inflammatory activities in the extravascular compartments where it increases resistance to bacteria. In breast milk, for example, sCD14 has been associated with reduced occurrence of gastrointestinal infections in infants (Labéta et al., 2000). Moreover, sCD14 isolated from mouse, human, and bovine subjects have been involved in activation of B cell activity (Filipp et al., 2001). Therefore, it has been hypothesized that consumption of cow milk containing sCD14 might confer similar beneficial effects (Lee et al., 2003a). In a bovine model of intramammary *Escherichia coli* infection, co-injection of recombinant bovine sCD14 with the bacteria accelerates the recruitment of neutrophils and clearance of bacteria (Lee et al., 2003b).

6.3 Tissue distribution and factors affecting sCD14 expression

Expression of sCD14 in human subjects has been detected in the lung, heart, thymus, and liver; however, expression in the liver is much greater than the other tissues. Therefore, liver is considered to be the major source of sCD14 in circulation. To our best knowledge, no information about sCD14 expression in cattle liver has been reported so far.

Another important source of sCD14 are immune cells. Thus, human monocytes express high levels of CD14 (~10^5 receptor/cell) whereas mCD14 expression on neutrophils is much lower (~3 x 10^3 receptors/cell). Expression of mCD14 on tissue macrophages can vary depending upon their origin. In cattle CD14 is expressed at 99,500-134,600 receptors, on the cell membrane of monocytes and to a lesser extent, at 1,900-4,400 receptors on neutrophils (Antal-Szalmas et al., 1997; Paape et al., 1996). An intracellular pool of CD14 exists in bovine PMN and is capable of translocating to the cell surface as mCD14 (Paape et al., 1996). Research conducted by Sohn et al. (2007) indicated that mCD14 expressed on bovine neutrophils is a source of plasma sCD14 in cattle. Moreover, they showed that sCD14 is shed from bovine neutrophils after stimulation by LPS.

A third major source of sCD14 is the mammary gland, which in cows is at concentrations around 1-6 μg/mL (Bannerman et al., 2003; Bannerman et al., 2004; Lee et al., 2003a,b). Interestingly, the cellular source of sCD14 in human milk was shown to be mammary epithelial cells, which secrete in culture a slightly smaller form of sCD14 than that released by monocytes (Labéta et al., 2000). Apparently, there is no research in dairy cows to indicate the source of CD14 in the mammary gland. Interestingly, Sohn et al. (2004) reported that in bovine milk the molecular mass of sCD14 ranges between 53 and 58 kDa, very similarly with the forms found in the blood plasma.

Various infectious diseases have been shown to increase sCD14 in the serum (Kitchens et al., 2001). For example, circulatory sCD14 increased in respiratory tract secretions of patients suffering from acute respiratory distress syndrome, and in cerebrospinal fluid of patients with bacterial meningitis.

Concentration of sCD14 in the milk, from healthy quarters of dairy cows, was reported to be at 6.90 μg/mL (Lee et al. 2003a,b). Intra-mammary inflammation, induced by LPS challenge, increases milk SCC in dairy cows, which in turn increases concentrations of sCD14 in the milk from the infected quarters. In addition, stage of lactation also affects concentration of sCD14 in bovine milk with higher levels observed during 0–4 d postpartum than other periods of lactation (Bannerman et al., 2004; Lee et al., 2003a). However, in normal human breast milk much greater concentrations of sCD14 (14.84 μg/mL) have been reported (Labéta et al., 2000).

6.4 Utilization of sCD14 for treatment of bacterial mastitis

Intramammary injection of recombinant bovine sCD14 together with low concentrations of LPS in lactating dairy cows induced recruitment of neutrophils when compared to either LPS or CD14 alone (Wang et al., 1997). Moreover, administration of a high concentration of LPS in the mammary gland causes an increase of sCD14 in the milk, attributed to shedding of mCD14 from recruited neutrophils, and might play a role in modulating the inflammatory responses during coliform mastitis in cows (Paape et al., 2002). Furthermore, recombinant bovine sCD14 was able to lower the severity of intrammmary gland infection by *E. coli* in a mouse model of mastitis (Leet et al., 2003a) and also decrease the severity of infection in dairy cows after intramammary challenge with *E. coli* (Leet et al., 2003b).

7. Ceruloplasmin

7.1 Structure

Ceruloplasmin (Cp; or ferroxidase) is a protein of the α-2 globulin fraction of the bovine serum. This protein belongs to the family of multicopper oxidases. Serum Cp is synthesized mainly in the liver hepatocytes (Løvstad, 2006). However, the protein is expressed in other tissues as indicated in the next section of this review. Dooley et al. (1981) were the first to characterized bovine Cp. It is the product of an intragenic triplication and is comprised of three homologous domains (Yang et al., 1986). In humans, Cp is a single polypeptide chain of 1,046 amino acids (Endo et al., 1982), whereas bovine Cp is comprised of 1,063 amino acids (Zimin et al., 2009). Early studies estimated bovine Cp at a MW of 100 kDa (Dooley et al., 1981), whereas more recent comparative studies between bovine and human Cp indicated MWs of 125.1 and 129.8 kDa, respectively (Boivin et al., 2001). Bovine Cp includes six copper atoms as an integral part of the native protein (Zgirski & Frieden, 1990). Liver hepatocytes produce apo-Cp that has no copper (Cu) in it (Macintyre et al. 2004). Subsequently, 7 Cu atoms are added to the protein (Mukhopadhyay et al. 1997), which establishes a more stable product, holo-Cp (Terada et al. 1995). Almost 90% of Cp in blood is in the form of holo-CP (Matsuda et al., 1974).

7.2 Functions

Ceruloplasmin contains more than 95% of plasma Cu and might play a role in Cu homeostasis (Martinez-Subiela et al., 2007). However, its role in Fe homeostasis has overshadowed its Cu-related function. Therefore, the main reported function of Cp is ferroxidation or facilitation of oxidation of Fe^{2+} to Fe^{3+} and its subsequent binding to apo-ferritin (Fleming et al., 1991). The ferroxidase activity of Cp is required for proper Fe homeostasis and lack of Cp leads to internalization and degradation of ferroportin, an Fe exporter (De Domenico et al., 2007). Furthermore, genetic defects of the Cp gene cause aceruloplasminemia, a rare disease with clinical manifestations, including retinal degeneration, diabetes mellitus, and neurological symptoms, which include ataxia, involuntary movements, and dementia (Miyajima, 2003). Humans with aceruloplasminemia also show Fe accumulation in various organs including the retina, liver, and brain, but there is no evidence of Cu deficiency or abnormalities in Cu metabolism (Jeong & David, 2003). It has also been reported that Cp may play a role in scavenging reactive oxygen species (Healy & Tipton, 2007).

7.3 Tissue distribution and factors that affect its expression

7.3.1 Tissue distribution

Serum concentration of Cp increases during inflammation, infection, and trauma largely as the result of increased gene transcription in hepatocytes, mediated by the inflammatory cytokines (Gitlin, 1988). Although the liver is the predominant source of serum Cp, extrahepatic expression of Cp gene has been demonstrated in many other tissues including spleen, lung, testis, brain, uterus, yolk sac, and placenta (Aldred et al., 1987, Thomas & Schreiber, 1989; Thomas et al., 1989). Ceruloplasmin also was detected in the milk and mammary gland of dairy cows (Tabrizi et al., 2008).

7.3.2 Stage of lactation and breed

The half-life of serum Cp is around 5.5 days, and studies demonstrate little or no exchange of Cu bound to Cp following its synthesis (Gitlin & Janeway, 1960; Sternlieb et al., 1961). Interestingly, failure to incorporate Cu during synthesis results in the secretion of an unstable apo-Cp moiety devoid of ferroxidase activity (Holtzman et al., 1970). In the normal adult human about 10% of the total circulating Cp is found as the apoprotein, which is rapidly catabolized with a half-life of about 5 h (Matsuda, 1974). Consistent with these data, an increase in the hepatic Cu pool results in a sustained increase in the concentration of Cp in the serum, whereas a decrease, as occurs in nutritional Cu deficiency, results in a marked decrease in serum Cp (Holtzman et al., 1966; Olivares & Uauy, 1996). Under normal circumstances the hepatic Cu pool is not rate-limiting for holo-Cp synthesis, as concentration of Cp in the serum concentration increases rapidly during infection, trauma, and pregnancy while the ratio of apo- to holo-Cp is maintained (Matsuda et al., 1974).

The basal oxidase activity of Cp in the plasma of female Angus calves, Holstein dairy cows, and steers (Angus and Angus x Simmental) was estimated at 1.31, 60, and 21.9 μg/mL, respectively (Cerone et al., 2000, Hansen et al., 2008, Nazifi et al., 2009); whereas the basal concentration of Cu was approximately 0.75 and 1.14 μg/mL in calves and steers, respectively (Cerone et al., 2000, Hansen et al., 2008).

A recent study of Hussein et al. (2011) reported concentrations of Cp in the serum of dairy cows during different stages of lactation (3–1 wk prepartum; 0–1 wk; 3–5 wk, and 15–18 wk postpartum) and showed greater concentration during 0-1 wk postpartum. Interestingly, these authors found that the activity of Cp is lower in the serum and in EDTA-treated plasma compared to heparinized plasma. They recommended heparinized plasma as the best way to preserve blood for measurement of Cp in dairy cow (Hussein et al., 2011).

A study involving supplementation of Cu in steers showed that concentration of Cp in plasma was increased in association with liver Cu. They found that 10 mg of Cu/kg of DM increased plasma and liver Cu, and concentration of Cp compared with steers supplemented with 5 mg of Cu/kg of DM. In addition, the same study demonstrated that feeding steers copper glycinate was associated with greater plasma Cp than with copper sulfate (19.0 vs. 14.6 μg/mL) (Hansen et al., 2008).

7.3.3 Ceruloplasmin during disease states

Ceruloplasmin has been evaluated as a marker of animal health and welfare (Skinner, 2001). Several studies in cattle indicate its diagnostic use (Sheldon et al., 2002, Szczubiał et al.,

2008). During administration of LPS (2.5 mg/kg body weight) in steers there is a decrease in concentration of Cp in the serum 2–3 h after LPS infusion (Carroll et al., 2009). The latter authors suggested that the decline in serum Cp might be related to Fe redistribution in the host blood, to lower Fe circulation in blood in order to prevent bacteria from that essential nutrient (Weinberg, 1984).

In another study involving infection of the mammary gland, with *Staphylococcus aureus* in dairy cows, it was demonstrated an increased concentration of Cp in the mammary gland in infected quarters compared to the healthy ones. Studies in young animals have shown that concentration of Cp in the serum increases during induced pneumonic pasteurellosis, with the highest concentration observed 2 and 4 h after the inoculation (Fagliari et al., 2003).

In a recent investigation Chassagne et al. (1998) suggested a breakpoint level of Cp over 143 µg/mL (oxydase units) in dairy cows as a reliable threshold to detect early mastitis cases. They showed that 83.5% of the cows that had lower than 49 Cp oxidase units in the serum were unaffected by mastitis versus 16.5% that were affected. Interestingly the same authors showed that high precalving plasma ceruloplasmin oxidase activity was a risk factor for early clinical mastitis.

In sheep and cattle, serum Cp has been used to a limited extent to investigate Cu deficiency (Lorentz & Gibb, 1975, Mills et al., 1976). This was based on the fact that Cu deficient animals injected with Cu show an increased Cp activity and blood Cu concentrations thereafter (Bingley & Anderson, 1972, Lorentz & Gibb, 1975). Another study by Cerone et al. (2000) demonstrated that in Cu deficient (Cu $<$ 0.35 µg/mL) calves, plasma activity of Cp was lower (i.e. 0.62 µg/mL) compared to control calves (i.e. Cu $<$ 0.75 µg/mL; Cp = 1.31 µg/mL).

The low level of plasma Cp might lead to decrease antimicrobial activity of phagocytes (Boyne & Arthur, 1981). It is anticipated that the Cp might deliver Cu to enzymes such as lysyl oxidase; ceruloplasmin might transport Cu to maintain the activity of leukocyte enzymes involved in the respiratory burst (Cerone et al., 2000).

A recent study demonstrated variations in Cp levels during intramammary administration of antibiotics alone (cefotaxime = 250 mg; 6 doses in total) or in combination with proteolytic enzymes (wobenzym drg and 100 mg of cefotaxime; 5 doses in total) in cows with clinical mastitis (Bakeš & Illek, 2006). In fact, concentration of Cp in the plasma before therapy was 25.77 µg/mL in both control and treated animals; however, concentration of Cp increased to 37.22 and 31.49 µg/mL after the treatment with antibiotics alone or in combination with proteolytic enzymes, respectively. Interestingly, the study of Bakeš & Illek (2006) showed that the enzyme therapy lowers the need for the use of antibiotics in dairy cows.

Another study involving bovine *Tropical Theileriosis* demonstrated alterations in the blood APP, including Cp in serum. The cut-off point for concentration of Cp in the plasma of Holstein dairy cows to be recognized as affected by the disease was suggested to be greater than 64 µg/mL, with 80% sensitivity for detection (Nazifi et al., 2009).

In conclusion, the potential to use serum Cp as a biomarker of disease state in dairy cattle is not very well established yet. Although, it was reported by several investigations that concentrations of Cp increase during administration of endotoxin (Conner et al., 1989), clinical mastitis (Tabrizi et al., 2008), or *Tropical Theileriosis* (Nazifi et al., 2009) further research is warranted to evaluate the functions and benefits of measuring Cp in cattle health.

8. Lactoferrin

8.1 Strucuture

Lactoferrin (Lf) is an 80 kDa non-heme Fe-binding glycoprotein of the transferrin family that is expressed in most biological fluids and is a major component of the mammalian innate immune system (Susana et al., 2009). Although the overall structure of Lf is very similar to that of transferrin they differ in their relative affinities for Fe and the propensity for release of Fe (Moore et al., 1997). The bovine Lf is a simple polypeptide chain comprised of 689 amino acid residues, and folded into 2 symmetrical lobes (N and C lobes), each of which is divided into 2 domains (Moore et al., 1997; Susana et al., 2009). Each lobe has a binding site for Fe^{3+} that lies between these 2 domains (Kurokawa et al., 1995). Furthermore, the Fe-binding sites comprise 4 protein ligands that provide 3 negative charges to balance the positive charge of Fe^{3+}. Lactoferrin might be in an open conformation (Fe-free), or a closed one, as a Fe-saturated molecule (Baker & Baker, 2005). Additionally, bovine Lf binds Fe more weakly than human transferrin (Aisen & Leibman, 1972) and it releases Fe more readily (Legrand et al., 1990).

8.2 Functions

Several different functions have been attributed to Lf including regulation of cellular growth and differentiation, intestinal Fe homeostasis, and host defense against microbial infection and inflammation (Ward et al., 2002). In this review we will focus on the anti-microbial functions of Lf related to its function as an APP. Lactoferrin possesses several antimicrobial activities that contribute to the innate immune responses at the mucosal layers. Most bacterial pathogens are dependent on Fe for their metabolic activities, growth, and proliferation. Lactoferrin, by its Fe-binding capability, sequesters this essential metal affecting growth of Fe-requiring pathogenic bacteria including enteropathogenic *E. coli* (Brock 1980). Interestingly, removal of Fe favors the growth of bacteria with low Fe requirements such as lactic acid producing bacteria, which are beneficial to the host (Petschow et al. 1999). Antimicrobial activities have also been described for Lf, which are independent of the Fe status of the protein. In this regard, a direct bactericidal activity has been described for Lf, which is due to a cationic domain located in the N-terminus of the molecule (Bellamy *et al.* 1992). Recent findings indicate that Lf binds to surface molecules (receptors) expressed on many microorganisms, causing cell death. Most interestingly, it was shown that Lf prevents interaction between Gram-negative bacteria outer cell wall component LPS and cations like Ca^{2+} and Mg^{2+}. The latter initiates the release of LPS from the cell wall, making bacteria vulnerable to external antimicrobial attacks (Coughlin et al., 1983; Ellison et al., 1988). Lactoferrin causes similar harm to Gram-positive bacteria based on its binding to anionic molecules on the bacterial surface, such as LTA, which subsequently decrease the negative charge on the cell wall favoring the contact between lysozyme and the underlying peptidoglycan over which it exerts an enzymatic effect (Leitch & Willcox, 1999). Lactoferrin aborts the viral infection at an early stage, by binding to certain viral antigens. This phenomenon is explained by binding of Lf to the glucosaminoglycans of eucaryotic cells; which prevents penetration of viral particles into cells (Yi et al., 1997). The protective effect of Lf is exerted by its suppression of major pro-inflammatory cytokines such as TNFα, IL-1β, and IL-6 (Machnicki et al., 1993; Haversen et al., 2002), and in increasing the amount of anti-inflammatory IL-10.

8.3 Tissue distribution and factors that affect lactoferrin expression

8.3.1 Tissue distribution

Synthesis of Lf can be continuous as part of exocrine fluids, under control of hormones such as in the reproductive tract and mammary gland (Teng et al., 2002), or at certain stages of neutrophil differentiation (Masson et al., 1969). Lactoferrin is secreted in the apo-form from epithelial cells in most exocrine fluids such as saliva, bile, pancreatic and gastric fluids, tears, and milk (Montreuil et al., 1960). In milk, Lf is synthesized mostly by glandular epithelial cells; its concentration in humans may vary from 1-7 mg/mL (milk and colostrum). In bovine milk, average concentration of Lf is at 30 μg/mL. Prolactin has been shown to affect the amount of Lf synthesized in the mammary gland (Green & Pastewka, 1978), whereas estrogens affect its production in the reproductive mucosa (Pentecost & Teng, 1987; Walmer et al., 1992; Teng et al., 2002). Synthesis of Lf in the endometrium is influenced by both estrogens and epidermal growth factor (Nelson et al., 1991). In neutrophils, Lf is synthesized during their differentiation and is subsequently stored in specific granules, whereas in mature neutrophils the production of Lf ceases (Masson et al., 1969). During inflammation and disease conditions, concentration of Lf in biological fluids may increase greatly and constitute a potential biomarker of inflammatory states. This is particularly obvious in blood, where concentrations of Lf range from 0.4-2 μg/mL, under normal conditions, to 200 μg/mL during septicemia.

8.3.2 Lactoferrin in plasma, milk, and cervical mucus

Concentrations of Lf in milk vary from 0.1–1.0 mg/mL in healthy cows; however, it can rapidly increase in cows with sub-clinical and clinical mastitis and this concentration is positively correlated with SCC (Kawai et al., 1999; Hagiwara et al., 2003). Concentration of Lf is usually 100-fold greater during drying off and early mammary involution periods than during lactation (Kutila et al., 2003).

Health status of the cows is a very important factor influencing the amount of Lf in the milk secretions. For example, Harmon et al. (1975) induced *E. coli* infection in a bovine mammary gland, which resulted in a 30-fold increase in the concentration of Lf in the mammary secretion, by 90 h post-inoculation. Furthermore, they observed that during acute mastitis, Lf levels in the milk increased up to 30-fold with the greatest production of Lf occurring in the infected quarter.

Concentrations of Lf in the cervical mucus of dairy cows range from 50 to 600 μg/mL, with a mean of 250 μg/mL (Rao et al., 1973). Interestingly, concentrations of Lf in the bovine and human cervical mucus are of the same order of magnitude. In samples collected from 7 women during mid-cycle, concentrations of Lf (Masson, 1970) ranged from 80 to 1,000 μg/mL with a mean of 350 μg/mL. Although it is not clear what is the source of Lf in the cervical gland it is likely that the cervical glands might secrete Lf in response to the bacterial presence in the reproductive tract.

Interestingly, a considerable variation in Lf content is also seen in the milk from different agricultural management systems. The concentration of Lf in the organic milk samples was found to be 0.03 mg/mL, or 1.5 times greater, compared to the 0.02 mg/mL in the conventional milk. The increased concentration of Lf in the organic milk is related to various factors like type of immunity boostings and other management interventions in organic dairy farms. Furthermore, a high concentration of Lf in organic milk strongly emphasizes the anti-microbiological functions of this APP in raw milk. It is well established that Lf prevents the supply of Fe for pathogens, such as coliforms, thus inhibiting their growth and proliferation (Zagorska, 2007).

8.3.3 Age-and breed-related changes of lactoferrin in milk

Various studies have indicated that concentrations of Lf in different body fluids vary in relation with the gender and age of the animals (Bennett & Mohla, 1976; Bezwoda et al., 1985; Antonsen et al., 1993). For example, Tsuji et al. (1990) demonstrated that Lf content in the milk of 2 breeds of dairy cows (Holstein and Jersey) and 2 breeds of beef cattle (Japanese Black and Japanese Brown) was different among the breeds and cows of the same breed. They also showed that multiparous dairy cows had 2- to 3-fold greater Lf content in the colostrum than primiparous ones. The highest Lf content in the colostrum of dairy cows was observed in the second lactation; however, no differences were observed after the third lactation. Lactoferrin content among individual cows was variable, especially in dairy breeds. The highest concentration of Lf in milk was 11.77 mg/mL and the lowest was not detectable. Average Lf content in colostrum of dairy breeds was 2 mg/mL and in the colostrum of beef breeds was 0.5 mg/mL. The authors suggested that the reason for lower Lf content in the milk of beef cows is that they produce less milk than dairy cows.

8.4 Lactoferrin supplements against endotoxin-related diseases

Published studies indicate that the use of Lf as a supplement and its effects on immunity have been quite promising. When Lf is fed to adult animals and human infants, it increases markedly the beneficial microbiota such as *Bifidus* and decreases the number of pathogenic bacteria such as *E. coli, streptococcus,* and *clostridium* (Kruzel et al., 1998). In one study, administration of endotoxin in mice was associated with septic shock, whereas when mice were fed Lf the lethal effects of endotoxin subsided to a great extent (Zhang et al., 1999). In another study with baby piglets, Lf fed alleviated the severe effects of endotoxin when they were injected with *E. coli* and it was found that only 17 pigs died compared to 74 pigs in the control group (Lee et al., 1999). In addition, 2 human studies, using healthy human volunteers, demonstrated that ingestion of Lf, derived from cow's milk, had positive immunoregulatory effects. These effects were specific to each individual and were related to the initial profile of the immune system of each person. Those data suggested that cow's Lf might be used to improve the immune status of the patients (Zimecki et al., 1998). In another similar human study, it was demonstrated that administration of Lf influenced the primary activation of the host defense system (Yamauchi et al., 1998).

Moreover, Griffiths et al. (2004) examined the effects of oral supplementation of newborn Balb/c mice with *bifidobacteria* (*B. infantis, B. bifidum*) and Fe-free apo-lactoferrin (bovine and human) on gut microbial environment and endotoxin concentration in the ileocecal filtrates as well as mucosal immunity. They observed that oral administration of mice with *bifidobacteria* and/or apo-lactoferrin resulted in lower concentration of endotoxin compared to saline controls. These data suggest that Lf can also be used as a preventive tool against endotoxin-related diseases in other species including dairy cattle. In addition, since antimicrobial properties of Lf have been documented against both Gram-positive and Gram-negative bacteria Lf can be used against infections from those groups of bacteria (Sanchez et al., 1992; Chierici & Vigi, 1994). Lactoferrin content also varies considerably within breed. In beef breeds, half of the cows had values of Lf at nearly zero level (Tsuji et al., 1990).

9. Calcitonin gene-related peptide

9.1 Structure

Calcitonin gene-related peptide (CGRP) is a 37 amino acid neuropeptide generated by the splicing of the RNA transcript of calcitonin gene (Amara et al., 1982). By using NMR and distance geometry studies, Breeze et al. (1991) reported that CGRP sequence comprises an N-terminal disulfide bridge-linked loop between Cys2 and Cys7, followed by an alpha-helix in residues Val8-Arg18, and a poorly defined turn-type conformation between residues Ser19-Gly21. In a more recent study, an investigation conducted with NMR and molecular modeling techniques proposed a structure for CGRP characterized by a rigid N-terminal disulfide-bonded loop leading into helix segments between amino acids Val8-Leu16 compared to Val8-Arg18 and a gamma-turn between amino acids Ser19 and Gly21 (Boulanger et al., 1995). Two available isoforms of CGRP, from most species, have been reported including alpha-CGRP and beta-CGRP, derived from different genes (Amara et al., 1985). Both alpha- and beta-CGRP exhibit similar functional activities and differ with 1 and 3 amino acids from each other (Morris et al., 1984). The amino acid sequence of bovine CGRP shows a homology with other CGRPs identified so far. It is different by only 1 amino acid with rat alpha-CGRP and porcine CGRP and by 3 and 4 amino acids from human alpha- and beta-CGRP, respectively (Collyear et al., 1991).

9.2 Functions

Although CGRP is involved in multiple functions in various tissues including gastrointestinal, cardiovascular, respiratory, endocrine, and central nervous systems we will focus our review on the role of CGRP in the APR. In fact, CGRP was reported to be associated with the APR by Russwurm et al. (2001). Concentrations of CGRP in the plasma increase during sepsis and septic shock in humans (Joyce et al., 1990; Arnalich et al., 1995) and during endotoxicosis in rats (Tang et al., 1997). A recent study of 61 patients with sepsis demonstrated that CGRP levels were greater in non-survivors than in survivors as early as day one of sepsis and remained increased in non-survivors throughout the entire disease state (Beer et al., 2002).

As an APP, CGRP may affect various metabolic, immunological, and biochemical processes of the host. For example, injection of CGRP in rodents is associated with increased concentrations of plasma glucose, lactate, and decreased plasma Ca (Young et al. 1993). Therefore, the increase of CGRP in plasma has been reported in various disease states, thus suggesting an important role of CGRP as a potential biomarker in predicting inflammatory conditions and diseases.

With regard to its immune roles CGRP was shown to stimulate eosinophil infiltration into tissues (Davies et al. 1992). Interestingly, CGRP also promotes adhesion of T cells to fibronectin, a glycoprotein component of the extracellular matrix, which plays a role in migration of T cells to the inflammed sites (Nong et al., 1989). Additionally, CGRP has been identified as a factor that inhibits capacities of macrophages to activate T-cells. It also prevents the inflammatory damage of the liver cells, inhibiting production of TNF-α (Kroeger et al., 2009). Besides its anti-inflammatory properties, recent data show that CGRP stimulates the release of pro-inflammatory cytokines. For example, exposure of BEAS-2B cell line to CGRP, at a range of concentrations, caused synthesis of IL-6, IL-8, and TNF-α 2 h after exposure and the release of their proteins 6 h after exposure (Veronesi et al. 1999).

Only a few studies have looked at the effects of CGRP in cows. In conscious hypophysectomized calves, this peptide caused a significant fall in adrenal vascular resistance and promoted steroidogenesis on the adrenal cortex in the absence of exogenous adrenocorticotrophin (ACTH) (Bloom et al., 1989). In fact, this experiment showed that CGRP produced a substantial rise in cortisol output, which rose steadily to a peak mean value of 409 pg/min/kg within 10 min, in the absence of exogenous ACTH.

9.3 Tissue distribution and factors that affect its release

9.3.1 Tissue distribution

To the best of our knowledge, there is no information about expression of CGRP in cattle tissues. Research in other species indicates that CGRP is highly expressed throughout the central and peripheral nervous systems and exhibits functional roles in various systems including gastrointestinal, cardiovascular, respiratory, endocrine, and central nervous (Brain & Grant, 2004). In another study in hamsters, infected with *E. coli* to cause sepsis, CGRP was expressed in multiple tissues including stomach, small intestines, colon, pancreas, heart, muscle, skin, visceral fat, testis, brain, spine, lungs, liver, kidneys, adrenal gland, spleen, white blood cells, peripheral macrophages, and thyroid glands versus expression only in thyroid glands, lungs, brain, colon, and spine in control animals (Domenech et al., 2001).

9.3.2 Disease states

There is a scarcity of data regarding the role of CGRP during inflammatory conditions in dairy cows and other ruminant species. In a study conducted by our team, to understand the etiology and pathogenesis of milk fever in dairy cows, we compared concentrations in the plasma of different variables including CGRP. Data from this study showed that dairy cows affected by milk fever had lower concentrations of CGRP in the plasma (38 vs 65 pg/dL) than control counterparts, and this effect was associated with lowered concentrations of Ca and P in the plasma (Ametaj et al., 2003). Interestingly, low plasma CGRP were associated with lowered concentrations of plasma Ca around calving date, particularly in the sick cows.

In another study conducted by us, in relation with the cause and pathology of fatty liver in dairy cows, we reported that cows with fatty liver had lower concentrations of CGRP in the plasma (ca. 20 pg/mL) throughout the study. On the other hand, cows that were not affected by fatty liver had greater concentrations of CGRP in the plasma on d 4 prepartum (45 vs 28 pg/mL) and during d 3, 8, 12, and 14 after calving. Moreover, concentration of plasma CGRP in control cows decreased by d 14 to levels similar to those observed in cows with fatty liver (ca. 25 pg/mL) and remained at that approximate concentration to the end of the study (Ametaj et al., 2005a,b). Although the functions of CGRP in dairy cows are not clear yet, it is possible that CGRP is involved in the metabolism of glucose and Ca in transition dairy cows. This hypothesis is supported by studies in rodents where injection of CGRP is associated with increased concentrations of glucose and lactate in the plasma (Young et al. 1993). Our data also demonstrated greater concentrations of glucose and lactate in the plasma of control cows, at several time-points, after partutrition versus fatty liver cows. Interestingly, Hinshaw et al. (1974) reported that intravenous administration of glucose helped removal of TAG from the liver and lessened the lethal effects of endotoxemia. Indeed, in our study we found an inverse correlation between total lipids in the liver at d 8 and 12 after parturition and plasma CGRP, and with plasma glucose and lactate at different postpartal times. These correlations raise the possibility that CGRP may help prevent fatty liver by increasing concentration and supply of glucose.

10. Ferritin

10.1 Structure

Ferritin was discovered in 1937 from horse spleen by French scientist Laufberger (1937), who coined the term "ferritin" from the Latin "ferratus" meaning "bound with Fe" after observation of the Fe content in the newly isolated protein (Laufberger, 1937). Ferritin is the principal Fe storage protein with 387-464 kDa. It contains a protein shell encasing an inner cavity where variable amounts of Fe are stored as a ferrihydrite mineral (Koorts & Viljoen, 2007). Structurally, a spherical protein coat of ferritin molecule, the apoferritin, surrounds an Fe core of hydroxyphosphate (Farrant, 1954). The apoferritin comprises 24 subunits that are composed of various combinations of 2 types of subunits, termed L (lever) and H (heart), having molecular weights of 19 and 21 kDa, respectively (Suryakala & Deshpande, 1999; Orino & Watanabe, 2008). The amount of core Fe ranges from 0 to 4,500 Fe atoms per molecule and reflects somatic Fe reserves, although naturally occurring ferritin contains less tha 3,000 Fe atoms/molecule (Theil, 1987; Harrison & Arosio, 1996). Ferritin isomers vary with each other in-terms of H to L subunits ratio depending on tissue type and developmental stage and in their metabolic properties (Wang et al., 2010). The H subunit contains the enzyme ferroxidase essential for incorporation of Fe, whereas the L subunit is devoid of ferroxidase and is primarily involved in Fe nucleation and physicochemical stability (Lawson et al., 1991; Levi et al., 1992). Serum ferritin is composed primarily of the L subunit type and relatively poor in Fe, whereas the ration of H/L subunits ranges from 0.03 to 0.27 (Kakuta et al., 1997).

Ferritin from cattle contains a major and a minor protein band, which contains high aspartate, glutamate, and glycine and lower methionine and histidine (Suryakala & Deshpande, 1999). Furthermore, bovine ferritin has comparatively higher concentrations of proline, threonine, and valine than equine or human ferritins (Cetinkaya et al., 1985). Although sequence identities of amino acids between mammalian ferritin H and L subunits are relatively low (50–56%), they are highly conserved among the corresponding subunits (H: 88–99%; L: 78–92%; Orino & Watanabe, 2008). $PO_{4(-3)}$/Fe ratio of 0.26 and two values of 16.9 and 10.8 S20w were noted for bovine liver ferritin (Suryakala & Deshpande, 1999). Additionally, ferritin molecule contains 20% neutral carbohydrates. Iron content of liver protein is 9.58% in cattle and the Fe:protein ratio of bovine ferritin has been reported to be at 0.161 (Suryakala & Deshpande, 1999). Using quantitative immunoprecipitation techniques concentration of Fe in serum ferritin was from 0.16 to 0.96 mg/mL (Suryakala & Deshpande, 1999), and the Fe content of ferritin was at 20%, regardless of its protein concentration in bovine fetal sera (Kakuta et al., 1997). For measurement of serum ferritin, antibody-driven reactions such as radioimmunoassay or enzyme linked immunosorbent assay (ELISA) are the commonly used assays. The purified ferritin from cattle liver cross-reacts with anti-buffalo liver and anti-equine spleen ferritins (antisera) by immunogel diffusion and immunoelectrophoresis (Suryakala & Deshpande, 1999).

10.2 Functions

Different studies have shown that extracellular ferritin can function as an Fe transporter to provide Fe to various cells (Wang et al. 2010). Sibille et al. (1988) calculated that one Kuppfer

cell could accumulate over 160,000 Fe molecules/minute via an efficient carrier mechanism. Moreover, ferritin plays a major role in intracellular Fe storage (Harrison et al., 1986). The survival of a bacterium within a host depends on its ability to extract nutrients from surrounding environment. Indeed Fe is an essential component or cofactor of many enzyme systems in bacterium, hence, it is a very important nutrient for bacteria to survive. However, because of its hydrophobic nature, most of the Fe in the host tissues is bound to high-affinity binding proteins like transferrin and lactoferrin while free Fe is very low (at 10^{-18} M). To scavenge Fe from these binding proteins, bacteria have evolved various kinds of highly developed and efficient mechanisms. For example, some highly virulent bacteria, such as *E. coli* and *Klebsiella* species, secrete siderophores or siderochromes, which serve as high affinity extracellular Fe chelating molecules. Similarly, mycobacteria produce mycobactin and exochelin, both Fe-binding proteins, to acquire Fe from the environment (Momotani et al. 1986). Other species of bacteria express receptors for transferring lactoferrin on their surfaces and internalize Fe this way. Still few others extract bounded Fe by proteolytic cleavage. In response to bacterial infection, host antimicrobial defense mechanisms involve sequestration of Fe away from the pathogens (Squires, 2004; Kannon, 2006). To make a host's internal environment more hostile to an invading microorganism, pro-inflammatory cytokines such as IL-1β inhibit synthesis of hepatic transferrin concurrently stimulating synthesis of ferritin in various cells throughout the body (Rogers et al., 1990). Interestingly, Gray et al. (2002) found activation of regulatory T cells by H ferritin subunit, resulting in IL-10 production. Similarly, TNF-α induces ferritin secretion in cultured human hepatocyte (Torti & Torti, 2002). The overall result is a redistribution of Fe from extracellular to intracellular compartments, thus rendering Fe less accessible to invading pathogenic bacteria (Squires, 2004; Kannon, 2006).
Superoxide radicals (O^{2-}), produced by enhancement of mitochondrial cytochrome P450 by toxins or pro-oxidants, or NADPH oxidase by phagocytes (Vignais, 2002), play key roles in oxidative stress by releasing Fe^{2+} from ferritin after donating an electron to Fe^{3+} (McCord, 1996; Orino & Watanabe, 2008). Oxidative stress mediated by reactive oxygen species (ROS) is major factor which is directly linked to inflammatory, malignant, and metabolic diseases in domestic and farm animals (Orino & Watanabe, 2008). However, oxidative stress mediated damage depends on the level of cellular Fe content, cell type, and total body Fe status because through the Fenton reaction an excess Fe^{2+} pool produces the most harmful free radicals (i. e., hydroxyls). There is an emerging body of evidence indicating that ferritin plays a protective role against oxidative stress. For instance, mouse ferritin H or L subunits are over-expressed in HeLa cells, and this lowers production of cellular ROS by pro-oxidants (Orino et al., 2001; Orino & Watanabe, 2008).

10.3 Tissue distribution and factors that affect its expression

10.3.1 Tissue distribution

Ferritin is widely distributed in almost each system of the body, which includes blood, spleen, liver, kidney, bone marrow, heart, pancreas, intestines, and placenta although its concentration is comparatively greater in the liver, spleen, and bone marrow (Harrison et al., 1986; Cetinkaya et al., 1985; Suryakala & Deshpande, 1999). Ferritin is distributed intracellularly in cytosol, mitochondria, and nucleus (Cai et al., 1997; Levi & Arosio, 2004; Surguladze et al., 2005); however because of the water-soluble nature, a small amount leaks into the extracellular fluid (Orino & Watanabe, 2008). In the circulatory system, it generally circulates in relatively low concentrations, at < 1 μg/mL. Circulating ferritin can be classified into two types: (1) serum ferritin, of which the source and secretion mechanisms remain to be elucidated, and (2) tissue ferritin, which probably leaks from damaged tissues (Orino & Watanabe, 2008). Ferritin is also isolated from other extracellular fluids, such as synovial fluid (Ota & Katsuki, 1998) and milk (Orino et al., 2004). Most of the serum ferritin remains in equilibrium with tissue ferritin, and it is directly proportional to Fe stores under normal conditions. The percentage of ferritin Fe to total serum Fe ranges from 8.8 to 28.5% in bovine fetus (Kakuta et al., 1997). Concentration of ferritin in the serum increases markedly with Fe supplementation in calves (Miyata et al., 1984). In cattle, various studies have shown that the normal concentration of serum ferritin ranges between 33-55 ng/mL (Smith, 1997). Moreover, serum ferritin levels between 10-30 ng/mL indicate Fe deprivation, whereas those of more than 80 ng/mL suggest Fe overload (Suttle, 2010)

10.3.2 Stage of lactation, breed, and age

Furugouri et al. (1982) reported that from a relatively baseline concentration during late gestation (35 ng/mL), ferritin gradually increases strating at 3 d prepartum and reaches its peak level at 2 wk postpartum (75 ng/mL). Subsequently, up to 10 wk postpartum it declines gradually, and thereafter remains almost unchanged (40 ng/mL). Although, concentration of ferritin in the serum is associated with gender in humans (Urushizaki, & Kohgo, 1980), no such differences are recorded in cattle (Miyata & Fourgouri, 1984; Atyabi et al., 2006), which might be attributed to absence of menstruation and blood loss in cows. On the other hand, serum ferritin in calves is as low as 14 ng/mL during the first wk and rises to 33 ng/mL at 1 mo of age; however, no further change is observed up to 25 mo of age (Miyata & Furogouri et al., 1987). Grazing has also been reported to be associated with serum ferritin concentration in cattle (Miyata et al., 1986). There are no studies in cattle to show an effect of breed and parity on concentrations of serum ferritin, however, such differences among human races and an inverse relationship between human parity and serum ferritin has been reported (Lazebnik et al., 1989).

Synthesis of feritin is controlled at both transcriptional and translational levels. In fact, this is regulated by Fe, at a translational level through interaction between Fe regulatory protein and conserved Fe responsive element (IRE, 28 bp) in the 50-untranslated region of ferritin H and L subunit mRNAs (Klausner & Harford, 1989; Torti & Torti, 2002; Orino & Watanabe, 2008). Contrary to this well-defined regulatory mechanism, transcriptional regulation of ferritin gene by oxidative stress (Wasserman & Fahl, 1997; Tsuji et al., 2000), cytokines (Torti et al., 1988; Wei et al., 1990), oncogenes (Tsuji et al., 1993), and hormones (Yokomori et al., 1991; Leedman et al., 1996) is Fe-independent and less evident (Orino & Watanabe, 2008).

10.3.3 Ferritin during disease states

Serum ferrtin is a true indicator of Fe-deficiency anemia and is reflected by lower than normal concentration of serum ferritin. Increased serum ferritin suggests pathologies associated with increased storage of Fe such as hemolytic anemia, megaloblastic anemia, or anemia of chronic disease in animals. Similarly, concentration of ferritin in the serum gradually increases with advancement of anemia in calves infected with *Theileria sergenti*. Serum ferritin also is increased during hepatic disease and neoplastic disorders (Roperto et al., 2010). Interestingly in steers fed a diet with lower calories there was an increase of serum ferritin within a 5 mo period (Furugouri, 1984). Underfeeding in cattle has been reported to lower hepatic glucose-6-phosphate dehydrogenase and superoxide dismutase activities, which result in depletion of antioxidant defense mechanisms and eventually give rise to a

state of oxidative stress and peroxidation. Serum ferritin is overproduced in conditions such as uncontrolled cellular proliferation, excessive production of toxic oxygen radicals, and during infectious and inflammatory states (Orino & Watanabe, 2008). Increased circulatory ferritin, during those states, reflects elevated total body Fe storage; however, these stores are sequestered and are not available for hematopoiesis, a process, which contributes to the widely recognized anemia of inflammation (Wang et al., 2010). Practical implication of meaurement of serum ferritin is to differentiate between true Fe deficiency (ferritin decreases) from the anemia of inflammation (ferritin is normal or increases). It is worth mentioning that true Fe deficiency could be missed if serum ferritin is elevated by a concomitant inflammatory condition. For example, concentration of ferritin is not recommended as a marker for the size of Fe stores in the early stages of lactation due to inflammation that accompanies parturtion (Furugouri et al., 1982). Thus, it is imperative to monitor serum ferritin in association with other APP (Smith, 1997).
The study of Orino et al (2004) showed that ferritin in the bovine milk is an indicator of intramammary infection as the concentrations of ferritin in the milk of mastitic cows (134.2 ± 28.7 ng/mL) were significantly greater than those of non-infected lactating cows (7.2 ± 1.2 ng/mL). The latter authors suggested that serum ferritin is an indicator of disease status and also may be a prognostic indicator of the disease (Orino & Watanabe, 2008).

11. Conclusions

Research on APP in cattle started several decades ago and the number of publications during the last 5-10 years has increased noticeably. There is an increasing body of evidence to support utilization of APP as biomarkers of inflammation in cattle. Different investigators have reported enhanced concentrations of APP in various metabolic and infectious diseases including fatty liver, milk fever, downer cow syndrome, milk fat depression, mastitis, metritis, laminitis, grain-induced ruminal acidosis and several infectious and viral diseases. However, it's more appropriate to conclude that APP might be used to indicate a general inflammatory state in the host and not a specific disease. Therefore, increased presence of APP in various fluids of the host should be used to suggest breaching of immune barriers of the host by bacterial, viral, fungal cells or their toxic products. Several APP have just begun to be tackled by bovine researchers; however, more research is warranted to establish the role(s) that APP play in host innate immunity.

12. Acknowledgment

We acknowledge the financial support of different funding organizations that have supported our research activities in the area of innate immunity during the last 8 years including Alberta Livestock Industry Development Fund, Alberta Livestock and Meat Agency, Alberta Milk, and National Science and Engineering Research Council of Canada.

13. References

Agrawal, A. & Volanakis, J. E. (1994). Probing the C1q-binding Site on Human C-reactive Protein by Site-directed Mutagenesis. *Journal of Immunology,* Vol.152, No.11, (June 1994), pp. 5404–5410, ISSN 0022-1767

Agrawal, A.; Shrive, A. K.; Greenhough, T. J. & Volanakis, J. E. (2001). Topology and Structure of the C1q-Binding Site on C-reactive Protein. *Journal of Immunology*, Vol.166, No.6, (March 2001), pp. 3998–4004, ISSN 0022-1767

Agrawal, A.; Simpson, M. J.; Black, S.; Carey, M. P. & Samols, D. (2002). A C-reactive Protein Mutant that Does not Bind to Phosphocholine and Pneumococcal C-polysaccharide. *Journal of Immunology*, Vol.169, No.6, (September 2002), pp. 3217–3222, ISSN 0022-1767

Aisen, P. & Leibman, A. (1972). Lactoferrin and Transferrin: a Comparative Study. *Biochimica et Biophysica Acta*, Vol.257, No.2, (February 1972), pp. 314-323, ISSN 0006-3002

Åkerstedt, M.; Waller, K. M.; Larsen, L. B.; Forsbäck, L. & Sternesjö, A. (2008). Relationship between Haptoglobin and Serum Amyloid A in Milk Quality. International Dairy Journal, Vol.18, No.6, (June 2008), pp. 669-674, ISSN 0958-6946

Åkerstedt, M.; Forsbäck, L.; Larsen, T. & Svennersten-Sjaunja, K. (2011). Natural Variation in Biomarkers Indicating Mastitis in Healthy Cows. *The Journal of Dairy Research*, Vol.78, No.1, (February 2011), pp. 88-96, ISSN 0022-0299

Alayash A. I. (2004). Oxygen Therapeutics: Can We Tame Hemoglobin? *Nature Reviews. Drug Discovery*, Vol.3, No.2, (February 2004), pp. 152-159, ISSN 1474-1776

Aldred, A. R.; Grimes, A.; Schreiber, G. & Mercer, J. F. (1987). Rat Ceruloplasmin. Molecular Cloning and Gene Expression in Liver, Choroid Plexus, Yolk Sac, Placenta, and Testis. *The Journal of Biological Chemistry*, Vol.262, No.6, (February 1987), pp. 2875-2878, ISSN 0021-9258

Alsemgeest, S. P.; Kalsbeek, H. C.; Wensing, T.; Koeman, J. P.; van Ederen, A. M. & Gruys, E. (1994). Concentrations of Serum Amyloid A (SAA) and Haptoglobin as Parameters of Inflammatory Diseases in Cattle. *Veterinary Quarterly*, Vol.16, No.1, (March 1994), pp. 21-32, ISSN 0165-2176

Alsemgeest, S. P.; Jonker, F. H.; Taverne, M. A.; Kalsbeek, H. C.; Wensing, T. & Gruys, E. (1995). Serum Amyloid A (SAA) and Haptoglobin (HP) Plasma Concentrations in Newborn Calves. *Theriogenology*, Vol.43, No.2, (January 1995), pp. 381-387, ISSN 0093-691X

Amara, S. G.; Jonas, V.; Rosenfeld, M. G.; Ong, E. S. & Evans, R. M. (1982). Alternative RNA Processing in Calcitonin Gene Expression Generates mRNAs Encoding Different Polypeptide Products. *Nature*, Vol.298, No.5871, (June 1982), pp. 240-244, ISSN 0028-0836

Amara, S. G.; Arriza, J. L.; Leff, S. E.; Swanson, L. W.; Evans, R. M. & Rosenfeld, M. G. (1985). Expression in Brain of a Messenger RNA Encoding a Novel Neuropeptide Homologous to Calcitonin Gene-related Peptide. *Science*, Vol.229, No.4718, (September 1985), pp. 1094-1097, ISSN 0036-8075

Ametaj, B. N.; Goff, J. P.; Horst, R. L.; Bradford, B. J. &Beitz, D. C. (2003). Presence of Acute Phase Response in Normal and Milk Fever Dairy Cows around Parturition, *Acta Veterinaria Scandinavica*, Vol.44, Supplement 1, (March 2003), pp. 66

Ametaj, B. N.; Bradford, B. J.; Bobe, G.; Nafikov, R. A.; Lu, Y.; Young, J. W. & Beitz, D. C. (2005a). Strong Relationships between Mediators of the Acute Phase Response and Fatty Liver in Dairy Cows. *Canadian Journal of Animal Science*, Vol.85, No.2, (June 2005), pp. 165-175, ISSN 1918-1825

Ametaj, B. N. (2005b). A New Understanding of the Causes Fatty Liver in Dairy Cows. *Advances in Dairy Technology*, Vol.17, pp. 97-112

Ametaj, B. N.; Koenig, K. M.; Dunn, S. M.; Yang, W. Z.; Zebeli, Q. & Beauchemin, K. A. (2009). Backgrounding and Finishing Diets are Associated with Inflammatory Responses in Feedlot Steers. *Journal of Animal Science*, Vol.87, No.4, (April 2009), pp. 1314-1320, ISSN 1525-3163

Ametaj, B. N.; Zebeli, Q. & Iqbal, S. (2010). Nutrition, Microbiota, and Endotoxin-Related Diseases in Dairy Cows. *Revista Brasileira de Zootecnia*, Vol.39, pp. 433-444, ISSN 1806-9290

Antal-Szalmas, P.; Van Strijp, J. A. G.; Weersink, A. J. L.; Verhoef, J. & Van Kessel, K. P. M. (1997). Quantitation of Surface CD14 on Human Monocytes and Neutrophils. *Journal of Leukocyte Biology*, Vol.61, No.6, (June 1997), pp. 721-728, ISSN 0741-5400

Antonsen, S.; Wiggers, P.; Dalhoj, J. & Blaabjerg, O. (1993). An Enzyme Linked-immunosorbent Assay for Plasma-Lactoferrin. Concentrations in 362 Healthy, Adult Blood Donors. *Scandinavian Journal of Clinical and Laboratory Investigation*, Vol.53, No.2, (April 1993), pp. 133–144, ISSN 0036-5513

Arnalich, F.; Sanchez, J. F.; Martinez, M.; Jimenez, M.; Lopez, J.; Vazquez, J. J. & Hernanz, A. (1995). Changes in Plasma Concentrations of Vasoactive Neuropeptides in Patients with Sepsis and Septic Shock. *Life Sciences*, Vol.56, No.2, (December 1994), pp. 75-81, ISSN 0024-3205

Arredouani, M.; Matthijs, P.; Van Hoeyveld, E.; Kasran, A.; Baumann, H.; Ceuppens, J. L. & Stevens, E. (2003). Haptoglobin Directly Affects T Cells and Suppresses T Helper Cell Type 2 Cytokine Release. *Immunology*, Vol.108, pp. 144-151, ISSN 0019-2805

Arredouani, M. S.; Kasran, A.; Vanoirbeek, J. A.; Berger, F.G.; Baumann, H. & Ceuppens, J. L. (2005). Haptoglobin Dampens Endotxin-induced Inflammatory Effects both In Vitro and In Vivo. *Immunology*, Vol.114, No.2, (February 2005), pp. 263-271, ISSN 0019-2805

Arthington, J. D.; Eichert, S. D.; Kunkle, W. E. & Martin, F. G. (2003). Effect of Transportation and Commingling on the Acute Phase Protein Response, Growth, and Feed Intake of Newly Weaned Beef Calves. *Journal of Animal Science*, Vol.81, No.5, (May 2003), pp. 1120-1125, ISSN 0021-8812

Atyabi, N.; Gharagozloo, F. & Nassiri, S. M. (2006). The Necessity of Iron Supplementation for Normal Development of Commercially Reared Suckling Calves. *Comparative Clinical Pathology*, Vol.15, No.3, (November 2006), pp. 165-168, ISSN 1618-5641

Badolato, R.; Wang, J. M.; Murphy, W. J.; Lloyd, A. R.; Michiel, D. F.; Bausserman, L. L.; Kelvin, D. J. & Oppenheim, J. J. (1994). Serum Amyloid A is a Chemoattractant: Induction of Migration, Adhesion, and Tissue Infiltration of Monocytes and Polymorphonuclear Leukocytes. *The Journal of Experimental Medicine*, Vol.180, No.1, (July 1994), pp. 203-209, ISSN 0022-1007

Badolato, R.; Johnston, J. A.; Wang, J. M.; McVicar, D.; Xu, L. L.; Oppenheim, J. J. & Kelvin, D. J. (1995). Serum Amyloid A Induces Calcium Mobilization and Chemotaxis of Human Monocytes by Activating a Pertussis Toxin-sensitive Signaling Pathway. *The Journal of Immunology*, Vol.155, No.8, (October 1995), pp. 4004–4010, ISSN 0022-1767

Baigrie, R. J.; Lamont, P. M.; Dallamn, M. & Morris, P. J. (1991). The Release of Interleukin-1B (IL-1) Precedes that of Interleukin-6 (IL-6) in Patients Undergoing Major

Surgery. *Lymphokine Cytokine Research,* Vol.10, No.4, (August 1991), pp. 253-256, ISSN 1056-5477

Baker, E. N. & Baker, H. M. (2005). Molecular Structure, Binding Properties and Dynamics of Lactoferrin. *Cell and Molecular Life Sciences,* Vol.62, No.22, (November 2005), pp. 2531-2539, ISSN 1420-682X

Bakeš, J. & Illek, J. (2006). Plasma Ceruloplasmin and Fibrinogen during Enzyme Therapy of Mastitis in Dairy Cows. *Acta Veterinaria Brno,* Vol.75, pp. 241-246, ISSN 0001-7213

Bannerman, D. D.; Paape, M. J.; Hare, W. R. & Sohn, E. J. (2003b). Increased Levels of LPS-binding Protein in Bovine Blood and Milk Following Bacterial Lipopolysaccharide Challenge. *Journal of Dairy Science,* Vol.86, No.10, (October 2003), pp. 3128-3137, ISSN 0022-0302

Bannerman, D. D.; Paape, M. J.; Lee, J. W.; Zhao, X.; Hope, J. C. & Rainard, P. (2004). Escherichia Coli and Staphylococcus Aureus Elicit Differential Innate Immune Responses Following Intramammary Infection. *Clinical and Diagnostic Laboratory Immunology,* Vol.11, No.3, (May 2004), pp. 463-472, ISSN 1071-412X

Bannerman, D. D.; Chockalingam, A.; Paape, M. J. & Hope, J. C. (2005). The Bovine Innate Immune Response during Experimentally-induced Pseudomonas Aeruginosa Mastitis. *Veterinary Immunology and Immunopathology,* Vol.107, No.3-4, (September 2005), pp. 201-215, ISSN 0165-2427

Baumann, H. & Gauldie, J. (1994). The Acute Phase Response. *Immunology Today,* Vol.15, No.2, (February 1994), pp. 74-80, ISSN 0167-5699

Bazil, V.; Baudys, M.; Hilgert, I.; Stefanova, I.; Low, M. G.; Zbrozek, J. & Horejsi, V. (1989). Structural Relationship between the Soluble and Membrane-bound Forms of Human Monocyte Surface Glycoprotein CD14. *Molecular Immunology,* Vol.26, No.7, (July 1989), pp. 657-662, ISSN 0161-5890

Beer, S.; Weighardt, H.; Emmanuilidis, K.; Harzenetter, M. D.; Matevossian, E.; Heidecke, C. D. & Holzmann, B. (2002). Systemic Neuropeptide Levels as Predictive Indicators for Lethal Outcome in Patients with Postoperative Sepsis. *Critical Care Medicine,* Vol.30, No.8, (August 2002), pp. 1794-1798, ISSN 0090-3493

Bellamy, W.; Takase, M.; Yamauchi, K.; Wakabayashi, H.; Kawase, K. & Tomita, M. (1992). Identification of the Bactericidal Domain of Lactoferrin. *Biochimica et Biophysica Acta,* Vol.1121, No.1-2, (May 1992), pp. 130–136, ISSN 0167-4838

Benditt, E. P. & Meek, R. L. (1989). Expression of the Third Member of the Serum Amyloid A Gene Family in Mouse Adipocytes. *The Journal of Experimental Medicine,* Vol.169, No.5, (May 1989), pp. 1841-1846, ISSN 0022-1007

Bennett, R. M. & Mohla, C. (1976). A Solid-phase Radio-immunoassay for the Measurement of Lactoferrin in Human Plasma: Variations with Age, Sex and Disease. *The Journal of Laboratory and Clinical Medicine,* Vol.88, No.1, (July 1976), pp. 156–166, ISSN 0022-2143

Benson, M. D. & Aldo-Benson, M. (1979). Effect of Purified Protein SAA on Immune Response *In Vitro*: Mechanisms of Suppression. *The Journal of Immunology,* Vol.122, No.5, (May 1979), pp. 2077-2082, ISSN 0022-1767

Bergsten, C.; Hancock, D. D.; Gay, J. M.; Gay, C. C. & Fox, L. K. (1998). Claw Diseases: the Most Common Cause of Dairy Lameness Diagnoses, Frequencies and Risk Groups in a University Herd, *Proceedings of the 31st Annual Convention of the American*

Association of Bovine Practitioners, pp. 188-194, Spokane, Washington, USA, September 24-26, 1998

Bezwoda, W. R.; Baynes, R. D.; Khan, Q. & Manssor, N. (1985). Enzyme Linked Immunosorbent Assay for Lactoferrin. Plasma and Tissue Measurements. *Clinica Chimica Acta; International Journal of Clinical Chemistry*, Vol.151, No.1, (September 1985), pp. 61-69, ISSN 0009-8981

Bingle, C. D. & Craven, C. J. (2004). Meet the Relatives: a Family of BPI- and LBP-Related Proteins. *Trends in Immunology*, Vol.25, No.2, (February 2004), pp. 53-55, ISSN 1471-4906

Bingley, J. B. & Anderson, N. (1972). Clinically Silent Hypocuprosis and the Effect of Molybdenum Loading on Beef Calves in Gippsland, Victoria. *Australian Journal of Agricultural Research*, Vol.23, No.5, pp. 885-904

Black, S.; Agrawal, A. & Samols, D. (2003). The Phosphocholine and the Polycation-binding Sites on Rabbit C-reactive Protein are Structurally and Functionally Distinct. *Molecular Immunology*, Vol.39, No.16, (June 2003), pp. 1045-1054, ISSN 0161-5890

Black, S.; Kushner, I. & Samols, D. (2004). C-Reactive Protein. *Journal of Biological Chemistry*, Vol.279, No.47, (November 2004), pp. 48487-48490, ISSN 0021-9258

Bloom, S. R.; Edwards, A. V. & Jones, C. T. (1989). Adrenal Responses to Calcitonin Gene-related Peptide in Conscious Hypophysectomized Calves. *The Journal of Physiology*, Vol.409, (February 1989), pp. 29-41, ISSN 0022-3751

Boivin, S.; Aouffen, M.; Fournier, A. & Mateescu, M. A. (2001). Molecular Characterization of Human and Bovine Ceruloplasmin Using MALDI-TOF Mass Spectrometry. *Biochemical and Biophysical Research Communications*, Vol.288, No.4, (November 2001), pp. 1006-1010, ISSN 0006-1291X

Boosalis, M. G.; Snowdon, D. A.; Tully, C. L. & Gross, M. D. (1996). Acute Phase Response and Plasma Carotenoid Concentrations in Older Women: Findings from the Nun Study. *Nutrition*, Vol.12, No.7-8, (July 1996), pp. 475-478, ISSN 0899-9007

Boulanger, Y.; Khiat, A.; Chen, Y.; Senecal, L.; Tu, Y.; St-Pierre, S. & Fournier, A. (1995). Structure of Human Calcitonin Gene-related Peptide (hCGRP) and of its Antagonist hCGRP 8-37 as Determined by NMR and Molecular Modeling. *Peptide Research*, Vol.8, No.4, (July- August 1995), pp. 206-213, ISSN 1040-5704

Bowman, B. H. & Kurosky, A. (1982). Haptoglobin: the Evolutionary Product of Duplication, Unequal Crossing Over, and Point Mutation. *Advances in Human Genetics*, Vol.12, No.189-261, pp. 453-454, ISSN 0065-275X

Boyne, R. & Arthur, J. R. (1981). Effects of Selenium and Copper Deficiency on Neutrophil Function in Cattle. *Journal of Comparative Pathology*, Vol.91, No.2, (April 1981), pp. 271-276, ISSN 0021-9975

Bradford, B. J.; Mamedova, L. K.; Minton, J. E.; Drouillard, J. S. & Johnson, B. J. (2009). Daily Injection of Tumor Necrosis Factor-{Alpha} Increases Hepatic Triglycerides and Alters Transcript Abundance of Metabolic Genes in Lactating Dairy Cattle. *The Journal of Nutrition*, Vol.139, No.8, (August 2009), pp. 1451-1456, ISSN 1541-6100

Brain, S. D. & Grant, A. D. (2004). Vascular Actions of Calcitonin Gene-Related Peptide and Adrenomedullin. *Physiological Reviews*, Vol.84, No.3, (July 2004), pp. 903-936, ISSN 0031-9333

Breeze, A. L.; Harvey, T. S.; Bazzo, R. & Campbell, I. D. (1991). Solution Structure of Human Calcitonin Gene-related Peptide by 1H NMR and Distance Geometry with

Restrained Molecular Dynamics. *Biochemistry*, Vol.30, No.2, (January 1991), pp. 575-582, ISSN 0006-2960

Brinckerhoff, C. E.; Mitchell, T. I.; Karmilowicz, M. J.; Kluve-Beckerman, B. & Benson, M. D. (1989). Autocrine Induction of Collagenase by Serum Amyloid A-like and beta2 Microglobulin-like Proteins. *Science*, Vol.243, No.4891, (February 1989), pp. 655-657, ISSN 0036-8075

Brock, J. H. (1980). Lactoferrin in Human Milk: its Role in Iron Absorption and Protection against Enteric Infection in the Newborn Infant. *Archives of Disease in Childhood*, Vol.55, No.6, (June 1980), pp. 417–421, ISSN 0003-9888

Busby, W. H. Jr. & Travis, J. C. (1978). Structure and Evolution of Artiodactyla Haptoglobins. *Comparative Biochemistry and Physiology B*, Vol.60, No.4, pp. 389-396, ISSN 0010-406X

Cai, C. X.; Birk, D. E. & Linsenmayer, T. F. (1997). Ferritin as a Developmentally Regulated Nuclear Protein of Avian Corneal Epithelial Cells. *The Journal of Biological Chemistry*, Vol.272, No.9, (May 1997), pp. 12831-12839, ISSN 0021-9258

Carroll, J. A.; Reuter, R. R.; Chase, C. C., Jr.; Coleman, S. W.; Riley, D. G.; Spiers, D. E.; Arthington, J. D. & Galyean, M. L. (2009). Profile of the Bovine Acute-phase Response Following an Intravenous Bolus-dose Lipopolysaccharide Challenge. *Innate Immunity*, Vol.15, No.2, (April 2009), pp. 81-89, ISSN 1753-4259

Carter, K. & Worwood, M. (2007). Haptoglobin: a Review of the Major Allele Frequencies Worldwide and their Association with Disease. *International Journal of Laboratory Hematology*, Vol.29, No.2, (April 2007), pp. 92-110, ISSN 1751-5521

Cerone, S. I.; Sansinanea, A. S.; Streitenberger, S. A.; Garcia, M. C. & Auza, N. J. (2000). Cytochrome C Oxidase, Cu, Zn-superoxide Dismutase, and Ceruloplasmin Activities in Copper-deficient Bovines. *Biological Trace Element Research*, Vol.73, No.3, (March 2000), pp. 269-278, ISSN 0163-4984

Cetinkaya, N.; Lengemann, F. W. & Kogan, P. (1985). Isolation, Purification and Characterization of Bovine Spleen Ferritin. *Comparative Biochemistry and Physiology - Part B: Biochemistry & Molecular Biology*, Vol.80, No.4, (April 1985), pp. 773-778, ISSN 1096-4959

Chan, J. P.; Chang, C. C.; Hsu, W. L.; Liu, W. B. & Chen, T. H. (2010). Asociation of Increased Serum Acute Phase Protein Concentrations with Reproductive Performance in Dairy Cows with Postpartum Metritis. *Veterinary Clinical Pathology*, Vol.39, No.1, (March 2010), pp. 72-78, ISSN 0275-6382

Chassagne, M.; Barnouin, J. & Chacornac, J. P. (1998). Biological Predictors for Early Clinical Mastitis Occurrence in Holstein Cows Under Field Conditions in France. *Preventive Veterinary Medicine*, Vol.35, No.1, (April 1998), pp. 29-38, ISSN 0167-5877

Chen, Y. C.; Wang, S. Y. & King, C. C. (1999). Bacterial Lipopolysaccharide Inhibits Dengue Virus Infection of Primary Human Monocytes/Macrophages by Blockade of Virus Entry via a CD14-dependent Mechanism. *Journal of Virology*, Vol.73, No.4, (April 1999), pp. 2650-2657, ISSN 0022-538X

Chiba, T.; Han, C. Y.; Vaisar, T.; Shimokado, K.; Kargi, A.; Chen, M. H.; Wang, S.; McDonald, T. O.; O'Brien, K. D.; Heinecke, J. W. & Chait, A. (2009). Serum Amyloid A3 does not Contribute to Circulating SAA Levels. *Journal of Lipid Research*, Vol.50, No.7, (July 2009), pp. 1353-1362, ISSN 0022-2275

Chierici, R. & Vigi, V. (1994). Lactoferrin in Infant Formulae. *Acta Paediatrica Supplement*, Vol.402, (September 1994), pp. 83–88, ISSN 1651-2227

Chow, J. C.; Young, D. W.; Golenbock, D. T.; Christ, W. J. & Gusovsky, F. (1999). Toll-Like Receptor-4 Mediates Lipopolysaccharide-induced Signal Transduction. *The Journal of Biological Chemistry*, Vol.274, No.16, (April 1999), pp. 10689-10692, ISSN 0021-9258

Coetzee, G. A.; Strachan, A. F.; van der Westhuyzen, D. R.; Hoppe, H. C.; Jeenah, M. S. & de Beer, F. C. (1986). Serum Amyloid-containing Human High Density Lipoprotein 3: Density, Size, and Apolipoprotein Composition. *Journal of Biological Chemistry*, Vol.261, No.21, (July 1986), pp. 9644-9651, ISSN 0021-9258

Collyear, K.; Girgis, S. I.; Saunders, G.; MacIntyre, I. & Holt, G. (1991). Predicted Structure of the Bovine Calcitonin Gene-related Peptide and the Carboxy-terminal Flanking Peptide of Bovine Calcitonin Precursor. *Journal of Molecular Endocrinology*, Vol.6, No.2, (April 1991), pp. 147-52, ISSN 0952-5041

Conner, J. G.; Eckersall, P. D.; Wiseman, A.; Bain, R. K. & Douglas, T. A. (1989). Acute Phase Response in Calves Following Infection with Pasteurella Haemolytica, Ostertagia Ostertagi and Endotoxin Administration. *Research in Veterinary Science*, Vol.47, No.2, (September 1989), pp. 203-207, ISSN 0034-5288

Coughlin, R. T.; Tonsager, S. & McGroaty, E. J. (1983). Quantitation of Metal Cations Bound to Membranes and Extracted Lipopolysaccharide of *Escherichia Coli*. *Biochemistry*, Vol.22, No.8, (April 1983), pp. 2002–2007, ISSN 0006-2960

Davies, D.; Medeiros, M. S.; Keen, J.; Turner, A. J. & Haynes, L. W. (1992). Endopeptidase-24.11 Cleaves a Chemotactic Factor from α-calcitonin Gene-related Peptide. *Biochemical Pharmacology*, Vol.43, No.8, (April 1992), pp. 1753-1756, ISSN 006-2952

de Beer, M. C.; Yuan, T.; Kindy, M. S.; Asztalos, B. F.; Roheim, P. S. & de Beer, F. C. (1995). Characterization of Constitutive Human Serum Amyloid A Protein (SAA4) as an Apolipoprotein. *Journal of Lipid Research*, Vol.36, No.3, (March 1995), pp. 526-534, ISSN 0022-2275

de Domenico, I.; Ward, D. M.; di Patti, M. C.; Jeong, S. Y.; David, S.; Musci, G. & Kaplan, J. (2007). Ferroxidase Activity is Required for the Stability of Cell Surface Ferroportin in Cells Expressing GPI- Ceruloplasmin. *The EMBO Journal*, Vol.26, No.12, (June 2007), pp. 2823–2831, ISSN 0261-4189

Domenech, V. S.; Nylen, E. S.; White, J. C.; Snider, R. H.; Becker, K. L.; Landmann, R. & Müller, B. (2001). Calcitonin Gene-related Peptide Expression in Sepsis: Postulation of Microbial Infection-specific Response Elements within the Calcitonin I Gene Promoter. *Journal of Investigative Medicine*, Vol.49, No.6, (November 2001), pp. 514-521, ISSN 1081-5589

Dooley, D. M.; Cote, C. E.; Collbaugh, T. S. & Jenkins, P. L. (1981). Characterization of Bovine Ceruloplasmin. *FEBS letters*, Vol.131, No.2, (August 1981), pp. 363-365, ISSN 0014-5793

Dubuc, J.; Duffield, T. F.; Leslie, K. E.; Walton, J. S. & LeBlanc, S. J. (2010). Risk Factors for Postpartum Uterine Diseases in Dairy Cows. *Journal of Dairy Science*, Vol.93, No.12, (December 2010), pp. 5764-5771, ISSN 0022-0302

Eckersall, P. D.; Young, F. J.; McComb, C.; Hogarth, C. J.; Safi, S.; Weber, A., McDonald, T.; Nolan, A. M. & Fitzpatrick, J. L. (2001). Acute Phase Proteins in Serum and Milk from Dairy Cows with Clinical Mastitis. *The Veterinary Record*, Vol.148, No.2, (January 2001), pp. 35-41, ISSN 0042-4900

Eckersall, P. D.; Young, F. J.; Nolan, A. M.; Knight, C. H.; McComb, C.; Waterston, M. M.; Hogarth, C. J.; Scott, E. M. & Fitzpatrick, J. L. (2006). Acute Phase Proteins in Bovine Milk in an Experimental Model of Staphylococcus Aureus Subclinical Mastitis. *Journal of Dairy Science*, Vol.89, No.5, (May 2006), pp. 1488-1501, ISSN 0022-0302

Eckhardt, E. R.; Witta, J.; Zhong, J.; Arsenescu, R.; Arsenescu, V.; Wang, Y.; Ghoshal, S.; de Beer, M. C.; de Beer, F. C. & de Villiers, W. J. (2010). Intestinal Epithelial Serum Amyloid A Modulates Bacterial Growth In Vitro and Pro-inflammatory Responses in Mouse Experimental Colitis. *BiomMed Central Gastroenterology,* Vol.10, (November 2010), pp. 133-141, ISSN 1471-230X

Edwards, K. M.; Gewurz, H.; Lint, T. F. & Mold, C. (1982). A Role for C-Reactive Protein in the Complement-mediated Stimulation of Human Neutrophils by Type 27 *Streptococcus Pneumoniae. Journal of Immunology,* Vol.128, No.6, (June 1982), pp. 2493-2496, ISSN 0022-1767

Ellison, R. T.; Giehl, T. J. & Laforce, F. M. (1988). Damage of the Membrane of Enteric Gram-negative Bacteria by Lactoferrin and Transferrin. *Infection and Immunity,* Vol.56, No.11, (November 1988), pp. 2774–2781, ISSN 0019-9567

Elsbach, P. & Weiss, J. (1998). Role of the Bactericidal/Permeability-increasing Protein in Host Defence. *Current Opinion in Immunology*, Vol.10, No.1, (February 1998), pp. 45-49, ISSN 0952-7915

Emmanuel, D. G. V.; Madsen, K. L.; Churchill, T. A.; Dunn, S. M. & Ametaj, B. N. (2007a). Acidosis and Lipopolysaccharide from *Escherichia Coli* B:055 Cause Hyperpermeability of Rumen and Colon tissues. *Journal of Dairy Science,* Vol.90, No.12, (December 2007), pp. 5552-5557, ISSN 1525-3198

Emmanuel, D. G.; Jafari, A.; Beauchemin, K. A.; Leedle, J. A. & Ametaj, B. N. (2007b). Feeding Live Cultures of *Enterococcus Faecium* and *Saccharomyces Cerevisiae* Induces an Inflammatory Response in Feedlot Steers. *Journal of Animal Science*, Vol.85, No.1, (January 2007), pp. 233-239, ISSN 1525-3163

Emmanuel, D. G. V.; Dunn, S. M. & Ametaj, B. N. (2008). Feeding High Proportions of Barley Grain Stimulates an Inflammatory Response in Dairy Cows. *Journal of Dairy Science,* Vol.91, No.2, (February 2008), pp. 606-614, ISSN 1525-3198

Endo, M.; Suzuki, K.; Schmid, K.; Fournet, B.; Karamanos, Y.; Montreuil, J.; Dorland, L.; van Halbeek, H. & Vliegenthart, J. F. (1982). The Structures and Microheterogeneity of the Carbohydrate Chains of Human Plasma Ceruloplasmin. A Study Employing 500-Mhz 1H-NMR Spectroscopy. *The Journal of Biological Chemistry*, Vol.257, No.15, (August 1982), pp. 8755-8760, ISSN 0021-9258

Eriksen, N. & Benditt, E. P. (1980). Isolation and Characterization of the Amyloid-related Apoprotein (SAA) from Human High Density Lipoprotein. *Proceedings of the National Academi of Sciences of the United States of America*. Vol.77, No.11, (November 1980), pp. 6860-6864, ISSN 0027-8424

Fagliari, J. J.; Weiss, D. J.; McClenanhan, D. & Evanson, O. A. (2003). Serum Protein Concentrations in Calves with Experimentally Induced Pneumonic Pasteurellosis. *Arquivo Brasileiro de Medicina Veterinária e Zootecnia,* Vol.55, No.4, (August 2003), ISSN 0102-0935

Farrant, J. L. (1954). An Electron Microscopic Study of Ferritin. *Biochemica et Biophysica Acta,* Vol.13, No.15 (March 1954), pp. 569-576, ISSN 0304-4165

Fenton, M. J. & Golenbock, D. T. (1998). LPS-Binding Proteins and Receptors. *Journal of Leukocyte Biology*, Vol.64, No.1, (July 1998), pp. 25-32, ISSN 0741-5400

Filipp, D.; Alizadeh-Khiavi, K.; Richardson, C.; Palma, A.; Paredes, N.; Takeuchi, O.; Akira, S. & Julius, M. (2001). Soluble CD14 Enriched in Colostrum and Milk Induces B Cell Growth And Differentiation. *Proceedings of the National Academy of Sciences of the United States of America*, Vol.98, No.2, (January 2001), pp. 603-608, ISSN 0027-8424

Fitzgerald, K. A.; Rowe, D. C. & Golenbock, D. T. (2004). Endotoxin Recognition and Signal Transduction by the TLR4/MD2-complex. *Microbes and infection/Institut Pasteur*, Vol.6, No.15, (December 2004), pp. 1361-1367, ISSN 1286-4579

Fleming, R. E.; Whitman, I. P. & Gitlin, J. D. (1991). Induction of Ceruloplasmin Gene Expression in Rat Lung during Inflammation and Hyperoxia. *The American Journal of Physiology*, Vol.260, No.2, (February 1991), pp. L68-74, ISSN 0002-9513

Frey, E. A.; Miller, D. S.; Jahr, T. G.; Sundan, A.; Bazil, V.; Espevik, T.; Finlay, B. B. & Wright, S. D. (1992). Soluble CD14 Participates in the Response of Cells to Lipopolysaccharide. *Journal of Experimental Medicine*, Vol.176, No.6, (December 1992), pp. 1665–1671, ISSN 0022-1007

Friedrichs, W. E.; Navarijo-Ashbaugh, A. L.; Bowman, B. H. & Yang, F. (1995). Expression of Inflammatory Regulation of Haptoglobin Gene in Adipocytes. *Biochemical and Biophysical Research Communications*, Vol.209, No.1, (April 1995), pp. 250-256, ISSN 0006-291X

Furlaneto, C. J. & Campa, A. (2000). A Novel Function of Serum Amyloid A: a Potent Stimulus for the Release of Tumor Necrosis Factor-alpha, Interleukin-1, and Interleukin-8 by Human Blood Neutrophil. *Biochemical and Biophysical Research Communications*, Vol.268, No.2, (February 2000), pp. 405-408, ISSN 0006-291X

Furugouri, K.; Miyata, Y. & Shijimaya, K. (1982). Ferritin in Blood Serum of Dairy Cows. *Journal of Dairy Science*, Vol.65, No.8, (August 1982), pp. 1529-1534, ISSN 0022-0302

Furugouri, K. (1984). Ferritin, Iron and Total Iron-Binding Capacity of The Serum From Holstein Young Steers in Prolonged Undernutrition. *Japanese Journal of Veterinary Science*, Vol.46, No.6, (1984), pp. 859-865, ISSN 0021 5295

Gabay, C. & Kushner, I. (1999). Acute Phase Proteins and other Systemic Responses to Inflammation. *The New England Journal of Medicine*, Vol.340, No.6, (February 1999), pp. 448-454, ISSN 0028-4793

Gallay, P.; Heumann, D.; Le Roy, D.; Barras, C. & Glauser, M. P. (1994). Mode of Action of Anti-Lipopolysaccharide-Binding Protein Antibodies for Prevention of Endotoxemic Shock in Mice. *Proceedings of the National Academy of Sciences of the United States of America*, Vol.91, No.17, (August 1994), pp. 7922-7926, ISSN 0027-8424

Gauldie, J.; Richards, C.; Harnish, D.; Lansdorp, P. & Baumann, H. (1987). Interferon beta 2/B-cell Stimulatory Factor Type 2 Shares Identity with Monocyte-derived Hepatocyte-stimulating Factor and Regulates the Major Acute Phase Protein Response in Liver Cells. *Proceedings of the National Academy of Sciences of the United States of America*, Vol.84, No.20, (October 1987), pp. 7251-7255, ISSN 0027-8424

Gitlin, D. & Janeway, C. A. (1960). Turnover of the Copper and Protein Moieties of Ceruloplasmin. *Nature*, Vol.185, No.4714, (March 1960), pp. 693, ISSN 0028-0836

Gitlin, J. D.; Gitlin, J. I. & Gitlin, D. (1977). Localizing of C-Reactive Protein in Synovium of Patients with Rheumatoid Arthritis. *Arthritis and Rheumatism*, Vol.20, No.8, (November-December 1977), pp. 1491-1499, ISSN 0004-3591

Gitlin, J. D. (1988). Transcriptional Regulation of Ceruloplasmin Gene Expression during Inflammation. *The Journal of Biological Chemistry*, Vol.263, No.13, (May 1988), pp. 6281-6287, ISSN 0021-9258

Gordon, A. H. & Koj, A. (1985). *The Acute-phase Response to Injury and Infection: the Roles of Interleukin-1 and other Mediators*, Elsevier, ISBN 978-044-4806-48-2, Amsterdam, Netherlands

Gray, C. P.; Arosio, P. & Hersey, P. (2002). Heavy Chain Ferritin Activates Regulatory T cells by Induction of Changes in Dendritic Cells. *Blood*, Vol.99, No.9, (May 2002), pp.3326-3334, ISSN 0006-4971

Green, M. R. & Pastewka, J. V. (1978). Lactoferrin is a Marker for Prolactin Response in Mouse Mammary Explants. *Endocrinology*, Vol.103, No.4, (March 1978), pp. 1510–1513, ISSN 0013-7227

Griffiths, E. A.; Duffy, L. C.; Schanbacher, F. L.; Qiao, H.; Dryja, D.; Leavens, A.; Rossman, J.; Rich, G.; Dirienzo, D. & Ogra, P. I. (2004). In Vivo Effects of *Bifidobacteria* and Lactoferrin on Gut Endotoxin Concentration and Mucosal Immunity in Balb/c Mice. *Digestive Diseases and Sciences*, Vol.49, No.4, (April 2004), pp. 579–589, ISSN 0163-2116

Grönlund U.; Hultén C.; Eckersall P. D.; Hogarth C. & Persson Waller K. (2003). Haptoglobin and Serum Amyloid A in Milk and Serum during Acute and Chronic Experimentally Induced Staphylococcus Aureus Mastitis. *The Journal of Dairy Research*, Vol.70, No.4, (November 2003), pp. 379-386, ISSN 0022-0299

Gupta, D.; Kirkland, T. N.; Viriyakosol, S. & Dziarski, R. (1996). CD14 is a Cell-activating Receptor for Bacterial Peptidoglycan. *Journal of Biological Chemistry*, Vol.271, No.38, (September 1996), pp. 23310-23316, ISSN 0021-9258

Guzelbektes, H.; Sen, I.; Ok, M.; Constable, P. D.; Boydak, M. & Coskun, A. (2010). Serum Amyloid A and Haptoglobin Concentrations and Liver Fat Percentage in Lactating Dairy Cows with Abomasal Displacement. *Journal of Veterinary Internal Medicine*, Vol.24, No.1, (January-February 2010), pp. 213-219, ISSN 0891-6640

Hagiwara, S.; Kawai, K.; Anri, A. & Nagahata, H. (2003). Lactoferrin Concentrations in Milk from Normal and Subclinical Mastitic Cows. *The Journal of Veterinary Medical Science*, Vol.65, No.3, (March 2003), pp. 319–323, ISSN 1573-7446

Hamann, J.; Kruger, M.; Kretschmar, M.; Nipp, B. & Gyodi, P. (1997). C-reactive Protein in Milk of Healthy and Subclinically Diseased Bovine Udder Quarters. *Milchwissenschaft*, Vol. 52, pp. 546–550

Hansen, S. L.; Schlegel, P.; Legleiter, L. R.; Lloyd, K. E. & Spears, J. W. (2008). Bioavailability of Copper from Copper Glycinate in Steers Fed High Dietary Sulfur and Molybdenum. *Journal of Animal Science*, Vol.86, No.1, (January 2007), pp. 173-179, ISSN 1525-3163

Harmon, R. J.; Schanbacher, F. L.; Ferguson, L. C. & Smith, K. L. (1975). Concentration of Lactoferrin in Milk of Normal Lactating Cows and Changes Occurring during Mastitis. *American Journal of Veterinary Research*, Vol.36, No.7, (July 1975), pp. 1001-1007, ISSN 0002-9645

Harris, H. W.; Rockey, D. C. & Chau, P. (1998). Chylomicronsalterthe Hepaticdis-tribution and Cellular Response to Endotoxin in Rats. *Hepatology*, Vol.27, No.5, (May 1998), pp. 1341-1348, ISSN 0270-9139

Harris, H. W.; Brady, S. E. & Rapp, J. H. (2002). Hepatic Endosomal Trafficking of Lipoprotein-bound Endotoxin in Rats. *The Journal of Surgical Research*, Vol.106, No.1, (July 2002), pp. 188-195, ISSN 0022-4804

Harrison, P. M.; Treffry, A. & Lilley, T. H. (1986). Ferritin as an Iron-Storage Protein: Mechanisms of Iron Uptake. *Journal of Inorganic Biochemistry*, Vol.27, No.4, (August 1986), pp. 287-293, ISSN 0162-0134

Harrison, P. M. & Arosio, P. (1996). The Ferritins: Molecular Properties, Iron Storage Function and Cellular Regulation. *Biochimica et Biophysica Acta*, Vol.1275, No.3, (July 1996), pp. 161–203, ISSN 0304-4165

Haversen, L.; Ohlsson, B. G.; Hahn-Zoric, M.; Hanson, L. A. & Mattsby-Baltzer, I. (2002). Lactoferrin Down-Regulates the LPS-induced Cytokine Production in Monocytic Cells via NF-Kappa B. *Cellular Immunology*, Vol.220, No.2, (December 2002), pp. 83–95, ISSN 0008-8749

Haziot, A.; Ferrero, E.; Kontgen, F.; Hijiya, N.; Yamamoto, S.; Silver, J.; Stewart, C. L. & Goyert, S. M. (1996). Resistance to Endotoxin Shock and Reduced Dissemination of Gram-negative Bacteria in CD14-deficient Mice. *Immunity*, Vol.4, No.4, (April 1996), pp.407-414, ISSN 1074-7613

Haziot, A.; Lin, X. Y.; Zhang, F. & Goyert, S. M. (1998). The Induction of Acute Phage Proteins by Lipopolysaccharide Uses a Novel Pathway that is CD14-independent. *The Journal of Immunology*, Vol.160, No.6, (March 1998), pp. 2570-2572, ISSN 0022-1767

Healy, J. & Tipton, K. (2007). Ceruloplasmin and What it Might Do. *Journal of Neural Transmission*, Vol.114, No.6, (June 2007), pp. 777-781, ISSN 0300-9564

Heegaard, P. M.; Godson, D. L.; Toussaint, M. J.; Tjørnehøj, K.; Larsen, L. E.; Viuff, B. & Rønsholt, L. (2000). The Acute Phase Response of Haptoglobin and Serum Amyloid A (SAA) in Cattle Undergoing Experimental Infection with Bovine Respiratory Syncytial Virus. *Veterinary Immunology and Immunopathology*, Vol.77, No.1-2, (November 2000), pp. 151-159, ISSN 0165-2427

Hershkoviz, R.; Preciado-Patt, L.; Lider, O.; Fridkin, M.; Dastych, J.; Metcalfe, D. D. & Mekori, Y. A. (1997). Extracellular Matrix-anchored Serum Amyloid A Preferentially Induces Mast Cell Adhesion. *American Journal of Physiology*. Vol.273, No. 1, (July 1997), pp. C179-C187, ISSN 0363-6143

Hinshaw, L. B.; Peyton, M. D.; Archer, L. T.; Black, M. R.; Coalson, J. J. & Greenfield, L. J. (1974). Prevention of Death in Endotoxin Shock by Glucose Administration. *Surgery, Gynecology & Obstetrics*, Vol.139, No.6, (December 1974), pp.851-859, ISSN 0039-6087

Hiss, S.; Mielenz, M.; Bruckmaier, R. M. & Sauerwein, H. (2004). Haptoglobin Concentrations in Blood and Milk after Endotoxin Challenge and Quantification of Mammary Hp mRNA Expression. *Journal of Dairy Science*, Vol.87, No.11, (November 2004), pp.3778-3784, ISSN 0022-0302

Hoblet, K. H. & Weiss, W. (2001). Metabolic Hoof Horn Disease. Claw Horn Disruption. *The Veterinary Clinics of North America. Food Animal Practice*, Vol.17, No.1, (March 2001), pp. 111-127, ISSN 0749-0720

Hoffman, J. S. & Benditt, E. P. (1983). Plasma Clearance Kinetics of the Amyloid-related High Density Lipoprotein Apoprotein, Serum Amyloid Protein (apoSAA) in the Mouse. Evidence for Rapid apoSAA Clearance. *The Journal of Clinical Investigation*, Vol.71, Vol.4, (April 1983), pp. 926-934, ISSN 0021-9738

Holtzman N. A.; Elliott D. A.; Heller R. H. (1966). Copper Intoxication. Report of a Case with Observations on Ceruloplasmin. *The New England Journal of Medicine*, Vol.275, No.7, (August 1966), pp. 347–352, ISSN 0028-4793

Holtzman, N. A. & Gaumnitz, B. M. (1970). Studies on the Rate of Release and Turnover of Ceruloplasmin and Apoceruloplasmin in Rat Plasma. *The Journal of Biological Chemistry*, Vol.245, No.9, (May 1970), pp. 2354–2358, ISSN 0021-9258

Horadagoda, A.; Eckersall, P. D.; Hodgson, J. C.; Gibbs, H. A. & Moon, G. M. (1994). Immediate Responses in Serum TNF-α and Acute Phase Protein Concentrations to Infection with Pasteurella Haemolytica A1 in Calves. *Research in Veterinary Science*, Vol.57, No.1, (July 1994), pp.129-132, ISSN 0034-5288

Horadagoda, N. U.; Eckersall, P. D.; Andrew, L.; Gallay, P.; Heumann, D. & Gibbs, H. A. (1995). Characterisation of Bovine Lipopolysaccharide Binding Protein and the In Vivo Acute Phase Response to Pasteurella Haemolytica Type A. *Veterinary Immunology and Immunopathology*, Vol.49, No.1-2, (November 1995), pp.61-74, ISSN 0165-2427

Horadagoda, N. U.; Knox, K. M.; Gibbs, H. A.; Reid, S. W.; Horadagoda, A.; Edwards, S. E. & Eckersall, P. D. (1999). Acute Phase Proteins in Cattle: Discrimination between Acute and Cronic Inflammation. *The Veterinary Record*, Vol.144, No.16, (April 1999), pp. 437-441, ISSN 0042-4900

Hussein, H.; Staufenbiel, R.; Müller, A.; El-Sebaie, A. & Abd-El-Salam, M. (2011). Ceruloplasmin Activity in Holstein Dairy Cows: Effects of Lactation Stages and Anticoagulants. *Comparative Clinical Pathology*, Vol.20, No.1, (February 2011), pp. 1-6, ISSN 1618-5641

Huzzey, J. M.; Duffield, T. F.; LeBlanc, S. J.; Veira, D. M.; Weary, D. M. & von Keyserlingk, M. A. G. (2009). Haptoglobin as an Early Indicator of Metritis. *Journal of Dairy Science*, Vol.92, No.2, (February 2009), pp. 621-625, ISSN 0022-0302

Ikeda, A.; Takata, M.; Taniguchi, T.; Tarumi, O. & Sekikawa, K. (1997). Molecular Cloning of Bovine CD14 Gene. *The Journal of Veterinary Medical Science*, Vol.59, No.8, (August 1997), pp. 715-719, ISSN 0916-7250

Iqbal, S.; Zebeli, Q.; Mazzolari, A.; Dunn, S. M. & Ametaj, B. N. (2010). Feeding Rolled Barley Grain Steeped in Lactic Acid Modulated Energy Status and Innate Immunity in Dairy Cows. *Journal of Dairy Science*, Vol.93, No.11, (November 2010), pp. 5147-5156, ISSN 1525-3198

Jacobsen, S.; Niewold, T. A.; Kornalijnslijper, E.; Toussaint, M. J. & Gruys, E. (2005). Kinetics of Local and Systemic Isoforms of Serum Amyloid A in Bovine Mastitic Milk. *Veterinary Immunology and Immunopathology*, Vol.104, No.1-2, (March 2005), pp.21-31, ISSN 0165-2427

Jafari, A.; Emmanuel, D. G.; Christopherson, R. J.; Thompson, J. R.; Murdoch, G. K.; Woodward, J.; Field, C. J. & Ametaj, B. N. (2006). Parenteral Administration of Glutamine Modulates Acute Phase Response in Postparturient Dairy Cows. *Journal of Dairy Science*, Vol.89, No.12, (December 2006), pp. 4660-4668, ISSN 1525-3198

Jawor, P.; Steiner, S.; Stefaniak, T.; Baumgartner, W. & Rząsa, A. (2008). Determination of Selected Acute Phase Proteins during the Treatment of Limb Diseases in Dairy Cows. *Veterinarni Medicina*, Vol.53, No.4, (April 2008), pp. 173-183, ISSN 0375-8427

Jeong, S. Y. & David, S. (2003). Glycosylphosphatidylinositol-anchored Ceruloplasmin is Required for Iron Efflux from Cells in the Central Nervous System. *The Journal of Biological Chemistry*, Vol.278, No.29, (July 2003), pp. 27144–27148, ISSN 0021-9258

Joyce, C. D.; Fiscus, R. R.; Wang, X.; Dries, D. J.; Morris, R. C. & Prinz, R. A. (1990). Calcitonin Gene-related Peptide Levels are Elevated in Patients with Sepsis. *Surgery*, Vol.108, No.6, (December 1990), pp. 1097-1101, ISSN 0039-6060

Juan, T. S.; Hailman, E.; Kelley, M. J.; Busse, L. A.; Davy, E.; Empig, C. J.; Narhi, L. O.; Wright, S. D. & Lichenstein, H. S. (1995). Identification of a Lipopolysaccharide Binding Domain in CD14 between Amino Acids 57 and 64. *Journal of Biological Chemistry*, Vol.270, No.10, (March 1995), pp. 5219-5224, ISSN 0021-9258

Kakuta, K.; Orino, K.; Yamamoto, S. & Watanabe, K. (1997). High Levels of Ferritin and its Iron in Fetal Bovine Serum. *Comparative Biochemistry and Physiology - Part A: Molecular & Integrative Physiology*, Vol.118, No.1, (September 1997), pp. 165-169, ISSN 1096-4940

Kalmovarin, N.; Friedrichs, W. E.; O'Brien, H. V.; Linehan, L. A.; Bowman, B. H. & Yang, F. (1991). Extrahepatic Expression of Plasma Protein Genes during Inflammation. *Inflammation*, Vol.15, No.5, (October 1991), pp. 369-379, ISSN 0360-3997

Kannon, J. G. (2006). Cytokines and Eicosanoids, In: *Modern nutrition in health and disease*, B. Caballero & R. J. Cousins, (Ed.), 655-666. Lippincott Williams & Wilkins, ISBN 978-07817-413-30, Philadelphia, USA

Kaplan, M. H. & Volanakis, J. E. (1974). Interaction of C-Reactive Protein Complexes with the Complement System. I. Consumption of Human Complement Associated with the Reaction of C-Reactive Protein with Pneumococcal C-polysaccharide and with the Choline Phosphatides, Lecithin and Sphingomyelin. *Journal of Immunology*, Vol.112, No.6, (June 1974), pp. 2135-2147, ISSN 0022-1767

Katoh, N. & Nakagawa, H. (1999). Detection of Haptoglobin in the High density Lipoprotein and the Very High-density Lipoprotein Fractions from Sera of Calves with Experimental Pneumonia and Cows with Naturally Occurring Fatty Liver. *Journal of Veterinary Medical Science*, Vol.61, No.2, (February 1999), pp. 119-124, ISSN 0916-7250

Kauf, A. C.; Rosenbusch, R. F.; Paape, M. J. & Bannerman, D. D. (2007). Innate Immune Response to Intramammary Mycoplasma Bovis Infection. *Journal of Dairy Science*, Vol.90, No.7, (July 2007), pp. 3336-3348, ISSN 1525-3198

Kawai, K.; Hagiwara, S.; Anri, A. & Nagahata, H. (1999). Lactoferrin Concentration in Milk of Bovine Clinical Mastitis. *Veterinary Research Communications*, Vol.23, No.7, (July 1999), pp. 391–398, ISSN 1573-7446

Khafipour, E.; Krause, D. O. & Plaizier, J. C. (2009). A Grain-based Subacute Ruminal Acidosis Challenge Causes Translocation of Lipopolysaccharide and Triggers Inflammation. *Journal of Dairy Science*, Vol.92, No.3, (March 2009), pp. 1060-1070, ISSN 1525-3198

Khemlani, L. S.; Yang, Z. & Bochsler, P. N. (1994). Identification and Characterization of a Bovine Lipopolysaccharide-binding Protein. *Journal of Leukocyte Biology*, Vol.56, No.6, (December 1994), pp. 784-791, ISSN 0741-5400

Kitchens, R. L.; Thompson, P. A.; Viriyakosol, S.; O'Keefe, G. E. & Munford, R. S. (2001). Plasma CD14 Decreases Monocyte Responses to LPS by Transferring Cell-bound LPS to Plasma Lipoproteins. *Journal of Clinical Investigation,* Vol.108, No.3, (August 2001), pp. 485-493, ISSN 0021-9738

Kitchens, R. L. & Thompson, P. A. (2005). Modulatory Effects of sCD14 and LBP on LPS-host Cell Interactions. *Journal of Endotoxin Research,* Vol.11, No.4, (August 2005), pp. 225-229, ISSN 0968-0519

Klausner, R. D. & Harford, J. B. (1989). Cis-Trans Models for Post-Transcriptional Gene Regulation. *Science,* Vol.246, No.4932, (November 1989), pp. 870–872, ISSN 0193-4511

Koj, A. (1985). Biological Functions of Acute-phase Proteins. In: *The Acute-phase Response to Injury and Infection: the Roles of Interleukin-1 and other Mediators.* Gordon, A. H. & Koj, A., pp. 145-160, Elsevier, ISBN: 978-044-4806-48-2, Amsterdam

Koj, A. (1998). Termination of Acute-phase Response: Role of some Cytokines and Anti-inflammatory Drugs. *General Pharmacology,* Vol.31, No.1, (July 1998), pp. 9-18, ISSN 0306-3623

Koorts, A. M. & Viljoen, M. (2007). Ferritin and Ferritin Isoforms II: Protection Against Uncontrolled Cellular Proliferation, Oxidative Damage and Inflammatory Processes. *Archives of Physiology and Biochemistry,* Vol.113, No.2, (April 2007), pp. 55-64, ISSN 1381-3455

Kroeger, I.; Erhardt, A.; Abt, D.; Fischer, M.; Biburger, M.; Rau, T.; Neuhuber, W. L. & Tiegs, G. (2009). The Neuropeptide Calcitonin Gene-related Peptide (CGRP) Prevents Inflammatory Liver Injury in Mice. *Journal of Hepatology,* Vol.51, No.2, (August 2009), pp. 342-53, ISSN 0168-8278

Kruzel, M. L.; Harari, Y.; Chen, C. Y. & Castro, G. A. (1998). The Gut. a Key Metabolic Organ Protected by Lactoferrin during Experimental Systemic Inflammation in Mice. *Advances in Experimental Medicine and Biology,* Vol.443, No.1, (October 1998), pp. 167-173, ISSN 0065-2598

Kujala, M.; Orro, T. & Soveri, T. (2010). Serum Acute Phase Proteins as a Marker of Inflammation in Dairy Cattle with Hoof Diseases. *The Veterinary Record,* Vol.166, No.8, (February 2008), pp. 240-241, ISSN 0042-4900

Kurokawa, H.; Mikami, B. & Hirose, M. (1995). Crystal Structure of Diferric Hen Ovotransferrin at 2.4 A Resolution. *Journal of Molecular Biology,* Vol.254, No.2, (November 1995), pp. 196-207, ISSN 0022-2836

Kurosky, A.; Barnett, D. R.; Lee, T. H.; Touchstone, B.; Hay, R. E.; Arnott, M. S.; Bowman, B. H. & Fitch, W. M. (1980). Covalent Structure of Human Haptoglobin: a Serine Protease Homolog (Amino Acid Sequence/Plasminogen/Prothrombin/Protein Evolution). *Proceedings of the National Academy of Sciences of the United States of America,* Vol.77, No.6, (June 1980), pp. 3388-3392, ISSN 0027-8424

Kushner, I. (1982). The Phenomenon of the Acute Phase Response. *Annals of the New York Academy of Sciences,* Vol.389, pp. 39-48, ISSN 0077-8923

Kushner I. & Mackiewicz A. (1987). Acute Phase Proteins as Disease Markers. *Disease Markers,* Vol.5, No.1, (March 1987), pp. 1-11, ISSN 0278-0240

Kutila, T.; Pyörälä, S. & Kaartinen, L. (2003). Lactoferrin and Citrate Concentrations at Drying-off and during Early Mammary Involution of Dairy Cows. *Journal of*

Veterinary Medicine Series A, Vol.50, No.7, (January 2003), pp. 350–353, ISSN 0931-184X

Labéta, M. O.; Vidal, K.; Nores, J. E.; Arias, M.; Vita, N.; Morgan, B. P.; Guillemot, J. C.; Loyaux, D.; Ferrara, P.; Schmid, D.; Affolter, M.; Borysiewicz, L. K.; Donnet-Hughes, A. & Schiffrin, E. J. (2000). Innate Recognition of Bacteria in Human Milk is Mediated by a Milk-derived Highly Expressed Pattern Recognition Receptor, Soluble CD14. *Journal of Experimental Medicine,* Vol.191, No.10, (May 2000), pp. 1807-1812, ISSN 0022-1007

Larson, M. A.; Wei, S. H.; Weber, A.; Weber, A. T. & McDonald, T. L. (2003). Induction of Human Mammary-associated Serum Amyloid A3 by Prolactin or Lipopolysaccharide. *Biochemical and Biophysical Research Commununication*, Vol.301, No.4, (February 2003), pp. 1030-1037, ISSN 0006-291X

Larson, M. A.; Weber, A.; Weber, A. T. & McDonald, T. L. (2005). Differential Expression and Secretion of Bovine Serum Amyloid A3 (SAA3) by Mammary Epithelial Cells Stimulated with Prolactin or Lipopolysaccharide. *Veterinary Immunology and Immunopathology*, Vol.107, No.3-4, (September 2005), pp. 255-264, ISSN 0165-2427

Larson, M. A.; Weber, A. & McDonald, T. L. (2006). Bovine Serum Amyloid A3 Gene Structure and Promoter Analysis: Induced Transcriptional Expression by Bacterial Components and the Hormone Prolactin. *Gene*, Vol.380, No.2, (October 2006), pp. 104-110, ISSN 0378-1119

Laufberger, V. (1937). Sur la Cristallisation de la Ferritine. *Bulletin de la Société de chimie biologique,* Vol.19, (1937), pp. 1575-1582, ISSN 0037-9042

Lawson, D. M.; Artymiuk, P. J.; Yewdall, S. J.; Smith, J. M. A.; Livingstone, J. C.; Treffry, A.; Luzzago, A.; Levi, S.; Arosio, P.; Cesareni, G.; Thomas, C. D.; Shaw, W. V. & Harrison, P. M. (1991). Solving the Structure of Human H Ferritin By Genetically Engineering Intermolecular Crystal Contacts. *Nature,* Vol.349, No.6309, (February 1991), pp. 541–544, ISSN 0028-0836

Lazebnik, N.; Kuhnert, B. R. & Kuhnert, P. M. (1989). The Effect of Race on Serum Ferritin during Parturition. *Journal of American College of Nutrition,* Vol.8, No.6, (December 1989), pp. 591-596, ISSN 0731-5724

Lee, J. W.; Paape, M. J.; Elsasser, T. H. & Zhao, X. (2003a). Elevated Milk Soluble CD14 in Bovine Mammary Glands Challenged with Escherichia Coli Lipopolysaccharide. *Journal of Dairy Science,* Vol.86, No.7, (July 2003), pp. 2382-2389, ISSN 0022-0302

Lee, J. W.; Paape, M. J.; Elsasser, T. H. & Zhao, X. (2003b). Recombinant Soluble CD14 Reduces Severity of Intramammary Infection by Escherichia Coli. *Infection and Immunity*, Vol.71, No.7, (July 2003), pp. 4034-4039, ISSN 0019-9567

Lee, W. C.; Hsiao, H. C.; Wu, Y. L.; Lin, J. H.; Lee, Y. P.; Fung, H. P.; Chen, H. H.; Chen, Y. H. & Chu, R. M. (2003c). Serum C-Reactive Protein in Dairy Herds. *Canadian Journal of Veterinary Research,* Vol.67, No.2, (May 2003c), pp. 102-107, ISSN 0830-9000

Lee, W. J.; Farmer, J. L.; Hilty, M. & Kim, Y. B. (1999). The Protective Effects of Lactoferrin Feeding Against Endotoxin Lethal Shock in Germfree Piglets. *Infection and Immunity,* Vol.66, No.4, (April 1999), pp. 1421-1426, ISSN 0019-9567

Leedman, P. J.; Stein, A. R.; Chin, W. W. & Rogers, J. T. (1996). Thyroid Hormone Modulates the Interaction Between Iron Regulatory Proteins and the Ferritin Mrna Iron-Responsive Element. *Journal of Biological Chemistry,* Vol.271, No.20, (May 1996), pp. 12017–12023, ISSN 0021-9258

Legrand, D.; Mazurier, J.; Colavizza, D.; Montreuil, J. & Spik, G. (1990). Properties of the Iron-binding Site of the N-terminal Lobe of Human and Bovine Lactotransferrins. *Biochememistry Journal,* Vol.266, No.2, (March 1990), pp. 575-581, ISSN 0264-6021

Leitch, E. C. & Willcox, M. D. (1999). Elucidation of the Antistaphylococcal Action of Lactoferrin and Lysozyme. *Journal of Medical Microbiology,* Vol.48, No.9, (September 1999), pp. 867–871, ISSN 0022-2615

Levi, S.; Yewdall, S. J.; Harrison, P. M.; Santambrogio, P.; Cozzi, A.; Rovida, E.; Albertini, A. & Arosio, P. (1992). Evidence That H- And L-Chains have Co-operative Roles in the Iron-uptake Mechanism of Human Ferritin. *Biochemical Journal,* Vol.288, No.2, (December 1992), pp. 591–596, ISSN 0264-6021

Levi, S. & Arosio, P. (2004). Mitochondrial Ferritin. *International Journal of Biochemistry & Cell Biology,* Vol.36, No.10, (October 2004), pp. 1887-1889, ISSN 1357-2725

Lim, S. K.; Kim, H.; Lim, S. K.; Bin Ali, A.; Lim, Y. K.; Wang, Y.; Chong, S. M.; Costantini, F. & Baumman, H. (1998). Increased Susceptibility in Hp Knockout Mice during Acute Hemolysis. *Blood,* Vol.92, No.6, (September 1998), pp. 1870-1877, ISSN 0006-4971

Lorentz, P. P. & Gibb, F. M. (1975). Caeruloplasmin Activity as an Indication of Plasma Copper Levels in Sheep. *New Zealand Veterinary Journal,* Vol.23, No.1-2, (January-February 1975), pp. 1-3, ISSN 0048-0169

Løvstad, R. A. (2006). A Kinetic Study on the Phenothiazine Dependent Oxidation of NADH by Bovine Ceruloplasmin. *Biometals,* Vol.19, No.1, (February 2006), pp. 1-5, ISSN 0966-0844

Machnicki, M.; Zimecki, M. & Zagulski, T. (1993). Lactoferrin Regulates the Release of Tumour Necrosis Factor Alpha and Interleukin 6 In Vivo. *International Journal of Experimental Pathology,* Vol.74, No.5, (October 1993), pp. 433–439, ISSN 0959-9673

Macintyre, G.; Gutfreund, K.; Martin, W.; Camicioli, R. & Cox, D. (2004). Value of an Enzymatic Assay for the Determination of Serum Ceruloplasmin. *The Journal of Laboratory & Clinical Medicine,* Vol.144, No.6, (December 2004), pp. 294–301, ISSN 0022-2143

Mack, D. R.; McDonald, T. L.; Larson, M. A.; Wei, S. & Weber, A. (2003). The Conserved TFLK Motif of Mammary-associated Serum Amyloid A3 is Responsible for Up-regulation of Intestinal MUC3 Mucin Expression In Vitro. *Pediatric Research,* Vol.53, No.1, (January 2003), pp. 137-142, ISSN 0031-3998

Mackiewicz, A. (1997). Acute Phase Proteins and Transformed Cells. *International Review of Cytology,* Vol.170, pp. 225-300, ISSN 0074-7696

Maeda, N.; Yang, F.; Barnett, D. R.; Bowman, B. H. & Smithies, O. (1984). Duplication within the Haptoglobin Hp2 Gene. *Nature,* Vol.309, No.5964, (May 1984), pp. 131-135, ISSN 0028-0836

Maliszewski, C. R. (1991). CD14 and Immune Response to Lipopolysaccharide. *Science,* Vol.252, No.5010, (May 1991), pp. 1321–1322, ISSN 0036-8075

Maliszewski, C. R.; Ball, E. D.; Graziano, R. F. & Fanger, M. W. (1985). Isolation and Characterization of My23, a Myeloid Cell-derived Antigen Reactive with the Monoclonal Antibody AML-2-23. *Journal of Immunology,* Vol.135, No.3, (September 1985), pp. 1929-1936, ISSN 0022-1767

Malle, E.; Steinmetz, A. & Raynes, J.G. (1993). Serum Amyloid A (SAA): an Acute Phase Protein and Apolipoprotein. *Atherosclerosis*, Vol.102, Vol.2, (September 1993), pp. 131-146, ISSN 0021-9150

Malle, E.; Bollmann, A.; Steinmetz, A.; Gemsa, D.; Leis, H. J. & Sattler, W. (1997). Serum Amyloid A (SAA) Protein Enhances Formation of Cyclooxygenase Metabolites of Activated Human Monocytes. *FEBS Letters*, Vol.419, Vol.2-3, (December 1997), pp. 215-219, ISSN 0014-5793

Martin, F.; Santolaria, F.; Batista, N.; Milena, A.; Gonzalez-Reimers, E.; Brito, M. J. & Oramas, J. (1999). Cytokine Levels (IL-6 and INF-gamma), Acute Phase Response and Nutritional Status as Prognostic Factors in Lung Cancer. *Cytokine*, Vol.11, No.1, (January 1999), pp. 80-86, ISSN 1043-4666

Martinez-Subiela, S.; Tecles, F. & Ceron, J. J. (2007). Comparison of two Automated Spectrophotometric Methods for Ceruloplasmin Measurement in Pigs. *Research in Veterinary Science*, Vol.83, No.1, (August 2007), pp. 12-19, ISSN 0034-5288

Masson, P. L.; Heremans, J. F. & Schonne, E. (1969). Lactoferrin, an Iron-binding Protein in Neutrophilic Leukocytes. *The Journal Experimental Medicine*, Vol.130, No.3, (September 1969), pp. 643- 658, ISSN 0022-1007

Masson, P. (1970). In: *La Lactoferrine*, Editions Arscia, pp. 93-146, Bruxelles. Belgium

Matsuda I.; Pearson, T. & Holtzman N. A. (1974). Determination of Apoceruloplasmin by Radioimmunoassay in Nutritional copper deficiency, Menkes' kinky hair syndrome, Wilson's disease, and umbilical cord blood. *Pediatric Research*, Vol.8, No.10, (October 1974), pp. 821–24, ISSN 0031-3998

McCord, J. M. (1996). Effects of Positive Iron Status at a Cellular Level. *Nutrition Reviews*, Vol.54, No.3, (March 1996), pp. 85–88, ISSN 0029-6643

McDonald, T. L.; Larson, M. A.; Mack, D. R. & Weber, A. (2001). Elevated Extrahepatic Expression and Secretion of Mammary-asociated Serum Amyloid A 3 (M-SAA3) into Colostrum. *Veterinary Immunology and Immunopathology*, Vol.83, No.3-4, (December 2001), pp. 203-211, ISSN 0165-2427

McGinley, M. D.; Narhi, L. O.; Kelley, M. J.; Davy, E.; Robinson, J.; Rohde, M. F.; Wright, S. D. and Lichenstein, H. S. (1995). CD14: Physical Properties and Identification of an Exposed Site that is Protected by Lipopolysaccharide. *Journal of Biological Chemistry*, Vol.270, No.10, (March 1995), pp. 5213-5218, ISSN 0021-9258

Meek, R. L.; Eriksen, N. & Benditt, E. P. (1992). Murine Serum Amyloid A3 is a High-densityapolipoprotein and is Secreted by Macrophages. *Proceedings of the National Academy of Sciences of the United States of America*, Vol.89, No.17, (September 1992), pp. 7949-7952, ISSN 0027-8424

Meijer, G. A.; van der Meulen, J. & van Vuuren, A. M. (1993). Glutamine is a Potentially Limiting Amino Acid for Milk Production in Dairy Cows: A Hypothesis. *Metabolism: Clinical and Experimental*, Vol.42, No.3, (March 1993), pp. 358-364, ISSN 0026-0495

Mills, C. F.; Dalgarno, A. C. & Wenham, G. (1976). Biochemical and Pathological Changes in Tissues of Friesian Cattle during the Experimental Induction of Copper Deficiency. *The British Journal of Nutrition*, Vol.35, No.3, (May 1976), pp. 309-331, ISSN 0007-1145

Miyajima, H. (2003). Aceruloplasminemia, an Iron Metabolic Disorder, *Neuropathology*, Vol.23, No.4, (December 2003), pp. 345–350, ISSN 0919-6544

Miyata, M. & Furugouri, K. (1984). Serum Ferritin Concentration of Dairy Bulls: Determinations by Radioimmunoassy and Enzyme Immunoassy. *Japanese Journal of Veterinary* Science, Vol.46, No.6, (December 1984), pp. 783-789, ISSN 0021-5295

Miyata, M. & Furugouri, K. (1987). The Relationship between Serum Ferritin Concentration and Tissue Non-Heme Iron or Tissue Ferritin in Dairy Cattle. *Japanese Journal of Veterinary* Science, Vol.49, No.6, (December 1987), pp. 1157-1159, ISSN 0021-5295

Miyata, Y.; Furugouri, K. & Shijimaya, K. (1984). Developmental Changes in Serum Ferritin Concentration of Dairy Calves. *Journal of Dairy Science*, Vol. 67, No.6, (June 1984), pp. 1256-1263, ISSN 0022-0302

Miyata, Y.; Furugouri, K.; Shijimaya, K. & Ando, S. (1986). Effect of Growth Rate and Grazing on Ferritin [Iron-Protein Complex], Iron and Total Iron-Binding Capacity of Serum From Holstein Steers. *Japanese Journal of Zootechnical Science*, Vol.57, No.6, (January 1986), pp. 36-44, ISSN 0021-5309

Mold, C.; Gresham, H. D. & Du Clos, T. W. (2001). Serum Amyloid P Component and C-Reactive Protein Mediate Phagocytosis through Murine FcγRs. *Journal of Immunology*, Vol.166, No.2, (January 2001), pp. 1200–1205, ISSN 0022-1767

Molenaar, A. J.; Harris, D. P.; Rajan, G. H.; Pearson, M. L.; Callaghan, M. R.; Sommer, L.; Farr, V. C.; Oden, K. E.; Miles, M. C.; Petrova, R. S.; Good, L. L.; Singh, K.; McLaren, R. D.; Prosser, C. G.; Kim, K. S.; Wieliczko, R. J.; Dines, M. H.; Johannessen, K. M.; Grigor, M. R.; Davis, S. R. & Stelwagen, K. (2009). The Acute Phase Protein Serum Amyloid A is Expressed in the Bovine Mammary Gland and Plays a Role in Host Defense. *Biomarkers*, Vol.14, No.1, (February 2009), pp. 26-37, ISSN 1354-750X

Momotani, E.; Furugouri, K.; Obara, Y.; Miyata, Y.; Ishikawa, Y. & Yoshino, T. (1986). Immunohistochemical Distribution of Ferritin, Lactoferrin, and Transferrin in Granulomas of Bovine Paratuberculosis. *Infection and Immunity*, Vol.52, No.2, (May 1986), pp. 623-627, ISSN 0019-9567 001-9567

Montreuil, J.; Tonnelat, J. & Mullet, S. (1960). Preparation and Properties of Lactosiderophilin (Lactotransferrin) of Human Milk. *Biochimica et Biophysica Acta*, Vol.45, (December 1960), pp. 413–421, ISSN 0006-3002

Moore, S. A.; Anderson, B. F.; Groom, C. R.; Haridas, M. & Baker, E. N. (1997). Three-dimensional Structure of Diferric Bovine Lactoferrin at 2.8 A resolution. *Journal of Molecular Biology*, Vol.274, No.2, (November 1997), pp. 222-236, ISSN 0022-2836

Morimatsu, M.; Sakai, H.; Yoshimatsu, K.; Minowa, O.; Yamamoto, S.; Yatomi, K.; Fujinaga, T. & Naiki, M. (1989). Isolation and Characterization of C-reactive Protein and Serum Amyloid P Component from Bovine Serum. *The Japanese Journal of Veterinary Science*, Vol.51, No.4, (August 1989), pp.723-732, ISSN 0021-5295

Morimatsu, M.; Watanabe, A.; Yoshimatsu, K.; Fujinaga, T.; Okubo, M. & Naiki, M. (1991). Elevation of Bovine Serum C-reactive Protein and Serum Amyloid P Component Levels by Lactation. *The Journal of Dairy Research*, Vol.58, No.3, (August 1991), pp.257-261, ISSN 0022-0299

Morris, H. R.; Panico, M.; Etienne, T.; Tippins, J.; Girgis, S. I. & MacIntyre, I. (1984). Isolation and Characterization of Human Calcitonin Gene-related Peptide. *Nature*, Vol.308, No.5961, (April 1994), pp. 746-748, ISSN 0028-0836

Moshage, H. (1997). Cytokines and the Hepatic Acute Phase Response. *The Journal of Pathology*, Vol.181, No.3, (March 1997), pp. 257-266, ISSN 0022-3417

Mukesh, M.; Bionaz, M.; Graugnard, D. E.; Drackley, J. K. & Loor, J. J. (2010). Adipose Tissue Depots of Holstein Cows are Immune Responsive: Inflammatory Gene Expression In Vitro. *Domestic Animal Endocrinology*, Vol.38, No.3, (April 2010), pp. 168-178, ISSN 0739-7240

Mukhopadhyay, C.; Mazumder, B. & Lindley, P. (1997). Identification of the Prooxidant Site of Human Ceruloplasmin: a Model for Oxidative Damage by Copper bound to Protein Surfaces. *Proceedings of the National Academy of Sciences of the United States of America*, Vol.94, No.21, (October 1997), pp. 11546–11551, ISSN 0027-8424

Nazifi, S.; Razavi, S. M.; Esmailnejad, Z. & Gheisari, H. (2009). Study on Acute Phase Proteins (Haptoglobin, Serum Amyloid A, Fibrinogen, and Ceruloplasmin) Changes and their Diagnostic Values in Bovine Tropical Theileriosis. *Parasitology Research*, Vol.105, No.1, (July 2009), pp. 41-46, ISSN 1432-1955

Nelson, K. G.; Takahashi, T.; Bossert, N. I.; Walmer, D. K. & Mclachlan, J. A. (1991). Epidermal Growth Factor Replaces Estrogen in the Stimulation of Female Genital-tract Growth and Differentation. *Proceedings of the National Academy of Sciences of the United States of America*, Vol.88, No.1, (January 1991), pp. 21–25, ISSN 0027-8424

Nielsen, B. H.; Jacobsen, S.; Andersen, P. H.; Niewold, T. A. & Heegaard, P. M. (2004). Acute Phase Protein Concentrations in Serum and Milk from Healthy Cows, Cows with Clinical Mastitis and Cows with Extramammary Inflammatory Conditions. *The Veterinary Record*, Vol.154, No.12, (March 2004), pp.361-365, ISSN 0042-4900

Nijsten, M. W. N.; Hack, C. E.; Helle, M.; ten Duis, H. J.; Klasen, H. J. & Aarden, L. A. (1991). Interleukin-6 and its Relation to the Humoral Immune Response and Clinical Parameters in Burned Patients. *Surgery*, Vol.109, No.6, (June 1991), pp. 761-767, ISSN 0039-6060

Nikunen, S.; Hartel, H.; Orro, T.; Neuvonen, E.; Tanskanen, R.; Kivela, S. L.; Sankari, S.; Aho, P.; Pyorala, S.; Saloniemi, H. & Soveri, T. (2007). Association of Bovine Respiratory Disease with Clinical Status and Acute Phase Proteins in Calves. *Comparative Immunology, Microbiology and Infectious Diseases*, Vol.30, No.3, (May 2007), pp. 143-151, ISSN 0147-9571

Nong, Y. H.; Titus, R. G.; Ribeiro, J. M. & Remold, H. G. (1989). Peptides Encoded by the Calcitonin Gene Inhibit Macrophage Function. *The Journal of Immunology*, Vol.143, No.1, (July 1989), pp. 45-49, ISSN 0022-1767

Ohtsuka, H., Kudo, K.; Mori, K.; Nagai, F.; Hatsugaya, A.; Tajima, M.; Tamura, K.; Hoshi, F.; Koiwa, M, & Kawamura S. (2001). Acute Phase Response in Nturally Occuring Coliform Mastitis. *The Journal of Veterinary Medical Science*, Vol.63, No.6, (June 2001), pp. 675-678, ISSN 1347-7439

Ohzato, H.; Yoshizaki, K.; Nishimoto, N.; Ogata, A.; Tagoh, H.; Monden, M.; Gotoh, M.; Kishimoto, T. & Mori, T. (1992). Interleukin-6 as a New Indicator of Inflammatory Status: Detection of Serum Levels of Interleukin-6 and C-Reactive Protein after Surgery. *Surgery*, Vol.111, No.2, (February 1992), pp.201-209, ISSN 0039-6060

Olivares, M. & Uauy, R. (1996). Copper as an Essential Nutrient. *American Journal of Clinical Nutrition*, Vol.63, No.5, (May 1996), pp. 791S–796S, ISSN 0002-9165

Orino, K.; Lehman, L.; Tsuji, Y.; Ayaki, H.; Torti, S.V. & Torti, F. M. (2001). Ferritin and the Response to Oxidative Stress. *Biochemical Journal*, Vol.357, No.1, (July 2001), pp. 241–247, ISSN 0264-6021

Orino, K.; Watanbe, S.; Ohtsuka, H.; Kohiruimaki, M. & Watanbe, K. (2004). Technical Note: Measurement of Ferritin in Bovine Milk and its Clinical Significance. *Journal of Dairy Science*, Vol.89, No.10, (October 2004), pp. 3842-3845, ISSN 0022-0302

Orino, K. & Watanabe, K. (2008). Molecular, Physiological and Clinical Aspects of the Iron Storage Protein Ferritin. *The Veterinary Journal,* Vol.178, No.2, (November 2008), pp. 191-201, ISSN 1090-0233

Orro, T.; Jacobsen, S.; LePage, J. P.; Niewold, T.; Alasuutari, S. & Soveri, T. (2008). Temporal Changes in Serum Concentrations of Acute Phase Proteins in Newborn Dairy Calves. *Veterinary Journal*, Vol.176, No.2, (May 2008), pp. 182-187, ISSN 1090-0233

Ota, T. & Katsuki, I. (1998). Ferritin Subunits in Sera and Synovial Fuids From Patients with Rheumatoid Arthritis. *Journal of Rheumatology,* Vol.25, No.12, (December 1998), pp. 2315–2318, ISSN 0315-162X

Paape, M. J.; Lilius, E. M.; Wiitanen, P. A.; Kontio, M. P. & Miller, R. H. (1996). Intramammary Defense Against Infections Induced by *Escherichia Coli* in Cows. *American Journal of Veterinary Research,* Vol.57, No.4, (April 1996), pp. 477-482, ISSN 0002-9645

Paape, M. J.; Rautiainen, P. M.; Lilius, E. M.; Malstrom, C. E. & Elsasser, T. H. (2002). Development of Anti-Bovine TNF-alpha mAb and ELISA for Quantitating TNF-alpha in Milk after Intramammary Injection of Endotoxin. *Journal of Dairy Science,* Vol.85, No.4, (April 2002), pp. 765-773, ISSN 0022-0302

Pedersen, L. H.; Aalbaek, B.; Rontved, C. M.; Ingvartsen, K. L.; Sorensen, N. S.; Heegaard, P. M. & Jensen, H. E. (2003). Early Pathogenesis and Inflammatory Response in Experimental Bovine Mastitis due to Streptococcus Uberis. *Journal of Comparative Pathology,* Vol.128, No.2-3, (February 2003), pp.156-164, ISSN 0021-9975

Pentecost, B. T. & Teng, C. T. (1987). Lactotransferrin is the Major Estrogen Inducible Protein in Mouse Uterine Secretions. *The Journal of Biological Chemistry,* Vol.262, No.21, (July 1987), pp. 10134–10139, ISSN 0021-9258

Petschow, B. W.; Talbott, R. D. & Batema, R. P. (1999). Ability of Lactoferrin to Promote the Growth of *Bifidobacterium* spp. *In Vitro* is Independent of Receptor Binding Capacity and Iron Saturation Level. *Journal of Medical Microbiology,* Vol.48, No.6, (June 1999), pp. 541–549, ISSN 0022-2615

Poitou, C.; Divoux, A.; Faty, A.; Tordjman, J.; Hugol, D.; Aissat, A.; Keophiphath, M.; Henegar, C.; Commans, S. & Clément, K. (2009). Role of Serum Amyloid a in Adipocyte-macrophage Cross Talk and Adipocyte Cholesterol Efflux. *The Journal of Clinical Endocrinology and Metabolism,* Vol.94, No.5, (May 2009), pp. 1810-1817, ISSN 0021-972X

Preciado-Patt, L.; Hershkoviz, R.; Fridkin, M. & Lider, O. (1996). Serum Amyloid A Binds Specific Extracellular Matrix Glycoproteins and Induces the Adhesion of Resting CD4+ T cells. *The Journal of Immunology,* Vol.156, No.3, (February 1996), pp. 1189-1195, ISSN 0022-1767

Pugin, J.; Heumann, I. D.; Tomasz, A.; Kravchenko, V. V.; Akamatsu, Y.; Nishijima, M.; Glauser, M. P.; Tobias, P. S. & Ulevitch, R. J. (1994). CD14 is a Pattern Recognition Receptor. *Immunity,* Vol.1, No.6, (September 1994), pp. 509-516, ISSN 1074-7613

Quaye, I. K. (2008). Haptoglobin, Inflammation and Disease. *Transactions of the Royal Society of Tropical Medicine and Hygiene,* Vol.102, No.8, (August 2008), pp. 735-742, ISSN 0035-9203

Rahman, M. M.; Lecchi, C.; Avallone, G.; Roccabianca, P.; Sartorelli, P. & Ceciliani, F. (2010). Lipopolysaccharide-Binding Protein: Local Expression in Bovine Extrahepatic Tissues. *Veterinary Immunology and Immunopathology*, Vol.137, No.1-2, (September 2010), pp. 28-35, ISSN 1873-2534

Rao, K. S.; Roberts, T. K.; Masson, P. L. & Heremans, J. F. (1973). Lactoferrin, as a Major Soluble Protein of Bovine Oestrus Cervical Mucus. *Journal of Reproduction and Fertility*, Vol.32, No.1, (January 1973), pp. 89-92, ISSN 0022-4251

Rogers, J. T.; Bridges, K. R.; Durmowicz, G. P.; Glass, J.; Auron, P. E. & Munro, H. N. (1990). Translational Control during the Acute Phase Response. Ferritin Synthesis in Response to Interleukin-1. *The Journal of Biological Chemistry*, Vol.265, No.24, (August 1990), pp. 14572-14578, ISSN 0021-9258

Roperto, S.; Borzacchiello, G.; Brun, R.; Costanzo, F.; Faniello, M. C.; Raso, C.; Rosati, A.; Russo, V.; Leonardix, L.; Saracinok, D.; Turco. M. C.; Uttaro, C. & Roperto, F. (2010). Ferritin Heavy Chain (FHC) is Up-regulated in Papillomavirus-associated Urothelial Tumours of the Urinary Bladder in Cattle. *Journal of Comparative Pathology*, Vol.142, No.1, (January 2010), pp. 9-18, ISSN 0021-9975

Russwurm, S.; Stonans, I.; Stonane, E.; Wiederhold, M.; Luber, A.; Zipfel, P. F.; Deigner, H. P. & Reinhart, K. (2001). Procalcitonin and CGRP-1 mRNA Expression in Various Human Tissues. *Shock*, Vol.16, No.2, (August 2001), pp. 109-112, ISSN 1073-2322

Sacks, G. P.; Seyani, L.; Lavery, S. & Trew, G. (2004). Maternal C-reactive Protein Levels are Raised at 4 Weeks Gestation. *Human Reproduction*, Vol.19, No.4, (April 2004), pp. 1025–1030, ISSN 0268-1161

Sadrzadeh, S. M.; Graf, E.; Panter, S. S.; Hallaway, P. E. & Eaton, J. W. (1984). Hemoglobin. a Biologic Fenton Reagent. *Journal of Biological Chemistry*, Vol.259, No.23, (December 1984), pp. 14354-14356, ISSN 0021-9258

Saeed, S. A.; Ahmad, N. & Ahme, S. (2007). Dual Inhibition of Cyclooxygenase and Lipooxygenase by Human Haptoglobin: its Polymorphism and Relation to Hemoglobin Binding. *Biochemical and Biophysical Research Communications*, Vol.353, No.4, (February 2007), pp. 915-920, ISSN 0006 291X

Salvatore, A.; Cigliano, L.; Bucci, E. M.; Corpillo, D.; Velasco, S.; Carlucci, A.; Pedone, C. & Abrescia, P. (2007). Haptoglobin Binding to Apolipoprotein A-I Prevents Damage from Hydroxyl Radicals on its Stimulatoory Activity of the Enzyme Lecithin-cholesterol Acyl-transferase. *Biochemistry*, Vol.46, No.39, (October 2007), pp. 11158-11168, ISSN 0006-2960

Samols, D.; Agrawal, A. & Kushner, I. (2002). Acute Phase Proteins. In: *Cytokine Reference On-Line*, J. J. Oppenheim & Feldman, M. (Ed.), Academic Press, Harcourt, London, UK,

Sanchez, L.; Calvo, M. & Brock, J. H. (1992). Biological Role of Lactoferrin. *Archives of Disease in Childhood*, Vol.67, No.5, (May 1992), pp. 657–661, ISSN 1468-2044

Savedra, R. J. r.; Delude, R. L.; Ingalls, R. R.; Fenton, M. J. & Golenbock, D. T. (1996). Mycobacterial Lipoarabinomannan Recognition Requires a Receptor that Shares Components of the Endotoxin Signaling System. *The Journal of Immunology*, Vol.157, No.6, (September 1996), pp. 2549-2554, ISSN 0022-1767

Schrödl, W.; Krueger, M.; Hien, T. T.; Fuldner, M. & Kunze, R. (1995). [C-reactive Protein as a new Parameter of Mastitis]. *Tierarztliche Praxis*, Vol.23, No.4, (August 1995), pp.337-341, ISSN 0303-6286

Schrödl, W.; Fuerll, B.; Reinhold, P.; Krueger, M. & Schuett, C. (2001). A Novel Acute Phase Marker in Cattle: Lipopolysaccharide Binding Protein (LBP). *Journal of Endotoxin Research*, Vol.7, No.1, (February 2001), pp. 49-52, ISSN 1753-4259, ISSN 0968-0519

Schrödl, W.; Jaekel, L. & Krueger, M. (2003). C-reactive Protein and Antibacterial Activity in Blood Plasma of Colostrum Fed Calves and the Effect of Lactulose. *Journal of Dairy Science*, Vol.86, No.10, (October 2003), pp. 3313-3320, ISSN 0022-0302

Schumann, R. R.; Rietschel, E. T. & Loppnow, H. (1994). The Role of CD14 and Lipopolysaccharide-Binding Protein (LBP) in the Activation of Different Cell Types by Endotoxin. *Medical Microbiology and Immunology*, Vol.183, No.6, (December 1994), pp. 279-297, ISSN 0300-8584

Schumann, R. R.; Leong, S. R.; Flaggs, G. W.; Gray, P. W.; Wright, S. D.; Mathison, J. C.; Tobias, P. S. & Ulevitch, R. J. (1990). Structure and Function of Lipopolysaccharide Binding Protein. *Science*, Vol.249, No.4975, (September 1990), pp. 1429-1431, ISSN 0036-8075

Schutt, C.; Schilling, T.; Grunwald, U.; Schonfeld, W. & Kruger, C. (1992). Endotoxin Neutralizing Capacity of Soluble CD14. *Research in Immunology*, Vol.143, No.1, (January 1992), pp. 71-78, ISSN 0021-9258

Shah, C.; Hari-Dass, R. & Raynes, J. G. (2006). Serum Amyloid A is an Innate Immune Opsonin for Gram-Negative Bacteria. *Blood*, Vol.108, No.5, (September 2006), pp. 1751-1757, ISSN 0006-4971

Shearer, J. K.; Bray, D. R.; Umphrey, J. E.; Elliott, J. B. (1996). Factors Influencing the Incidence of Lameness in Dairy Cattle, *Proceedings of the 33rd Annual Florida Dairy Production Conference*, pp. 40-51, Gainesville, Florida, USA, April 9-10, 1996

Sheldon, I. M.; Noakes, D. E.; Rycroft, A. & Dobson, H. (2001). Acute Phase Protein Responses to Uterine Bacterial Contamination in Cattle after Calving. *The Veterinary Record*, Vol.148, No.6, (February 2001), pp. 172-175, ISSN 0042-4900

Sheldon, I. M.; Noakes, D. E.; Rycroft, A. N. & Dobson, H. (2002). Effect of Postpartum Manual Examination of the Vagina on Uterine Bacterial Contamination in Cows. *The Veterinary Record*, Vol.151, No.18, (November 2002), pp. 531-534, ISSN 0042-4900

Shrive, A. K.; Cheetham, G. M. T.; Holden, D.; Myles, D. A. A.; Turnell, W. G.; Volanakis, J. E.; Pepys, M. B.; Bloomer, A. C. & Greenhough, T. J. (1996). Three Dimensional Structure of Human C-Reactive Protein. *Nature Structural and Molecular Biology*, Vol.3, No.4, (April 1996), pp. 346-354, ISSN 1072-8368

Sibille, J. C.; Kondo, H. & Aisen, P. (1988) Interactions between Isolated Hepatocytes and Kupffer Cells in Iron Metabolism: a Possible Role for Ferritin as an Iron Carrier Protein. *Hepatology*, Vol.8, No.2, (March-April 1988), pp. 296–301, ISSN 0270-9139

Skinner, J. G. (2001). International Standardization of Acute Phase Proteins. *Veterinary Clinical Pathology*, Vol.30, No.1, pp. 2-7, ISSN 0275-6382

Smith, B. I.; Donovan, G. A.; Risco, C. A.; Young, C. R. & Stanker, L. H. (1998). Serum Haptoglobin Concentrations in Holstein Dairy Cattle with Toxic Puerperal Metritis. *The Veterinary Record*, Vol.142, No.4, (January 1998), pp. 83-85, ISSN 0042-4900

Smith, J. E. (1997). Iron Metabolism and its Disorders, In: *Clinical biochemistry of domestic animals*, J. J. Kaneko, J. W. Harvey, & M. Bruss, (Ed.), 223- 240. Academic Press Limited, ISBN 0-12-396305-2, California, USA

Smith, B. I.; Kauffold, J. & Sherman, L. (2010). Serum Haptoglobin Concentrations in Dairy Cattle with Lameness due to Claw Disorders. *The Veterinary Journal*, Vol.186, No.2, (November 2010), pp. 162-165, ISSN 1090-0233

Sohn, E. J.; Paape, M. J.; Peters, R. R.; Fetterer, R. H.; Talbot, N. C. & Bannerman, D. D. (2004). The Production and Characterization of Anti-bovine CD14 Monoclonal Antibodies. *Veterinary Research*, Vol.35, No. 5, (September 2004), pp.597-608, ISSN 0928-4249

Sohn, E. J.; Paape, M. J.; Bannerman, D. D.; Connor, E. E.; Fetterer, R. H. & Peters, R. R. (2007). Shedding of Scd14 by Bovine Neutrophils Following Activation with Bacterial Lipopolysaccharide Results in Down-regulation Of IL-8. *Veterinary Research*, Vol.38, No.1, (January-February 2007), pp. 95-108, ISSN 0928-4249

Squires, R. A. (2004) Host Pathogen Interactions. In: *Veterinary pathophysiology*, R. H. Dunlop & C. Malbert, (Ed.), 79-110. Blackwell Publishing Ltd., ISBN 978-0-8138-2826-8, Oxford, UK

Steel, D. M. & Whitehead, A. S. (1994). The Major Acute Phase Reactants: C-reactive Protein, Serum Amyloid P Component and Serum Amyloid A Protein. *Immunology Today*. Vol.15, No.2, (February 1994), pp. 81-88, ISSN 0167-5699

Sternlieb, I.; Morell, A. G.; Tucker, W. D.; Greene, M. W. & Scheinberg, I. H. (1961). The Incorporation of Copper into Ceruloplasmin *In Vivo*: Studies with Copper^{64} and Copper^{67}. *The Journal of Clinical investigation*, Vol.40, No.10, (October 1961), pp. 1834-1840, ISSN 0021-9738

Suojala, L.; Orro, T.; Jarvinen, H.; Saatsi, J. & Pyorala, S. (2008). Acute Phase Response in two Consecutive Experimentally Induced E. Coli Intramammary Infections in Dairy Cows. *Acta Veterinaria Scandinavica*, Vol.50, No.1, (June 2008), pp. 18, ISSN 1751-0147

Surguladze, N.; Patton, S.; Cozzi, A.; Fried, M. G. & Connor, J. R. (2005). Characterization of Nuclear Ferritin and Mechanism of Translocation. *Biochemical Journal*, Vol.388, No.3, (June 2005), pp. 731-740, ISSN 0264-6021

Suryakala, S. & Deshpande, V. (1999). Purification and Characterization of Liver Ferritins from Different Animal Species. *Veterinary Research Communications*, Vol.23, No.3, (May 1999), pp. 165-181, ISSN 0165-7380

Susana, A.; Chavez, G.; Gallegos, S. A. & Cruz, Q. R. (2009). Lactoferrin: Structure, Function and Application. *International Journal of Antimicrobial Agents*, Vol.33, No.4, pp. 301.e1-301.e8, ISSN 1872-7913

Suttle, N. F. (2010). *Mineral Nutrition in Livestock*, 4th edition, 334-354. CABI, ISBN 978-1-84593-472-9, Oxfordshire, UK

Szczubiał, M.; Dąbrowski, R.; Kankofer, M.; Bochniarz, M. & Albera, E. (2008). Concentration of Serum Amyloid a and Activity of Ceruloplasmin in Milk from Cows with Clinical and Subclinical Mastitis. *The Bulletin of the Veterinary Institute in Pulawy*, Vol.52, No.2, pp. 391–395

Tabrizi, A. D.; Batavani, R. A.; Rezaei, S. A. & Ahmadi, M. (2008). Fibrinogen and Ceruloplasmin in Plasma and Milk from Dairy Cows with Subclinical and Clinical Mastitis. *Pakistan Journal of Biological Sciences*, Vol.11, No.4, (February 2008), pp. 571-576, ISSN 1028-8880

Takahashi, E.; Kuwayama H.; Kawamoto, K.; Matsui, T. & Inokuma, H. (2009). Detection Serum amyloid A Isoforms in Cattle. *Journal of Veterinary Diagnostic Investigation*, Vol.21, No.6, (November 2009), pp. 874-877, ISSN 1040-6387

Teng, C. T.; Beard, C. & Gladwell, W. (2002). Differential Expression and Estrogen Response of Lactoferrin Gene in the Female Reproductive Tract of Mouse, Rat and Hamster. *Biology of Reproduction*, Vol.67, No.5, (November 2002), pp. 1439–1449, ISSN 0006-3363

Tang, Y.; Han, C.; Fiscus, R. R. & Wang, X. (1997). Increase of Calcitonin Gene-related Peptide (CGRP) Release and mRNA levels in Endotoxic Rats. *Shock*, Vol.7, No.3, (March 1997), pp. 225-229, ISSN 1073-2322

Terada, K.; Kawarada, Y.; Miura, N.; Yasui, O.; Koyama, K. & Sugiyama, T. (1995). Copper Incorporation into Ceruloplasmin in Rat Livers. *Biochimica et Biophysica Acta*, Vol.1270, No.1, (January 1995), pp. 58–62, ISSN 0925-4439

Teran, E.; Escudero, C.; Moya, W.; Flores, M.; Vallance, P. & Lopez- Jaramillo, P. (2001). Elevated C-reactive Protein and Proinflammatory Cytokines in Andean Women with Pre-eclampsia. *International Journal of Gynaecology & Obstetrics*, Vol.75, No.3, (December 2001), pp. 243–249, ISSN 0020-7292

Theil, E. C. (1987). Ferritin: Structure, Gene Regulation, and Cellular Function in Animals, Plants, and Microorganisms. *Annual Review of Biochemistry*, Vol.56, (July 1987) pp. 289-315, ISSN 0066-4154

Thomas, T. & Schreiber, G. (1989). The Expression of Genes Coding for Positive Acute-phase Proteins in the Reproductive Tract of the Female Rat. High Levels of Ceruloplasmin mRNA in the Uterus. *FEBS letters*, Vol.243, No.2, (January 1989), pp. 381-384, ISSN 0014-5793

Thomas, T.; Schreiber, G. & Jaworowski, A. (1989). Developmental Patterns of Gene Expression of Secreted Proteins in Brain and Choroid Plexus. *Developmental Biology*, Vol.134, No.1, (July 1989), pp. 38-47, ISSN 0012-1606

Thompson, D.; Pepys, M. B. & Wood, S. P. (1999).The Physiological Structure of Human C-Reactive Protein and its Complex with Phosphocholine. *Structure*, Vol.7, No.2, (February 1999), pp. 169-177, ISSN 0969-2126

Tillet, W. S. & Francis, T. J. (1930). Serological Reactions in Pneumonia with a Non-protein Somatic Fraction of Pneumococcus. *Journal of Experimental Medicine*, Vol.52, No.4, (September 1930), pp. 561-571, ISSN 0022-1007

Tobias, P. S.; Soldau, K.; Iovine, N.; Elsbach, P. & Weiss, J. (1997). Lipopolyseccharide (LPS) Binding Proteins BPI and LBP form Different Complexes with LPS. *Journal of Biological Chemistry*, Vol.272, No.30, (July 1997), pp. 18682-18685, ISSN 0021-9258

Tobias, P. S.; Tapping, R. I. & Gegner, J. A. (1999). Endotoxin Interactions with Lipopolysaccharide-responsive Cells. *Clinical Infectious Diseases*, Vol.28, No.3, (March 1999), pp. 476-481, ISSN 1058-4838

Torti, F. M. & Torti, S. V. (2002). Regulation of Ferritin Genes and Protein. *Blood*, Vol.99, No.10, (May 2002), pp. 3505–3516, ISSN 0006-4971

Torti, S. V.; Kwak, E. L.; Miller, S. C.; Miller, L. L.; Ringold, G. M.; Myambo, K. B.; Young, A. P. & Torti, F. M. (1988). The Molecular Cloning and Characterization of Murine Ferritin Heavy Chain, A Tumor Necrosis Factor-Inducible Gene. *Journal of Biological Chemistry*, Vol.263, No.25, (September 1998), pp. 12638–12644, ISSN 0021-9258

Tourlomoussis, P.; Eckersall, P. D.; Waterson, M. M. & Buncic, S. (2004). A Comparison of Acute Phase Protein Measurements and Meat Inspection Findings in Cattle. *Foodborne Pathogens and Disease*, Vol.1, No.4, (December 2004), pp. 281-290, ISSN 1535-3141

Travis, J. C. & Sanders, B. G. (1972). Haptoglobin Evolution: Polymeric Forms of Haptoglobin in the Bovidae and Cervidae Families. *The Journal of Experimental Zoology*, Vol.180, No.1, (April 1972), pp. 141-148, ISSN 0022-104X

Tsuji, Y.; Kwak, E.; Saika, T.; Torti, S. V. & Torti, F. M. (1993). Preferential Repression of the H Subunit of Ferritin by Adenovirus E1A in NIH-3T3 Mouse Fbroblasts. *Journal of Biological Chemistry*, Vol.268, No.10, (April 1993), pp. 7270–7275, ISSN 0021-9258

Tsuji, Y.; Ayaki, H.; Whitman, S. P.; Morrow, C. S.; Torti, S. V. & Torti, F. M. (2000). Coordinate Transcriptional and Translational Regulation of Ferritin in Response to Oxidative Stress. *Molecular and Cellular Biology*, Vol.20, No.16, (August 2000), pp. 5818–5827, ISSN 0270-7306

Turk, R.; Juretić, D.; Geres, D.; Bacić, G.; Milesević, M.; Flegar-Mestrić, Z.; Turk, N. & Svetina, A. (2008). Bovine Platelet-activating Factor Acetylhydrolase (PAF-AH) Activity Related to Fertility. *Animal Reproduction Science*, Vol.105, No.3-4, (May 2008), pp. 344-353, ISSN 0378-4320

Uhlar, C. M.; Burgess, C. J.; Sharp, P. M. & Whitehead, A. S. (1994). Evolution of the Serum Amyloid A (SAA) Protein Superfamily. *Genomics*, Vol.19, No.2, (January 1994), pp. 228-235, ISSN 0888-7543

Uhlar, C. M. & Whitehead, A. S. (1999). Serum Amyloid A, the Major Vertebrate Acute Phase Reactant. *European Journal of Biochemistry*, Vol.265, No.2, (October 1999), pp. 501-523, ISSN 0014-2956

Ulevitch, R. J. & Tobias, P. S. (1995). Receptor-dependent Mechanisms of Cell Stimulation by Bacterial Endotoxin. *Annual Review of Immunology*, Vol.13, pp. 437-457, ISSN 0732-0582

Urushizaki, I. & Kohgo, Y. (1980). [Structural and Immunological Characteristics of Ferritin (author's transl)]. *The Japanese Journal of Clinical Hematology*, Vol.21, No.8, (August 1980), pp.1084-1089, ISSN 0485-1439

van der Westhuyzen, D. R.; de Beer, F. C. & Webb N. R. (2007). HDL Cholesterol Transport during Inflammation. *Current Opinion in Lipidology*, Vol.18, No.2, (April 2007), pp. 147-151, ISSN 0957-9672

Veronesi, B.; Carter, J. D.; Devlin, R. B.; Simon, S. A. & Oortgiesen, M. (1999). Neuropeptides and Capsaicin Stimulate the Release of Inflammatory Cytokines in a Human Bronchial Epithelial Cell Line. *Neuropeptides*, Vol.33, No.6, (December 1999), pp. 447-456, ISSN 0143-4179

Vignais, P. V. (2002). The Superoxide-Generating NADPH Oxidase: Structural Aspects and Activation Mechanism. *Cellular and Molecular Life Sciences*, Vol.59, No.9, (September 2002), pp. 1428–1459, ISSN 1420-682X

Vigushin, D. M.; Pepys, M. B. & Hawkins, P. N. (1993). Metabolic and Scintigraphic Studies of Radioiodinated Human C-reactive Protein in Health and Disease. *Journal of Clinical Investigation*, Vol.91, No.4, (April 1993), pp. 1351–1357, ISSN 0021-9738

Volanakis, J. E. & Kaplan, M. H. (1971). Specificity of C-Reactive Protein for Choline Phosphate Residues of Pneumococcal C-polysaccharide. *Proceedings of the Society for*

Experimental Biology and Medicine, Vol.136, No.2 (February 1971), pp. 612-614, ISSN 0037-9727

Volanakis, J. E. & Wirtz, K. W. A. (1979). Interaction of C-Reactive Protein with Artificial Phosphatidylcholine Bilayers. *Nature,* Vol.281, No.5727, (September 1979), pp. 155-157, ISSN 0028-0836

Volanakis, J. E. (2001). Human C-reactive Protein: Expression, Structure, and Function. *Molecular Immunology,* Vol.38, No.2-3, (August 2001), pp. 189-197, ISSN 0161-5890

Walmer, D. K.; Wrona, M. A.; Hughes, C. I. & Nelson, K. G. (1992): Lactoferrin Expression in the Mouse Reproductive Tract during the Natural Estrous Cycle: Correlation with Circulating Estradiol and Progesterone. *Endocrinology,* Vol.131, No.3, (September 1992), pp. 1458–1466, ISSN 0013-7227

Wang, W.; Knovich, M. A.; Coffman, L. G.; Torti, F. M. & Torti, S. V. (2010). Serum Ferritin: Past, Present and Future. *Biochimica et Biophysica Acta,* Vol.1800, No.8, (August 2010), pp. 760-769, ISSN 0006-3002

Wang, Y.; Paape, M. J.; Leino, L.; Capuco, A. V. & Narva, H. (1997). Functional and Phenotypic Characterization of Monoclonal Antibodies to Bovine L-selectin. *American Journal of Veterinary Research,* Vol.58, No.12, (December 1997), pp. 1392-1401, ISSN 0002-9645

Ward, P. P.; Uribe-Luna, S. & Conneely, O. M. (2002). Lactoferrin and Host Defense. *Biochemistry and Cell Biology,* Vol.80, No.1, pp.95-102, ISSN 0829-8211

Wasserman, W. W. & Fahl, W. E. (1997). Functional Antioxidant Responsive Elements. *Proceedings of the National Academic Sciences of the United States of America,* Vol.94, No.10, (May 1997), pp. 5361–5366, ISSN 0027-8424

Weber A.; Weber A. T.; McDonald T. L. & Larson M. A. (2006). Staphylococcus Aureus Lipotechoic Acid Induces Differential Expression of Bovine Serum Amyloid A3 (SAA3) by Mammary Epithelial Cells: Implications for Early Diagnosis of Mastitis. *Veterinary Immunology and Immunopathology,* Vol.109, No.1-2, (January 2006), pp. 79-83, ISSN 0165-2427

Wei, Y.; Miller, S. C.; Tsuji, Y.; Torti, S. V. & Torti F. M. (1990). Interleukin 1 Induces Ferritin Heavy Chain in Human Muscle Cells. *Biochemical and Biophysical Research Communications,* Vol.169, No.1, (May 1990), pp. 289–296, ISSN 0006-291X

Weinberg, E. D. (1984). Iron Withholding: a Defense Against Infection and Neoplasia. *Physiological Reviews,* Vol.64, No.1, (January 1984), pp. 65-102, ISSN 0031-9333

Wenz, J. R.; Fox, L. K.; Muller, F. J.; Rinaldi, M.; Zeng, R. & Bannerman, D. D. (2010). Factors Associated with Concentrations of Select Cytokine and Acute Phase Proteins in Dairy Cows with Naturally Occurring Clinical Mastitis. *Journal of Dairy Science,* Vol.93, No.6, (June 2010), pp. 2458-2470, ISSN 0022-0302

Wicher, K. B. & Fries, E. (2007). Convergent Evolution of Human and Bovine Haptoglobin: Partial Dublication of the Genes. *Journal of Molecular Evolution,* Vol.65, No.4, (October 2007), pp. 373-379, ISSN 0022-2844

Winter, P.; Fuchs, K.; Walshe, K. & Colditz, I. G. (2003). Serum Amyloid A in the Serum and Milk of Ewes with Mastitis Induced Experimentally with Staphylococcus Epidermidis. *The Veterinary Record,* Vol.152, No.18, (May 2003), pp.558-562, ISSN 0042-4900

Wolf, M.; Kettyle, E.; Sandler, L.; Ecker, J. L.,; Roberts, J. & Thadhani, R. (2001). Obesity and Preeclampsia: the Potential Role of Inflammation. *Obstetrics & Gynecology*, Vol.98, No.5, (November 2001), pp. 757–762, ISSN 0029-7844

Wurfel, M. M.; Hailman, E. & Wright, S. D. (1995). Soluble CD14 Acts as a Shuttle in the Neutralization of Lipopolysaccharide (LPS) by LPS-Binding Protein and Reconstituted High Density Lipoprotein. *The Journal of Experimental Medicine*, Vol.181, No.5, (May 1995), pp. 1743-1754, ISSN 0022-1007

Yamauchi, K.; Wakabayashi, H.; Hashimoto, S.; Teraguchi, S.; Hayasawa, H. & Tomita, M. (1998). Effects of Orally Administered Bovine Lactoferrin on the Immune System of Healthy Volunteers. *Advances in Experimental Medicine and Biology*, Vol.443, pp. 261-265, ISSN 0065-2598

Yang, W. Z.; Ametaj, B. N.; Benchaar, C.; He, M. L. & Beauchemin, K. A. (2010). Cinnamaldehyde in Feedlot Cattle Diets: Intake, Growth Performance, Carcass Characteristics, and Blood Metabolites. *Journal of Animal Science*, Vol.88, No.3, (March 2010), pp. 1082-1092, ISSN 1525-3163

Yang, R. Z.; Lee, M. J.; Hu, H.; Pollin, T. I.; Ryan, A. S.; Nicklas, B. J.; Snitker, S.; Horenstein, R. B.; Hull, K.; Goldberg, N. H.; Goldberg, A. P.; Shuldiner, A. R.; Fried, S. K. & Gong, D. W. (2006). Acute Phase Serum Amyloid A: an Inflammatory Adipokine and Potential Link between Obesity and its Metabolic Complications. *PLoS Medicine*, Vol.3, No.6, (June 2006), pp. e287, ISSN 1549-1277

Yang, F.; Brune, J. L.; Baldwin, W. D.; Barnett, D. R. & Bowman, B. H. (1983). Identification and Characterization of Human Haptoglobin cDNA. *Proceedings of the National Academy of Sciences of the United States of America*, Vol.80, No.19, (October 1983), pp. 5875-5879, ISSN 0027-8424

Yang, F.; Naylor, S. L.; Lum, J. B.; Cutshaw, S.; McCombs, J. L.; Naberhaus, K. H.; McGill, J. R.; Adrian, G. S.; Moore, C. M. & Barnett, D. R. (1986). Characterization, Mapping, and Expression of the Human Ceruloplasmin Gene. *Proceedings of the National Academy of Sciences of the United States of America*, Vol.83, No.10, (May 1986), pp. 3257-3261, ISSN 0027-8424

Yang, F.; Friedrichs, W. E.; Navarijo-Ashbaugh, A. L.; deGraffenried, L. A.; Bowman, B. H. & Coalson, J. J. (1995). Cell Type-specific and Inflammatory-induced Expression of Haptoglobin Gene in Lung. *Laboratory Investigation*, Vol.73, No.3, (September 1995), pp. 433-440, ISSN 0023-6837

Yi, M.; Kaneko, S.; Yu, D. Y. & Murakami, S. (1997). Hepatitis C Virus Envelope Proteins Bind Lactoferrin. *The Journal of Virology*, Vol.71, No.8, (August 1997), pp. 5997-6002, ISSN 0022-538X

Yokomori, N.; Iwasa, Y.; Aida, K.; Inoue, M.; Tawata, M. & Onaya, T. (1991). Transcriptional Regulation of Ferritin Messenger Ribonucleic Acid Levels by Insulin in Cultured Rat Glioma Cells. *Endocrinology*, Vol.128, No.3, (March 1991) pp. 1474–1480, ISSN 0013-7227

Young, A. A.; Rink, T. J. & Wang, M. W. (1993). Dose Response Characteristics for the Hyperglycemic, Hyperlactemic, Hypotensive and Hypocalcemic Actions of Amylin and Calcitonin Gene-related Peptide-I (CGRP alpha) in the Fasted, Anaesthetized Rat. *Life Sciences*, Vol.52, No.21, (March 1993), pp. 1717-1726, ISSN 0024-3205

Zagorska, J. (2007). The Evaluation of Organic Milk Quality. *PhD Thesis, Latvia University of Agriculture, Faculty of Food technology.*

Zebeli, Q. and Ametaj, B. N. (2009). Relationships between Rumen Lipopolysaccharide and Mediators of Inflammatory Response with Milk Fat Production and Efficiency in Dairy Cows. *Journal of Dairy Science,* Vol.92, No.8, (August 2009), pp. 3800-3809, ISSN 0022-0302

Zeng, R.; Bequette, B. J.; Vinyard, B. T. & Bannerman, D. D. (2009). Determination of Milk and Blood Concentrations of Lipopolysaccharide-Binding Protein in Cows with Naturally Acquired Subclinical and Clinical Mastitis. *Journal of Dairy Science,* Vol.92, No.3, (March 2009), pp. 980-989, ISSN 1525-3198

Zgirski, A. & Frieden, E. (1990). Binding of Cu(II) to Non-prosthetic Sites in Ceruloplasmin and Bovine Serum Albumin. *Journal of Inorganic Biochemistry,* Vol.39, No.2, pp. 137-148, ISSN 0162-0134

Zhang G. H.; Mann, D. M. & Tsai, C. M. (1999). Neutralization of Endotoxin In Vitro and In Vivo by a Human Lactoferrin-Derived Peptide. *Infection and Immunity,* Vol.67, No.3, (March 1999), pp. 1353-1358, ISSN 0019-9567

Zimecki, M.; Wlaszczyk, A.; Cheneau, P.; Brunel, A. S.; Mazurier, J.; Spik, G. & Kubler, A. (1998). Immunoregulatory Effects of a Nutritional Preparation Containing Bovine Lactoferrin Taken Orally by Healthy Individuals. *Archivum Immunologiae Et Therapiae Experimentalis (Warszawa),* Vol.46, No.4, pp. (April 1998), 231-240., ISSN 0004-069X

Zimin, A. V.; Delcher, A. L.; Florea, L.; Kelley, D. R.; Schatz, M. C.; Puiu, D.; Hanrahan, F.; Pertea, G.; Van Tassell, C. P.; Sonstegard, T. S.; Marcais, G.; Roberts, M.; Subramanian, P.; Yorke, J. A. & Salzberg, S. L. (2009). A Whole-genome Assembly of the Domestic Cow, *Bos taurus*. *Genome Biology,* Vol.10, No.4, (April 2009), pp. R42, ISSN 1465-6914

Zimlichman S.; Danon A.; Nathan I.; Mozes G. & Shainkin-Kestenbaum R. (1990). Serum Amyloid A, an Acute Phase Protein, Inhibits Platelet Activation. *The Journal of Laboratory and Clinical Medicine,* Vol.116, No.2, (August 1990), pp. 180-186, ISSN 0022-2143

14

Inflammatory Response and Acute Phase Proteins in the Transition Period of High-Yielding Dairy Cows

Erminio Trevisi[1], Massimo Amadori[2], Ivonne Archetti[2], Nicola Lacetera[3] and Giuseppe Bertoni[1]
[1]*Istituto di Zootecnica, Università Cattolica del Sacro Cuore, Piacenza*
[2]*Laboratory of Cellular Immunology, Istituto Zooprofilattico Sperimentale della Lombardia e dell'Emilia-Romagna, Brescia*
[3]*Dipartimento di Produzioni Animali, Università della Tuscia, Viterbo*
Italy

1. Introduction

Dairy cows undergo tremendous adaptive changes during the transition from late gestation to early lactation (Drackley et al., 2005). The importance of the periparturient period in determining health, productivity and profitability has been accurately described by Grummer (1995), Goff & Horst (1997), Drackley (1999) and Drackley et al. (2005).

Many are in fact the metabolic and microbial diseases typical of this period: milk fever, metritis, rumen acidosis, lameness (Drackley, 1999). Furthermore, the well known reduction of immune competence increases the susceptibility to mastitis and other infections. The risk of diseases seems to be increased as much as milk yield is genetically increased (Müller et al., 1999). This could be due to the metabolic stress consequences of high milk yield compared with nutrients intake, which is likely the cause of an impairment of the defence systems (Pond & Newsholme 1999). Another possibility, suggested by Drackley et al. (2005), is that multiple stressors, as much as they are severe and prolonged, can divert enough resources (energy, amino acids, etc.) and cause immune system depression. This mechanism could account for the increase of risks in case of poor management, heat stress conditions, excessive rain and mud, etc.

The hypothesis of multiple stressors combined with the general observation that many cows, in the same farm, are able to meet the challenge of the transition period, suggests that a genetic component is important for metabolic adaptation and, contemporaneously, that an improved management of farms could reduce the risks of affections. Therefore, according to Goff & Horst (1997), "the well-being and profitability of the cow could be greatly enhanced by understanding those factors that account for the high disease incidence in periparturient cows". Regarding these aspects, particularly intriguing are the following issues:

- how do some metabolic diseases increase the risk (Erb & Gröhn, 1988) of further metabolic and microbial diseases?

- how is the immune system depressed, considering that signs of disregulated responses can be detected even before calving, when energy balance is still positive?
- which role is played by the dry matter intake (DMI) as well as the energy efficiency in early lactation and which mechanisms determine their changes? Namely, why is DMI more or less depressed in the last days of the "dry" period before calving and, thereafter, its rate of increase is often not related to milk yield?

1.1 Inflammation in the periparturient period

Unfortunately, we do not have an answer to all the above questions; yet, there is evidence that inflammatory phenomena could provide a suitable conceptual framework for several of them:

- Cappa et al. (1989) showed the appearance of clinically overt inflammatory problems after calving (30% in a farm and 100% in another one);
- Bertoni et al. (1997) showed a positive relationship between haptoglobin at day in milk (DIM) 15 and both days open (calving to conception) and culling rates of cows, particularly in case of high genetic merit (Calamari et al., 1997);
- Trevisi et al. (1998) showed that early lactating cows with a lower liver synthesis activity were less fertile (137 vs. 89 days from calving to conception). The low liver activity was indexed by lower levels of albumin, Retinol Binding Protein - RBP - and lipoproteins. Probably, this activity is linked to inflammatory disorders because concomitantly high haptoglobin and globulin levels were also observed;
- Trevisi et al. (2001) evaluated the inflammatory response after calving on the basis of the blood levels of albumin, vitamin A (RBP index) and total cholesterol (lipoprotein index) and developed a composite Liver Activity Index (LAI): the lower the index, the higher the inflammatory condition (as shown by +APP changes).
- Bertoni et al. (2008) retrospectively separated parturient cows of 5 herds in accordance **with** LAI values in the 1st month of lactation. Results were very interesting, in fact cows with low LAI values (the lower quartile of the cows under study) showed:
    - higher frequency of clinical symptoms (42% vs 5% for LO-LAI and UP-LAI groups respectively) and often more than one disease case per cow;
    - less milk yield and reduced fertility;
    - higher haptoglobin peaks after calving, confirming the more severe inflammation, also observed in cows without clinical symptoms;
    - a larger energy deficiency, despite the lower milk yield, as confirmed by the more accentuated losses of body condition score (BCS) and the higher levels of beta-hydroxy-butyrate. Interestingly, the worse negative energy balance (NEB) could be due to a lower DMI, as suggested by the lower plasma levels of urea; in fact, uremia is related to total protein intake and therefore - in a population fed the same Total Mixed Ratio (TMR) – to DMI;
    - a lower energy efficiency utilization, as likely result of the increased maintenance cost necessary to support immune system activity (Trevisi et al., 2007; Trevisi et al. 2010b);
- Trevisi et al. (2010c) showed that cows with a higher inflammatory response after calving are characterized by pronounced differences of inflammatory markers in the previous dry period too [e.g. higher levels of sialic acid and Reactive Oxygen Metabolites (ROM) and lower ones of RBP, cholesterol, haemolytic complement].

The occurrence of inflammatory conditions in periparturient dairy cows and their consequences were also confirmed *ex iuvantibus.* Consistent results have been obtained by the authors following administration of acetylsalicylate (i.m. or by os) in apparently healthy cows at calving time, to prevent and/or to treat possible sub-clinical inflammatory conditions. In fact, the incidence of clinical disorders and the severity of the inflammatory response after calving were reduced in treated cows and, most important, milk yield and fertility were significantly improved (Bertoni et al., 2004; Trevisi & Bertoni, 2008; Trevisi et al., 2008a). Analogous results were also observed using both phytoextracts (showing immunomodulatory and antinflammatory properties) and anti-Endotoxin serum. Namely, diet supplementation with *Echinacea angustifolia*, over 3-4 weeks around calving, seems able to attenuate some typical adverse effects of inflammation around calving and to improve energy metabolism (Trevisi et al., 2008b). Nevertheless, the presence of some contradictory aspects (e.g. marked post calving rise of plasma haptoglobin) suggests the need for further investigations. Treatment with an anti-Endotoxin serum immediately before calving did not reduce the prevalence of disease cases in the transition period, but attenuated the response to the disease stress and anyway improved reproductive activity and conception rates (Bertoni et al., 2003).

In other trials, treatments with antibiotics immediately before calving (Bertoni et al., 2003) failed to improve performance and to reduce disease prevalence at the beginning of lactation. Furthermore, the anticipation of acetylsalicylate treatments before calving did not show encouraging results, in that the incidence of health disorders was not reduced and the attenuation of inflammation appeared less evident in comparison to acetylsalicylate treatments after calving (Trevisi et al., 2008). Moreover, oral, low-dose treatments with IFN-α (a cytokine that exerts anti-inflammatory effects in monogastric species) in late gestation also failed to reduce inflammation after calving. Contrariwise to the supposed effect, IFN-α caused an increased inflammatory response after calving, with consequent reduction of milk yield and a worsening of performance, suggesting a pro-inflammatory effect in ruminants; the possible causes of this phenomenon were illustrated by the authors in a previous study (Trevisi et al., 2009).

The above displayed results clearly suggest that calving time is accompanied by more or less serious inflammatory conditions, often without clinical symptoms. Furthermore, these conditions could negatively affect metabolism, health and reproductive activity of cows. The possible mechanism is the liver synthesis deviation (from usual to acute phase proteins), reduction of DMI and energy efficiency, thus negative energy balance (NEB) and its consequences (immune system impairment, delay of reproductive resumption, etc.). Nevertheless, it remains a major question: which is (are) the cause(s) of these inflammations?

1.2 Possible causes of inflammation in dairy cattle, with particular attention to the transition period

Inflammation is a well known condition - described by Celsus (50 BC) - characterized by "rubor et tumor cum calore et dolore". It was suggested to be caused by tissue damage and infections, although many types of injury produce a similar inflammatory response (Hunter, 1794; cited by Grimble, 2001). It is in fact noteworthy that different types of injuries (e.g. trauma, burns, exposure to noxious chemicals, etc.), as well as various stresses (e.g. oxidation, heat, intense physical exercise etc.) in addition to autoimmune diseases, cancer, some toxic substances, can be responsible for an inflammatory response (figure 1).

Moreover, very peculiar is the possibility of endotoxins (LPS) and/or bacteria passing through the digestive channel wall, when its barrier function is damaged for different reasons: excessive fermentation, ischemia-reperfusion etc. (Rowlands and Gardiner, 1998).
Inflammation process is also termed as acute-phase response (Richard and Gauldie, 1995), and comprises immediate events localized at sites of damage as well as an activation of systemic phenomena mediated by cytokines. A counter-regulatory system plays a critical role during APR in preventing the host from mounting an excessive defence response (Kapcala, 1999), which would be dangerous. A large variety of leukocyte and non-leukocyte cell types are able to synthesize either pro-inflammatory cytokines (e.g. IL-1, IL-6 and TNF-α), which promote local and systemic responses (Cousins, 1985; Dinarello, 1997; Elsasser et al., 1997; Gruys et al., 1999), or anti-inflammatory cytokines (e.g. IL-4, IL-10), which depress the activity of the former to avoid dangerous side effects (Grimble, 2001). Thereafter, some cytokines initiate the cascade of inflammatory mediators targeting the endothelium, and causing the release of eicosanoids (prostaglandins, leukotrienes, lipoxins, etc.) by activation of the cyclo-oxygenase-2. Eicosanoids are the main mediators of inflammation and justify the typical clinical symptoms of this process.
Inflammation can be triggered by several factors that often occur in the transition period (Drackley, 1999). In this phase, any type of disorder, although apparently modest or originated from apparently not so dangerous agents (e.g. common parasites or infections, modest lesions or injuries, little diet mistakes, grouping and movement of cows, deficiency in housing), could be conducive to more severe affections in the whole transition period if the usual homeostatic adaptation strategies fail. Peculiar causes of inflammation during the transition period could be the following:

- mammary gland differentiation and proliferation;
- uterus and placenta interactions;
- physical effort during the calving as well as possible traumas consequent to difficult or abnormal calving (dystocia);
- immunosuppression, as possible reason of more frequent infections.

Moreover, different clinically adverse events could interact and progressively magnify each other, allowing for the development of secondary forms before or after calving (i.e. respiratory affections, ketosis and/or liver lipidosis, metritis, laminitis, mastitis etc.). Furthermore, any activating stimulus of inflammation causes an up-regulation of inflammatory gene expression, mostly through activation of Nuclear Factor–kB (NF-kB), a transcription factor associated with inflammation (Lindström & Bennett, 2005), and in particular to the expression of the relevant pro-inflammatory genes. Consequently, NF-kB up-regulates the release of pro-inflammatory cytokines as well as the release of several other proteins related to inflammation (e.g. monocyte chemoattractant Protein-1, the inducible isoform of cyclo-oxygenase, an inducible form of nitric oxide synthase, NOS-2, with higher nitric oxide production, adhesion molecule ICAM-1; Elewaut et al., 1999). Thus, pro-inflammatory cytokines would be responsible of their further synthesis and, hence, of the amplification of inflammation itself. Therefore, inhibitors of NFkB (e.g. cortisol, antioxidants, ω3 fatty acids, etc.) are useful to stop inflammation.

1.2.1 Mammary gland

In the last 2 weeks of pregnancy, in coincidence with mammary gland development a small rise of body temperature (about +0.3-0.5°C) and sometime a slight rise of plasma haptoglobin levels are usually observed; this could be one of the first signals of inflammation onset. It is also known that mammary development is a process with features in common to the inflammation (e.g. edema, rash), and that it is tightly modulated by systemic hormones and local secreted factors like beta-1 integrin, epidermal growth factor receptor, matrix metalloproteinases etc. The possible relationship between these two phenomena (development of mammary gland and inflammation) has not been investigated yet, but it seems intriguing (see also section 4.2).

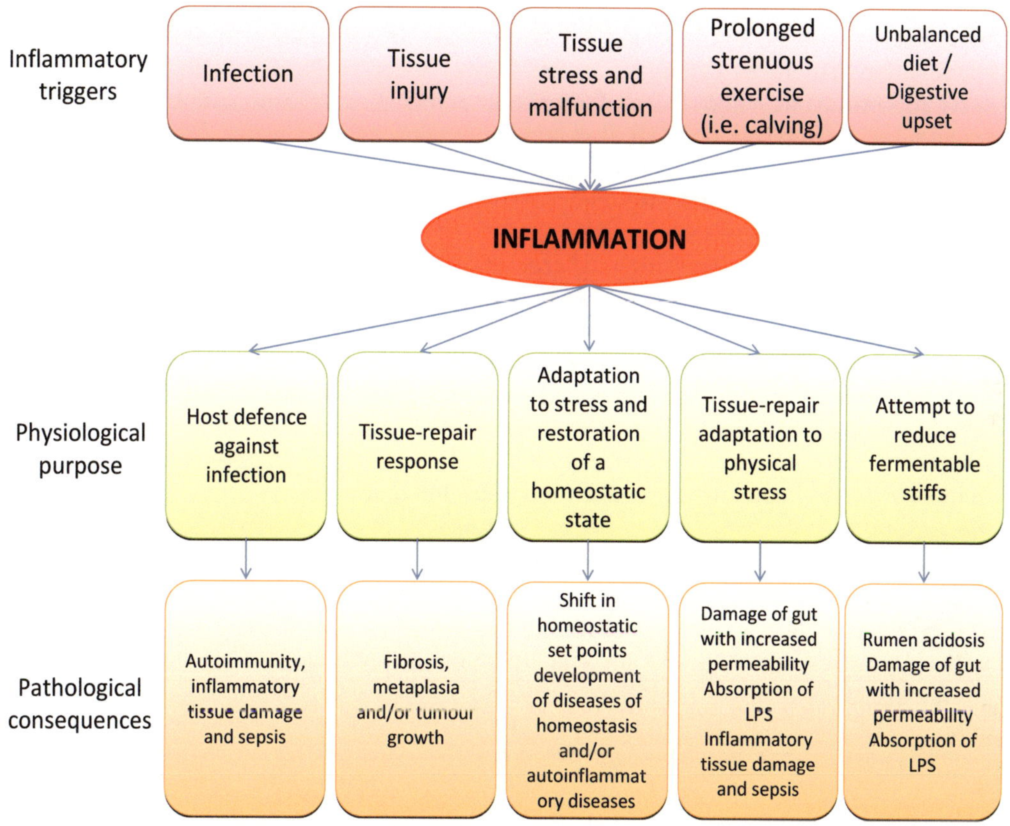

Fig. 1. Cause, physiological and pathological outcomes of inflammation (adapted from Medzhitov, 2008)

1.2.2 Uterus and placenta

As previously reported (Trevisi & Bertoni, 2008), the inflammation is considered a key feature of both preterm and term labour in humans (Lindström & Bennett, 2005), with an influx of inflammatory cells into the uterus and elevated levels of pro-inflammatory cytokines observed during parturition. Some years before, Simpson et al. (1998) identified a basal production of both pro-inflammatory and anti-inflammatory cytokines at parturition. During its whole life, placenta seems able to produce cytokines to improve its function (Hauguel-de Mouzon & Guerre-Millo, 2006), and the anti-inflammatory cytokine IL-10 seems important to counteract inflammation associated to preterm parturition (Hanna et al., 2006). Both inflammation and labour seem associated to the activity of NF-kB and thus to the expression of the relevant pro-inflammatory genes, as above reported.

Interestingly, Sibai et al. (1993) observed that "low-dose aspirin decreases the incidence of preeclampsia among nulliparous women" as possible consequence of lower thromboxane production. This result confirms the possibility to modulate the production of pro-inflammatory mediators around calving and, therefore, the inflammatory response itself; more research is undoubtedly needed to improve this basic knowledge.

1.2.3 Physical effort

Strenuous exercise is accompanied by an increase in circulating proinflammatory and inflammation-responsive cytokines, which shows some similarities with the response to sepsis and trauma as suggested by Pedersen et al. (1998). The same authors observed that sequential release of TNF-α, IL-1β, IL-6 and IL-1 receptor antagonist (IL-1ra) in the blood is comparable to that observed in relation to bacterial diseases. In particular, Lambert (2009) suggests that prolonged and strenuous exercise, can cause the impairment of intestinal mucosa integrity, increasing its permeability. The exhausting exercise can in fact determine several consequences, like high glucocorticoid levels, reduced blood flow rate, hyperthermia, hypoxia, oxidative and nitrosative stress as well as absorption of lipopolisaccharides, which promote the release of pro-inflammatory cytokines. According to Lambert (2009) data, such intestinal dysfunction is a non-rare condition in pigs. We are not aware of specific data on dairy cows, but prolonged physical activity can occur in case of difficult calving (or dystocia). This physical challenge, accompanied by other disturbances typical of calving time (e.g. trauma, psychological stress, digestive upset, etc.) could induce a release of pro-inflammatory cytokines and, thus, inflammation.

1.2.4 Infectious diseases linked to immunosuppression

As previously demonstrated, there exists a strict correlation between the occurrence of infections and a state of substantial immunosuppression in transition dairy cows. Several studies documented impairment of the ability of lymphocytes and neutrophils to respond to infectious challenges in periparturient dairy cows, which is likely to provide an explanation for the high incidence of infections (namely, metritis and environmental mastitis) during the early lactation period (Kehrli et al., 1999; Lacetera et al., 2005; Goff, 2006; Mulligan & Doherty 2008).

Immunosuppression goes along with marked changes in the endocrine, nutritional and metabolic status that are much more dramatic than at any other time in the life cycle of a dairy cow. The most common causes are:

- increased concentrations of circulating cortisol for several hours around parturition;
- metabolic disturbances [e.g., NEB, hypocalcemia, etc.];
- frequent inadequate feed intake despite an increased energy requirement for the developing conceptus and the impending lactogenesis;
- reduced intake of immunomodulating nutrients (vitamins A and E, selenium, copper and zinc);
- digestive disturbances due to sudden dietary changes;
- oxidative stress with risk of damage for membranes of immune cells;
- environmental stressors deriving from the usual management of dry and lactating dairy cows.

The above events contribute to immunosuppression in the transition period, as shown in previous studies (Grummer, 1995; Burton et al., 2005; Goff, 2006; Spears and Weiss, 2008).

However, most of them occur at calving time or immediately thereafter. Thus, there are probably further causes of immunosuppression, considering that signs of a disregulated innate immune response start 2-3 weeks before calving.

In this scenario, convincing evidence suggests that periparturient immunosuppression can be partly accounted for by the negative energy balance and related phenomena (e.g. fatty liver syndrome), which act as major contributing factors (Breukink & Wensing, 1997; Lacetera et al., 2005). Several studies have thus been performed to establish possible cause-and-effect relationships between NEB and impairment of the immune response in periparturient dairy ruminants. Recently, Wathes et al. (2009) reported that several inflammatory response genes were upregulated in cows undergoing conditions of severe NEB, whereas Moyes et al. (2010) reported that the majority of genes involved in the acquired immune response were down-regulated in NEB cows. Previous studies indicated that ketotic ruminants are immunosuppressed as well. Also, the hypothesis was tested that immunosuppression under NEB conditions might be due to increased concentration of some metabolites [namely, ketone bodies and nonesterified fatty acids (NEFA)] (Suriyasathaporn et al., 1999; Lacetera *et al.*, 2004). In particular, studies on NEFA indicated that concentrations of plasma NEFA mimicking intense lipomobilization altered (a) the ability of lymphocytes to proliferate or secrete immunoglobulin M and interferon-γ in response to polyclonal stimuli (mitogens) (Lacetera *et al.*, 2004), as well as (b) the viability and oxidative burst of polymorphonuclear (PMN) cells (Scalia et al., 2006). Furthermore, some authors recently suggested that plasma concentrations of NEFA may be possible diagnostic markers of impaired immunity and higher risk of infections around parturition (Moyes et al., 2009; Ospina et al., 2010). In particular, Ospina et al (2010) indicated that prepartum and postpartum serum NEFA higher than 0.3 or 0.6 mmol/l, respectively, were associated with increased risk for displaced abomasum, clinical ketosis, retained placenta and metritis.

In addition to that, evidence of a distinct worsening of inflammatory conditions and signs of transient immunosuppression in the periparturient period were consistently detected by the authors in field studies on cohorts of Frisian cattle. Thus, decreased levels of blastogenic response of lymphocytes to mitogens and lower levels of hemolytic complement around parturition went along with APR and altered hematological values, persistent hypoalbuminemia and hyperalphaglobulinemia (see a few results in figure 2). Such a shift from the reference values should be traced back to the peculiar adaptation strategies of these animals to NEB and perhaps to the serious metabolic stress of high-yield lactation.

1.3 Inflammation and energy balance

As well known, "Nature has accorded a high priority to the functions of pregnancy and milk secretion, allowing them to proceed at the expense of other metabolic processes even to the point that a disease state is created" (Bauman & Currie, 1980). Namely, as previously stressed (Bertoni et al., 2009) and except for the case of very serious diseases, milk yield in the first weeks of lactation is pursued much more quickly and independently from feed intake (Figure 3); as a result, NEB is unavoidable. For this reason post-calving cows are characterized by shortage of some metabolic fuels (e.g. glucose and aminoacids), drained by the mammary glands for milk syntheses, and by an increase of metabolites due to lipid mobilization (e.g. NEFA, BHBA). Therefore, what can be avoided is simply an excessive NEB, mainly through a good DMI, because energy concentration cannot be modified to a large extent avoid health disorders. Thus, as suggested by Villa-Godoy et al. (1988), the severity of NEB does not seem a consequence of the high milk yield at the beginning of lactation, but a result of poor DMI, which can be caused by diseases (and inflammation) and not only by physical factors.

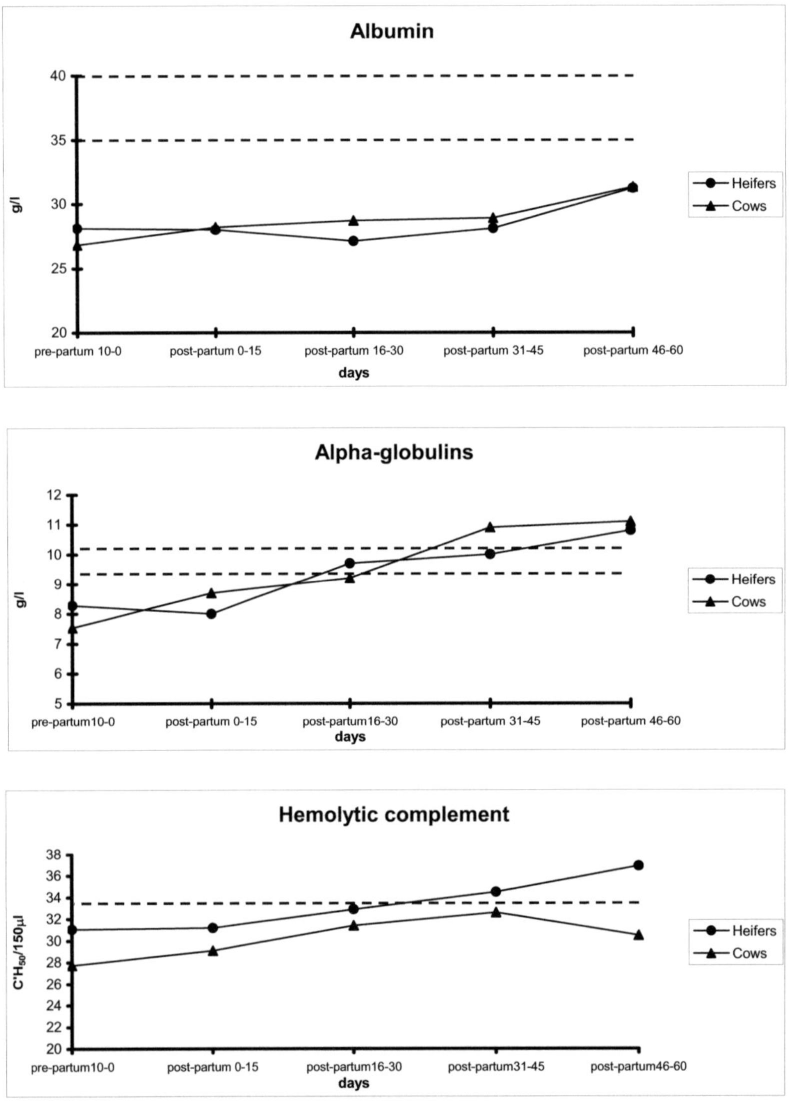

----- limits of normal values. Only the lower one is indicated for hemolytic complement

LEGEND

This study was performed on 30 healthy, high-yielding Italian Frisian dairy cattle (10 heifers and 20 cows), from two herds with a record of very good productive and reproductive performances. Blood samples in vacuum tubes were always collected from the same animals at 10-day intervals from the last two weeks of the dry period until day 60 after parturition. At each time point animals were within a 10-day range with respect to the date of parturition. The tests were carried out as previously described (Amadori et al., 1997).

Fig. 2. Time-course of some serum protein fractions and haemolytic complement.

In general, feed intake is affected by both physical and metabolic factors, but the former appear the limiting ones in early lactation. Nevertheless, in transition cows, other factors could also account for a reduction of DMI. In fact, cows often show marked rises of body temperature (>39.5°C) in the days following calving. These rises of temperature are mainly consequences of common malaise conditions immediately after parturition, linked to inflammatory phenomena, thus to a release of pro-inflammatory cytokines. As previously suggested, inflammation is also recurrent without disease, because pro-inflammatory mediators, which induce fever as well as anorexia and muscle catabolism (Elsasser et al., 2000), can be released for other causes (figure 1). Unfortunately, NEB is worsened since the metabolic changes induced by cytokines increase the availability of energy for a higher immune system activity. Puigserver et al. (2001) have in fact demonstrated that inflammation is coupled with the increase of cellular respiration and expression of genes linked to mitochondrial uncoupling (e.g. body temperature rise). In accordance with that, cows with more severe inflammation after calving are likely to suffer from a reduced efficiency in the use of Net Energy (Trevisi et al., 2007 and Trevisi et al., 2010); coupled with lower DMI, this means a worsening of usual NEB.
The severe NEB, quite common in early lactating cows, is really dangerous as cause of metabolic diseases (ketosis) and immunosuppression; furthermore it has been associated to a reproductive failure for a negative (toxic) effect on follicles and oocytes (Kruip et al., 1999; Jorritsma et al., 2004).

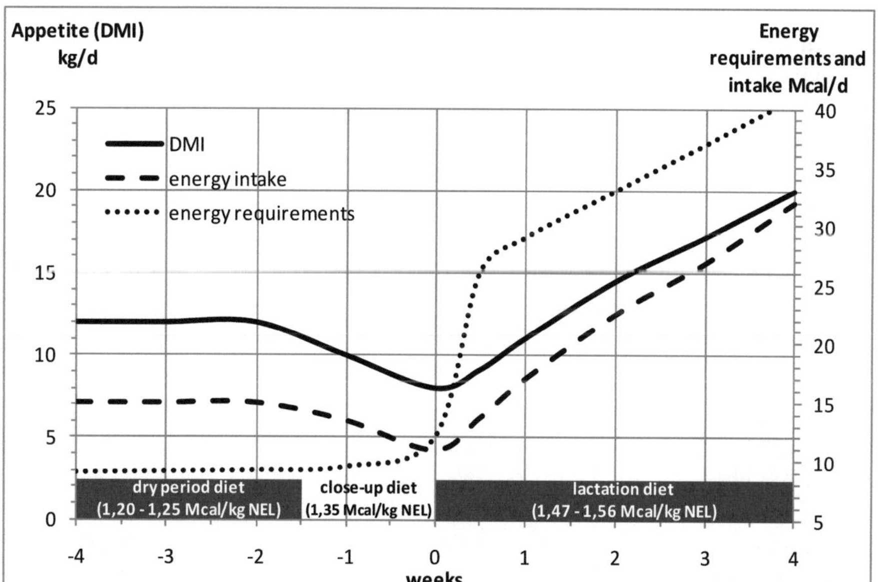

Fig. 3. Average levels of appetite and energy requirements (energy mobilization was not considered) in the transition of high yielding dairy cows. In brackets the suggested net energy for lactation concentrations (NEL) of diets of 3 stages.

2. Mechanisms of the acute phase response (APR) in the liver

The negative effect of inflammation at calving time can be also mediated by the liver diversion of activities due to the acute phase response (APR); the increased synthesis of haptoglobin and several other positive APP causes a lower synthesis of usual liver proteins, for this reason called negative -APP (albumin, lipoproteins, retinol binding protein etc.).

2.1 Inflammation and liver changes

As above explained, some of the inflammation effects - anorexia, catabolic conditions, fever (with an increase in feed energy wastage; Klasing, 2000), adipose mobilization and maybe more the significant disturbance of liver synthesis activity - can be particularly pernicious in the peripartum period. Altogether, they can increase the risk of metabolic diseases, such as ketosis and liver lipidosis, but indirectly of the infectious ones as well (Goff & Horst, 1997). Looking at liver, pro-inflammatory cytokines promote the liver synthesis of several plasma proteins (Powanda, 1980; Cousins, 1985; Elsasser *et al.*, 1997; Gruys *et al.*, 1999; Murata et al., 2004; Peterson *et al.*, 2004; Gruys *et al.*, 2005) including the positive acute phase proteins (+APP: i.e. haptoglobin, SAA, ceruloplasmin, C-reactive protein, a1-antitrypsin). Unfortunately, this increased synthesis partly competes with the production of the usual liver proteins, which are to some degree reduced at the same time (Fleck, 1989; Wan *et al.*, 1989). Thus, several of these proteins, named the negative APP (-APP), are affected (i.e. albumins, "carriers" of vitamins and hormones, lipoproteins, some specific enzymes as paraoxonase, etc.) (Gruys *et al.*, 2005). The functions of -APP are essential to the metabolic integrity of the animal and their synthesis is therefore highly maintained.

2.2 Indices to evaluate the consequences of acute phase reactions during the early lactation period

From the above considerations, -APP seem appropriate indices to detect consequences of an inflammatory condition in the peripartum period. In fact, changes of –APP (e.g. low levels or retarded increases) are prolonged in comparison to the rise of +APP. Moreover, in our experience the association between +APP response after calving and acute inflammatory phenomena is not always very clear and marked. Therefore, we have recently proposed two composed indices based on levels of some –APP observed in the first month of lactation, with the aim to evaluate the changes on liver activity synthesis caused by inflammatory events occurred around caving: the Liver Activity Index (LAI, Trevisi et al., 2001a) and the Liver Functionality Index (LFI; Bertoni et al., 2006).

LAI includes the average blood level at 7th, 14th and 28th DIM of some proteins synthesized by the liver: albumin, lipoproteins (indirectly measured as total cholesterol), and Retinol-binding Protein (RBP, measured as retinol, as the retinol level in the plasma is strictly related to RBP synthesized by the liver). Data of these 3 blood parameters were transformed into units of standard deviation obtained for each cow as follows: the mean value of the herd population of each plasma parameter (albumin, total cholesterol, and RBP) was subtracted from each cow value at 7, 14, and 28 DIM and divided by the corresponding standard deviation . Thus, the final LAI of each cow is the result of the arithmetical mean of the 3 partial values obtained from the 3 selected blood indices of 3 bleedings. At the end, LAI values represent a good estimation of the consequences of an inflammatory challenge which occurs at calving time, or around it, in each cow checked within a defined herd; therefore, LAI allows to retrospectively rank cows of the same herd from low to good adaptation to some very important risky situations during the transition period.

LFI has the same aim, but includes albumin, lipoproteins (indirectly measured as total cholesterol) and bilirubin (as indirect measure of the enzymes, synthesized by the liver, which operate its clearance). LFI is an index of the relevant changes between DIM 3 (V3) and 28 (V28), standardized in accordance with the optimal pattern of changes of the 3 parameters, obtained from healthy cows at the same stage of lactation. For each parameter, LFI calculation is done in 2 steps (table 1). Briefly, the 1st one considers the effects occurred at 3rd DIM (V3) and changes between 3rd and 28th (V28) DIM. For albumin and cholesterol these two effects equally concur (50%) to the partial LFI result (Alb-I and Chol-I), while for bilirubin the effect at DIM 3 represents 67% of the total partial LFI index. In the 2nd step, these partial indices were standardized in accordance with the average values observed in "healthy" cows, as defined by the upper LAI quartiles (Bertoni et al., 2008) (e.g. subtracting the correspondent mean value and dividing by the correspondent standard deviation). Ultimately, LFI was obtained by adding the values of the three partial indices. In table 1 are also included two examples of LFI calculation, belonging to 2 cows, with a low and with a high LFI index.

Respect to LAI, LFI allows to evaluate the same consequences of an inflammatory challenge, occurring at calving time or around it, but the retrospective ranking can include cows belonging to different herds. Anyhow it is interesting that the two indices are well correlated (Trevisi et al., 2010b). Therefore, considering that the determination of LFI is easier and cheaper than LAI, and that LFI allows for a comparison between herds, LFI appears a more reliable index to measure the success/failure of cow adaptation in the transition period.

Step 1	Albumin (Alb-I) sub-index = 50% V3 + 50% (V28-V3)
	Cholesterol (Chol-I) sub-index = 50% V3 + 50% (V28-V3)
	Bilirubin (Bil-I) sub-index = 67% V3 + 33% (V3-V28)
Step 2	**LFI = (Alb-I - 17,71)/1,08 + (Chol-I -2,57)/0,43 - (Bil-I -6,08)/2,17**

COW 1 (low LFI)

		V3	V28			partial LFI indexes
albumin	g/L	30.00	33.00	Step 1	Alb-I = 0,5 * 30 + 0,5 * (33-30) =	16.50
cholesterol	mmol/L	1.50	3.75		Chol-I = 0,5 * 1,5 + 0,5 * (3,75-1,50) =	1.88
bilirubin	mcmol/L	15.50	3.50		Bil-I = 0,67 * 15,5 + 0,33 * (15,5-3,5) =	14.35
						LFI
				Step 2	LFI = [(16,5 - 17,71) / 1,08] + [(1,88 - 2,57) / 0,43] - [(14,35 - 6,08) / 2,17]	**-6.52**

COW 2 (high LFI)

		V3	V28			partial LFI indexes
albumin	g/L	35.00	38.00	Step 1	Alb-I = 0,5 * 35 + 0,5 * (38-35) =	19.00
cholesterol	mmol/L	1.80	5.50		Chol-I = 0,5 * 1,8 + 0,5 * (5,5 - 1,80) =	2.75
bilirubin	mcmol/L	6.00	1.50		Bil-I = 0,67 * 6,0 + 0,33 * (8,0 - 1,5) =	6.17
						LFI
				Step 2	LFI = [(19,0 - 17,71) / 1,08] + [(2,75 - 2,57) / 0,43] - [(6,17 - 6,08) / 2,17]	**1.57**

Table 1. Example of the calculation of LFI index.

2.2.1 Practical use of LAI and LFI indices

Inflammatory phenomena at calving time are well related to more severe health problems - sometime without strong reduction of milk yield reduction – as well as to the reduction of performance and fertility (Bionaz et al., 2007; Bertoni et al., 2008). Therefore, by monitoring LAI or more conveniently LFI, it is possible to identify subjects that need more attention and proper therapies. In fact, these indexes, if determined in all the transition subjects in a herd, measure the extent of inflammatory consequences and are useful to show their presence in cows not affected by clinical symptoms. In accordance with the low LAI and LFI as well as some other indices (clinical, metabolic, productive, BCS, etc.,) we can observe two different types of cows at the end of the first month of lactation:

i. subjects that continue to suffer from inflammatory phenomena, indicated - for example - by high plasma haptoglobin level. These cows require an accurate diagnosis, mainly concerning uterus, mammary gland, foot integrity and functioning, etc.;
ii. subjects that have solved inflammatory events occurred around calving, but maintain inadequate liver function, which demands some support to accelerate liver recovery.

Finally, all the subjects under these conditions are at risk for fertility.

2.2.2 APR changes with prognostic value

In any case, in consideration of the adopted procedures both LAI and LFI are not able to detect in advance cows at risk in the peripartum period. Therefore, of remarkable usefulness would be the identification of parameters showing differences in the period that precedes calving, and, therefore, with a predictive meaning at calving time.

Interestingly, by ranking cows at the end of the 1st month of lactation for LAI or LFI values, we detected important changes in some markers before calving. Cows with low LAI (Trevisi et al., 2010c) are characterized - even without any symptom - by slightly lower plasma levels of some -APP (e.g. RBP, lipoprotein, albumin) and haemolytic complement, as well as higher levels of syalic acid and ROMs in the last month of pregnancy. In other experiments (Trevisi et al., 2010a; Trevisi et al., 2010b), cows with lower LFI showed - again before calving and without clinical symptoms - higher levels of IL-6, ceruloplasmin, bilirubin, NEFA, ROM and lower ones of RBP and lysozyme. Most of the differences observed in the latter experiences were marked in comparison to previous research and reached statistical significance. Despite these results are been obtained in cows with extremely low levels of LFI, they confirm what appears in several experiences: animals which previously suffered for inflammations are more responsive to new inflammatory challenges; it is difficult to establish if higher susceptibility is innate or acquired.

In general, these results suggest that before calving we can observe two different conditions:

- subjects that show inflammatory phenomena without clinical symptoms, which could be detected by the rise of +APP (e.g. haptoglobin), pro-inflammatory cytokines (e.g. IL-6), lipomobilization (e.g. increase of NEFA) and oxidative stress (e.g. rise of ROM);
- subjects that only present residual signals of previous inflammatory events, which could be detected mainly by the slightly lower levels of some –APP (e.g. lipoprotein, albumin and RBP), but also lysozyme.

In the first case (subclinical inflammations), the approach will be an attempt to identify the possible cause of health disorders (e.g. mastitis, lameness, etc.) with further and detailed investigations, followed by appropriate therapy. In the second case, the subjects should be followed with more attention at calving time because they are likely to be more susceptible to any inflammatory challenge; these animals are eligible for treatments with anti-inflammatory molecules (e.g. acetyl-salicylic acid) immediately after parturition.

2.3 From APR to a metabolic stress: Causes and effects

As previously suggested (Figure 1), the APR can take place in the absence of detectable infections even before calving, thus increasing the risk of possible traumas and related tissue damage at calving time. Thus, the observed response does not fit into conventional models of APR, which implies that the origin of such a response should be set into an alternative conceptual framework. In this respect, we have to consider that APR is part of an ancestral, overlapping set of immune, stress and inflammatory responses aimed at the neutralization of stimuli perturbing immune system homeostasis (Ottaviani & Franceschi, 1998). In this scenario, the effector mechanisms are remarkably similar for both infectious and non-infectious stimuli. In fact, a pro-inflammatory cytokine like IL-1 induces activation of the hypothalamo-pituitary-adrenocortical (HPA) axis as well as stimulation of cerebral noradrenaline; the effects of IL-1 are remarkably similar to those observed following either LPS administration (reminiscent of infectious stress) - that cause the release of pro-inflammatory cytokines - or acute, non-infectious stressing events in laboratory animals, such as electric shock or restraint (Dunn et al., 1999). Therefore, an innate immune response can be mounted in different forms and extent by the host after exposure to both infectious and non-infectious stimuli.

Not surprisingly, acute inflammation (e.g. cellular damage) also triggers innate immune responses, which are very similar to those observed after an infectious stress. Nevertheless, at ordinary calving cows do not suffer from severe metabolic stress; therefore, this does not seem the cause of inflammatory conditions, but a consequence and a possible amplification factor. On the other hand, compelling evidence shows that some cytokines promote the metabolic stress, on which a potent regulation can be also exerted by orally (e.g. IFN-alpha; Trevisi et al., 2009) or parenterally administered cytokines. Some major findings deserve utmost attention:

- there is an up-regulation of several genes related to metabolic and physiologic functions after oral delivery of human IFN-alpha in cattle (Namangala et al., 2006), which implies a connection with metabolic stress;
- the IL-6 gene plays a crucial homeostatic role in hepatocytes of transition cows during inflammation and ketosis; under these conditions IL-6 can exert important effects on metabolic and energy production pathways, while inducing APR at the same time (Loor et al., 2007).

2.4 Effector mechanisms of the APR

Which rational link can be surmised between metabolic stress, inflammatory cytokines and APR? One of the likely associations between metabolic stress and innate immunity could be traced back to the lymphoid stress-surveillance system, i.e. to the network of lymphocyte populations (mainly $\gamma\delta$ T cells) which recognize neo-antigens like MIC on stressed cells (Hayday A.C., 2009), i.e. cells exposed to events as diverse as heat shock, infections, DNA damage, etc. Also in cattle, MIC proteins are ligands for the activating NK cell receptor NKG2D, expressed on NK cells, CD8+$\alpha\beta$ T cells and $\gamma\delta$ T cells; stimulation of these cells with recombinant MIC causes an IFN-γ response (Guzman et al., 2010); this is likely to trigger and sustain inflammatory cascades by activating macrophages for a sustained release of ROM and reactive nitrogen intermediates (RNIs) (Schreiber & Schreiber, 2003).

Levels of oxidative stress are actually increased in the periparturient period, but it often occurs only after calving (Bertoni et al., 2008; Sordillo et al., 2009), as consequences of inflammatory conditions that precede metabolic stress. Interestingly, this condition seems more evident in high-yielding dairy cows that are more susceptible to inflammatory events that occur at calving time. In this scenario, major negative outcomes of metabolic performance (oxidative stress, tissue hypoxia, accumulation of toxic metabolites, etc.) could easily give rise to activation of the lymphoid stress-associated surveillance system, thus worsening the inflammation.

On the other hand, an inflammatory response could be directly triggered by both hypoxia and accumulation of ROM in tissues and organs. In particular, by a specific hypoxia-inducible transcription factor (HIF-1), hypoxia induces the synthesis of vascular endothelial growth factor (VEGF), which increases the permeability of blood vessels in co-operation with NO and CO generated by endothelial nitric oxide synthetase (eNOS); in turn, the activity of HIF-1 is stimulated by IL1-β, Tumor Necrosis Factor (TNF)-α and NO even under normoxic conditions (see Hellwig-Bürgel et al., 2005 for review). Again these conditions are common after calving, therefore the metabolic stress does not seem the primer of inflammation in the periparturient cows, but it confirms an important role in the worsening and in the reiteration of inflammation at this stage.

Owing to the above, the induction of inflammatory conditions underlying APR in periparturient cows can be accounted for by activation of both lymphoid and myeloid effector cells, with possible complementation / synergisms of the relevant final effects, to be investigated in further studies. In addition, the opening of the calving canal in periparturient cows and the exposure of uterus to contaminating environmental bacteria can account for a short-term APR.

3. Risk factors underlying high APR in the periparturient period

A few parameters underlying inadequate homeostatic regulation of the inflammatory / AP responses were revealed in some studies of ours and other authors. These can be conveniently divided into factors underlying the very onset of APR (points 1, 2) and its subsequent, abnormal amplification (points 3,4):

1. The prepartum levels of serum lysozyme. These are significantly lower in subjects which develop lower levels of –APP in the first month of lactation (Trevisi et al., manuscript submitted). Interestingly, lysozyme at certain concentrations can exert *in vitro* a significant down-regulation of IL-8, TNF-alpha and caspase-1 responses (Trevisi et al., manuscript submitted). The lysozyme gene is located on chromosome BTA5 in a region where quantitative trait loci (QTL) for milk production have been mapped. The role of lysozyme in controlling post-partum inflammation makes the lysozyme gene a possible candidate for the QTL effect, since lysozyme can affect animal health and welfare in this delicate period and therefore milk production during the entire lactation.
2. Dehydroepiandrosterone (DHEA). This hormone plays an important role in the regulation of inflammatory cytokines like IL-6, as shown by the aging models in humans (Daynes et al., 1993); a major control of the TNF-alpha response has been described as well (Danenberg et al., 1992). Owing to the above, low levels of such a hormone in the dry period may be conducive to the development of an IL-6 and ceruloplasmin response in this phase, as observed by the authors in previous studies. (Trevisi et al., manuscript submitted).
3. The intra ed extracellular Heat Shock Protein 72 kDa (HSP72) complex. In the authors' experience (Catalani et al., 2010a), the HSP72 response is an important component of

the adaptation strategy of periparturient dairy cows to negative energy balance and lipomobilization after calving. In a global view, the crucial functions of HSP72 in the control of both TNF-alpha and a fundamental cellular alarmin like High Motility Group Box-1 (HMGB-1) (Tang et al., 2007) are probably the foundation of the strong and long-lasting HSP72 response of cows after calving. Beyond that, the HSP72 response is conducive to induction and differentiation of immuno-regulatory Treg cells (CD4+, CD25+), aimed at containing and restricting the inflammatory responses of the host (Van Eden et al., 2005). Therefore, a defective HSP72 response could outline a risk condition for cows in the post calving period.

4. Some undefined factors underlying the blast response of lymphocytes to bacterial LPS. In the authors' experience (Catalani et al., 2010b) there is a general tendency to a reduction of the blast response of bovine peripheral blood mononuclear cells (PBMC) to LPS after calving; yet, low and high responders in this assay tend to maintain such a feature on a different scale; most important, high responder cows show the least number of disease cases in first weeks of lactation, with a possible association to Single Nucleotide Polymorphisms (SNPs) of the Toll Like Receptor 4 gene to be verified in a large number of animals (see Catalani et al., 2010b). Interestingly, Treg cells induced by the aforementioned HSP72 complex could play a role in the overall reduction of the blast response to LPS, as also suggested by the significant negative correlation between the two variables.

Interestingly, circumstantial evidence in the authors' labs on thousands of cow serum samples (Table 2) indicated that high-yielding Frisian dairy cows show much lower serum lysozyme contents (< 1 μg/ml) compared with other dairy and beef cattle breeds; also, the lower lysozyme contents are correlated in our experience with higher peripheral blood granulocyte counts, lower albumin/globulin ratios and persistent monocytosis (data not shown). In this scenario, the IL-6 response observed in some dairy cattle before and after calving (Trevisi et al., manuscript submitted) can contribute to a functional differentiation of monocytes to macrophages (Chomarat et al., 2000), i.e. cells with a higher pro-inflammatory potential.

4. Hypotheses and acceptable speculations

4.1 The crucial role of the late pregnancy period

We have already addressed in a previous section the issue of possible prognostic factors in cow pregnancy. This tenet was actually suggested by accumulated evidence, showing that a high and long-lasting APR in the periparturient period stems from a major failure of the cows' homeostatic control circuits. Thus, the combined effects of some genetic and environmental factors before calving should activate the aforementioned lymphoid and myeloid surveillance systems; the observed features of defective homeostatic control of the inflammatory response could contribute all together to high and long-lasting APR after calving, associated to a poor outcome of the transition period. In addition, on the basis of the accumulated data (as explained in section 2.2.2 "APR changes with prognostic value"), the authors believe that a defective homeostatic response takes place first before lactation onset, i.e. before the expected phase of serious metabolic stress. In particular, the time-course of both IL-6 and some APP (e.g. ceruloplasmin for +APP and albumin for –APP) responses indicates that relevant *noxae* should be searched in the late pregnancy, non-lactating period. In this respect, the aforementioned early risk factors for APR occurrence (lysozyme,

	Albumin (mg/ml)	Lysozyme (µg/ml)	*Haptoglobin* (mg/dL HbBC)
Beef cattle (all)			
Average	30.27	2.28	10.25
Standard deviation	3.69	2.40	13.17
n	459	465	465
Male dairy cattle *			
Average	29.94	1.47	7.84
Standard deviation	3.08	1.31	8.91
n	24	24	24
Cattle with haptoglobin > 100 mg/dL HbBC **			
Average	26.52	1.70	146.20
Standard deviation	3.74	1.60	41.15
n	7	7	7
Beef cattle <350 KG			
Average	28.34	2.07	12.20
Standard deviation	4.29	1.66	13.51
n	62	63	63
Beef cattle 350-500 KG			
Average	30.12	2.44	10.94
Standard deviation	3.41	2.70	14.79
n	262	263	263
Beef cattle > 500 KG			
Average	30.69	2.05	9.29
Standard deviation	3.60	1.93	9.86
n	99	99	99

* 18 Frisian and 6 Brown cattle < 3 years old

** Cattle with high haptoglobin serum levels were set apart to illustrate the correlation with low albumin concentrations (negative APR)

Total protein was assessed by the biuret reagent on a Synchron CX5 multi-analyzer (Beckman-Coulter). Serum albumin was determined by electrophoresis on an agarose gel and densitometric examination of protein bands (Hydrasis apparatus, SEBIA). Reference value for adult healthy cattle: 30-35 mg/ml.

Haptoglobin was investigated as previously described (Makimura & Suzuki, 1982). Reference value for healthy cattle: < 10 mg/dL of Haemoglobin Binding Capacity (HbBC).

Serum lysozyme concentration was measured by the lyso-plate-assay (Osserman & Lawlor, 1966). Reference values for healthy cattle: 1-3 µg/ml.

Table 2. Clinical chemistry values of beef and non-lactating dairy cattle.

DHEA) could play a role vis-à-vis a physiological pro-inflammatory stimulation before calving. In turn, the ensuing, disregulated inflammatory conditions in the late pregnancy period could pave the way to high APR and related incidence of disease cases after calving, as indirectly shown *ex iuvantibus* by the good results of oral acetylsalicylic acid treatments after calving (Bertoni et al., 2004; Trevisi & Bertoni, 2008). Also, a seriousinflammatory condition of peri-parturient dairy cows is related to a lesser production performance (Bertoni et al., 2008), as repeatedly confirmed in our experience by the lower daily milk yields of cows with ongoing APR under conditions of controlled dry matter uptake.

4.2 Physiological events in late pregnancy and APR

Which kind of event could actually trigger an inflammatory response way before stressing events like mammary gland edema, placenta expulsion, calving and lactation onset? The first possibility is obviously represented by subclinical infections, which go undetected by stockmen and practitioners. In particular, reference is made to mastitis cases of the "dry" period, leading to infected mammary gland quarters at lactation onset (Bradley & Green, 2000; Green et al., 2002). Subclinical viral infections due to poor or no vaccine prophylaxis, as well as neglected podal lesions could undoubtedly play a role, too. However, whenever subclinical microbial infections can be reasonably ruled out, which otherwise innocuous, physiological, pro-inflammatory condition can trigger in some individuals IL-6 and acute phase responses because of poor homeostatic control? A strong case can be probably made for a contribution of the massive leukocyte infiltration into the mammary gland at this stage, aimed at removal of apoptotic cells and cell debris (Oliver & Sordillo, 1989). In fact, the process of active involution is most likely completed by 21 days after cessation of milking; later on, during steady state involution, fluid volume is maintained at very low levels with the highest concentrations of both macrophages and granulocytes; at this stage, the activity of phagocytic cells is no more compromised like in early involution because of the attempt to eliminate milk components and cellular debris (Nickerson, 1989). As a result, the observed IL-6 and APR in the "dry" period may be coincident with the highest pro-inflammatory potential of leukocytes infiltrating the mammary gland. Also, as described in a previous chapter, inflammation underlies both preterm and term labour, with an elevated levels of pro-inflammatory cytokines during parturition (Lindström & Bennett, 2005). Finally, inflammatory stimuli in the central nervous system can induce cytokines in the periphery by increasing sympathetic outflow; this has been demonstrated for IL-6 as well (Johnson, 1997), and it may hold true for the IL-6 response in cattle both before and after calving. Regardless of the triggering event, the authors believe that a primary, disregulated inflammatory response 4-5 weeks before calving is likely to determine sort of negative imprinting of the innate immune response; in turn, the latter is going to trigger after calving a high and long-lasting APR to the physiological, combined stimuli of calving and exposure of uterus to contaminating environmental bacteria. As explained in the previous paragraphs, such an APR after calving is strongly predictive of disease occurrence and early removal from the herd, this latter feature being obviously affected by the actual precocity of clinical diagnosis and pharmacological treatments.

4.3 Management of the periparturient period

It is a strategic period as well known, but its importance may be even greater in high-yielding cows which appear more susceptible to inflammation (Table 3).

1.	Ensure proper body condition at dry off and during dry period to provide reserve energy to meet requirements for milk production and reproduction in early lactation, but avoiding any excess: ideal BCS 3.0-3.3 points (Edmonson et al., 1989).
2.	Prevent new intramammary infections by proper dry-off procedure: e.g. by combining the usual antibiotic treatment in mammary gland with an intramuscular antibiotic treatment, with a large-spectrum to have also a systemic coverage against bacteria;
3.	Prevent virus and bacteria infections: vaccination against main viruses (IBR, BVD, PI3, rota-coronaviruses, *E. coli*, leptospira) and perhaps antiparasite treatments around dry-off period;
4.	Prevent hoof problems: to ensure hoof care (trimming) around dry-off period (within 10 days before or after dry-off)
5.	Prevent digestive upsets: proper diet distribution; proper diet composition during the whole dry period to cover energy (about 1.3 Mcal/kg dry matter as Net Energy), vitamin and mineral requirements and to guarantee about 12% of crude protein in dry matter; a very short (8-10 d) and light close-up period (addition of about 1.5-2.0 kg/d of cereals or lactation concentrate to usual TMR);
6.	Ensure comfortable housing: appropriate size of free-stall cubicles, clean and dry pen, thermo neutral conditions, no overcrowding; reduced changes of groups etc.;
7.	Proper feeding and housing will prevent any kind of metabolic diseases that however must be quickly treated;
8.	Well monitored calving: without hurry and possibly trauma and avoiding isolation;
9.	Frequent checks before and after calving to verify health status: rectal temperature, gynaecological visit, good rumen fill, normal utilization of stored fat, high milk production;
10.	Stimulate and maintain aggressive appetite during the dry period and early lactation (by specific supplements, if needed).

Table 3. Decalogue of correct dry period and calving management in dairy cows (to reduce inflammatory conditions)

5. Conclusions

Our results suggest that any cow in the transition period can incur in inflammatory phenomena of different seriousness and quite often without clinical symptoms. The consequences of this are a worsening of negative energy balance either for a lower dry matter intake and for some waste of energy and nutrients; furthermore, the acute phase response causes a deviation of liver synthesis and in turn a reduction of several protein-enzymes which are responsible for liver functions. The inflammation phenomenon is triggered by pro-inflammatory cytokines as well as by eicosanoids; their release can occur for many different reasons: infections, tissue damage, stress conditions, heavy physical effort, etc.. This means that several and quite different can be the causes of inflammation, so that several have to be the ways to prevent it: infectious and metabolic disease control, reduction of distocya as risk of tissue damage and physical effort, reduction of stress factors (heat, poor housing , digestive disorders which allow the absorption of endotoxins etc.); specific rules for the dry and transition periods should be established and aimed at avoiding or reducing inflammatory conditions around calving.

From a practical point of view, the consequences of inflammation at calving time are reduction of performance: milk yield, BCS, fertility, but also an increased risk of new diseases for an impairment of the immune system and liver functions (also due to higher fat lipidosis). Worthwhile could be the possibility to detect - before calving - at risk animals which could be treated to reduce the inflammation consequences (i.e. by acetylsalicylate immediately after calving); also useful could be the possibility to recognize in early lactation the cows which suffered for severe and prolonged inflammations with different levels of seriousness after calving. These latter cows could be in fact treated to stop inflammation, to promote liver recovery and to improve the reproductive activity. Blood samples 2-3 weeks before calving or immediately after it and at the end of 1st month of lactation can allow for prediction of these situations, in accordance with the acute phase protein changes.

6. Acknowledgements

The co-operation of Dr. L. Bertocchi and Dr. G. Tadeo (IZSLER, Brescia, Italy) and Dr. F. Piccioli-Cappelli, Dr. P. Grossi and Dr. S. Cogrossi (Istituto di Zootecnica, Università Cattolica S. Cuore, Piacenza, Italy) in field surveys on cattle is gratefully acknowledged. This study was financially co-supported by the Italian Ministry of Health (Project IZSLER PRF 2006201) and Università Cattolica del S. Cuore.

7. References

Amadori, M., Archetti, I.L., Frasnelli, M., Bagni, M., Olzi, E., Caronno, G. & Lanteri, M. (1997). An immunological approach to the evaluation of welfare in Holstein Frisian cattle. *Journal of Veterinary Medicine* Series B, Vol. 44, pp. 321-327, ISSN 0514-7166.

Bauman, D.E. & Currie, W.B. (1980). Partitioning of nutrients during pregnancy and lactation: a review of mechanisms involving homeostasis and homeorhesis. *Journal of Dairy Science*, 63: 1514-1529, ISSN: 0022-0302

Bertoni, G., Calamari, L., Maianti, M.G. & Cappa, V. (1997). Factors others then milk yield that affect the reproductive traits of dairy cows. *Livestock Production Science* (1997) 50, 99-100, ISSN 1871-1413

Bertoni, G., Trevisi, E. & Librandi, F. (2003). Treatments with antibiotics or with Anti-Endotoxin serum before calving: effects on milk yield and fertility. XV Congresso Nazionale A.S.P.A., Parma, 18-20 giugno 2003. *Italian Journal of Animal Science*, vol. 2 (suppl. 1): 163-165, ISBN 88-86817-02-9

Bertoni G., Trevisi, E. & Piccioli-Cappelli, F. (2004). Effects of Acetyl-salycilate used in post-calving of dairy cows. *Veterinay. Research Communication* 28 (Suppl.1):217-219, ISSN: 0165-7380

Bertoni, G., Trevisi, E., Ferrari, A.R. & Gubbiotti, A. (2006). The dairy cow performances can be affected by inflammations occurring around calving. *Book of Abstract of the 57th EAAP Meeting*, 17-20 September 2006, Antalya, Turkey, 325, ISBN: 978-90-8686-003-6

Bertoni, G., Trevisi, E., Han, X. & Bionaz, M. (2008). Effects of Inflammatory Conditions on Liver Activity in the Puerperium and Consequences for Performance in Dairy Cows. *Journal of Dairy Science*, 91:3300-3310, ISSN 0022-0302

Bertoni, G., Trevisi, E. & Lombardelli, R. (2009). Some new aspects of nutrition, health conditions and fertility of intensively reared dairy cows. *Italian Journal of Animal Science*, vol. 8, 491-518, 2009, ISSN: 15944077

Bionaz, M., Trevisi, E., Calamari, L., Librandi, F., Ferrari, A. & Bertoni, G. (2007). Plasma Paraoxonase, Health Problems, Inflammatory Conditions and Liver Function in Transition Dairy Cows. *Journal of Dairy Science* 90:1740-1750, ISSN: 0022-0302

Bradley, A.J. & Green, M.J. (2000). A Study of the Incidence and Significance of Intramammary Enterobacterial Infections Acquired During the Dry Period. *Journal of Dairy Science* 83:1957-1965, ISSN 0022-0302.

Breukink, H.J & Wensing, T. (1997). Pathophysiology of the liver in high yielding dairy cows and its consequences for health and production. *Israel Journal of Veterinary Medicine*, 52, pp. 66-72. ISSN: 0334-9152

Burton, J.L., Madesn, S.A., Chang, L.-C, Weber, P.S.D., Buckham, K.R., R.van Dorp, Hickey, M.-C. & Earley, B. (2005). Gene expression signatures in neutrophils exposed to glucocorticoids: a new paradigm to help explain 'neutrophil dysfunction' in periparturient dairy cows. *Veterinary. Immunology and Immunopathology*, 105, pp. 197-219, ISSN: 0165-2427

Calamari, L., Maianti, M.G. & Bertoni, G. (1997) - Relazioni fra potenzialità produttiva, problemi nel puerperio e fertilità nella vacca da latte. *9° Meeting Nazionale "Studio dell'efficienza riproduttiva degli animali di interesse zootecnico"*, Bergamo, 16 maggio 1997: 99-103.

Cappa, V., Trevisi, E. & Bertoni, G. (1989). Variazioni ematiche e produttive nel 1° mese di lattazione in bovine di allevamenti con o senza problemi "post-partum". *Zootecnica e Nutrizione Anim*ale, 15: 645-660, ISSN: 0390-0487

Catalani, E., Amadori, M., Vitali, A., Bernabucci, U., Nardone, A. & Lacetera, N. (2010a). The Hsp72 response in peri-parturient dairy cows: relationships with metabolic and immunological parameters. *Cell Stress and Chaperones*, Vol. 15, pp. 781-790, ISSN 1355-8145.

Catalani, E., Amadori, M., Vitali, A., Nardone, A., Bernabucci, U.& Lacetera, N. (2010b). Relationships between lipopolysaccharide responsiveness, genetic characteristics and incidence of infections in peri-parturient dairy cows. *Proceedings 9th International Veterinary Immunology Symposium (IVIS)*, Tokyo. Japan, August 16-20, Pp. 138 (abs.).

Chomarat, P., Banchereau, J., Davoust, J. & Palucka, A.K. (2000). IL-6 switches the differentiation of monocytes from dendritic cells to macrophages. *Nature immunology*, Vol. 1, pp. 510-514, ISSN 1529-2908.

Cousins, R.J. (1985). Absorption, transport and hepatic metabolism of copper and zinc: special reference to metallothionein and ceruloplasmin. *Physiological Review*, 65(2): 238-309, ISSN: 0031-9333

Danenberg, H.D., Alpert, G., Lustig, S. & Ben-Nathan, D. (1992). Dehydroepiandrosterone protects mice from endotoxin toxicity and reduces tumor necrosis factor production. *Antimicrobial agents and chemotherapy*, Vol. 36, pp. 2275-2279, ISSN 0066-4804.

Daynes, R.A., Araneo, B.A., Ershler, W.B., Maloney, C., Li, G.Z. & Ryu, S.Y. (1993). Altered regulation of IL-6 production with normal aging. Possible linkage to the age-associated decline in dehydroepiandrosterone and its sulfated derivative. *Journal of immunology*, Vol. 150, pp. 5219-5230, ISSN 0022-1767.

Dinarello, C.A. (1997). Proinflammatory and anti-inflammatory cytokines as mediators in the pathogenesis of septic shock. *Chest*, 112:321S-329S, ISSN: 0012-3692

Drackley, J.K. (1999). Biology of dairy cows during the transition period: the final frontier? *Journal of Dairy Science*, 82: 2259-2273, ISSN: 0022-0302

Drackley, J.K., Dann, H.M., Douglas, G.N., Guretzky, N.A., Litherland, N.B., Underwood, J.P. & Loor, J.J. (2005). Physiological and pathological adaptations in dairy cows that may increase susceptibility to periparturient diseases and disorders. *Italian Journal of Animal Science* 4:323-344, ISSN: 15944077

Dunn, A.J., Wang, J. & Ando, T. (1999). Effects of cytokines on cerebral neurotransmission. Comparison with the effects of stress. *Advances in Experimental Medicine and Biology*, Vol. 461, pp. 117-127, ISSN 0065-2598.

Elewaut, D., Didonato, J.A., Kim, J.M., O'Neill, D., Truong, F., Eckmann, L. & Kagnoff, M.F. (1999). Nuclear factor-kappa B is a central regulator of the intestinal epithelial cell innate immune response induced by infection with enteroinvasive bacteria. *Journal of Immunology*, 163:1457-1466, ISSN: 0022-1767

Elsasser, T.H., Kahl, S., Steele, N.C. & Rumsey, T.S. (1997). Nutritional modulation of somatotropic axis-cytokine relationships in cattle: a brief review. *Comparative biochemistry and physiology*, 116A(3): 209-221, ISSN: 0300-9629

Elsasser, T.H., Klasing, K.C., Filipov, N. & Thompson, F. (2000). The metabolic consequences of stress: targets for stress and priorities of nutrient use. In: *The biology of animal stress. Basic principles and implications for animals welfare*, edited by G.P. Moberg and J.A Mench, CABI Publishing. Pages 77-110, ISBN 978-0851993591

Erb, H.N. & Grohn, Y.T. (1988). Epidemiology of metabolic disorders in the periparturient dairy cows. *Journal of Dairy Science*. 71:2556-2571, ISSN: 0022-0302

Fleck, A. (1989). Clinical and nutritional aspects of changes in acute phase proteins during inflammation. *Proceedings of the Nutrition Society*, 48: 347-354, ISSN: 0029-6651

Goff, J.P. (2006). Major advances in our understanding of nutritional influences on bovine health. *Journal of Dairy Science*, 89, 1292-1301. ISSN: 0022-0302

Goff, J.P., Horst, R.L. (1997). Physiological changes at parturition and their relationship to metabolic disorders. *Journal of Dairy Science*, 80:1260-1268. ISSN: 0022-0302

Green, M.J., Green, L.E., Medley G.F., Schukken Y.H. & Bradley A.J. (2002). Influence of Dry Period Bacterial Intramammary Infection on Clinical Mastitis in Dairy Cows. *Journal of Dairy Science*, 85:2589-2599, ISSN: 0022-0302

Grimble, R.F. (2001). Stress proteins in disease: metabolism on a knife edge. *Clinical Nutrition*, 20(6): 469-476, ISSN: 0261-5614

Grummer, R.R. (1995). Impact of changes in organic nutrient metabolism on feeding the transition cow. *Journal of Animal Science* 73, pp. 2820-2833, ISSN: 0021-8812

Gruys, E., Toussaint, M.J., Landman, W.J., Tivapasi, M., Chamanza, R. & VanVeen, L. (1999). Infection, inflammation and stress inhibit growth. Mechanisms and non-specific assessment of the processes by acute phase proteins. In: *Production diseases in farm animals*, edited by Th. Wensing, Wageningen Pers, 72-87, ISBN 9789076998572

Gruys, E., Toussaint, M.J., Niewold, T.A. & Koopmans, S.J. (2005). Acute phase reaction and acute phase proteins. *Journal of Zhejiang University-SCIENCE B (Biomedicine & Biotechnology)*., 6(11):1045-1056, ISSNs 1673-565X

Guzman, E., Birch, J.R. & Ellis S.A. (2010). Cattle MIC is a ligand for the activating NK cell receptor NKG2D. *Veterinary Immunology and Immunopathology*, Vol. 136, pp. 227-234. doi: 10.1016/j.vetimm.2010.03.012, ISSN 0165-2427.

Hauguel-de Mouzon, S. & Guerre-Millo, M. (2006). The placenta cytokine network and inflammatory signals. *Placenta*, 27:794-798, ISSN: 0143-4004

Hanna, N., Bonifacio, L., Weinberger, B., Reddy, P., Murphy, P., Romero, R. & Sharma S. (2006). Evidence for interleukin-10-mediated inhibition of cyclooxygenase-2 expression and prostaglandin production in preterm human placenta. *American Journal of Reproductive Immunology*, 55: 19-27, ISSN:1600-0897

Hayday, A.C. (2009). γδ T cells and the lymphoid stress-surveillance response. *Immunity*, Vol. 31, No. 2, (August 2009), pp 184-196, ISSN 1074-7613.

Hellwig-Bürger, T., Stiehl, D.P., Wagner, A.E., Metzen, E. & Jelkmann, W. (2005). Hypoxia-Inducible Factor-1 (HIF-1): a novel transcription factor in immune reactions. *Journal of Interferon & Cytokine Research*, Vol. 25, pp. 297-310, ISSN 1079-9907.

Johnson, R.W. (1997). Inhibition of growth by pro-inflammatory cytokines: an integrated view. *Journal of Animal Science*, Vol. 75, pp. 1244-1255, ISSN 0021-8812.

Jorritsma, R., César, M.L., Hermans, J.T., Krintwagen, C.L.J.J., Vos, P.L.A.M. & Kruip, T.A.M. (2004). Effects of non-esterified fatty acids on bovine granulosa cells and developmental potential of oocytes in vitro. *Animal Reproduction Science* 81:225-235, ISSN: 0378-4320

Kapcala, P.L. (1999). Inflammatory stress and the immune system. In "Military strategies for sustainment of nutrition and immune function *and Immune Function*", National Academy Press, Washington, D.C., pp. 409-436, ISBN 9780309063456

Kehrli, M.E. Jr., Kimura, K., Goff, J.P., Stabel, J.R. & Nonnecke, B.J. (1999). Immunological dysfunction in periparturient cows - What role does it play in postpartum infectious diseases? *Proc. Annu. Conf. Am. Assoc. Bovine Pract.*, pp. 24-28. ISSN: 0095-1137

Klasing, K.C. (2000). Dietary approaches to protecting animal health. In: *"Agenda 2000: the food revolution"*, Alltech's European ed., Nicholasville, KY, USA, pp 9-19.

Kruip, T.A.M., Meijer, G.A., Rukkwamsuk, T. & Wensing, T. (1999). Investigation into the mechanisms of reduction in fertility of high yielding cows. In: Th. Wensing (ed.) Production diseases in farm animals. Wageningen Pers, Wageningen, The Netherlands, pp 183-190, ISBN 90-74134-60-2

Lacetera, N., Scalia, D., Franci, O., Bernabucci, U., Ronchi, B. & Nardone, A. (2004). Effects of nonesterified fatty acids on lymphocyte functions in dairy heifers. *Journal of Dairy Science* 87, pp.1012-1014. ISSN: 0022-0302

Lacetera, N., Scalia, D., Bernabucci, U., Ronchi, B., Pirazzi, D. & Nardone, A. (2005). Lymphocyte functions in overconditioned cows around parturition. *Journal of Dairy Science* 88, pp. 2010-2016. ISSN: 0022-0302

Lambert, G.P. (2009). Stress-induced gastrointestinal barrier dysfunction and its inflammatory effects. *Journal of Animal Science*, 87(E. Suppl.):E101-E108, ISSN: 0021-8812

Lindström, T.M. & Bennett P.R. (2005). The role of nuclear factor kappa B in human labour. *Reproduction* 130: 569-581, ISSN: 1470-1626

Loor, J.J., Everts, R.E., Bionaz, M., Dann, H.M., Morin, D.E., Oliveira, R., Rodriguez-Zas, S.L., Drackley, J.K. & Lewin, H.A. (2007). Nutrition-induced ketosis alters metabolic and signaling gene networks in liver of periparturient dairy cows. *Physiological Genomics*, Vol. 32, pp. 105-116, ISSN 1094-8341.

Medzhitov, R. (2008). Origin and physiological roles of inflammation. *Nature*, vol. 454, pp. 428-435. ISSN 0028-0836

Moyes, K.M., Larsen, T., Friggens, N.C., Drackley, J.K., & Ingvartsen, K.L. (2009). Identification of potential markers in blood for the development of subclinical and clinical mastitis in dairy cattle at parturition and during early lactation. *Journal of Dairy Science* 92, pp. 5419-5428. ISSN: 0022-0302

Moyes, K.M., Drackley, J.K., Morin, D.E., Rodriguez-Zas, S.L., Everts.3, R.E., Lewin, H.A. & Loor, J.J. (2010). Mammary gene expression profiles during an intramammary challenge reveal potential mechanisms linking negative energy balance with impaired immune response. *Physioogical Genomics* 41, pp. 161-170. ISSN: 1094-8341

Müller-Decker, K. (1999). Ciclooxygenases. In *"Prostaglandins, Leukotriens and other eicosanoids"* Eds. Marks F., Fürstenberger, Wiley-VCH, Germany. Pages 65-88, ISBN 3-527-29360-4

Mulligan, F.J. & Doherty, M.L. (2008). Production diseases of the transition cow. *Veterinary Journal* 176, pp. 3-9. ISSN: 1090-0233

Murata, H., Shimada, N. 6 Yoshioka M. (2004). Current research on acute phase proteins in veterinary diagnosis: an overview. *Veterinary Journal*, 168:28–40, ISSN: 1090-0233

Namangala, B., Inoue, N., Kohara, J., Kuboki, N., Sakurai, T., Hayashida, K. & Sugimoto, C. (2006). Evidence for the immunostimulatory effects of low-dose orally delivered human IFN-alpha in cattle. *Journal of Interferon & Cytokine Research*, Vol. 26, pp. 675-681, ISSN 1079-9907.

Nickerson, S.C. (1989). Immunological aspects of mammary involution. *Journal of Dairy Science*, Vol. 72, No. 6, pp. 1665-1678, ISSN 0022-0302.

Oliver, S.P. & Sordillo L.M. (1989). Approaches to the manipulation of mammary involution. *Journal of Dairy Science*, Vol. 72, No. 6, pp. 1647-1664, ISSN 0022-0302.

Ospina, P.A., Nydam, D.V., Stokol, T. & Overton, T.R. (2010). Evaluation of nonesterified fatty acids and β-hydroxybutyrate in transition dairy cattle in the northeastern United States: Critical thresholds for prediction of clinical diseases. *Journal of Dairy Science* 93, pp. 546-554. ISSN: 0022-0302

Ottaviani, E. & Franceschi, C. (1998). A new theory on the common evolutionary origin of natural immunity, inflammation and stress response: the invertebrate phagocytic immunocyte as an eye-witness. *Domestic Animal Endocrinology*, Vol. 15, pp. 291-296, ISSN 0739-7240.

Pedersen, B.K., Ostrowski, K., Rohde, T., Bruunsgaard, H. (1998). The cytokine response to strenuous exercise. *Canadian Journal of Physiology and Pharmacology* 76(5): 505–511. doi:10.1139/cjpp-76-5-505. ISSN 0008-4212

Petersen, H.H., Nielsen, J.P. & Heegaard, P.M. (2004). Application of acute phase protein measurements in veterinary clinical chemistry. *Veterinary Research*, 35: 163-187, ISSN 0928-4249

Pond, C.M. & Newsholme, E.A. (1999). Coping with metabolic stress in wild and domesticated animals. In: Oldham, J.D., Simm, G., Groen, A.F., Nielsen, B.L., Pryce, J.E., Lawrence, T.L.J. (Eds.), *"Metabolic Stress in Dairy Cows"*, Vol. 24. British Society of Animal Science, pp. 9 – 20, Occasional publication.

Powanda, M.C. (1980). Host metabolic alterations during inflammatory stress as related to nutritional status. American Journal of Veterinary Research, 41(11): 1905-1911, ISSN:0002-9645

Puigserver, P., Rhee, J., Lin, J., Wu, Z., Yoon, J.C., Zhang, C-Y., Krauss, S., Mootha, V. K., Lowell, B.B. & Spiegelman, B.M. (2001). Cytokine stimulation of energy expenditure through p38 MAP kinase activation of PPARg coactivator-1. *Molecular cell*, 8(5):971-982, ISSN:1097-2765

Richards, C.D. & Gauldie, J. (1995). Role of Cytokines in acute-phase response. In *"Human Cytokines: Their Role in Disease and Therapy"*, edited by Aggarwal B.B. and Puri K.R., Blackwell Science, Cambridge (USA). Pages 253-263 ISBN 9780865423527

Rowlands, B.J. & Gardiner, K.R. (1998). Nutritional modulation of gut inflammation. *Proceedings of the Nutrition Society*, 57: 395-401, ISSN: 0029-6651

Scalia, D., Lacetera, N., Bernabucci, U., Demeyere, K., Duchateau, L. & Burvenich, C. (2006). In vitro effects of non-esterified fatty acids on bovine neutrophils oxidative burst and viability. *Journal of Dairy Science* 89, pp. 147-154. ISSN: 0022-0302

Schreiber, G.H. & Schreiber, R.D. (2003). Interferon-γ. In: *The Cytokine Handbook,* A.W. Thomson & M.T. Lotze, (Eds.), Fourth edition, Vol. 1, 567-601. Academic Press, London, UK, ISBN 978-0-12-689663-3.

Sibai, B.M., Caritis, S.N., Thom, E., Klebanoff, M., McNellis, D., Rocco, L., Paul, R.H., Romero, R., Witter, F., Rosen, M. & Depp R. (1993). Prevention of preeclampsia with low-dose aspirin in healthy, nulliparous pregnant women. *The New England Journal of Medicine*, 329: 1213-1218, ISSN 0028-4793

Simpson, K.L., Keelan, J.A. & Mitchell, M.D. (1998). Labor-associated changes in intelreukin-10 production and its regulation by immunomodulators in human choriodecidua. *Journal of Clinical Endocrinology and Metabolism* 83: 4332-4337, ISSN: 0021-972X

Sordillo, L.M., Contreras, G.A. & Aitken, S.L. (2009). Metabolic factors affecting the inflammatory response of periparturient dairy cows. *Animal Health Research Reviews* 10:53–63. doi:10.1017/S1466252309990016, ISSN 1466-2523.

Spears, J.W. & Weiss, P.W. (2008). Role of antioxidants and trace elements in health and immunity of transition dairy cows. *Veterinary Journal* 176, pp. 70-76. ISSN: 1090-0233

Suriyasathaporn, W., Daemen, A. J. J. M., Noordhuizen-Stassen, E. N., Dieleman, S. J., Nielen, M. & Schukken, Y. H. (1999). β-Hydroxybutyrate levels in peripheral blood and ketone bodies supplemented in culture media affect the in vitro chemotaxis of bovine leukocytes. *Veterinary Immunology and Immunopathology* 68:177–186, ISSN: 0165-2427

Tang, D., Kang, R., Xiao, W., Jiang, L., Liu, M., Shi, Y., Wang, K., Wang, H., & Xiao, X. (2007). Nuclear heat shock protein 72 as a negative regulator of oxidative stress (hydrogen peroxide)-induced HMGB1 cytoplasmic translocation and release. *Journal of Immunol*ogy, Vol. 178, pp. 7376-7384, ISSN 0022-1767.

Trevisi, E., Calamari, L., Iamartino, N. & Bertoni, G. (1998). Sintesi epatiche nel post-parto della bovina: possibili cause di variazione e relazione con la fertilità. *Proc. X Meeting Nazionale su "Studio della efficienza riproduttiva degli animali di interesse zootecnico"*. Bergamo, 12.06.1998, 10: 37-41.

Trevisi, E., Calamari, L. & Bertoni, G. (2001). Definition of a liver activity index in the transition dairy cow and its relationship with the reproductive performance. *Proc. X Int. Symp. of Veterinary Laboratory Diagnosticians*, 4-7 July, Salsomaggiore-Parma, Italy, 118-119.

Trevisi, E., Gubbiotti, A. & Bertoni, G. (2007). Effects of inflammation in peripartum dairy cows on milk yield, energy balance and efficiency. 2nd International Symposium on Energy and Protein Metabolism and Nutrition, Vichy (France), 9-13 Septembre. In *"Energy and protein metabolism and nutrition - Eaap 124"*, edited by: I. Ortigues-Marty, pp. 395-396 ISBN 978-90-8686-041-8.

Trevisi, E., Bakudila, A.M. & Bertoni, G. (2008a). Modulazione dell'evento infiammatorio nel periparto della bovina da latte mediante la somministrazione di acido acetilsalicilico. *Buiatria. Journal of the Italian Association for Buiatrics* 3 (2): 61-68.

Trevisi, E., Piccioli-Cappelli, F., Bani, P. & Bertoni, G. (2008b). Effects of Polinacea™ extract in periparturient dairy cows. *Book of Abstracts of the 59th Annual Meeting of the European Association for Animal Production*, Vilnius, Lithuania, 24-27 August, p. 147, ISBN: 978-90-8686-074-6

Trevisi, E. & Bertoni, G. (2008). Attenuation with acetylsalicylate treatments of inflammatory conditions in periparturient dairy cows. In *"Aspirin and health research progress"*, Nova Science Publishers, Hauppauge, NY, USA. pp 23-37, ISBN 9781604561647

Trevisi, E., Amadori, M., Bakudila, A. & Bertoni G. (2009). Metabolic changes in dairy cows induced by oral, low-dose interferon-alpha treatment. *Journal of Animal Science*, Vol. 87 (9), pp. 3020-3029, ISSN 0021-8812.

Trevisi, E., Amadori, M., Cogrossi, S. & Bertoni G. (2010a). Metabolic stress and interleukin-6 response in high-yielding, periparturient dairy cows. 9th IVIS (International Veterinary Immunology Symposium), August 16-20, 2010, Tokyo, Japan, Page 138.

Trevisi, E., Ferrari, A., Piccioli-Cappelli, F., Grossi, P. & Bertoni, G. (2010b). An additional study on the relationship between the inflammatory condition at calving time and net energy efficiency in dairy cows. In: *"Energy and Protein Metabolism and Nutrition. EAAP publication No. 127"*. Wageningen Academic Publishers. Pp 489-490, ISBN 978-90-8686-153-8.

Trevisi, E., Zecconi, A., Bertoni, G. & Piccinini, R. (2010c). Blood and milk immune and inflammatory responses in periparturient dairy cows showing a different liver activity index. *Journal of Dairy Research* 77: 310-317, ISSN: 0022-0299

Van Eden, W., Van Der Zee, R. & Prakken B. (2005). Heat-shock proteins induce T-cell regulation of chronic inflammation. *Nature Reviews Immunology*, Vol. 5, pp. 318-330, ISSN 1474-1733.

Villa-Godoy, A., Hughes, T.L., Emery, R.S., Chapin, L. & Fogwell, R.L. (1988). Association between energy balance and luteal function in lactating dairy cows. *Journal of Dairy Science* 71:1063-1072, ISSN: 0022-0302

Wan, J.M., Haw, M. P. & Blackburn, G.L. (1989). Nutrition, immune function and inflammation: an overview. Symposium on "The interaction between nutrition and inflammation", *Proceedings of the Nutrition Society*, 48: 315-335, ISSN 0029-6651.

Wathes, D.C., Cheng, Z., Chowdhury, W., Fenwick, M.A., Fitzpatrick, R., Morris, D.G., Patton, J. & Murphy, J.J. (2009). Negative energy balance alters global gene expression and immune responses in the uterus of postpartum dairy cows. *Physiological Genomics* 39, 1-13, ISSN: 1094-8341

15

Acute Phase Proteins in Cattle

Jawor Paulina and Stefaniak Tadeusz
*Wroclaw University of Environmental and Life Sciences,
Department of Immunology, Pathophysiology and
Veterinary Prevention, Wroclaw
Poland*

1. Introduction

The acute phase response (APR) is a reaction of an organism to homeostatic disturbances, that could be due to an infection, tissue injury, neoplastic growth or immunological disorders. At the site of injury there is a local reaction - the aggregation of platelets, clot formation, dilatation and leakage of blood vessels, and the accumulation and activation of granulocytes and mononuclear cells. Activated cells release acute phase cytokines including, interleukin-6 (IL-6), interleukin-1 beta (IL-1b) and tumor necrosis factor-alpha (TNF-a) – in order of importance. Due to specific receptors present on different target cells, these cytokines may act a systemic reaction - fever, leucocytosis, an increase in erythrocyte sedimentation rate, an increase in secretion of ACTH and glucocorticoids, activation of complement and clotting cascades, a decrease in serum levels of iron and zinc, a negative nitrogen balance, and dramatic changes in the concentration of some plasma proteins called acute phase proteins (APPs) (Heinrich et. al., 1990). The APPs belong to the group of proteins that become increased in concentration by 25% or more during inflammation (Kushner 1982, as cited in Whicher et al., 1991).

In cattle, inflammation is not always followed by a leukocyte population increase. The normally low neutrophil-to-lymphocyte ratio (0.5 in cows) compared with other species (3.5 in dogs, 1.8 in cats) may predispose ruminants to a delayed granulopoietic response because of a slower acceleration of myelopoiesis, preventing rapid leucocytosis (Taylor, 2006). Moreover, in cattle, the detection of inflammatory processes is more difficult to assess, because the symptoms of diseases are not easily detectable. Also, loose-housing systems make it even more difficult to observe individual cows and to recognize sick animals.

The APPs are sensitive factors that allow the early and precise detection of inflammation in ruminants (Kent, 1992). The most frequently investigated proteins in cattle are: haptoglobin (Hp), serum amyloid A (SAA), fibrinogen (Fb), ceruloplasmin, alpha 1-antitrypsin and alpha 1-acid glycoprotein (α_1-AGP) (Conner et al., 1986; Dowling et al., 2002; Eckersall & Conner, 1988; Horadagoda et al., 1993). The liver is the major organ responsible for the synthesis of acute phase proteins (Miller et al., 1951). In cattle some proteins may be extra-hepatically synthesized, e.g. Hp and SAA may also be produced in the mammary gland (Hiss et al., 2004; Molenaar et al., 1999, as cited in Molenaar et al., 2005). Proteins that increase in concentration during the inflammatory process are positive reacting proteins (e.g. Hp, Fb and SAA) and proteins that decrease in concentration are negative reacting proteins (e.g.

albumin, transferrin). Changes in APP levels (Hp and Fb) are slower and more prolonged compared to other changes that occur during the acute phase response, such as fever development, white blood cell count and decreased zinc concentration (Godson et al., 1995). Serum amyloid A and Hp may be used to discriminate between acute and chronic inflammatory conditions and were found to be better discriminators than haematological tests e.g. number of leucocytes, percentage of neutrophils and band neutrophils (Horadagoda et al., 1999). A significantly higher proportion of cattle with acute inflammation were found to have higher values of SAA and Hp than those with chronic inflammation (Horadagoda et al., 1999). The possibility of using APPs as markers of inflammation has triggered broad research in terms of cattle diseases. The usefulness of acute phase proteins for diagnosis and prognosis during the course of the most frequently occurring disturbances in cows (dystocia, retained placenta, metritis, abdominal disorders, mastitis and limb diseases) and calves (respiratory tract and diarrhoea) and in herd health monitoring will be discussed.

2. Acute phase proteins in cattle diseases

2.1 Peripartum reproductive disorders (dystocia, retained placenta, metritis)

Transition from a dry period to lactation demands a tremendous effort from cows. Not all cows are capable of coping with this challenge and, as a result, they suffer from health problems. Normal calving induces an acute phase reaction. Parturition increases the Hp concentration but not the concentration of α_1-acid glycoprotein in cows (Uchida et al. 1993). Contrary to findings by Uchida et al. (1993), Cairoli et al. (2006) found an increase α_1-AGP concentrations between two weeks before and two weeks after parturition. The SAA concentration increases after delivery and the highest concentration was reached at 48 hours (Uchida et al., 1993). The increase in SAA concentration was related to tissue damage in the cow after passage of the calf through the cervix and expulsion of the placenta. Similar to Uchida et al. (1993), in a study by Chan et al. (2010), the SAA in healthy cows reached the highest concentration within 3 days after delivery (66±15 mg/l). Haptoglobin was detectable in the serum of all animals within 3 days after calving, and of these, 95.8% had concentrations higher than >130.9 mg/l. By the third week after parturition the serum Hp concentrations in healthy cows had decreased to ≤130.9 mg/l, while serum SAA concentrations decreased to ≤51.9 mg/l during the first week after parturition. The possibility that the synthesis of APPs may be influenced by hormones such as cortisol or prostaglandin cannot be excluded (Alsemgeest et al., 1993).

In relation to peripartum reproductive disorders, acute phase proteins were examined as markers of the inflammatory process and predictors of the outcome of disease. It seemed that the APPs were not useful markers of predicting dystocia. In cows with dystocia followed by Caesarean section, the mean concentrations of Hp and Fb before surgery were within the reference ranges (0.07 and 6.3 g/l, respectively) (Hirvonen & Pyörälä, 1998). Also, in a study by Schönfelder et al. (2005), the Hp concentrations in cows with too large (relatively or absolutely) foetus, before Caesarean section, were similar to those in cows with regularly sized calves (median 0.1 vs. 0.009 g/l, respectively). It seems that conditions more serious than the foetus being too large must be present to induce increased Hp concentrations. In cows with torsio uteri, which led to a Caesarean section, the median Hp concentration before surgery was 2.1 g/l (Schönfelder et al., 2005).

The serum Hp concentrations during other postpartum reproductive disorders were ambiguous in the literature. In a study by Skinner et al. (1991), the mean Hp serum concentration in cows with severe metritis was 1.04 g/l (range from 0.56 to 1.61 g/l). Cows with a retained placenta (RP) and without metritis had lower mean Hp concentrations 0.76 g/l (range 0.21-1.2 g/l). On the contrary, low Hp concentrations were found in cows with toxic puerperal metritis (Smith et al., 1998). The mean concentration on diagnosis day was 0.19±0.15 g/l. Because the cows were carefully watched for signs of metritis after parturition, it is possible that low serum Hp concentrations in some of the animals were due to early diagnosis of the disease, and blood samples were taken before Hp had increased. Hirvonen et al. (1999b) also showed that plasma Hp concentrations remained low or moderate in most cows with acute postpartum metritis, and that in one cow (out of 14) the Hp concentration was not even detectable. In RP cows, just 1 out of 5 showed an Hp concentration above 0.1 g/l. The α_1-AGP levels were increased in cows with acute postpartum metritis, but their levels did not correlate with the severity of the disease. The highest concentrations of α_1-AGP were noted in the plasma of cows with metritis and also dystocia and/or RP. In a study by Chan et al. (2010), cows with acute puerperal metritis had significantly higher Hp concentrations than those in the healthy group throughout the 6 months after delivery, but the higher concentrations of SAA in the metritis group were significantly different in a shorter period (between 4 days and 2 months postpartum). The highest Hp concentration was found in the period of 0-3 days postpartum (1.1 ±0.43 g/l), whereas for SAA it was 4-7 days postpartum (85±23 mg/l). The Hp concentration may be also used to evaluate the efficiency of therapy (Mordak, 2008). Cows with RP were divided into two groups with or without manual removal of the membrane. Cows with manual extraction were further divided into groups where the placenta had either been easily removed or there had been problems and remains of the placenta were left in the uterus. Cows without placenta removal were divided into groups where the placenta had been expelled within 4 days or after 4 days. Ten days after calving the highest Hp concentration was found in the group where the placenta had been expelled after 4 days (2.22±0.36g/l), and the lowest was found in cows where the placenta had been easily removed manually (0.9±0.3 g/l). For cows where placental removal was not complete or where they had been expelled within 4 days, the Hp concentrations were not statistically different (1.83±0.2 vs. 1.53±0.27 g/l, respectively). Regarding Hp concentration on the tenth day, these results suggest that situations where the membranes are easily removed manually are the most beneficial for cows, but Hp concentrations at that time were still higher than those in cows serum without RP (0.46±0.19 g/l).

In spite of the ambiguous results for APP concentrations during postpartum health disturbances, it can clearly be seen that high APP concentrations postpartum are negatively associated with health. Cows exhibiting Hp serum concentrations higher than 1 g/l at 15 days of lactation had an increased risk of early culling (Bertoni et al., 1997). Also Hirvonen et al. (1999b) found that cows with Hp concentrations >0.7 g/l were later culled, due to poor body condition and low fertility.

In recent years, it has become more popular to use APPs as predictors or risk factors for diseases. In heifers with RP, Hp was detectable in the last week before delivery and the mean Hp concentration was 0.9 ± 0.01 g/l. The mean SAA concentration was 20.3 ± 8.86 mg/l. The differences in Hp and SAA levels between heifers with and without RP were statistically significant (Krakowski & Zdzisinska, 2007). Huzzey et al. (2009a) showed that the Hp concentration might be used as an early predictor of metritis. Cows with Hp concentrations ≥1 g/l at day 3 postpartum were 6.7 times more likely to develop severe or mild metritis. Also, Dubuc et al. (2010) showed that Hp concentration ≥ 0.8 g/l in the first week postpartum are a risk factor not only for metritis, but also for purulent vaginal discharge and cytological endometritis, as well.

The determination of APPs, especially haptoglobin, seems to be very useful during the peripartum period. Early detection of animals at risk and monitoring the efficiency of therapy and prognosis are very crucial, not only for economic reasons, but also with regard to animal welfare issues.

2.2 The most common abdominal disorders and surgical interventions

The concentrations of APPs have been described in cases of traumatic pericarditis and reticuloperitonitis, abomasal displacement (DA), abomasal volvulus and caesarean sections. McSherry et al. (1970) examined the plasma concentrations of fibrinogen in 160 sick cows. Many diseases were found to be associated with elevated plasma Fb levels, but pericarditis and peritonitis tended to produce the most consistent changes. Pericarditis, which was traumatic in origin, was detected in eight cows where the Fb concentrations were in the range of 9.25-16.75 g/l (McSherry et al., 1970). Also, Makimura and Usui (1990), in cattle with traumatic pericarditis, examined the concentrations of Hp, mucoprotein and sialic acid. Although in most cases the Hp concentration was increased at the same time as the other APPs, in animals with concurrent *Theileria sergenti* parasitic infection, the Hp concentration was lower than expected. This showed that in the cases of latent or apparent haemolytic disorders, diagnosis of inflammatory disorders with Hp estimation may be difficult. In the diagnosis of traumatic pericarditis, albumins also seem to be very useful. In a study by Yoshida (1991), cows with pericarditis had decreased levels of serum albumins (21.9 ±3.8 g/l), and the lowest concentration was found in cases with purulent type of traumatic pericarditis.

In a study on plasma Fb concentrations (McSherry et al., 1970) among 44 cows with peritonitis, 34 had Fb above 8.0 g/l (range 8.4-31.25 g/l). In 70% of these animals Fb exceeded 10 g/l. In 30 cows peritonitis was due to traumatic reticulo-peritonitis. Hirvonen and Pyörälä (1998) reported that cows with traumatic reticulo-peritonitis had high Fb concentrations. The mean Fb concentration in eleven cows was 11.6 g/l and in ten exceeded 7 g/l. All cows with traumatic reticulo-peritonitis had preoperative Hp concentrations >0.55 g/l and the mean Hp concentration was 1.07 g/l. The fact to find both Fb and Hp high concentrations in traumatic reticulo-peritonitis, as well as significantly higher concentrations than in cows with other surgically-treated abdominal disorders (e.g. abomasal displacement, caesarean section), makes them an attractive parameters for evaluation in diagnostics of traumatic reticulo-peritonitis. After surgery, cows with traumatic reticulo-peritonitis showed only a small increase in Hp and Fb concentrations, followed by a steady decrease during the late hospitalization phase.

Displacement of the abomasum (DA) does not usually induce a significant Fb response. The Fb concentration was found to be in the range of 9.0-10.25 g/l in only three out of nine cows, and in the remaining cows it was between 3.1-8 g/l (McSherry et al., 1970). In a study by Hirvonen and Pyörälä (1998), in cows with abomasal displacement or volvulus, the mean plasma Fb concentration before surgery was 6.2 g/l. Fibrinogen was also found to be within the reference range in a study by Irmak and Turgut (2005). Cows with left DA had a mean

Fb concentration 3.8 g/l and cows with right DA had 3.7 g/l. Similar to the results of Hirvonen and Pyörälä (1998), in a study by Jawor et al. (2009) the mean Fb concentration in cows with DA was within the reference range (Table 1). In this study, blood samples were taken at three times. The first time (I) at cow arrival to the clinic (where the surgery was to be performed); the second (II) was at the third day of hospitalization; and the third sample (III) was taken just before the animal was returned to the owner, mostly on the seventh day. A right paralumbar fossa omentopexy was performed. Levels of Fb, Hp, SAA and albumin levels were also determined. In contrast to findings reported by Hirvonen and Pyörälä (1998), in our experience, the mean Hp concentration before surgery was higher (0,15 vs. 1.21 g/l respectively). The mean Hp concentration was elevated in all blood collections. Fibrinogen remained low throughout the whole observation period. Only the changes in SAA during post-operative monitoring were significant, specifically between blood collections I and III (Table 1).

APP concentrations		I n=8	II n=8	III n=8
Hp g/l	Mean (SD)	1.21 (±1.08)	1.10 (±0.63)	1.14 (±1.28)
	Median	0.81	1.17	0.79
Fb g/l	Mean (SD)	6.4 (±2.0)	5.95 (±1.08)	5.23 (±1.32)
	Median	6.24	5.95	5.48
SAA mg/l	Mean (SD)	138.59 (±34.7) a	122.86 (±38.6)	96.77 (±38.9) b
	Median	130.92	142.08	103.99

Table 1. Concentrations of Hp, Fb and SAA in cows with displaced abomasum (adapted from Jawor et al., 2009). I, II, III – blood-sampling. Values followed by different letters are significantly different at $P \leq 0.05$.

Abdominal surgery in cows induces an increase in Hp. In the study done by Hirvonen & Pyörälä, (1998) on abdominal surgery (DA, caesarean section, explorative laparotomy) a moderate Hp response, that peaked 2-3 days after surgery, was reported. In our study mean Hp and SAA concentration was lower after surgery. These differences in Hp changes might result from different initial concentrations - contrary to our results, the initial Hp concentration in study Hirvonen and Pyörälä (1998) in cows with abomasal pathology was low and APR driven by surgery is not major. A low concentration of albumin was detected in cows during the entire period of observation (I-26.5±6.9; II-24.9±2.6, III-25.0±4.6). Low concentrations of albumins together with high Hp and SAA levels confirmed a severe inflammatory state in the cows. The relatively quick change in SAA concentrations contrary to Hp and albumin, showed that during the monitoring of recovery process in cows with DA, the most accurate APP marker for post-surgery recovery process is SAA. Fibrinogen did not seem to be efficient enough for monitoring the cases of DA. However, Hirvonen and Pyörälä (1998) pointed out that Fb concentrations might be helpful in the postoperative monitoring of infectious complications, such as peritonitis.

In terms of DA, the Hp level determination before parturition may be a useful diagnostic tool to assess the risk of this disease (Huzzey et al., 2009b). During the week before parturition, the Hp serum concentration in cows developing DA postpartum was significantly higher as compared with healthy cows (0.5±0.02 vs. 0.2±0.02 g/l, respectively).

The odds for developing DA were 3.1-fold higher in cows with Hp concentration ≥0.8 g/l during week before parturition.
The determination of Hp may also be useful for caesarean sections (Balbierz et al., 1977). In uncomplicated cases, Hp appeared in the serum on the second day after surgery and remained elevated for 8-9 days. When complications occurred after surgery, the Hp concentration remained elevated for the whole observation period (18 days). The determination of Hp concentrations after surgery may be also used as a predictor of regenerative potential in cases of caesarean section after torsio uteri (Schönfelder et al., 2005). Cows that were fertile later had the highest Hp concentration on day 3 (median 3.21 g/l), which later decreased. In cows that did not become pregnant later, the Hp concentration increased from day 2 (median 0.74 g/l) and demonstrated prolonged inflammatory states, which probably caused infertility.
The determination of APPs in surgical procedures is a valuable tool for veterinary surgeons in monitoring the recovery process and the early detection of inflammatory complications. However, it must be remembered that surgical intervention induces a short increase in Hp and SAA levels, but not Fb levels.

2.3 Mastitis

Mastitis is recognized as being one of the most important reasons for culling dairy cows (Esslemont & Kossaibati 1997; Whitaker et al., 2000). The significant impact on health and milk production aroused researcher into APPs and mastitis. Up to now the evaluation of somatic cell count (SCC) has remained as the gold standard for determining udder health. However, research results have suggested that APPs might be interesting as either a valuable supplement even as an alternative to SCC. Changes in concentrations of Hp, Fb, ceruloplasmin, α-1 antitrypsin, acid soluble glycoproteins, α_1-proteinase inhibitor and SAA were investigated under field conditions and in experimentally induced mastitis.

2.3.1 APPs in serum

Haptoglobin, known as the haemoglobin reactive protein (HRP), in cows with mastitis was investigated by Spooner and Miller (1971). Out of 26 cows, Hp was detected in the sera of 24 cows with clinical summer mastitis (septic mastitis). Later, Conner et al. (1986) found that all cows with summer mastitis had significantly elevated concentrations of α-1 antitrypsin and ceruloplasmin in comparison to normal cows. In all cows with mastitis, Hp was elevated, whereas in healthy cows Hp was undetectable. Skinner et al. (1991) concluded that a haptoglobin concentration >0.4 g/l indicates significant infection and that a concentration of 0.2 g/l and above may indicate early or mild infection. Eckersall et al. (1988, as cited in Skinner et al., 1991) suggested that the prognosis for cattle with an Hp concentration > 1 g/l is poor, but a later study could not confirm this (Skinner et al., 1991). The experimental induction of mastitis explained some more details about the usefulness of APPs and characterized the APR during mastitis. After experimental induction of mastitis in 10 pregnant heifers with *Actinomyces pyogenes*, *Fusoacerium necrophorum* and *Peptostreptococcus indolicus*, changes in plasma Fb, serum Hp, acid-soluble glycoproteins (ASG) and the α_1-proteinase inhibitor (α_1-PI) were analysed (Hirvonen et al., 1996). Fibrinogen was found to be a reliable indicator for detecting the presence of bacterial infections in all heifers, but not as a prognostic indicator for mastitis, as there was no difference in the Fb response between animals who recovered and those who did not. Haptoglobin and ASG were most effective in indicating the severity of infection and in predicting the final outcome of the disease in the heifers. The Hp response was different between moderate and severely affected heifers. The maximum Hp response was reached in 2-3 days. In severely infected heifers, Hp was four times higher than in the moderately affected heifers. The Hp levels in severely infected heifers remained elevated 2 weeks after bacterial inoculation, whereas in the moderately infected animals Hp returned to normal 5 days after the bacterial challenge. The maximum values for ASG were reached within 3-5 days. The ASG values in severely infected animals remained high for 2 weeks after inoculation. Serum α_1-PI levels increased in severely affected heifers (maximum activities were reached in 3 days), but in moderately affected animals there was no clear response by this APP after the challenge. The WBC response was similar in all animals and had no predictive value for the severity of the disease in this study. These differences were not so evident in later studies. Hirvonen et al. (1999a) found that the differences between severely versus moderately or mildly affected cows with *E. coli* were present for SAA (which is more sensitive) but not for haptoglobin. Eckersall et al. (2001) showed that although serum Hp concentrations were higher in cows suffering from mastitis compared to healthy cows, no difference was observed between the cows suffering from mild and moderate mastitis. These differences might have been due to the different pathogens used and the numbers of bacteria inoculated, isolated from udders in these studies or individual ability for APPs synthesis (Jacobsen et al., 2004). Ohtsuka et al. (2001) showed that in naturally occurring coliform mastitis the Hp concentration was different in cows with severe (n=7) and mild mastitis (n=11) on days 3 and 9 after diagnosis, but not on day 6. The concentrations of Hp and SAA from different studies are compared in Table 2.

	Eckersall et al. (2001)		Grönlund et al. (2003)		Nielsen et al. (2004)	Jawor (2007)
	mild (n=16)	moderate (n=13)	acute (n=6)	chronic (n=5)	(n=10)	(n=11)
Hp (mg/ml)	0.47	0.74	0.965	0.07	0.79	1.27
SAA (µg/ml)	13.8	29.9	262	7.2	752*(739)**	69.86

Table 2. Median Hp and SAA serum concentrations in mastitis (*mean, **standard deviation).

2.3.2 APPs in milk

Milk seems to be a better than serum material for testing APPs during mastitis. It is easier and quicker to obtain a large number of milk samples without stressing the animals. Mazur (1980), using agar electrophoresis, showed the presence of HRP in cows' whey. The highest frequency of HRP was detected in the whey obtained from quarters with progressed inflammatory lesions and a significantly increased number of somatic cells (Mazur A. & Mazur O., 1981). Increased milk concentrations of Hp and SAA in cows with mastitis were shown by Eckersall et al. (2001). In cows' milk from infected quarters with moderate mastitis, concentrations of SAA but not Hp were significantly greater than in cows with mild mastitis. In milk SAA seems to have a greater potential for the detection of mastitis than Hp since it had higher sensitivity, specificity and efficiency in differentiating between cows with mastitis and healthy cows (Eckersall et al., 2001). Since the concentrations of APPs in milk also significantly increased with increasing somatic cell count, this suggests

that milk APPs may indicate the severity of an infection (Nielsen et al., 2004). In cases of chronic subclinical mastitis, only milk SAA levels were significantly higher than pre-infection and healthy control quarters (Grönlund et al. 2003). Later studies showed that whilst increased concentrations of APPs in milk were noticed in cows with chronic subclinical mastitis, the contents of Hp and SAA varied markedly (Grönlund et al., 2005). Haptoglobin and/or SAA were detected in 83% of the examined composite milk samples (pooled milk from quarters). Since cows had to have detectable levels of Hp or SAA in at least two udder quarters for elevated levels to be found in the composite samples, analysis at the quarter level is preferable. The important findings were that almost all udder quarter samples from healthy control cows had undetectable levels of Hp and SAA, and that Hp and/or SAA concentrations above 0.3 and 0.9 mg/l (the detection limit in this study), respectively, indicated an abnormal udder quarter.
Although methods for determining levels of Hp in milk have been described (Eckersall et al., 2001; Grönlund et al., 2003; Hiss et al., 2004) tests which allow a quick and simple determination are necessary. Akerstedt et al. (2006) described an optical biosensor for Hp determination in milk. It was based on the strong interaction between Hp and haemoglobin. This assay has the potential to be useful in screening for Hp in milk samples. It could be used for the semi-quantitative determination in milk from cows with no observable signs of mastitis. The local production of Hp and SAA in the udder during acute mastitis makes these APPs sensitive and rapid markers of acute inflammation. Up till now there are no commercially available methods for their rapid testing. For broad milk testing for APPs presence at cow-side tests are necessary.

2.4 Lameness and limb diseases

Limb pathology in dairy herds is a serious problem. With increasing milk production the problem might become even more significant as high-yield milk cows are more predisposed to lameness (Green et al., 2002). The economic losses from lameness are due to the higher incidence of culling, the lower likelihood of pregnancy (Bicalho et al., 2007; Mendelez et al., 2003) and the lower milk production (Green et al., 2002; Rajala-Schultz et al., 1999).
In order to limit the losses related to lameness, it is important to detect lame cows as early as possible. A few papers were recently published on the estimation of APPs in lameness, and the efficiency of trimming and treatment. Kujala et al. (2010) investigated concentrations of Hp and SAA cows with sole ulcers and/or white line abscesses, without any other clinical symptoms. The blood from lame and healthy cows was taken on day 0 (diagnosis of lameness), and again from lame cows on days: 4, 7 or 8 and 14. No antibiotic treatment was used. The SAA concentrations were significantly elevated from day 0 until 7/8. There was no difference between SAA concentrations in the samples taken on day 14 from lame cows and healthy cows, and the cows were no longer lame as well. No significant differences were observed in the serum Hp concentrations between the groups. Serum amyloid A is known to be more sensitive APP in cattle than Hp (Heegard et al., 2000) and, according to the authors cited above, the local changes in the hooves were large enough to induce a general SAA response but not a response by Hp. Higher concentrations of haptoglobin were detected among 60 dairy cattle diagnosed with pododermatitis septica (PS), pododermatitis circumscripta (PC), interdigital necrobacillosis (IN) and papillomatous digital dermatitis (PPD) (Smith et al., 2010). Haptoglobin was measured after the initial diagnosis and on days 3 and 5 afterwards. Elevated levels (>0.37g/l) were found on day 1 in cows with PS, PC, IN

and PDD: 65.9%, 37.5%, 71.4% and 25.0% of the cows, respectively. Although the number of animals with an increased Hp concentration decreased after 5 days, still 14.3-50% of the cows with PS, PC and PPD had elevated Hp level in last blood sample. The decreasing Hp concentrations in cows with PS, IN and PDD indicated the effective treatment for these disorders (Smith et al., 2010). An investigation of albumin, Fb, Hp, seromucoid and ceruloplasmin levels in first lactation heifers was carried out to determine the presence of any relationships with the development of hoof horn haemorrhaging (Laven et al., 2004). None of seven examined proteins showed any relationship between changes and the development of hoof horn haemorrhaging after calving. It seems that more serious pathologies in hoofs such as - sole ulcers and interdigital necrobacillosis must be present to induce general APR.

The estimation of concentrations and the dynamics of changes in APP levels can be a valuable tool, supplementing the clinical assessment during treatment (Jawor et al., 2008). In our study we compared concentrations of Hp, SAA and Fb in healthy cows and cows with limb diseases. The cows were retrospectively divided into groups I - with systematic decreases in APP levels in successive blood collections (n=6) and II - with an increase in the concentration of one or more APPs in the second or third blood collection (n=8). Group III comprised healthy cows at different stages of lactation and dry cows (n=10). From groups I and II blood was taken for the first time (1) on the day of their arrival at the clinic, for the second time (2) between the third and sixth day of stay, and for the third time (3) when the animal was healthy enough to be sent back to its owner. Blood from healthy cows was only taken once. The mean initial concentrations and changes in levels during treatment are shown in Table 3.

		1			**2**			**3**	
	I	**II**	**III***	**I**	**II**	**III***	**I**	**II**	**III***
Hp g/l	2.4 ±0.6 **a**	1.2 ±0.7	0.1 ±0.1 **b**	0.8 ±0.4	0.9 ±0.5	0.1 ±0.1	0.1 ±0.1	0.3 ±0.2	0.1 ±0.1
SAA mg/l	219.7 ±30.4 **A**	153.7 ±24.3 **A**	24.4 ±7.8 **B**	124.5 ±6.5 **a**	127.1 ±29.0 **Aa**	24.4 ±7.8 **Bb**	79.1 ±22.4	86.1 ±17.8 **a**	24.4 ±7.8 **b**
Fb g/l	12.2 ±1.3 **A**	8.0 ±0.6 **Bc**	5.0 ±0.2 **Bb**	9.9 ±0.9 **A**	6.9 ±0.5 **Bc**	5.0 ±0.2 **Bb**	7.2 ±1.2	6.6 ±0.8	5.0 ±0.2

1,2,3 blood samples, I,II,III experimental groups. Values followed by different letters within the same blood collection were statistically different: small letters $P \leq 0.05$, capital letters $P \leq 0.01$. *cows from healthy group were sampled once

Table 3. Mean (±SEM) concentrations of haptoglobin, serum amyloid A and fibrinogen during the treatment of limb diseases (adapted from Jawor et al., 2008).

The highest concentrations of all investigated proteins were recorded at the beginning of the treatment. As the concentrations of APPs depend on the extent of underlying tissue damage (Heegaard et al., 2000), the very high concentrations of Hp, Fb, SAA at the beginning in group I suggested a very severe, acute inflammatory process. High, gradual decrease in this group shows that treatment process went without complications. An initial decrease in the concentrations of Hp, SAA and Fb between the first and second blood collections from five cows in Group II was also noticed. This proved that the treatment applied was appropriate and that it contributed towards reducing the inflammatory process in the cows, but, in cases

of further complications (e.g. wound infections, bronchitis, the occurrence of other inflammatory states of the limbs), we noticed increases in one or two of the APPs under examination at the next blood collection.
Although the APR is not specific and the problem cannot be recognized based only an increase in APPs, this may actually be advantageous to a veterinarian as a valuable indicator that the recovery process is not going correctly. The triple determination of APPs during treatment seems to be a valuable supplement to clinical findings. For practical purposes, we recommend at least two APP estimations. The first one should be performed at the beginning of treatment to evaluate the severity (chronic/acute) of the process and the extent of tissue damage. The second should be performed immediately before returning the cow to its owner. This estimation, in addition to other clinical parameters (such as a decrease in lameness, an increase in appetite and milk yield), is a good measure of the efficiency of the therapy. The additional estimation should be performed during treatment in following cases: there are doubts regarding the correctness of the treatment, when there is very little or no clinical improvement, or before making critical decisions, such as whether or not to amputate claw. Acute phase protein determination is also useful during the recovery period because the time between dressing changes after claw resection is gradually prolonged. During this period, apart from assessing how a cow is coping with putting weight onto an affected leg and her general behaviour under field conditions, there is no possibility of assessing the healing process.

2.5 Respiratory diseases in calves

In addition to diarrhea, respiratory tract diseases are one of the main health problems afflicting young dairy calves (Sivula et al., 1996; Svensson et al., 2003). To prevent disease outbreaks, early detection, isolation and treatment of diseased animals is important. Results from several different studies have shown that estimation of APPs is useful for detecting and monitoring respiratory diseases. In calves with respiratory tract diseases, the following APPs were examined: Hp, Fb, SAA, transferrin (Tf), lipopolysaccharide binding protein (LBP), α_1-acid glycoprotein (AGP), α_1-antitripsin (α_1-AT), seromucoid (Sm), ceruloplasmin (Cp), albumin, α_1-antichymotrypsin and α_2-macroglobulin.

2.5.1 APPs during experimental infections

Most of results regarding APPs in respiratory infections were obtained from experimental infections. Although scientists are not in agreement as to whether bacterial or viral infections mount a higher response, it has been shown that APR is induced faster after bacterial infections (Table 4). After intra-tracheal aerosol inoculation with *Mannheimia (Pasteurella) haemolytica,* the earliest detectable rise in Hp, Sm and α_1-AT in calves was after 24 h (Conner et al., 1989). However, bacterial infection did not cause a rise in ceruloplasmin levels. The highest concentrations of Hp, Sm and α_1-AT were reached on day 3 (1.0 g/l; 1.91 g/l; 1090 iu/l respectively). In this study, α_1-anitichymotripsin and α_2-macroglobulin were also shown to be acute phase reactants in calves. Horadagoda and Eckresall (1994) also inoculated calves intra-tracheally with *M. haemolytica* serotype A1. Within 10 hours post-inoculation, there was a small, insignificant increase in Hp. In contrast, SAA showed more dynamic changes: there was a progressive, linear change in SAA, and the mean concentration increased from close to the detection limit (3 mg/l) at inoculation, to 18 mg/l by 10 hours post-inoculation. These results indicate that SAA is more rapid than Hp in calves in response to infection with *M. haemolytica.* To assess the acute phase response in bovine respiratory disease (BRD), infection with Bovine Herpes Virus-1 (BHV-1) and *P. haemolytica* was performed on 49 animals (Godson et al., 1996). Calves were challenged on day 0 with BHV-1 and with *M. haemolytica* on day 4. Over the first 4 days post BHV-1 infection, only 10% of the animals developed Hp concentrations >0.1 g/l. On day 5 (24h post bacterial challenge) 43% of the calves displayed elevated Hp levels. The highest Hp concentrations (Table 4) were observed on day 8 (4 days post bacterial challenge), where 84% of the animals had Hp concentrations >0.1 g/l. Increased Hp concentrations were significantly associated with disease severity (e.g. fever, increased sickness index and weight loss). Godson et al. (1996) showed that Hp concentration measurements may serve as prognostic indicators, to assist determination of the severity of disease. Animals that subsequently died had significantly higher Hp concentrations on day 8, compared to those that recovered. Further examination of the acute phase response of calves to viral infection was performed by Heegaard et al. (2000). After experimental BRSV infection, most calves displayed elevated SAA concentrations, which were detectable at day 5 p.i and peaked at approximately day 5-8 p.i. The highest SAA concentrations ranged from 60-80 mg/l: 5-7 times the normal SAA concentrations in control animals. Hp showed a similar pattern of changes. The maximum Hp response was observed on day 6-7 p.i., and reached 8-10 g/l: approximately 500 times the detection limit of the assay (18 mg/l). Severe BRSV infections were found to correlate with haptoglobin concentrations > 1 g/l on day 7 p.i., and SAA concentrations ≥ 60 mg/l. In this study, the acute phase response induced by BRSV was generally the same or higher than previously reported for bacterial infections in calves. Serum amyloid A responded more rapidly to infection, but Hp concentrations correlated better with disease severity (fever and extent of lung consolidation) (Heegaard et al., 2000). In a study by Ganheim et al. (2003), calves were infected BVDV and/or *M. haemolytica.* In the group challenged with mixed infection, animals were first inoculated with virus, followed by bacteria 5 days later. After BVDV infection, concentrations of Hp, SAA and Fb reached a maximum level 8-9 days p.i. After inoculation with bacterial agent, the highest APP concentrations were reached 1-2.5 days p.i. In the BVDV/*M. haemolytica* infected group, APP response patterns were more complicated, with larger individual differences. In general, the magnitude of the response was similar, but the duration of elevated APP concentrations were longest in the mixed infection group, reflecting the duration of clinical symptoms. In a study by Grell et al. (2005), calves experimentally infected with BRSV displayed the highest Hp concentrations at approximately 7-9 days post-inoculation. Calves presenting with the most severe clinical symptoms (respiratory rate, rectal temperature) had the highest Hp levels, while calves presenting with the mildest clinical symptoms displayed the lowest levels of acute phase reaction; however, no statistical correlation was found, probably due to the small number of animals (n=6).

APPs were shown to be valuable proteins for the evaluation of a *P. multocida* A3 experimental infection model in calves (Dowling et al., 2002). In calves challenged with greater volumes (300 vs. 60 ml), plasma Hp levels were found to be significantly increased, regardless of the number bacteria (10^9 vs. 10^{10} cfu). It is possible that increased volume challenges affect a greater area of the lungs, especially if the initially slow response in Hp production provides more time for bacterial proliferation. Dowling et al. (2002) showed that α1-AGP might be particularly valuable protein; examination of α1-AGP concentrations for all treatments indicated that large volume challenges were associated with a greater increase from basal levels, than low volume challenges. Other experimental studies examined less popular APPs, such as LBP or transferrin (Tf). Single intratracheal inoculation of *Pasteurella haemolytica* A1 showed increased lipopolysaccharide binding protein (LBP) activity in calves (Horadagoda et al., 1995). Lipopolysaccharide binding protein activity increased after 12 hours, and by 36 h, there was a 4-fold increase in serum concentrations. Early reaction of LBP was reported in a study by Schroedl et al. (2001). Concentrations of LBP in experimental calves, that were intra-tracheally infected with *Mannheimia haemolytica,* increased 6 hours post-infection, with a peak response at 24 hours post-infection. Haptoglobin reactions were slower, with a significant increase occurring 12 hours post-infection, and a maximal response at approximately 48h post-infection. In terms of response time, LBP appears to be superior to Hp as an early marker of infection; however, its concentration only rose 7-fold, while, in contrast, Hp rose 300-fold. In calves, which died following infection, LBP levels were more elevated than in survivors; unfortunately, the number of animals was too small to draw any conclusions (Schroedl et al., 2001). A study by McNair et al. (1998) demonstrated that, the negative APP, Tf) could also be useful in calves. Although serum Tf levels remained within the reference range, in calves that were experimentally infected with *Histophilus somni,* its concentration was associated with lung lesions. In fact, the lowest Tf concentrations were measured in calves with extensive lesions, and there were significant differences between mean values (on days 1-6) between the group with no lesions and the group with extensive lesions.

Study	Infectious agent	Time to reach maximum level	Hp (mean or max range g/l)	Hp determination method
Conner et al. (1989)	*M. haemolytica*	3d	1,0	haemoglobin binding capacity
Godson et al. (1996)	BHV-1 and *M. haemolytica*	8d (4d after bacterial challenge)	1,1	ELISA
Heegard et al. (2000)	BRSV	6-7d	8-10*	ELISA
Schroedl et al. (2001)	*M. haemolytica*	2d	>4.5**	ELISA
Ganheim et al. (2003)	BVD and/or *M. haemolytica*	8.5-9.5 d (BVDV) 2-2.5 (*M. haemolytica*) 7- 10 (both agents)**	0.89-1.77* 1.1-2.0* 0.65-2.24*	measure of peroxidase activity Hp-Hb

Table 4. Comparison of maximal Hp concentrations and the number of days required to reach maximum Hp levels across several studies. *Highest individual concentrations; **approximate results read off from line graphs.

2.5.2 APPs in field studies

Studies on acute phase reactions in field conditions are more complicated, because the timing of initial infection is often unknown, and it is difficult to determine the phase of infection. Nikunen et al. (2007) studied concentrations of Fb, Hp, SAA, LBP and AGP in 84 calves suffering from respiratory disease. Among isolated pathogens from tracheobronchial lavage (including *Mycoplasma dispar* and other mycoplasmas, but not *M. bovis, P. multocida,*

Pasteurella sp., F. necrophorum and *A. pyogenes*) and seroconverted bovine viruses (e.g. adenovirus-7, adenovirus-3, coronavirus and parainfluenza virus-3), only *Pasteurella multocida* was associated with increased concentrations of all tested APPs. The higher concentration of APPs observed in calves with *P. multocida* suggests a strong pathogenic role for this bacteria. Although it was shown that APPs increase rapidly in experimentally infected cattle, this increase coincided with clinical signs, and the relative usefulness of APPs in actually predicting respiratory disease during the incubation period is not satisfactory. Svensson et al. (2007) showed that in calves, the discriminative ability of serum Hp levels for indicating the presence of clinical respiratory-tract diseases was poor overall, and no better than rectal temperature. Furthermore, Hp levels were significantly affected by sex and rectal temperature. When Hp and fever were combined, and either increased Hp or fever (>39.5 °C) was used for detecting respiratory disease, the best test performance was achieved in heifer calves at serum Hp concentrations >0.15 g/L, with a sensitivity of 72% and a specificity of 59%. Therefore serum Hp levels, when combined with rectal temperature, may be a valuable parameter in herd-level diagnostics, at least in heifer calves.

APPs may also be useful for determining the response to therapy and making the right treatment decisions. Carter et al. (2002) found that serum Hp concentrations in transported feedlot cattle were greater in calves treated more than once, than in calves not treated or treated only once. At the beginning of treatment, Hp concentrations were higher in calves requiring more than one treatment compared to calves with one treatment (0.76 vs. 0.55 g/l). In addition, Berry et al. (2004) showed that Hp concentrations are a useful tool for predicting the number of antimicrobial treatments required in newly received feedlot calves. Hp concentrations on day 0 and 7 were positively correlated with the number of treatments during the trial. Hp concentrations on those days increased with increasing numbers of antimicrobial treatments. Retrospective analysis of APPs concentrations in growing calves suffering from bronchopneumonia, showed that, both Hp and Fb could be used for identification of calves requiring an anti-inflammatory treatment (Humblet et al., 2004). Animals in this study were classified into two categories: animals requiring either no-treatment or antibiotics alone; and animals requiring both antibiotics and anti-inflammatory drugs (AI). Treatments were administered according to clinical symptoms. In blood samples taken before clinical examination, elevated APPs levels were observed. Hp and Fb thresholds for medical decisions (i.e. to use AI or not) were 25 mg/l and 2.7 g/l respectively. Hp and Fb were useful predictors of inflammation severity; most of the animals (80%) that received anti-inflammatory treatment after clinical examination presented pathological Hp and/or Fb values upon onset of disease. Hp alone was able to confirm> 75% of case decisions (i.e. whether diseased calves were treated or not).

APP concentrations may be useful for monitoring the treatment of respiratory disease in calves. In our study (Jawor and Stefaniak, 2006), blood was sampled 3 times: first (I), when the owner either sent the calf to the clinic or reported signs of disease; second (II), between 3 and 6 days later; and third (III), 13-17 days after the first sample was collected. In one case, a 3rd sample was not collected because of euthanasia. Blood samples were also collected once from clinically healthy calves. Changes in APPs concentrations are shown in Table 5. Mean Hp concentrations were only increased in the beginning, while concentrations of SAA (sample I) and Fp (samples I and II) were significantly different from healthy controls. Hp was undetectable in all calves in samples II and III, with one exception: increased Hp and SAA concentrations were found in one calf in the last blood sample collection (III). An increase in Hp and SAA levels following an earlier decrease is characteristic of secondary infection (Ganheim et al., 2003). Thus, the observed increase in Hp and SAA in the above mentioned calf was probably due to the presence of a secondary infection. Later, this calf was unsuccessfully treated several times and eventually died. After an initial decrease in SAA concentrations, an increase in SAA levels was observed in the serum of 3 calves in the last blood sample collection; although a simultaneously increase in Hp and Fb was observed in only one calf. Because SAA is known to be a more sensitive protein, it is hard to explain if this increase observed in 2 calves was caused by secondary infection or other factors, such as stress (Alsemgeest et al., 1995a). In 3 out of 7 calves from the healthy control group, SAA concentrations were higher than the 25.6 mg/l, basal level established by Ganheim et al. (2003). This may imply that, even in the absence of clinical symptoms, these calves were not perfectly healthy.

	Calves with bronchopneumonia			Control group
	I (n=8)	II (n=8)	III (n=7)	(n=7)
Hp g/l	0.3 (±0.4)	0.0 (±0.0)	0.0 (±0.1)	0.0 (±0.0)
SAA mg/l	95.7 (±46.1)[a]	62.0 (±42.5)	75.9 (±36.9)	31.3 (±20.9)[b]
Fb g/l	6.54 (±2.08)[a]	5.85 (±1.24)[a]	4.94 (±1.21)	3.13* (±0.37)[b]

Table 5. Mean (±SD) concentrations of Hp, SAA and Fb during treatment monitoring of calves with bronchopneumonia. Values followed by different letters are significantly different. $P \leq 0.05$ (adapted from Jawor and Stefaniak, 2006).

The decreasing concentrations of tested APPs observed in the majority of calves treated for bronchopneumonia suggests diminishing inflammatory processes. In contrast, high APP concentration after an initial decrease strongly suggest the presence of secondary infections, meaning that treatment should be continued.

Of the many APPs, Hp, SAA and Fb have been examined most thoroughly. Bovine SAA is a more sensitive indicator of acute disease than Hp, and reacts more rapidly than Hp, that could also reflect poor maintenance conditions. The wide use of APPs to determine the magnitude of inflammatory changes, to assist in choosing proper therapy, and to monitor its efficiency, should enable application of APPs for the determination of respiratory diseases in calves.

2.6 Diarrhea in calves

Very few studies have been conducted regarding APPs concentrations in calves with diarrhea. Moreover, most of these studies only assessed diarrhea as background for APPs investigations of other illnesses, such as respiratory diseases. For example, Svensson et al. (2007), during a study of the efficacy of serum Hp concentration, as indicator of respiratory-tract disease in calves, found that calves which had diarrhea within 10 days prior to blood collection had a median Hp concentration of 0.07 g/l. Hp concentrations in individual animals ranged from very low (similar to healthy calves) to high in some calves with respiratory diseases (80% central range 0.04-0.63 g/l). In experimental studies of *Salmonella* infection, production of ceruloplasmin (Cp) and Hp was investigated. In a study by Piercy (1979), calves infected with *S.* Dublin showed a significant increase in Cp between 3 and 4 days, and Cp concentrations decreased to normal levels by day 7. A similar pattern of changes was found for Hp levels in a study where calves were experimentally infected with a mixture of three *Salmonella* serotypes (*S.* Dublin, *S.* Enteritidis and *S.* Heidelberg) (Deignan et al., 2000). Median Hp levels significantly increased within 3 days of challenge (0.21 g/l) and decreased by day 5. Hp was shown to be a useful marker of infection severity. Serum Hp concentrations were found to significantly correlate with clinical measures of disease severity: fecal and morbidity scores. A positive correlation was also found between hp levels and body temperature.

The usefulness of assessment of Hp, SAA and Fb levels for calves treatment monitoring having diarrhea was evaluated in a study by Jawor (2007). In this study, blood samples were collected 3 times: first (I), when the calf was admitted to the Clinic for Ruminants (University of Veterinary Medicine Vienna, Austria); second (II), 3-4 days later; and third (III), 7-10 days after the beginning of treatment. In cases where the calf was either euthanized or returned to the owner, blood samples were collected only twice. The median age of the calves was 8 days (range 1-30 days). The mean concentration and ranges of examined APPs are shown in Table 6.

	I (n=10)	II (n=10)	III (n=6)
Hp g/l	0.14 (0-0.49)	0.02 (0-0.18)	0.02 (0-0.13)
SAA mg/l	156.8 (53.0-302.4) **A**	102.1 (54.6-142.1)	53.5 (15.0-105.1) **B**
Fb g/l	7.28 (4.3-14.7)	6.68 (4.8-9.2)	4.9 (3.4-6.2)

Table 6. Mean (range) concentrations of Hp, SAA and Fb during monitoring of the treatment of diarrhea in calves. Values followed by different letters are significantly different. $P \leq 0.01$ (adapted from Jawor 2007).

In a study by Okamoto et al. (1998), 35 of 73 calves with diarrhea (47.9%) had detectable serum Hp levels (ranging from 0.05 to 0.7 g/l). In Jawor (2007) study, 40% of calves had an Hp concentration >0.1 g/l. However, if calves with Hp levels ≥0.05 g/l were also included, then 60% of the animals had detectable Hp in blood sample I. Mean Hp concentrations were similar to those reported in a study by Okamoto et al. (1998), where calves had 0.16 g/l. During treatment, Hp concentrations decreased. Serum amyloid A levels were above the reference range (according to Ganheim et al., 2003) in all calves, for samples I and II, while the lowest SAA concentrations were measured in sample III. A high percentage of calves with increased Fb concentrations were observed (70% in I samples above 5 g/l) and very high mean Fb levels were detected at the beginning of treatment, while during treatment a gradual decrease was noted. Because the Fb increase associated with diarrhea may be due to dehydration, the index of total protein to Fb (Thomas, 2000) was calculated. This index (data not shown) indicates that the observed Fb increase may be due to inflammatory processes. SAA concentrations were elevated during the entire treatment period for most of the calves. In one calf, in III blood sample increased serum levels of all examined APPs was found. This was likely triggered by a respiratory infection, because the animal was observed to cough at the same time. Among Hp, SAA and Fb levels, only SAA showed significant changes during diarrhea treatment monitoring. The very high initial serum SAA concentrations and subsequent significant decrease during treatment suggests that this APP may be very useful in calves with diarrhea. The presence of increased SAA levels in sample III suggests that, either inflammation is still present or the time between sample I and sample III was too short. Taking into account the levels and changes observed for all three examined APPs in calves with diarrhea, SAA seems to be the most useful in calves with enteritis. Although Hp concentrations increased, this was not observed in all calves. Furthermore, Fb estimation required an additional determination of plasma proteins, to distinguish between a relative increase in hemo-concentration and an absolute Fb increase during inflammation.

3. Estimation of APPs in cows and calves for evaluating herd health

One of the main targets of milk producers is to keep healthy cows with a long-term high milk production. Herd health protection has not only ethical but also economic significance. Keeping healthy cows means providing their optimal reproduction levels and therefore milk production. Early detection of the risk of disease and the early introduction of appropriate actions should protect the majority of animals within a herd (Stefaniak, 2003).

Aim	Production group	Parameters/number of animals examined
Evaluation of health during rearing	Calves	Determination of Hp, SAA and Fb in 2nd and between 21-28 days of life, along with Ig determination in 25-30% of newborn calves
Evaluation of risk in cows during transition period and at the peak of lactation	Dairy cows	Hp, SAA, Fb (% of cows with elevated levels and their concentrations in individual cows, along with metabolic and mineral parameters)
Dairy herd health monitoring/improving the herd health programme	Cows in different stages of lactation and dry cows	Hp, Fb (% of animals with elevated levels and mean)
Udder health monitoring	Lactating dairy cows	Hp and SAA in milk samples from individual cows
Pre-slaughter examination	Feedlot steers	Confirmation of normal Hp and Fb levels in all of 5-10% of randomly examined animals assigned to slaughter

Table 7. Opportunity for using APPs in the health monitoring of cattle.

The two most important ways to achieve this are: first – to supervising programmes of herd health protection, and second – to detect the increasing danger of inflammation/diseases at an early stage or before they occur. Acute phase protein estimation may be used to help monitor the health and welfare of production animals on farms (Eckersall, 2000). Acute phase proteins in cattle are valuable tools since they are not only applicable for the monitoring of inflammatory processes, but they can also be used for any non-inflammatory conditions, such as parturition, metabolic diseases and stress (Murata et al., 2004), or for improving the pre-slaughter examination, thereby improving the safety of food for public health (Saini et al., 1998). Possible applications of APPs in the health monitoring of cattle are shown in Table 7. Cattle health monitoring during periods of increased disease risk (transition period in dairy cows, weaning of calves) by determination of APPs provides the possibility of early disturbance detection, facilitating decision making about the separation of endangered animals from the others, and minimizing the risk of disease transmission

(Stefaniak et al., 2003). The APPs are more useful for monitoring health than proinflammatory cytokines, because after the inflammatory stimulus, their concentrations remain elevated for longer time (Gruys et al., 2006). Therefore, the possibility of detecting their elevated levels in representative groups of clinically healthy cattle is more probable due to the typical dynamics of APPs during the acute phase response (Conner & Eckresall, 1988).

3.1 APP utilization for pre-slaughter cattle examination

Acute phase proteins may be used to monitor health of slaughter animals. In slaughtered cattle without evident disease activity Hp-values were unmeasurable, whereas in most cases with disease activity Hp values were elevated. Serum amyloid A values were found to be elevated in animals with overt lesions, but Hp appears to be a useful variable to discern cattle without disease activity from those with lesions (Gruys et al., 1993). Saini et al. (1998) proposed that a potential application of APPs might be in screening and separating healthy from diseased animals. In a group of 57 retained carcasses of ante-mortem normal cattle, 56% had elevated Hp levels. Standard pre-slaughter examination is sometimes unreliable. Over a 3-year period, the carcasses of 7.7% of ante-mortem clinically normal steers and 20.6% of culled normal cows were retained due to post-mortem found changes (Saini et al., 1998). In emergency slaughtered cattle it was found that Hp and AGP levels were raised, indicating that examination of the APPs could help in improving food safety (Hirvonen et al., 1997). Haptoglobin, SAA and AGP were estimated in the plasma of 81 cattle of which a detailed post-mortem examination confirmed the presence of inflammation, and the APP concentrations were compared between the cases classified as acute and chronic inflammatory lesions (Horadagoda et al., 1999). In the 81 animals with inflammation, it was apparent that SAA and Hp levels were raised in acute rather than chronic cases, whereas in the latter group AGP was more likely to be elevated. The author suggested that Hp and SAA have a high value for detecting acute inflammatory conditions, whereas AGP was a better marker for chronic inflammation in cattle (Horadagoda et al., 1999). Measurement of APPs in meat inspection has good perspectives but more rapid detection methods have to be developed.

3.2 APPs in evaluating herd health status

Estimation of APPs in calves and cows may be very helpful in herd health monitoring. In 175 heifer calves born within one year on a dairy farm of 390 cows, the mean Fb concentration in the blood plasma was 4.0 g/l at the 48th hour of life, and increased to 4.8 g/l by the 25th day. At the 48th hour of life, all of the calves with Ig levels greater than 15 g/l showed normal Fb concentrations, but in the other groups (Ig levels below 5 g/l, between 5-10 g/l and 10-15 g/l), few individuals had elevated Fb levels (4.54%, 1.20% and 3.64% respectively). By the 25th day of life the mean Fb levels were within reference range in all of the groups examined and the rates of calves showing elevated Fb levels were 18.2%, 12%, 3.6% and 13.3% in the respective groups divided according to the Ig level at the 48th hour of life (Furman et al., 2011). On the same farm, increased Hp concentrations (>0.1 g/l) were found in the serum of 32% of calves at the 48th hour of life. By the 25th day of life, 31% of the calves showed elevated Hp levels. Because Hp is not commonly detected in healthy cattle (Eckersall & Conner, 1988), it was surprising that a high rate of calves showed elevated Hp levels at the 48th hour and the 25th day of life. It was concluded that the calves had been in risk of an inflammatory process from first few hours of life, since the increase in Hp concentrations after infection with the bacterial agent occurs within 24 hours (Ganheim et al., 2003). The highest Hp levels, as well as the highest individual differences, occurred in the calves of the group showing failure of passive transfer (Ig levels below 5 g/l at the 48th hour of life). In the same calves at the 25th day of the rate of elevated Hp levels as well as the mean Hp level had increased. In contrast, in properly colostrum-protected calves (over 10 g Ig/l), the mean level and the rate of elevated serum Hp concentrations had decreased. This observation agreed with the higher intensity and frequency of respiratory and gastrointestinal tract morbidity in the calves poorly protected with colostrum. In study by Alsemgeest et al. (1995b) the Hp and SAA levels were normal in newborn calves. Diseases that appeared before the fourth day of life induced an increase in SAA levels in all diseased calves, but Hp levels were only raised in two out of eight individuals. The authors indicated that because the SAA concentration at birth is very low and increases rapidly in diseased calves, it might be used as marker of infection during the perinatal period. Stefaniak et al. (2003), during an examination of 75 clinically healthy calves aged 1-3 days from two dairy herds, found elevated Hp levels in two calves. Both calves had failure of passive transfer (serum IgG level below 5 g/l) and were from the same farm in which only 31% of the calves achieved serum IgG levels > 10g/l. The authors considered two probable reasons for this – either the inflammation occurred very early (possibly before birth), which might have caused the poor transfer of colostrum Ig, or a poor immune protection enabled early disease appearance. The results showed that in problem herds or in herds with low levels of colostrum protection the probability of a rise in APP levels occurred more frequently (Stefaniak et al., 2003).

Blood sampling during the first weeks after arrival in the herd would give an indication of the pressure of infections and/or stress during transportation and mixing and so they may not give a fair picture of the management conditions of the actual farm (Ganheim et al. 2007). Sampling at monthly intervals during the middle and later stages of the rearing period may be more relevant for determining the conditions on a specific farm. After experimental infection calves with BVDV and/or *M. haemolytica* basal levels of serum concentrations for haptoglobin, SAA and fibrinogen were established and may be used for evaluating calf health in herds (Ganheim et al., 2003). For Hp, SAA and Fb were 0.13 g/l, 25.6 mg/l. 6.45 g/l respectively. They suggested that such values might be useful as a diagnostic tool when screening herds of calves for subclinical or clinical disease to evaluate animal health. Detection of animals with supra-normal APPs values could be useful to identify animals that are, or have recently been, clinically or sub-clinically diseased.

Estimation of APP might be used as a tool for controlling the effectiveness of vaccination program. In a study by Stefaniak et al. (1997), nine calves were immunized with Somnuvac® vaccine at the fourth and eighth weeks of life. The calves were on a farm of 400 dairy cows with a high incidence of respiratory tract infection. Blood samples were taken at 4, 5, 8, 9, and 12 weeks of life. No elevated (over 0.2 g/l) Hp levels were observed and no clinical signs of disease occurred in the experimental group. Among nine control, non-immunized calves at 8, 9 and 12 weeks of life, every time one (but not the same) animal had increased Hp levels, and in two of them coughing and elevated body temperatures were found (>39.5 °C). The determination of Hp levels confirmed the protective influence of vaccination against respiratory tract inflammation in the endangered herds.

Changes in serum concentrations of Hp and SAA were evaluated every 15 days over 6-month period in dairy cattle in a study by Humblet et al. (2006). Blood samples were taken at three peripartum periods: P1, prepartum (from week 8/7 to parturition); P2, first week postpartum; and P3, from week 2 to week 15 or 16. At each visit the cows were clinically examined. There were no significant differences in Hp or SAA concentrations observed in healthy cows between the P1 and P3 periods. In more than 95% of the samples from healthy cows, the Hp and SAA levels were below the cut-off points (Hp ≤30 mg/l for P1 and P3, Hp <150 mg/l for P2; SAA ≤25 mg/l for P1 and P3, SAA <60 mg/l for P2). Only 73% of the diseased animals had Hp and SAA levels above the defined cut-off points. The highest sensitivity but lowest specificity in the diagnosis of disease status was for Hp and SAA in the P2 period. Poor sensitivity in other postpartum periods could be related to the higher incidence of chronic vs. acute inflammation. In the other periods the specificity of Hp and SAA was relatively high (90.8 and 89.2%), such that normal APP concentrations could more accurately be used to identify healthy animals. Due to an increase in the Hp concentration after parturition, Hp and SAA should be used with caution as markers of inflammation in the week following calving. A high percentage of false positive results based on SAA status (48.6% above the cut-off point) were found in healthy animals without increased Hp concentrations. Thus, in routine analysis, Hp would be more appropriate than SAA for detecting disease (Humblet et al., 2006).
Based on the results of Hp determination in 15 different Polish dairy herds during health monitoring in 2009-2010 (Table 8), we found that elevated levels (exceeding 0.2 g/l) occurred in 35% of cows in early lactation. At the peak of lactation the percentage of cows with elevated Hp concentrations decreased to 14.6% and at the end of lactation to 10.5% in the examined cows. In dry cows sampled between 60 and 10 days before parturition 11.7% also showed elevated Hp levels. The results indicate that elevated Hp levels occur relatively frequently in dairy herds, and that postpartum period is associated with the greatest incidence of increased Hp concentrations. Fibrinogen levels were estimated in 12 out of 15 of the abovementioned herds (Table 9). The mean Fb levels in the representative groups slightly exceeded 5 g/l and the incidence of elevated Fb concentrations (over 7 g/l) occurred more frequently in lactating cows (13.5-14.6%) than in dry cows (5.9%). It may be concluded that acute or chronic inflammatory cases associated with an Fb increase occur the most frequently during early lactation.

	Early lactation (n=82)	**Peak of lactation** (n=48)	**Late lactation** (n=57)	**Dry cows** (n=77)	**Total** (n=264)
No. of samples with elevated Hp concentrations	29	7	6	9	51
Rate (%)	35.37	14.58	10.53	11.69	19.32
Range within herds (%)	0 - 66.7	0 - 40	0 - 42.86	0 - 40	0 - 50

Table 8. The occurrence of elevated (>0.2 g/l) haptoglobin concentrations in 264 cows from representative groups of 15 dairy herds.

The determination of APPs may be an efficient way of monitoring dairy herd health. Stefaniak and Jawor (2007) determined the acid base balance, urea, total serum protein and its fractions, asparagine aminotransferase, total calcium, ionized calcium, inorganic phosphate, magnesium and Hp and Fb levels in representative groups of cows from two dairy farms with a loose-housing system. Farm A (600 Polish Holstein-Fresian cows; milk yield 10,700 kg) and farm B (170 Polish black and white and Polish red and white × Holstein-Fresian cows; milk yield 6500 kg) were sampled six times at two monthly intervals. Blood samples were taken from groups of cows: group I – 10 cows between 14 and 150 days in milk (DIM), group II – 10 cows more than 150 DIM, group III – 10 dry cows. After each monitoring period the results were discussed with the owner and a local veterinarian and recommendations were proposed. Repeated laboratory monitoring helped to normalize the analysed parameters. The course of Hp and Fb levels and the decreasing frequency of elevated concentrations indicated improvements in the cows' health. Any disturbances that occurred during herd monitoring mainly came from the owners' or farm workers' mistakes or a negligence at project completion. Herd health monitoring using APP measurement needs a close cooperation between the veterinarian and the owner.

Group	Mean % (range)				Mean concentration (g/l)
	<3 g/l	3-5 g/l	5-7 g/l	>7 g/l	
Early lactation (n=74)	2.7% (0-20)	31.08% (0-77.8)	52.7% (0-100)	13.51% (0-33.3)	5.53
Lactation peak (n=57)	3.51% (0-33.3)	31.58% (0-66.7)	50.88% (0-100)	14.04% (0-66.7)	5.32
Late lactation (n=55)	5.45% (0-33.3)	52.73% (0-100)	27.27% (0-100)	14.55% (0-66.7%)	5.16
Dry cows (n=68)	7.35% (0-50%)	45.59% (0-100)	41.18% (0-80)	5.88% (0-33,3)	5.01
Total (n=254)	4.74% (0-29.17)	37.94% (6.67-55.17)	44.66% (12.5-80)	12.65% (0-42.86)	5.26

Table 9. Fibrinogen concentrations in 254 representative cows from 12 dairy farms.

The determination of APP levels seems to be one of better methods allowing the health and welfare of animals in large herds, based on the examination of blood or milk samples obtained from representative groups of animals (Nikołajczuk & Molenda 2000). When the results from representative groups are within the reference range, they may provide a basis for considering the herd health status as "good". In our practice we simultaneously utilize Hp, Fb and albumin levels, and with this combination we can detect more cases of subclinical acute and chronic inflammation. For many years the estimation of APPs has provided an important source of knowledge about herd health. The determination of APPs along with other parameters during the metabolic monitoring of herds may provide a complete view of herd health.

4. Conclusions

Sick cattle have lower milk yields/body growth rates, causing significant direct and indirect economical losses. Because of the group housing systems, it is difficult to early diagnose an inflammation in individual animals. Despite these difficulties, handling strategies should focus on herd health protection and the early detection of threats, as well as the introduction of improved therapeutic procedures before animals become ill. The determination of APPs levels in blood and milk samples from representative groups of cows is an attractive method, that also enables determination of other biochemical parameters, providing an useful prognostic tool of the cows' health status and the degree of possible threats. Multiple estimations of such parameters in the same herd can provide information, which could be used to improve animal handling. Among the many available APPs for cattle diagnostics, the most commonly used and the most readily available are Hp, SAA and Fb. In addition to a rise in APP concentration, the degree of increase can be used to evaluate herd health. The finding that the concentration of some APPs, such as SAA and Hp, increase in stressful conditions, as well as in fatty liver syndrome, broaden the possible diagnostic applications of APPs in cattle.

A future diagnostic application of APPs is their use as part of pre-slaughter examination of slaughter animals. Such procedures should significantly improve the detection rate of animals suffering from subclinical inflammatory processes; which lead to significant losses because of confiscation of whole carcasses, or parts, showing signs of pathology/inflammation during postmortem/postslaughter examination. Implementation of such procedures on farms, before animals are transported to the slaughterhouse, would enable detection of ill animals for treatment, allowing them to be sent for slaughter after recovery.

In spite of the time required, the determination of APPs has potential importance when deciding whether to treat ill animals or send them for sanitary slaughter to rescue the meat value. The presence of strongly elevated APP concentrations before treatment, combined with poor prognosis, may be helpful in making decision about therapy i.e. do not start. Moreover, if treatment has begun, the determination of APPs might help in monitoring the course of the disease and the efficacy of the chosen therapy. The results of our studies indicate that appropriate time points for collecting blood samples for monitoring most of diseases in cattle are: immediately before starting treatment; and after 3 to 7 days of treatment. A stepwise decrease in APP concentrations, and a return to normal (or near normal) levels, confirms the positive effect of treatment.

There is a broad spectrum of possible applications of APP-based diagnostics for use with cattle. It is necessary to develop and optimise rapid field tests that allow determination of APPs in a short time period, after collection of blood or milk samples from animals.

5. References

Åkerstedt, M.; Björck, L.; Persson Waller, K. & Sternesjö, Å. (2006). Biosensor assay for determination of haptoglobin in bovine milk. *Journal of Dairy Research*, Vol.73, No.3, (August 2006), pp. 299-305

Alsemgeest, S.P.M.; Taverne, M.A.M.; Boosman, R.; Weyden, B.C. & Gruys, E. (1993). Peripartum acute-phase protein serum amyloid-A concentration in plasma of cows and fetuses. *American Journal of Veterinary Research,* Vol.54, No.1, (January 1993), pp.164-167

Alsemgeest, S.P.M.; Lambooy, I.E.; Wierenga, H.K.; Dieleman, S.J.; Meerkerk, B.; van Ederen, A.M. & Niewold, T.A. (1995a). Influence of physical stress on the plasma concentration of serum amyloid-A (SAA) and haptoglobin (Hp) in calves. *Veterinary Quarterly,* Vol.17, No.1, (March 1995) pp. 9-12

Alsemgeest, S.P.M.; Jonker, F.H.; Taverne, M.A.M.; Kalsbeek, H.C.; Wensing, T.& Gruys, E. (1995b). Serum amyloid-A (SAA) and haptoglobin (Hp) plasma concentrations in newborn calves. *Theriogenology,* Vol.43, No.2, (January 1995), pp. 381-387

Balbierz, H.; Nowacki, W.; & Russ, T. (1977). Some properties of the HRP factor (Hemoglobin Reacive Protein) in cattle (in Polish, abstract in English). Polskie Archiwum Weterynaryjne Vol.20, No.1, pp. 87-95

Bertoni, G.; Calamari, L.; Maianti, M.G. & Cappa, V. (1997). Factors other than milk yield that affect reproductive traits of dairy cows. *Livestock Production Science,* Vol.50, no.1, (October 1997), pp. 99-100

Berry, B.A.; Confer, A.W; Krehbiel, C.R.; Gill, D.R.; Smith ,R.A. & Montelongo, M. (2004). Effects of dietary energy and starch concentrations for newly received feedlot calves: II. Acute-phase protein response. *Journal of Animal Science,* Vol.82, No.3, (March 2004), pp. 845-850

Bicalho, R.C.; Vokey, F.; Erb, H.N. & Guard, C.L. (2007). Visual locomotion scoring in the first seventy days in milk: impact on pregnancy and survival. *Journal of Dairy Science,* Vol.90, No.10, (October 2007), pp. 4586-4591

Cairoli, F.; Battocchio, M.; Veronesi, M.C.; Brambilla, D.; Conserva, F.; Eberini, I.; Wait, R. & Gianazza, E. (2006). Serum protein pattern during cow pregnancy: acute-phase proteins increase in the peripartum period. *Electrophoresis,* Vol.27, No.8, (April 2006), pp. 1617-1625

Carter, J.N.; Meredith, G.L.; Montelongo, M.; Gill, D.R.; Krehbiel, C.R.; Payton, M.E. & Confer, A.W. (2002). Relationship of vitamin E supplementation and antimirobial treatment with acute-phase protein responses in cattle affected by naturally acquired respiratory tract disease. *American Journal of Veterinary Research,* Vol.63, No.8, (August 2002), pp. 1111-1117

Chan, J.P-W.; Chang, C-C.; Hsu, W-I.; Liu, W-B. & Chen, T-H. (2010). Association of increased serum acute-phase protein concentrations with reproductive performance in dairy cows with postpartum metritis. *Veterinary Clinical Pathology,* Vol.39, No.1, (March 2010), pp. 72-78

Conner, J.G;. Eckersall, P.D.; Doherty, M. & Douglas, T.A. (1986). Acute phase response and mastitis in the cow. *Research in Veterinary Science,* Vol.41, No.1, (July 1986) pp. 126-128

Conner, J.G. & Eckersall, P.D. (1988). Bovine acute phase response following turpentine injection. *Research in Veterinary Science,* Vol.44, No.1, (January 1988), pp. 82-88

Conner, J.G.; Eckersall, P.D.; Wiseman, A.; Bain, R.K. & Douglas, T.A. (1989). Acute phase response in calves following infection with *Pasteurella haemolytica, Ostertagia ostertagi* and endotoxin administration. Research in Veterinary Science, Vol.47, No.2, (September 1989), pp. 203-207

Deignan, T.; Alwan, A.; Kelly, J.; McNair, J.; Warren, T. & O'Farrelly, C. (2000). Serum haptoglobin: an objective indicator of experimentally-induced *Salmonella* infection in calves. *Research in Veterinary Science,* Vol.69, No.2, (October 2000), pp. 153-158

Dowling, A.; Hodgson, J.C.; Schock, A.; Donachie, W.; Eckersall, P.D. & McKendrick, I.J. (2002). Experimental induction of pneumonic pasteurellosis in calves by intratracheal infection with *Pasteurella multocida* biotype A:3. *Research in Veterinary Science*, Vol.73, No.1, (August 2002), pp. 37-44

Dubuc, J.; Duffield, T.F.; Leslie, K.E.; Walton, J.S. & Leblanc, S.J. (2010). Risk factors for postpartum uterine diseases in dairy cows. *Journal of Dairy Science*, Vol.93, No.12, (December 2010), pp. 5764-5771

Eckersall, P.D. & Conner, J.G. (1988). Bovine and canine acute phase proteins. *Veterinary Research Communications*, Vol.12, No.2-3, pp. 169-178

Eckersall, P. D. (2000). Recent Advances and Future Prospects for the Use of Acute Phase Proteins as Markers of Disease in Animals. *Revue de Médecine Vétérinaire*, Vol.151, No.7, pp. 577-584

Eckersall, P.D.; Young, F.J.; McComb, C.; Hogarth, C.J.; Safi, S.; Weber, A.; McDonald, T.; Nolan, A.M. & Fitzpatrick, J.L. (2001). Acute phase proteins in serum and milk from dairy cows with clinical mastitis. *The Veterinary Record*, Vol. 148, No.2, (January 2001), pp. 35-41

Esslemont, R.J. & Kossaibati, M.A. (1997). Culling in 50 dairy herds in England. *The Veterinary Record*, Vol.140, No.2 (January 1997), pp. 36-39

Furman-Fratczak, K.; Rzasa, A. & Stefaniak T. (2011). The influence of colostral immunoglobulin concentration in heifer calves' serum on their health and growth. *Journal of Dairy Science* (accepted for publication)

Ganheim, C.; Hulten, C.; Carlsson, U.; Kindahl, H.; Niskanen, R. & Waller, K.P. (2003). The acute phase response in calves experimentally infected with Bovine Viral Diarrhoea Virus and/or *Mannheimia Haemolytica*. *Journal of Veterinary Medicine B*, Vol.50, No.4, (May 2003), pp. 183 -190

Ganheim, C.; Alenius, S. & Persson Waller K. (2007). Acute phase proteins as indicators of calf herd health. *The Veterinary Journal*, Vol.173, No.3, (May 2007) pp. 645-651

Godson, D.L.; Baca-Estrada, M.E.; Van Kessel, A.G.; Hughes, H.P.; Morsy, M.A.; Van Donkersgoed, J.; Harland, R.J.; Shuster, D.E.; Daley, M.J. & Babiuk, L.A. (1995). Regulation of bovine acute phase responses by recombinant interleukin-1 beta. *Canadian Journal of Veterinary Research*, Vol.59, No.4, (October 1995), pp. 249-255

Godson, D.L; Campos, M.; Attah-Poku, S.K.; Redmond, M.J.; Cordeiro, D.M.; Sethi, M.S.; Harland, R.J. & Babiuk, L.A. (1996). Serum haptoglobin as an indicator of the acute phase response in bovine respiratory disease. *Veterinary Immunology and Immunopatholology*, Vol.51, No.3-4, (June 1996), pp. 277-292

Green, L.E.; Hedges, V.J.; Schukken, Y.H.; Biowey, R.W. & Packington, A.J. (2002). The impact of Clinical Lameness on Milk Yield of Dairy Cows. *Journal of Dairy Science*, Vol.85, No.9, (September 2002), pp. 2250-2256

Grell, N.S.; Tjørnehøj, K.; Larsen, L.E. & Heegard, P.M.H. (2005). Marked induction of IL-6, haptoglobin and INF-γ following experimental BRSV infection in young claves. *Veterinary Immunology and Immunopathology*, Vol.103, No.3-4, (February 2005), pp. 235-245

Grönlund, U.; Hulten, C.; Eckersall, P.D. & Hogarth, C. (2003). Haptoglobin and serum amyloid A in milk and serum during acute and chronic experimentally induced *Staphylococcus aureus* mastitis. *Journal of Dairy Research*, Vol.70, No.4, (November 2003), pp. 739-386

Grönlund, U.; Hallen Sandgren, C. & Persson Waller, K. (2005). Haptoglobin and serum amyloid A in milk from dairy cows with chronic sub-clinical mastitis. Veterinary *Research*, Vol.36, No.2, (March-April), pp.191-198

Gruys, E.; Ederen, A.M.; Alsemgeest, S.P.M.; Kalsbeek, H.C. & Wensing, T. (1993). Acute phase protein values in blood of cattle as indicator of animals with pathological process. *Archiv für Lebensmittelhygiene*, Vol.44, No.5, (September/October), pp.107-111

Gruys, E.; Toussaint, M.J.M.; Niewold, T.A.; Koopmans, S.J.; van Dijk, E. & Meloen, R.H. (2006). Monitoring health by values of acute phase proteins. *Acta Histochemica*, Vol.108, No.3, (May 2006), pp. 229–232

Heegaard, P.M.H.; Godson, D.L.; Toussaintc, M. J.M.; Tjùrnehùj, K.; Larsen, L. E.; Viuff, B. & Rùnsholt, L. (2000). The acute phase response of haptoglobin and serum amyloid A (SAA) in cattle undergoing experimental infection with bovine respiratory syncytial virus. *Veterinary Immunology and Immunopathology*, Vol.77, No.1-2, (November 2000), pp. 151-159

Heinrich, P.C.; Castell, J.V. & Andus, T. (1990). Interleukin-6 and the acute phase response. *Biochemistry Journal*, Vol.265, No.3, (February 1990), pp. 621-626

Hirvonen, J.; Pyörälä, S. & Jousimies-Somer, H. 1996. Acute phase response in heifers with experimentally induced mastitis. *Journal of Dairy Research*, Vol.63, No.3, (August 1996), pp. 351-360

Hirvonen, J.; Hietakorpi, S. & Saloniemi, H. (1997). Acute phase response in emergency slaughtered dairy cows. *Meat Science*, Vol.46, No.3, (July 1997), pp. 29-257

Hirvonen, J. & Pyörälä, S. (1998). Acute-phase response in dairy cows with surgically-treated abdominal disorders. *The Veterinary Journal*, Vol.155, No.1, (January 1998) pp. 53-61

Hirvonen, J.; Eklund, K.; Teppo, A.M.; Huszenicza, G.; Kulcsar, M.; Saloniemi, H. & Pyörälä, S. (1999a). Acute phase response in dairy cows with experimentally induced *Escherichia coli* mastitis. *Acta Vererinaria Scandinavica*, Vol. 40, No.1, pp. 35-46

Hirvonen, J.; Huszenicza, G.; Kulcsar, M. & Pyörälä, S. (1999b). Acute-phase response in dairy cows with acute postpartum metritis. *Theriogenology*, Vol.51, No.6, (April 1999) pp. 1071-1083

Hiss, S.; Mielenz, M.; Bruckmaier, R.M. & Sauerwein, H. (2004). Haptoglobin concentrations in blood and milk after endotoxin challenge and quantification of mammary hp mRNA expression. *Journal of Dairy Science*, Vol.87, No.11, (November 2004), pp. 3778-3784

Horadagoda, A.; Eckersall, P.D.; Alsemgeest, S.P.M. & Gibbs, H. A. (1993). Purification and quatnitative measurment of bovine serum amyloid-A. *Research in Veterinary Science*, Vol.55, No.3, (November 1993), pp. 317-325

Horadagoda, A. & Eckersall, P.D. (1994). Immediate responses in serum TNFα and acute phase protein concentrations to infection with Pasteurella haemolytica A1 in calves. *Research in Veterinary Science*, Vol.57, No.1, (July 1994), pp. 129-132

Horadagoda, N.U.; Eckersall, P.D.; Andrew, L.; Gallay, P.; Heumann, D. & Gibbs, H.A. (1995). Characterisation of bovine lipopolysaccharide binding protein and the in vivo acute phase response to Pasteurella haemolytica Type A. *Veterinary Immunology and Immunopathology*, Vol.49, No. 1-2 (November 1995), pp. 61-74

Horadagoda, N.U.; Knox, K.M.G.; Gibbs, H.A.; Reid, S.W.J.; Horadagoda, A.; Edwards, S.E.R. & Eckersall, P.D. (1999). Acute phase proteins in cattle: discrimination between acute and chronic inflammation. *The Veterinary Record*, Vo.144, No.16, (April 1999), pp. 437-441

Humblet, M.F.; Coghe, J.; Lekeux, P. & Godeau, J.M. (2004). Acute phase proteins assessment for an early selection of treatments in growing calves suffering from bronchopneumonia under field conditions. *Research in Veterinary Science*, Vol.77, No.1, (August 2004), pp. 41–47

Humblet, M.F.; Guyot, H.; Boudry, B.; Mbayahi, F.; Hanzen, C.; Rollin, F. & Godeau, J.M. (2006). Relationship between haptoglobin, serum amyloid A, and clinical status in a survey of dairy herds during a 6-month period. *Veterinary Clinical Pathology*, Vol.35, No.2, (June 2006), pp. 188-193

Huzzey, J.M.; Duffield, T.F.; LeBlanc, S.J.; Veira, D.M.; Weary, D.M. & Keyserlingk, M.A.G. (2009a). Haptoglobin as an early indicator of metritis. *Journal of Dairy Science*, Vol.92, No.2, (February 2009), pp. 621-625

Huzzey, J.M.; Overton, T.R.; Nydam, D.V. & Grant, R.J. (2009b). Peripartum measures of stress, inflammation and energy status as predictors for postpartum health disorders in transition dairy cows. *Journal of Animal Science*, 87, E-Supplement 2, 120. *Journal of Dairy Science*, 92, E-Supplelent 1, 120

Irmak, K. & Turgut, K. (2005). Disseminated intravascular coagulation in cattle with abomasal displacement. *Veterinary Research Communications*, Vol.29, No.1, (January 2005), pp. 61-68

Jacobsen, S.; Andersen, P.H.; Toelboell T. & Heegard, P.M.H. (2004). Dose dependency and individual variability of the lipopolysaccharide-induced bovine acute phase protein response. *Journal Dairy Science*, Vol.87, No.10, (October 2004), pp. 3330-3339

Jawor, P. & Stefaniak, T. (2006). Acute phase proteins in treatment of calves with respiratory tract inflammation (in Polish, English abstract). Folia Universitatis Agriculturae Stetinensis, Zootechnica Vol.48, No.250, pp. 51-56

Jawor, P. (2007). Determination of haptoglobin and fibrinogen during monitoring herd health and selected inflammatory states in cattle. Ph. D thesis (in Polish), Wroclaw University of Environmental and Life Sciences

Jawor, P.; Hauser, S.; Baumgartner, W.; Stefaniak, T. & Rzasa, A. (2008). Determination of selected acute phase proteins during the treatment of limb diseases in dairy cows. *Veterinarni Medicina*, Vol.53, No.4, (April 2008), pp.173-183

Jawor, P.; Stefaniak, T.; Steiner, S. & Baumgarnter, W. (2009). Dynamics of Selected Acute Phase Proteins In Surgical Abomasum Reposition In Cows. *Folia Veterinaria*, Vol.53, Supplementum LIII, (June 2009), pp.18-21

Kent J. (1992). Acute phase proteins: their use in veterinary diagnosis. *British Veterinary Journal*, Vol.148, No.4, (July-August 1992), pp. 279-282

Krakowski, L. & Zdzisińska, B. (2007). Selected cytokines and acute phase proteins in heifers during the ovarian cycle course and in different pregnancy periods. *Bulletin of the Veterinary Institute in Pulawy*, Vol.51, No.1, pp.31-36

Kujala, M.; Orro, T. & Soveri, T. (2010). Serum acute phase proteins as a marker of infammation in dairy cattle with hoof diseases. *The Veterinary Record*, Vol.166, No.8, (February 2010), pp. 240-241

Laven, R.A.; Livesey, C.T. & May, S.A. (2004). Relationship between acute phase proteins and hoof horn haemorrhages in postpartum first-lactation heifers. *The Veterinary Record*, Vol.154, No.13, (March 2004), pp. 389-395

Makimura, S. & Usui, M. (1990). Correlation between haptoglobin and sialic acid or mucoprotein in diseased bovine serum. *Japan Journal of Veterinary Medical Science*, Vol.52, No.6, (December 1990), pp. 1245-1250

Mazur, A. (1980). Determination of HRP (Hemoglobin Reactive Protein) in sera and whey of cows by simple agar-electrophoresis (in Polish, English abstract). Medycyna Weterynaryjna, Vol.36, No.11, pp. 699-700

Mazur, A. & Mazur, O. (1981). Hemoglobin Reactive Protein (HRP) in case of udder inflammation in cows (in Polish, English abstract). Medycyna Weterynaryjna, Vol.37, No.5, pp. 262-264

McNair, J.; Elliott, C.; Bryson, D.G. & Mackie, D.P. (1998). Bovine serum transferrin concentration during acute infection with *Haemophilus somnus*. *The Veterinary Journal*, Vol.155, No.3, (May 1998), pp. 251-255

McSherry, B.J.; Horney, F.D. & deGroot, J.J. (1970). Plasma fibrinogen levels in normal and sick cows. *Canadian Journal of comparative Medicine*, Vol.34, No.3, (July 1970), pp. 191-197

Melendez, P.; Bartolome, J.; Archbald, L.F. & Donovan, A. (2003). The association between lameness, ovarian cysts and fertility in lactating dairy cows. *Theriogenology* Vol.59, No.3-4, (February 2003), pp. 927-937

Miller, L.L.; Bly, C.G.; Watson, M.L. & Bale, W.F. (1951). The dominant role of the liver in plasma protein synthesis; a direct study of the isolated perfused rat liver with the aid of lysine-epislon-C14. *The Journal of Experimental Medicine*, Vol.94, No.5, (November 1951), pp. 431-453

Molenaar, A.; Harris, P.; Green, J.; Callaghan, M.; Kim, K.; Wieliczko, R.; Johannessen, K.; Dines, R.; Watson, R.; Arkus, V.; Dalziel, J.; Singh, K.; Rajan, G.; Pearson, M.; Farr, V.; Miles, M.; Oden, K.; Good, L.; McLaren, R.; Prosser, C.; Grigor, M.; Davis, S. & Stelwagen, K. (2005). Mammary serum amyloid A3, progress toward determining structure and function. *Proceedings of 5th International Colloquium on Animal Acute Phase Proteins*. Dublin, March 2005

Mordak, R. (2008). Usefulness of haptoglobin for monitoring the efficiency of therapy of fetal membrane retention in cows (in Polish, English abstract). *Medycyna Weterynaryjna* Vol.64, No.4A (April 2008), pp. 434-437

Murata, H.; Shimada, N. & Yoshioka M. (2004). Current research on acute phase proteins in veterinary diagnosis: an overview. *The Veterinary Journal*, Vol.168, No.1 (July 2004) pp. 28–40

Nielsen, B.H.; Jacobsen, S.; Andersen, P.H.; Niewold, T.A. & Heegaard, P.M.H. (2004). Acute phase protein concentrations in serum and milk from healthy cows, cows with clinical mastitis and cows with extramammary inflammatory conditions. *The Veterinary Record*, Vol.154, No.12 (March 2004), pp. 361-365

Nikołajczuk, M., Molenda. (2000) Application of the acute phase proteins in veterinary diagnostics (in Polish, English abstract). Zeszyty Naukowe Akademii Rolniczej we Wrocławiu. Vol.29, No.390 (October 2000), pp. 9-14

Nikunen, S.; Härtel, H.; Orro, T.; Neuvonen, E.; Tanskanen, R.; Kivelä, S.L.; Sankari, S. Aho, P.; Pyörälä, S.; Saloniemi, H. & Soveri, T. (2007). Association of bovine respiratory disease with clinical status and acute phase proteins in calves. *Comparative Immunology, Microbiology and Infectious Diseases*, Vol.30, No.3, (May 2007), pp. 143-151

Ohtsuka, H.; Kudo, K.; Mori, K.; Nagai, F.; Hatsugaya, A.; Tajima, M.; Tamura, K.; Hoshi, F.; Koiwa, M. & Kawamura, S. (2001). Acute phase response in naturally occurring coliform mastitis. *Journal of Veterinary Medical Science*, Vol.63, No.6 (June 2001), pp. 675-678

Okamoto, K.; Harada, M.; Akuzawa, M. & Deguchi, E. (1998). Peripheral blood lymphocyte blastogenesis and concentrations of serum haptoglobin and alpha 1-acid glycoprotein in normal calves and calves on the first onset of diarrhea. *Animal Science and Technology*, Vol.69, No.7 (July 1998), pp. 683-689

Piercy, D.W.T. (1979). Acute phase responses to experimental salmonellosis in calves and colibacillosis in chickens: serum iron and caeruloplasmin. *Journal of Comparative Pathology*, Vol.89, No.3, (July 1979) pp. 309-319

Rajala-Schultz, P.J.; Gröhn, Y.T. & McCulloch, C.E. (1999). Effects of Milk Fever, Ketosis and Lameness on Milk Yield in Dairy Cows. *Journal of Dairy Science*, Vol.82, No.2, (February 1999), pp. 288-294

Saini, P.K.; Riaz, M.; Webert, D.W.; Eckersall, P.D.; Young, C.R.; Stanker, L.H.; Chakrabarti, E. & Judkins J.C. (1998). Development of a simple enzyme immunoassay for blood haptoglobin concentration in cattle and its application in improving food safety. *American Journal of Veterinary Research*, Vol.59, No.9, (September 1998), pp. 1101-1107

Schönfelder, A.; Schrödl, W.; Krüger, M.; Richter, A. & Sobiraj, A. (2005). The change of acute phase protein haptoglobin in cattle during spontaneous labor and Caesarean section with or without torsio uteri intrapartum (in German). *Berliner und Munchener Tierarztliche Wochenschrift*, Vol.118, No.5-6, (May-June 2005), pp.240-246

Schroedl, W.; Fuerll, B.; Reinhold, P.; Krueger, M. & Schuett, C. (2001). A novel acute phase marker in cattle: lipopolisacharide binding protein (LBP). *Journal of Endotoxin Research*, Vol.7, No.1, pp. 49-52

Sivula, N.J.; Ames, T.R.; Marsh, W.E. & Werdin, R.E. (1996). Descriptive epidemiology of morbidity and mortality in Minnesota dairy heifer calves. *Preventive Veterinary Medicine*, Vol.27, No.3-4, (July 1996), pp. 155-171

Skinner, J.G.; Brown, R.A.L. & Roberts, L. (1991). Bovine haptoglobin response in clinically defined filed conditions. *The Veterinary Record*, Vol.128, No.7, (February 1991), pp. 147-149

Smith, B.I.; Donovan, G.A.; Risco, C.A.; Young, C.R. & Stanker, L.R. (1998). Serum haptoglobin concentrations in Holstein dairy cattle with toxic puerperal metritis. *The Veterinary Record*, Vol.142, No.4, (January 1998) pp. 83-85

Smith, B.; Kauffold, J. & Sherman, L. (2010). Serum haptoglobin concentrations in dairy cattle with lameness due to claw disorders. *The Veterinary Journal*, Vol.186, No.2, (November 2010) pp. 162-165

Spooner, R.L. & Miller, J.K. (1971). The measurement of haemoglobin reactive protein in ruminants as an aid to the diagnosis of acute inflammation. *The Veterinary Record*, Vol.88, No.1, (January 1971) pp. 2-4

Stefaniak, T.; Nowacki, W.; Molenda, J.; Sobiech, E. & Nikołajczuk M. (1997). Monitoring selected blood parameters in calves immunized with Somnuvac® vaccine in field conditions (in Polish, English abstract). *Medycyna Weterynaryjna,* Vol.53, No.11 (November 1997) pp. 668-673

Stefaniak, T. (2003). Acute phase proteins as a markers of animal welfare (in Polish). In: *Acute phase proteins in Animals,* Kostro K. & Gliński Z. (Ed.), 247-249, Wydawnictwo Akademii Rolniczej w Lublinie, Lublin, Poland

Stefaniak T., Galli J., Borkowski J., Jawor P. (2003). Utilization of acute phase proteins in health monitoring of young ruminants (in Polish, English abstract). *Folia Univsitatis Agriculturae Stetinensis,* 233, Zootechnica 45, pp. 81-86

Stefaniak, T.& Jawor, P. (2007). Large dairy herds health monitoring. *Proceedings of 13th International Conference "Production Diseases In Farm Animals",* p. 351, Leipzig, Germany, July 29th - August 4th 2007

Svensson, C.; Lundborg, K.; Emanuelson, U. & Olsson S.O. (2003). Morbidity in Swedish dairy calves from birth to 90 days of age and individual calf-level risk factors for infectious diseases. *Preventive Veterinary Medicine,* Vol.58, No.3-4, (May 2003) pp. 179–197

Svensson, C.; Liberg, P. & Hultgren, J. (2007). Evaluating the efficacy of serum haptoglobin concentration as indicator of respiratory-tract disease in dairy calves. *The Veterinary Journal,* Vol.174, No.2, (September 2007) pp. 288-294

Taylor, J.A. (2006). Leukocyte Responses in Ruminants, In: *Schalm's Veterinary Hematology* Ed.Feldman A.B.F., Zinkl J.G., Jain N.C. pp. 391-404 Ed. Blackwell Publishing Professional, Iowa, USA

Toussaint, M.J.M.; van Ederen, A.M. & Gruys, E. (1995). Implication of clinical pathology in assessment of animal health and in animal production and meat inspection. Comparative Haematology International, Vol.5, No.3, pp. 149-157

Tomas J.S. (2000). Overview of plasma proteins, In: *Schalm's Veterinary Hematology* Ed.Feldman A.B.F., Zinkl J.G., Jain N.C. pp. 891-898 Ed. Lippincott Williams & Wilkins, Canada

Uchida, E.; Katoh, N. & Takahashi, K. (1993). Appearance of haptoglobin in serum from cows at parturition. *Journal of Veterinary Medical Science,* Vol.55, No.5, (October 1993) pp. 893-894

Wither, T.; Bienvenu, J. & Price, C.P. (1991). Molecular biology, measurement and clinical utility of the acute phase proteins. *Pure and Applied Chemistry,* Vol.63, No.8, (October 1991) pp. 1111-1116

Yoshida, Y. (1991). Electrophoretic studies on serum proteins in cows with traumatic pericarditis. *Journal of Veterinary Medical Science,* Vol.53, No.1, (February 1991) pp. 5-11